U0279506

汉英气功学大辞典

Chinese-English Dictionary of Qigong

李照国　刘希茹　编著

上海科学技术出版社

图书在版编目(CIP)数据

汉英气功学大辞典/李照国,刘希茹编著.—上海:
上海科学技术出版社,2020.1
ISBN 978 - 7 - 5478 - 4659 - 9

Ⅰ.①汉… Ⅱ.①李… ②刘… Ⅲ.①气功学—词典
—汉、英 Ⅳ.①R214 - 61

中国版本图书馆 CIP 数据核字(2019)第 244285 号

汉英气功学大辞典

李照国　　刘希茹　　编著

上海世纪出版(集团)有限公司
上海 科 学 技 术 出 版 社 出版、发行
(上海钦州南路 71 号　邮政编码 200235　www. sstp. cn)
上海雅昌艺术印刷有限公司印刷
开本 889×1194　1/32　印张 22.5
字数 1 000 千字
2020 年 1 月第 1 版　2020 年 1 月第 1 次印刷
ISBN 978 - 7 - 5478 - 4659 - 9/R · 1962
定价:128. 00 元

内 容 提 要

随着中医的国际传播和发展,中医翻译已经逐步实现了统一化和标准化,这为气功学术语翻译规范化的实现奠定了基础。《汉英气功学大辞典》根据《易经》《黄帝内经》、道家、儒家和佛家的基本理论以及《中国气功辞典》的相关内容,选择了 7 000 余条气功术语、词语和名言,对每个术语、词语和名言进行汉英双解释义。按照每个术语的实际含义,先用现代汉语进行解释和说明,再按照中医名词术语国际标准化发展的基本原则和方法翻译为英文,双语释义便于国内外学者了解和掌握。

本辞典是对气功学基本概念、术语和用语的较为系统、完整、准确的翻译,可供从事中医学、气功学教育、对外交流等工作的读者阅读参考。

前　　言

气功者,国之瑰宝、民之隗宝、世之神宝! 自伏羲创建中华文明以来,气功即随之问世,并逐步发展为神州大地之少阳;自轩辕创建中华文化以来,气功即随之传世,并努力发展为百族交融之太阳;自诸子创建中华思想以来,气功即随之扬世,并全面发展为诸子百家之阳明;自三教融会贯通以来,气功即随之盛世,并深入发展为历朝历代之元阳!

中华文化之所以传承千秋万代而不绝,中华民族之所以朝朝代代而不灭,除中华文化思想的深入指导和中医理法方药的全面防治之外,亦与气功精气神力的养育密不可分。气功对中华民族历朝历代发展的影响,亦如春夏秋冬之温热凉寒,既有生长壮老已之实,更有生长化收藏之望,令历朝历代之国人坚信不疑!

2014 年教育部牵头启动"中华思想文化术语传播工程"以来,自那时起,国人一直在努力地全面恢复中华文化,一直在深入地对外传播和传扬中华文化,中华文明和文化终于令真正的国人仰观吐曜,终于令真诚的西人俯察含章!

为了真正全面恢复中华文化,继承和发展气功学亦至为必要。正是为了全面恢复中华文化,我们才比较完整准确地分析总结了气功学的传统理论和方法,并在《黄帝内经》和吕光荣主编的《中国气功辞典》等的基础上,确定了气功术语的内涵和定义,并按照中医国际传播和发展的基本原则和方法,将其翻译为英文,为对外传播和发展中医与中华文化而开辟了一条蹊径。

李照国

2019 年 4 月

编 写 说 明

一、名词术语的选择

本辞典根据《易经》《黄帝内经》、道家、儒家和佛家的基本理论以及吕光荣主编的《中国气功辞典》,选择了7 000余条术语、词语和名言,并对每一术语、词语和名言的来源和含义进行了简明扼要的分析总结,比较全面地介绍了气功的基本理论、方法和功效。

二、名词术语的翻译

气功学属于中国传统医学的一个领域,其术语按照中医名词术语国际标准化发展的基本原则和方法进行翻译。中医名词术语翻译的基本原则如下:第一是自然性原则,即借用西方的自然对应语翻译中医的相关术语;第二是简洁性原则,即以简明扼要的方式翻译中医术语,以便规范化;第三是民族性原则,即通过翻译体现中医是中华文化的杰出代表;第四是回译性原则,即翻译的中医名词术语在结构上应与中文形式相近,以便中外合璧;第五为规定性原则,即对中医名词术语的翻译在内涵上加以限定,使其不能另有解释;第六是统一性原则,即通过对中医名词术语翻译的基本统一,为其标准化的实现奠定基础。

翻译气功学术语时,我们基本上按照中医翻译的原则和标准进行逐一翻译。具体的翻译方法有五。

一是直译,这也是中医名词术语国际标准化的最为基本的原则和方法。按照民族性和回译性的基本原则,气功学的术语、名词和名言基本都是按照直译进行翻译。如"五心(指手、足心及心脏)"直译为 five hearts,其释义为"The term of five hearts refers to the palms, the soles and the heart."再如"身门(指耳、目、口为身之门)"直译为 body gate,其释义为"Body gate is a term of Qigong, referring to the ears, the eyes and the mouth."

二是音译,即按照民族性原则,对气功学中特有的中华文化概念采用音译,这也是中医国际标准化发展的一个基本原则。如"丹田(指炼丹、产丹的部位,为人身之本,真气汇聚之处)"音译为 Dantian,其释义为"Dantian is a term of Qigong, referring to the region for producing Dan (pill or cinnabar) in alchemy, which is the root of human body where genuine Qi concentrates. Dantian is divided into the upper Dantian (the region between the eyes), the middle Dantian (the region below the heart) and the lower Dantian (the region below the navel)."再如"水沟(为督脉的一个穴位,位于人中之中。这一穴位为气功运行的一个常见部位)"音译为 Shuigou (GV 26),其释义为"Shuigou (GV 26) is an acupoint in the governor meridian, located in the center of Renzhong (the region between the nose and the mouth). This acupoint is a region usually used for keeping the essential Qi in practice of Qigong."自明清以来中医已经传播到了西方乃至世界各地,其重要的概念和术语,基本都采用音译。如"阴、阳、气、推拿"的音译 Yin, Yang, Qi, Tuina,已经成为当今中医国际发展的标准译法。

三是音意结合,即对一个术语和名词中的某个特别的字予以音译,其他的字则采用意译。如"气海"(气海为气功学名词,"元阳在肾,肾为气之海")音意结合译为 Qi sea,其释义为"Qi sea, a term of Qigong, refers to the fact that the original Qi is in the kidney and the kidney is the sea of Qi.""气"音译为 Qi 已经成为中医名词术语的国际标准。再如"阴中之阳(指阴中有阳,与肝有关)"音意结合翻译为 Yang within Yin,其释义为"Yang within Yin means that there is Yang in Yin related to the liver."将"阴阳"音译为 Yin 和 Yang,也已经成为中医名词术语的国际标准。

四是直译意译结合。之所以将一些气功学术语和名词翻译为意译与直译结合的形式,就是因为英语语言中缺乏中国传统文化中的一些基本概念。如"九载功"(其作法为自然坐正,闭目,调气,收心,坚持九年,可使人体气、血、脉、肉、髓、筋、骨、发、形强健,返老还壮)译为 nine tranquil techniques,其中的"载"和"功",就属于意译。其释义为"The term of nine tranquil techniques is a dynamic exercise, marked by sitting upright, closing the eyes, regulating Qi, concentrating the heart in practicing Qigong. After conscientiously practicing Qigong for nine years, it will strengthen Qi, blood, meridians, muscles, marrow, sinews, bones, hair and body, and eventually prolonging life."

五是多发并举。之所以采用多发并举的译法,主要是为了通过气功学的基本名词术语体现中华传统文化的精气神。如"魂魄"一词,一般常译作 soul,因为英语语言中只有 soul 这一个词,没有"魂"和"魄"这两个词语。但在中医学和气功学中,"魂"和"魄"则是既独立又相关的两个重要概念,而非单一概念。如"肝藏魂""肺藏魄",就充分说明了这一点。如果将"魂"和"魄"统一译作 soul,即无法体现"肝"和"肺"的基本精神了。为了充分说明这一点,西方翻译中医的通俗派将"魂"译作 ethereal soul,将"魄"译作 corporeal soul。如此之译虽然不尽其意,但有一定的实际意义,特别是独立了"魂"和"魄",统一了英译。所以在翻译气功学的名词术语时,"魂"和"魄"也借此译作 ethereal soul 和 corporeal soul,以实现其国际传播的统一化。

三、译法的特别说明

"龙"是中华民族文化和圣祖的代表,而 dragon 则是古代西方人想象中的邪恶动物。把"龙"翻译为 dragon,显然是对中华民族的误解。所以在翻译中医四大经典(即《黄帝内经》《难经》《神农本草经》《伤寒杂病论》)时,我们一直将"龙"音译为 Loong,这也是明清时期西方一些传教士的音译方式,也是我国香港常规的音译方式,颇值借鉴。我们与西方对华友好的汉学家交流的时候指出,即便 dragon 是西方最为辉煌的动物,也不能将"龙"译为 dragon,因为"龙"是中华民族圣祖的代表。自远古以来的中国人,就是龙的传人。如果将"龙"译为 dragon,那么中国人就不是龙的传人,而是 dragon 的传人。作为 dragon 的传人,中国人自然就成为西方圣祖的传人,而不是中国人了。对此,西方对华友好的汉学家完全赞同,特别希望中国的学者能真正有中华的意识。当今对外传播和发展中医的学者更应有真正的中华意识。如果没有真正的中华意识,自然无法有中华文化的基础。在气功学中,与"龙"相关的术语比较多,我们均将其音译为 Loong。之所以将"龙"音译为 Loong 而没有音译为 Long,是因为 Long 与英语中的 long 结构一致,会影响"龙"的实际含义。

中医在国际传播和发展中,已经逐步形成了统一化和标准化的规范,即对某些概念、术语的翻译完全一致,为气功学术语翻译的统一化和标准化的实现奠定了基础。如"经脉"在国际上比较流行的译法有二,即

meridian 和 channel。将"经脉"译作 channel 应该是最为客观的，但由于在中医名词术语国际标准的制定中，将其统一译作 meridian，所以气功学所有的"经脉"，也都统一地译作 meridian。

在中医学中，"督脉、任脉、冲脉、带脉"之"脉"也指的是 channel 或 meridian。1982—1991 年世界卫生组织西太区制定针灸学经络和穴位的国际标准时，将"督脉、任脉、冲脉、带脉"之"脉"皆译作 vessel，显然是不符合实际的。所以翻译气功学的名词术语时，我们将"督脉、任脉、冲脉、带脉"之"脉"皆译作 meridian，以便完全统一气功学名词术语翻译的内涵和标准。

目　　录

A

阿赖耶识【ā lài yē shí】 为佛家气功习用语，"识有八种，谓阿赖耶识眼、耳、鼻、舌、身、意及意识"。原意为藏，即能藏一切法之意。气功中指神识、性灵。
intelligence and identification A common term of Qigong in Buddhism. "There are eight kinds of intelligence and identification, including the eyes, the ears, the tongue, the body, the mind and the consciousness". The original meaning is to store, indicating to store the information of every exercise. In Qigong, it refers to identification of the spirit and nature.

阿那波那【ā nà bō nà】 指心息调融的一种方法，即通过气功实践完善对人体心、脑、神、气的调和、静安和融合。
Ana Bona A method for regulating, concentrating, coordinating and tranquilizing the heart, the brain, the spirit and Qi in the human body.

阿字观【ā zì guān】 为佛家气功功法。① 指声观，即结跏趺坐，意识活动集中于阿音，息息不懈；② 指字观，坐法同上，意想身体之中，有一圆明月轮，其中开八叶白色莲花。
sense of Chinese character A An exercise of Qigong in Buddhism, ① referring to either the sense of sound, marked by sitting in lotus position, continuously concentrating the activity of consciousness in the sound of Chinese character A; ② or the sense of Chinese character A, marked by sitting in lotus position, concentrating consciousness in the body with the imagination of the moonshine and the growth of eight leaves in the lotus.

阿字数息观【ā zì shù xī guān】 为佛家气功功法。坐法为盘膝正坐，放松形体，现阿字于出入之息。
number and information sense of the Chinese character A An exercise of Qigong in Buddhism, marked by sitting upright with crossed legs, relaxing the body and respiring with the sound of Chinese character A.

哀伤神【āi shāng shén】 指哀伤能损伤脑神。
sorrow impairing the spirit Means that grief can injury the spirit in the brain.

哀乐失时【āi yuè shī shí】 指悲哀、欢乐违背常理，即精神失调。
sorrow and happiness wasting time Means that sorrow and happiness violate common sense, referring to disorder of the spirit.

爱【ài】 为佛家气功习用语。① 指贪爱、爱欲；② 指七情之一。
love Refers to: ① womanizer and love desire, the common term of Qigong in Buddhism; ② or one of the seven human emotions (i. e. joy, anger, sorrow, fear, love, hate and desire).

爱清子【ài qīng zǐ】 为南宋时的气功学家，其所撰写的气功专著较为详细地阐述了气功的理论与方法。
Ai Qingzi A master of Qigong in the

A

South Song Dynasty（1127 AD − 1279 AD），who wrote a monograph of Qigong to introduce the theory and practice of Qigong.

安般【ān bān】　为阿那波那的别称，指心息调融的一种方法。

Anban　A synonym of Ana Bona, which is a method for regulating and concentrating the heart.

安不忘危【ān bù wàng wēi】　指身体健康，但不能忘记生病危急之时。

quietness without neglecting peril　Refers to cultivating health without neglecting critical time of disease.

安禅【ān chán】　为佛家气功习用语，指打坐入定，即习练佛家气功。

defending dhyana　A common term of Qigong in Buddhism, referring to sitting for stabilizing the body, which is a way to practice Qigong in Buddhism.

安处【ān chù】　指环境阴阳和调，明暗适中，才能安居而处。

content circumstance　Refers to regulation of Yin and Yang in environment. Only when lightness and shade are moderate can practitioners live a peaceful life.

安处之道【ān chù zhī dào】　源自气功专论，阐述习练气功的环境。

peaceful situation way　Collected from a monograph of Qigong, mainly describing the environment for practicing Qigong.

安定【ān dìng】　指摄心归一。

calm　Refers to perfect tranquilization of the heart.

安精神【ān jīng shén】　指安定精神，稳定情绪。

calming spirit　Refers to stabilizing the spirit and emotion.

安昆仑【ān kūn lún】　指补脑安神。

tranquilization of the brain　Refers to tonifying the brain and stabilizing the spirit.

安乐【ān lè】　指形体安适，精神愉快，情绪稳定。

peace and happiness　Refers to suitable body, pleasant spirit and stable emotion.

安神【ān shén】　指收敛情志，集中精神，弃除杂念，达到精神内守。

concentrated spirit　Refers to restraining emotion, concentrating spirit and eliminating distracting thought in order to internally defend the spirit.

安神祖窍【ān shén zǔ qiào】　指意守玄牝，凝神内聚。

concentrating spirit and ancestral orifice　Refers to defending the nose and mouth with mind in order to concentrate the spirit and to accumulate internal aspects.

安时处顺【ān shí chù shùn】　指安于时世，顺乎自然，情绪即可以稳定。

natural living　Refers to being content with the present age and following the natural way in order to stabilize emotion.

安稳【ān wěn】　佛家气功习用语，指形体安定，情绪稳定，神形和调。

stability　A common term of Qigong in Buddhism, referring to stability of the body, quietness of emotion and regulation of the spirit and the body.

安心【ān xīn】　佛家气功习用语，指意想于一景、一事、一物而安住于此。

concentrated contemplation　Refers to thinking about one scene, one matter and one thing in order to peacefully stay there.

安心病处【ān xīn bìng chù】 指意守病灶。

contemplation of focus Refers to pay great attention to focus of infection.

安心神【ān xīn shén】 指慎戒外感风毒邪气，能于安定精神意识活动。

tranquilization of heart spirit Refers to cautiously relieving external contraction, wind toxin and evil Qi in order to stabilize the activities of the spirit and thought.

安元和气法【ān yuán hé qì fǎ】 为静功。其作法为，入净室中，端身正坐，调节呼吸，令气微微然。

exercise for defending origin and harmonizing Qi A static exercise, marked by entering a quiet room, sitting upright, regulating respiration and softening Qi.

安在紫房帏幕间【ān zài zǐ fáng wéi mù jiān】 指存思心神之意。紫房指心，帏幕为心包络。

tranquility in the heart and pericardium A celebrated dictum, referring to stability of the heart spirit. In this celebrated dictum, Zifang refers to the heart and Weimu refers to the pericardium meridian.

庵罗识【ān luó shí】 同七常住果，为佛家气功习用语，指佛家气功所要达到的理想境界。

An Luo's knowledge The same as seven ideal boundaries, is a common term of Qigong in Buddhism, referring to the ideal state of the spirit in Buddhism.

唵阿吽【ǎn ā hǒu】 佛家气功功法。其作法为，结跏趺坐，意想如来真实身诸相圆满，念唵字安像顶上、阿字安口上、吽字安心上，身像与唵、阿、声相合即可。

An A Hong The exercise of Qigong in Buddhism, marked by sitting in lotus position, imagining the genuine body of Tathagata, reciting the Buddhism concept An to keep it on the top of the head, reciting the Buddhism concept He to keep it on the lip of the mouth, reciting the Buddhism concept Hong to keep it in the heart. To practice Qigong in such an exercise, the body image should coordinated with the Buddhism concepts An, A and Sheng.

唵字法【ǎn zì fǎ】 佛家气功功法。其作法为，站式或坐式，口念晦字，意识活动集中于唵字，反复若干次。

exercise with Buddhism concept An An exercise of Qigong in Buddhism, marked by standing or sitting, reciting the Buddhism concept An, concentrating the activity of consciousness in the Buddhism concept An and repeating for several times.

按摩并六字诀【àn mó bìng liù zì jué】 为动静相兼功。其作法为，平明睡起，先醒心，后醒眠，两手搓热，熨眼数十遍，以睛左旋右转各九遍，闭目少顷，勿夫睁开，即除风火。披衣起坐，叩齿集神，次鸣天鼓，依呵、呼、呬、吹、嘘、嘻六字诀，吐浊吸清，按五行相生，循序而行一周。

formula of tuina with six Chinese characters An exercise combined with dynamic exercise and static exercise, marked by getting up in daybreak, waking the heart first for finally awakening, rubbing the hands hot, heating the eyes for ten times, turning and rotating the eyes for nine times, closing the eyes for a while to expel wind and fire; then dressing clothes and sitting, clicking the teeth, concentrating the spirit, pressing the ears to hear sound; then

A

reading the six Chinese characters Ke (breathing out), Hu (exhaling), Xi (sighing), Chui (blowing), Xu (breathing out slowly) and Xi (panting) to exhale turbid Qi and inhale clear Qi. According to the mutual promotion among the five elements (including wood, fire, earth, metal and water), such an exercise for practicing Qigong can be continued for one week.

按摩补五脏法【àn mó bǔ wǔ zàng fǎ】 为动功。其作法为,用两手掌擦热后拭摩两眼,有养肝明目去翳作用。

exercise of tuina for tonifying the five Zang-organs Includes the heart, the liver, the spleen, the lung and the kidney, which is a dynamic exercise, marked by rubbing the palms hot and then rubbing the eyes for nouri-shing the liver, improving eyesight and eliminating cataract.

按摩导引法【àn mó dǎo yǐn fǎ】 为动功,其方法多样。如两手相捉,如洗手法;两手浅相叉,翻复向胸;两手相叉,共按胜,左右同。

exercise of Daoyin for tuina A dynamic exercise with various methods, such as holding the hands like washing the hands; mildly crossing the hands and repeatedly turning to the chest; crossing the hands to press the fleshes from the left to the right and vice versa.

B

八背舍法【bā bèi shè fǎ**】** 即① 观想身外不净,使贪心不起;② 再观想身处不净,灭除贪心而巩固之;③ 观想青、赤、黄、白等色,意念集中,除去杂念、烦恼;④ 观想空无边处,定志不散;⑤ 意识在无边处静定;⑥ 意识在无所有处禅定;⑦ 意念在非想非非想处寂定;⑧ 灭想除受,意识活动虚静,解脱思想束缚,获得愉快安适。八背舍法,又名解脱法,为禅定而舍去烦恼、贪欲而得到理想境界。

eight relieving methods A static exercise, indicating to ① observe physical impurity in order to eliminate avarice; ② to observe physical impurity again to eliminate greediness; ③ to observe and to imagine green color, red color, yellow color and white color in order to concentrate consciousness and to eliminate distracting thought and annoyance; ④ to observe and to imagine vacuum in order to stabilize the will without any dispersion; ⑤ to tranquilize consciousness in the state of vacuum; ⑥ to tranquilize consciousness in the state of vacuum and dhyana; ⑦ to tranquilize consciousness in the state of silence without any idea; ⑧ to eliminate any idea and thought, to tranquilize the activity of consciousness and to relieve fettered thought in order to stabilize the body and to enjoy happiness. The term of eight relieving methods is also called exercise for relief, referring to relieving annoyance with the eight important ways, and eliminating annoyance and greed with dhyana meditation in order to reach the ideal state.

八不中道法【bā bù zhōng dào fǎ**】** 为静功,佛家气功功法。其作法为结跏趺坐,意识思维活动"必生不灭,不来不去,不增不灭",是稳定神形的气功自然方法。

eight psychological equilibriums A static exercise of Qigong practice in Buddhism, marked by sitting in lotus position, and keeping the activities of consciousness and thinking in the way of "non-production and non-extinction, non-coming and non-leaving, non-increasing and non-losing". Such a static exercise is a natural way for stabilizing the spirit and body.

八定法【bā dìng fǎ**】** 佛家气功功法,即安定身心、悟空清净、身处乐境、念空净界、与天一体、无边处定、观空处禅、意想寂静。此八定法指由浅入深、稳定情绪、协调形神的八种方法。

eight explicit methods An exercise of Qigong in Buddhism, including stabilizing the body and the heart, awaking to the nihility of life with tranquility, staying in a happy state, thinking in a vacuum state, integrating with the universe, corresponding with vacuum, staying in dhyana with sincerity and keeping mentality tranquilied. Such an exercise of Qigong in Buddhism refers to eight ways for deepening from shallow, stabilizing the emotion and regulating the spirit and body.

八段锦站功【bā duàn jǐn zhàn gōng**】** 动功,主要是调身、调气和调神的八种方法。其作法为,形神放松,准备作功;自然站势,以清晨或上午为好;双手托天理三焦,双手臂自然下垂,双手掌交叉,掌心向上;两手向前划弧,顺势翻掌心向上,手掌大、小鱼际向上托于头顶之上;双手自然下垂,掌心向下按,然后翻手使掌心向上置于下腹前,随即两手掌向相反方向翻掌;左手缓缓向左近乳处抬起,过头,并向上抬;右手掌向下,用力向下按,稍停后挽手;右手抬高,左手下按,方法同,按并单举十数次;然后形神放松,精神内守,头项向左、向右缓缓转动十数次;或意识活动集中于丹田。

eight-section of brocade in standing A dynamic exercise of Qigong practice for regulating the body, Qi and the spirit, marked by relaxing the body and the spirit for preparation, naturally standing up in early morning or in the late morning; pulling the triple energizer with both hands, naturally lowering the shoulders, crossing the fists and raising the palms; drawing the curves forward with both hands, raising the palms at the same time, lifting the major thenar and hypothenar with the palms to the top of the head; naturally lowering the hands and pressing the palms downward, putting the palms before the lower abdomen, then turning over the palms to the different directions; slowly lifting the left hand along the left breast to the head; lowering the right hand forcefully downward and then holding the hand later on; highly lifting the right hand and lowering the left in the same way with dozens of times respectively; then relaxing the body and the spirit, internally concentrating the essence and the spirit, and mildly turning the head and neck to the left and right and vice versa for dozens of times respectively; or concentrating the activity of consciousness in Dantian. Dantian is divided into the upper Dantian (the region between the eyes), the middle Dantian (the region below the heart) and the lower Dantian (the region below the navel).

八段锦坐功【bā duàn jǐn zuò gōng**】** 动功,主要是调身、调气和调神的八种方法。其作法为,起床或睡前,取盘膝坐,正身正头正腰,闭目冥心,宁思静神,两手轻握于下腹部前,上齿轻闭,两目垂帘,调匀呼吸,排除杂念,安定精神,意守丹田。

eight-section of brocade in sitting A dynamic exercise of Qigong practice with eight ways to regulate the body, Qi and the spirit, marked by sitting upright with crossed knees after getting up or before sleeping; straightening the body, the head and the waist; closing the eyes and concealing the heart, stabilizing mentality and tranquilizing the spirit; holding the hands mildly to the lower abdomen; softly closing the upper teeth and lowering eyes for quietness; fairly regulating respiration, eliminating distracting thought, stabilizing the spirit and concentrating the consciousness in Dantian. Dantian is divided into the upper Dantian (the region between the eyes), the middle Dantian (the region below the heart) and the lower Dantian (the region below the navel).

八方【bā fāng】　四方四隅。

eight directions　Refers to four directions with four corners.

八风【bā fēng】　八方之风及引起精神损伤的八种情志活动。

eight winds　Refers to either eight kinds of directional wind or eight emotional activities that damage the spirit.

八公【bā gōng】　八方气功养生名士，即苏飞、李尚、左吴、田由、雷被、毛被、五被、晋昌。

eight celebrities　Refers to eight important masters of Qigong, i.e. Su Fei, Li Shang, Zuo Wu, Tian You, Lei Bi, Mao Bi, Wu Bi and Jin Chang.

八卦【bā guà】　文明圣祖伏羲创建的易经中的八卦，即乾象征天、坤象征地、震象征雷、巽象征风、坎象征水、离象征火、艮象征山、兑象征泽。

Eight Trigrams　Refers to the eight original Trigrams in Yijing created by Fu Xi who was the ancestor of Chinese civilization. Among these Eight Trigrams, Qian Trigram symbolizes the sky, Kun Trigram symbolizes the earth, Zhen Trigram symbolizes thunder, Xun Trigram symbolizes wind, Kan Trigram symbolizes water, Li Trigram symbolizes fire, Gen Trigram symbolizes mountain and Dui Trigram symbolizes pool.

八卦朝元统要【bā guà cháo yuán tǒng yào】　源自气功专论，主要阐述八卦还元归根的核心是达到阴阳升降平衡。

balance of the Eight Trigrams in entering the origin　Collected from a monograph of Qigong, referring to the discussion about the ascent, descent and balance of Yin and Yang which is the essential for the Eight Trigrams to restore the origin and root.

八卦配偶【bā guà pèi ǒu】　指八卦阴阳两方面的卦象与脏腑配合，相互为用，奇偶配合相当。

compatibility in Eight Trigrams　Refers to the combination of Yin and Yang in the Eight Trigrams with the five Zang-organs (including the heart, the liver, the spleen, the lung and the kidney) and the six Fu-organs (the gallbladder, stomach, small intestine, large intestine, bladder and triple energizer).

八节【bā jié】　立春、立夏、立秋、立冬、春分、秋分、夏至、冬至八个节气。

eight solar terms　Refers to the beginning of spring, the beginning of summer, the beginning of autumn, the beginning of winter, the spring equinox, the autumn equinox, the summer solstice and the winter solstice.

八解脱法【bā jiě tuō fǎ】　为静功，即① 观想身外不净，使贪心不起；② 再观想身处不净，灭除贪心而巩固之；③ 观想青、赤、黄、白等色，意念集中，除去杂念、烦恼；④ 观想空无边处，定志不散；⑤ 意识在无边处静定；⑥ 意识在无所有处禅定；⑦ 意念在非想非非想处寂定；⑧ 灭想除受，意识活动虚静，解脱思想束缚，获得愉快安适。八背舍法，又名解脱法，为禅定而舍去烦恼、贪欲而得到理想境界。

eight resolving methods　A static exercise, indicating to ① observe physical impurity in order to eliminate avarice; ② to observe physical impurity again to eliminate greediness; ③ to observe and to imagine green color, red color,

B

yellow color and white color in order to concentrate consciousness and to eliminate distracting thought and annoyance; ④ to observe and to imagine vacuum in order to stabilize the will without any dispersion; ⑤ to tranquilize consciousness in the state of vacuum; ⑥ to tranquilize consciousness in the state of vacuum and dhyana; ⑦ to tranquilize consciousness in the state of silence without any idea; ⑧ to eliminate any idea and thought, to tranquilize the activity of consciousness and to relieve fettered thought in order to stabilize the body and to enjoy happiness. The term of eight relieving methods is also called exercise for relief, referring to relieving annoyance with the eight important ways, and eliminating annoyance and greed with dhyana meditation in order to reach the ideal state.

八戒【bā jiè】 佛家八条戒律，即一不杀生，二不盗，三不淫，四不妄语，五不饮酒，六不坐高大床上，七不著华璎珞，八不自歌舞作乐。

eight commandments Refers to eight laws in Buddhism for preventing fault and tranquilizing the spirit and body, i.e. ahimsa, no stealing, no obscenity, no nonsense, no drinking alcohol, no sitting on the bed, no pearl and jade necklace and no singing and dancing.

八景神【bā jǐng shén】 ① 指上部八景神：发神、脑神、眼神、鼻神、耳神、口神、舌神、齿神；② 指中部八景神：肺神、心神、肝神、脾神、左肾神、右肾神、胆神、喉神；③ 指下部八景神：肾神、大小肠神、胴（胰）神、胸神、膈神、两胁神、左阴右阳神、右阴左阳神。

eight organic spirits ① Refers to ei-

ther eight upper spirits, including hair spirit, brain spirit, eye spirit, nose spirit, ear spirit, mouth spirit, tongue spirit and tooth spirit; ② or eight middle spirits, including lung spirit, heart spirit, liver spirit, spleen spirit, left kidney spirit, right kidney spirit, gallbladder spirit and throat spirit; ③ or lower eight spirits, including kidney spirit, large and small intestines spirit, pancreas spirit, chest spirit, diaphragm spirit, left rib-side spirit and right rib-side spirit as well as left Yin spirit and right Yang spirit.

八觉【bā jué】 八种稳定情绪的方法，或八种杂念。

eight feelings Refers to either eight disciplines; or eight distracting thoughts.

八脉交会穴【bā mài jiāo huì xué】 指通向任脉、督脉、冲脉、带脉、阴蹻脉、阳蹻脉、阴维脉、阳维脉的八个穴位，即列缺、后溪、公孙、足临泣、照海、申脉、内关、外关。这些穴位为气功精气运行之重要部位。

confluence acupoints of the eight meridians Refers to the acupoints of Lieque (LU 7), Houxi (SI 3), Gongsun (SP 4), Zulinqi (GB 41), Zhaohai (KI 6), Shenmai (BL 62), Neiguan (PC 6) and Waiguan (TE 5) located on the eight meridians known as conception meridian, governor meridian, thoroughfare meridian, belt meridian, Yinqiao meridian, Yangqiao meridian, Yinwei meridian and Yangwei meridian. These acupoints are the regions usually used in practice of Qigong.

八难【bā nàn】 指八种难治之病。

eight difficulties Refers to eight incurable diseases.

八念法【bā niàn fǎ】 为动静功法。其作法为,选择闲静处,乃至山林旷野,结跏趺坐。八念为意念佛、意念法、念僧法、念戒法、念舍法、念天法、念息法、念病法。主要功能是稳定神形,治疗心悸、惊怖、烦躁、恼怒、忧思、恐惧的八种方法。

eight intentions A static exercise, marked by selecting a clear and quiet place like a mountain forest and wilderness, sitting with crossed legs. The eight intentions include Buddhism, consciousness, monk, exhortation, abandonment, celestial principles, concentration and cultivating health. Such a static exercise can stabilize the spirit and the body, and cure palpitation, terror, agitation, rage, anxiety and fear.

八琼【bā qióng】 指人体的脏腑及口中的唾液。

eight jades Refers to the five Zang-organs (including the heart, the liver, the spleen, the lung and the kidney), the six Fu-organs (including the gallbladder, the stomach, the small intestine, the large intestine, the bladder and the triple energizer) and saliva in the mouth.

八胜处方【bā shèng chǔ fāng】 为静功,属佛家气功功法。其作法为,盘膝正坐,观外色青、观外色黄、观外色赤、观外色白;观外界色少,除灭烦恼并巩固之;观外界色多,消除对色的烦恼。意识集中在所观想的目标,断除贪心,制伏烦恼,调节精神。

eight principal restraints A method of static exercise of Qigong in Buddhism, marked by sitting upright with crossed knees, observing green color, yellow color, red color and white color in the external world; observing less colors in the external world, which can eliminate annoyance and consolidate the mind; observing more colors in the external world, which can eliminating annoyance of colors. The effect of this static exercise is for concentrating the emotion on the ideal aims, eliminating greed, relieving annoyance and regulating essence and spirit.

八石【bā shí】 指朱砂、雄黄、云母、空青、硫黄、戎盐、硝石、雌黄八种矿物药物。

eight minerals Refers to eight mineral medicinals, including Zhusha (Cinnabaris, cinnabar), Xionghuang (Realgar, realgar), Yunmu (Muscovitum, muscovite), Kongqing (Mallache, hollow azurite), Liuhuang (Sulfur, sulphur), Rongyan (Halitum, halite), Xiaoshi (saltpeter) and Xionghuang (Realgar, realgar).

八识【bā shí】 指眼、耳、鼻、舌、身、意六识加第七传送识,第八阿赖耶识。

eight senses Refers to the eyes, ears, nose, tongue, body, emotion and two ways in Buddhism for normalizing movement and observation.

八识归元法【bā shí guī yuán fǎ】 为静功,通过调身、调气、调神,可治郁证、痛证、躁证、神病、真心痛、眩晕中风证、肺痨、瘿瘤、消渴证、心痹证及消化系统、泌尿系统疾病。

eight methods for entering the origin The term of eight methods for entering the origin is a static exercise, referring to eight ways of regulation, including regulation of the body, regulation of Qi, regulation of spirit, regu-

B

lation of activity and regulation of viscera in order to tonify the brain and to nourish essence as well as to treat stagnation, epilepsy, apoplexy, tuberculosis, thirst disease, heart impediment and disease in digestive system and urinary system.

八素【bā sù】 指能宁静、安详、修养精气神的八种方式。

eight purities Refers to eight ways to tranquilize, purify and cultivate the essence, Qi and the spirit.

八威【bā wēi】 指八方之神或八卦之神。

eight privileges Refers to the spirit in the eight directions and eight Trigrams.

八位胎藏【bā wèi tāi zàng】 即佛家所指胎儿在母胎中的八个时期。即受胎后七日曰间凝滑,受胎十四日后曰疱,受胎至二十一日曰聚血,受胎二十八日曰健南,受后三十五日肉团增长,受胎后四十二日生毛发爪齿,受胎四十九日眼耳鼻舌身四根圆满具备,受胎五十六日以后,在胎藏中,形象完备。

eight periods of conception Refers to eight times when embryo is in mother's womb, indicating that conception for seven days will concentrate pregnancy; conception for fourteen days will appear vesicle in the skin; conception for twenty-eight days will fortify the health; conception for thirty-five days will increase the fleshes; conception for forty-two days will increase the growth the hair and the teeth; conception of for forty-nine days will fulfill the growth of the eyes, the ears, the nose, the tongue and the body; conception for fifty-six days will well develop the embryo.

八仙【bā xiān】 指铁拐李、钟离权、张果老、何仙姑、吕洞宾、蓝采和、韩湘子、曹国舅。

eight immortals Refers to eight great masters, i.e. Tie Guanli, Zong Liquan, Zhang Guolao, He Xiangu, Lǚ Dongbin, Lan Caihe, Han Xiangzi and Cao Guojiu.

八邪【bā xié】 指邪见、邪思维、邪语、邪业、邪命、邪方便、邪念、邪定八种错误的见解。

eight evils Refers to heretical observation, heretical thought, heretical speech, heretical business, heretical life, heretical activity, heretical idea and heretical decision.

八叶莲华观【bā yè lián huá guān】佛家气功功法。其作法为,盘膝正坐,意守八叶莲花(心),能解脱诸烦恼的缠绕,和适情志活动。

meditation with eight leaves of lotus An exercise of Qigong in Buddhism, marked by sitting upright with crossed legs and keeping the consciousness in the eight leaves of lotus (referring to the heart). Such an exercise of Qigong in Buddhism can relieve annoyance and stabilize the activity of emotion.

八音【bā yīn】 指的是佛法中八种要音,即极好音、柔软音、和适音、尊慧音、不女音、不误音、深远音、不竭音。

eight sounds Refers to eight special sounds in Buddhism, i.e. best sound, soft sound, mild sound, intelligent sound, no female sound, no wrong sound, no deep sound and no exhausted sound, which can balance the organs, cultivating the spirit, promoting Qi and strengthening the body.

八圆【bā yuán】 为佛家气功术语，指的是能调节精神意识活动，和谐行为的八法，即教圆、理圆、智圆、断圆、行圆、位圆、因圆、果圆。

eight cycles A common term of Qigong in Buddhism, referring to the eight ways in Buddhism for regulating the activities of the spirit and consciousness as well as harmonizing the behavior. These eight cycles including tranquility cycle, rational cycle, wisdom cycle, elimination cycle, active cycle, continuous cycle, success cycle and result cycle.

八月节后导引法【bā yuè jié hòu dǎo yǐn fǎ】 为动功。其作法为，八月节后每日丑寅时，清静入座，两手按于两膝上旋转按摩，可除腰背疾患。

exercise of Daoyin after the feast days of August A dynamic exercise of Qigong, marked by quietly sitting in Chou (the period of the day from 1 a.m. to 3 p.m.) and Yin (the period of the day from 3 a.m. to 5 a.m.) with both hands pressing and kneading on the knees. Such a dynamic exercise can cure diseases located in the chest and back.

八月中导引法【bā yuè zhōng dǎo yǐn fǎ】 为动功。其作法为，八月中每日丑时，盘膝而坐，可除腰胁疾苦，明目。

exercise of Daoyin in the middle of August Dynamic exercise of Qigong practice, marked by sitting up with the crossed knees in Chou (the period of a day from 1 a.m. to 3 a.m. in the morning) every day in the August for relieving pain in the chest and improving the eyesight.

八灾患【bā zāi huàn】 为佛家气功习用语，指忧、喜、苦、乐、寻、伺、出息、入息等妨害禅定的八种因素。

eight disasters A common term of Qigong in Buddhism, referring to anxiety, happiness, bitterness, joy, search, watch, inhalation and exhalation which may impair transcendental meditation.

八斋戒【bā zhāi jiè】 指佛家八条戒律，即一不杀生，二不盗，三不淫，四不妄语，五不饮酒，六不坐高大床上，七不著华璎珞，八不自歌舞作乐。

eight fast commandments Refers to eight laws in Buddhism for preventing fault and tranquilizing the spirit and body, i.e. ahimsa, no stealing, no obscenity, no nonsense, no drinking alcohol, no sitting on the bed, no pearl and jade necklace and no singing and dancing.

八正【bā zhèng】 指八个节气的正气。

eight kinds of righteousness Refers to normal climates in eight stems.

八正道【bā zhèng dào】 指神形调和的八种正确方法和路径。

eight righteous ways Refers to eight correct ways for regulating the spirit and body.

白带【bái dài】 指妇女从阴道中经常流出白色黏液，伴腰酸腹痛，多因脾虚肝郁、湿热下注、带脉失约、任脉不固所致。

whitish vaginal discharge Marked by frequent effusion of mucus with aching waist and abdominal pain caused by spleen deficiency, liver stagnation, downward pouring of warmth and heat, disorder to the belt meridian and insecurity of the conception meridian.

白发【bái fà】 为气功适应证，多因肾气衰弱，血气亏虚，致头发失去荣养而变白色。

white hair　An indication of Qigong，usually caused by weakness of kidney Qi and deficiency of the blood and Qi.

白发候导引法【bái fà hòu dǎo yǐn fǎ**】** 动功，方法多样。如坐地上，伸直两脚，用两手按小腿，头弯到地，补骨髓，养精血。

exercise of Daoyin for white hair　A dynamic exercise with various methods，such as sitting on the ground，stretching the feet，pressing the shanks with both hands and lowering the head to the ground. Such a dynamic exercise can tonify the marrow and nourish the essence and the blood.

白虎【bái hǔ**】**　① 指二十八宿中西方的七宿；② 内丹书中指"心中元神谓之龙，肾中元精谓之虎"。

white tiger　Refers to ① either the seven constellations in the west among the twenty-eight constellations；② or "the original spirit in the heart called Loong and the original essence in the kidney called tiger" mentioned in the books about internal Dan（pills of immortality）.

白居易【bái jū yì**】**　唐代诗人，也是气功家。

Bai Juyi　A great poet and a great master of Qigong in the Tang Dynasty（618 AD－907 AD）.

白乐天【bái lè tiān**】**　唐代著名诗人，气功家白居易的另外一个称谓。

Bai Letian　Another name of Bai Juyi，the great poet and master of Qigong in the Tang Dynasty（618 AD－907 AD）.

白露八月节坐功【bái lù bā yuè jié zuò gōng**】** 动功。每日丑寅时正坐，两手按膝，转头推引，各三五次，叩齿、吐纳、咽液，可治风气留滞腰背、鼻阻、口歪斜、颈肿、喉痹不能言等症。

sitting exercise of White Dew in the feast days in the August　A dynamic exercise，marked by sitting in Chou（the period of a day from 1 a.m. to 3 a.m. in the morning）and Yin（the period of a day from 3 a.m. to 5 a.m. in the morning）with both hands pressing the knees，turning and stretching the head for three and five times respectively，clicking the teeth，breathing in and out as well as swallowing humor. Such a dynamic exercise can treat various diseases，such as retention of wind Qi in the waist and back，nasal obstruction，facial palsy，neck swelling and throat impediment.

白履忠【bái lǚ zhōng**】**　唐代气功家梁丘子的另外一个称谓。

Bai Lǚzhong　Another name of Liang Qiuzi，a great master of Qigong in the Tang Dynasty（618 AD－907 AD）.

白石【bái shí**】**　指齿象。

white stone　Refers to the manifestation of teeth.

白叟【bái sǒu**】**　宋代气功学家白玉蟾的另外一个称谓。

Bai Sou　Another name of Bai Yuchan，a great master of Qigong in the Song Dynasty（960 AD － 1279 AD）.

白心【bái xīn**】**　① 指清静自守；② 指清静之苦心，为佛家气功习用语。

white heart　A term of Qigong，① referring to either quietness and self-control；② or quietness with the earnest heart which is a common term of Qigong in Buddhism.

白雪【bái xuě**】**　为练功效验之一，指练功中微闭双目，双眼出现一片光明。

white snow　A term of Qigong，referring to one of the effects in practicing Qigong，characterized by subtly closing the eyes with brightness in the eyes.

白玉蟾【bái yù chán】　白玉蟾（1194—1229）为宋代的一位气功学家，著有多部气功专著。

Bai Yuchan　A great master of Qigong in the Song Dynasty（960 AD‐1279 AD），wrote several monographs of Qigong.

白玉蟾运气【bái yù chán yùn qì】　动功。其作法为，盘坐，以两手按肩，两眼朝左侧看，运气十二口，主治胸腹虚饱。

Bai Yuchan's regulation of Qi　A dynamic exercise，marked by sitting with crossed legs，pressing the shoulders with both hands，looking toward the left and directing Qi for twelve times. Such a dynamic exercise can relieve deficient fullness of the chest and the abdomen.

白元【bái yuán】　指肺神。

white origin　Refers to the lung spirit.

白云观【bái yún guàn】　宋元时期气功家丘处机遗骨埋葬处。

White Cloud Temple　A place where Qiu Chuji，a great master of Qigong in the late Song Dynasty（960 AD‐1127 AD）and the early Yuan Dynasty（1271 AD‐1368 AD），was buried.

白云子【bái yún zǐ】　唐代气功家张白的另外一个称谓。

Bai Yunzi　Another name of Zhang Bai，a great master of Qigong in the Tang Dynasty（618 AD‐907 AD）.

白浊白带导引法【bái zhuó bái dài dǎo yǐn fǎ】　动功。其作法为，各捏肾俞和气海两穴八十一次，擦亦八十一次，然后双手抱两膝，呼吸意念脐下，使气从

尾闾上升。

exercise of Daoyin for leukorrhagia　A dynamic exercise，marked by pinching Shenshu（BL 23）and Qihai（CV 6）for eighty-one times，rubbing Shenshu（BL 23）and Qihai（CV 6）for eighty-one times，holding the knees with both hands，inhaling deep below the navel，and promoting Qi to flow upwards from the coccyx.

百病生于气【bǎi bìng shēng yú qì】　指多种疾病的发生，与气机紊乱、功能活动失调及气虚有密切关系。

All diseases are caused by disorder of Qi.　This is a celebrated dictum，referring to the fact that all diseases are caused by disorder of Qi activity，dysfunction of all the organs and deficiency of Qi.

百骸【bǎi hái】　泛指全身骨骼。

skeleton　Refers to all the bones in the whole body.

百会【bǎi huì】　①指督脉中的一个穴位；②指气功常见意守部位；③指百神之会。这一穴位为气功运行的一个常见部位。

Baihui（GV 20）　Refers to ① either an acupoint in the governor meridian；② or the region where consciousness maintains in practicing Qigong；③ or convergence of hundred spirits. This acupoint is a region usually used for keeping the essential Qi in practice of Qigong.

百节【bǎi jié】　①指全身所有关节；② 也指全身各部。

hundred joints　Refers to ① either all the joints in the whole body；② or all parts in the whole body.

百疒所钟存无英【bǎi kē suǒ zhōng cún wú yīng】　意为练功时意念存想肺

神（七日后）可法除百般病证。

Treatment of all diseases depends on the liver spirit. This is a celebrated dictum, indicating to expel all diseases through contemplation of the liver spirit in practicing Qigong.

百劳【bǎi láo】 为大椎的一个别名，是督脉的一个穴位，位于后正中线，第七颈椎棘突下凹陷中。为气功学重要体表标志之一。此穴位为气功习练之处。

Bailao A synonym of Dazhui（GV 14）, an acupoint in the governor meridian, located in the back midline and in the depression of spinous process in the seventh cervical vertebra, which is the important symbol in Qigong. This acupoint is a region usually used in practice of Qigong.

百灵命宅【bǎi líng mìng zhái】 指脑，为诸神会聚之处。

lark life residence Refers to the brain where all spirits flock together.

百脉总枢【bǎi mài zǒng shū】 气血源头，为气功学术语，指神定息定，调息也在其中。

combination of all meridians The same as origin of Qi and blood which is a term of Qigong, referring to tranquilized spirit and respiration.

百窍关联【bǎi qiào guān lián】 源自气功专论，阐述全身各部的生理功能、病理变化及其联系，指出习练气功，能于调整各部的关系，祛邪治病。

connection of all orifices Collected from a monograph of Qigong, describing the physiological function, pathological changes and connection of all parts of the body, indicating that practicing Qigong can regulate all parts of the body and eliminate pathogenic factors to cure disease.

百窍关联总有神【bǎi qiào guān lián zǒng yǒu shén】 指身体各部经络、关窍、肌肉、骨骼、肢节的联系是神的作用。

Combination of all orifices must depend on the spirit. This is a celebrated dictum, referring to the effect of the spirit that enables the meridians, the orifices, the muscles, the bones and the limbs to combine with each other.

百日小静【bǎi rì xiǎo jìng】 指百日取得初步功夫，说明习练气功，贵在坚持。

mild quietness in hundred days Refers to preliminary benefit from hundred days of exercise, indicating importance of persistence in practicing Qigong.

百嶂内视胎息诀【bǎi zhàng nèi shì tāi xī jué】 为静功口诀，其习练主要是先调气，然后调节精神。

internal vision of fetal respiration in all fields A mnemonic rhyme of static exercise, referring to regulating Qi first and then regulating the spirit.

百字碑【bǎi zì bēi】 《百字碑》为气功学专论，由唐代吕岩所作，概括吕气功修练的全过程。吕岩为吕洞宾的另外一个称谓。

Baizi Bei （*Monument with Hundred Characters*） A monograph of Qigong entitled *Monument with Hundred Characters*, written by Lǚ Yan, summarizing the whole procedure of Qigong practice. Lǚ Yan was another name of Lǚ Dongbin.

搬运【bān yùn】 即习练周天功时，神运精气沿任、督脉运行谓之搬运。

transportation Refers to flow of the spirit and movement of the essence and Qi along the conception meridian and the governor meridian in practicing celestial circuit Qigong.

搬运捷法【bān yùn jié fǎ**】**　为静功。其作法为，每日五更起坐，两足相向，热摩涌泉无数，以汗出为度。

rapid exercise for transportation A static exercise, marked by sitting at the five watches (or periods) of the night, coinciding the feet with each other, rubbing Yongquan (KI 1) (an acupoint in the kidney meridian) hot for many times till sweating.

半跏趺坐【bàn jiā fū zuò**】**　为佛家调身法之一。

half sitting exercise One of the methods used in Buddhism for regulating and cultivating the body.

邦子入山寻大【bāng zǐ rù shān xún dà**】**　为静功。自然站立，放松形神，以左手指左方，头向右侧眼向右平视，运气二十四口，然后换右手，动作运气同前。主治瘫痪。

entering mountain to look for the great A static exercise, marked by naturally standing up, relaxing the body with the left hand and turning to the left, turning the head to the right side, looking the eyes horizontally to the right side, and directing Qi for twenty-four times; then changing the right hand with the same way to move. This static exercise can treat paralysis.

胞【bāo**】**　① 指眼睑；② 指子宫；③ 指膀胱。

bao Refers to ① either eyelid; ② or uterus; ③ or bladder.

胞胎元一【bāo tāi yuán yī**】**　指太极阴阳变化之初，亦指天、地、人混合于一元。元一即元气。用以说明气功阴阳变化作用。

fetal original one Refers the early changes of Yin and Yang, or integration of the sky, earth and man into one origin. Original one refers to original Qi, indicating the effect of the changes of Yin and Yang.

薄厥【báo jué**】**　为气功适应证，指因大怒等精神刺激而致阳气亢盛，血随气逆郁积头部，出现头痛、眩晕，甚则卒然昏厥，不省人事等的病证。

flopping syncope characterized by sudden fainting An indication of Qigong, usually caused by rage and spirit stimulation that exuberates Yang Qi and stagnates the blood in the head, causing headache, vertigo, syncope and unconsciousness.

宝精【bǎo jīng**】**　① 指习练气功，益气养精；② 指以精为宝，爱惜而不施泄。

precious essence Refers to ① either practice of Qigong for enriching Qi and nourishing essence; ② or taking the essence as treasure, making great efforts to protect it and to avoid dispersing it.

宝章【bǎo zhāng**】**　源自气功专论，指气功的经典著作。

precious canon Refers to the classic canons of Qigong.

宝志【bǎo zhì**】**　为南朝时期的僧人，亦有气功之力。

Bao Zhi A Buddhist in the North Dynasty (420 AD – 589 AD) who was also familiar with Qigong.

宝珠【bǎo zhū**】**　指玄珠，即丹。

jewel pearl Refers to supreme pearl which means Dan (pills of immortality).

保固神气【bǎo gù shén qì**】**　指习练气功，固涩肾精，保养精神、精气。

keeping and stabilizing spiritual Qi Refers to stabilizing the kidney essence in order to nourish the essence, spirit and spiritual Qi in practicing Qigong.

保和大和【bǎo hé dà hé】 指天能保持太和景象,有利于万物的生长。

keeping harmony and increasing harmony Refers to the fact the sky can keep supreme harmony, which is beneficial to the growth and development of all the things in the universe.

保命立基说【bǎo mìng lì jī shuō】 源自气功专论,主要阐述保固命根的道理及稳定精神、调节呼吸的方法。

idea about protecting life and establishing foundation Collected from a monograph of Qigong, mainly describing the principles for protecting and strengthening the root of life as well as the ways for stabilizing the spirit and regulating respiration.

保生要录【bǎo shēng yào lù】 《保生要录》为气功养生专著,由宋代蒲虔贯注,概要论述了气功养生法。

Baosheng Yaolu (*Important Record of Protecting Life*) A monograph of Qigong and life cultivation entitled *Important Record of Protecting Life*, explained by Pu Qianguan in the Song Dynasty (960 AD – 1279 AD), mainly discussing the exercises for practicing Qigong and cultivating life.

保守完固【bǎo shǒu wán gù】 指习练气功,默默堤防,动静之间完固不表,则气凝神存身享无穷之福。

exercise for keeping defense Refers to silent prevention and no manifestation of stability between dynamic exercise and static exercise in practicing Qigong, enabling the spirit to be concentrated and the body to be healthy.

保形以养神【bǎo xíng yǐ yǎng shén】 为气功学术语,形体是精神存在的基础,神依形存,形须神立。形体健全则神得以安宁,故保形以养神。

strengthening the body to nourish the spirit A term of Qigong, referring to the fact that the body is the foundation for the existence of the spirit, indicating that the spirit depends on the body to exist and the body also depends on the spirit to grow. Only when the body is healthy can the spirit be stabilized. So to protect the body is also the way to nourish the spirit.

葆光【bǎo guāng】 指潜藏的光明,为虚静而生智慧之意。

latent light Refers to hidden light, indicating that quietness and tranquility increase wisdom.

葆气养神【bǎo qì yǎng shén】 指气与神之间的致密关系。

protecting Qi and nourishing the spirit Refers to the close relation between Qi and the spirit.

抱朴【bào pǔ】 即怀抱纯朴,不受自然和社会因素的干扰。

free for desires Refers to the importance of purity and sincerity without disturbance of the natural world and the social factors.

抱朴子【bào pǔ zǐ】 《抱朴子》为医学、气功学和养生学专著,由晋代葛洪所著,强调气功与药物综合应用与临床。也指葛洪。

Bao Puzi (*Acme Purity and Perfection*) A monograph about traditional Chinese medicine, Qigong and life cultivation entitled *Acme Purity and Perfection*, written by Ge Hong in the Jin Dynasty (266 AD – 420 AD), emphasizing the importance of combined application of Qigong and medicine in clinical treatment. It also refers to Ge Hong, a great scientist of traditional Chinese medicine and a great master of Qigong in the Jin Dynasty (266 AD - 420 AD).

抱朴子守真法【bào pǔ zǐ shǒu zhēn fǎ】 为静功,指未定情绪;指淡泊自守;指排除杂念。《抱朴子》为医学、气功学和养生学专著。

Bao Puzi's exercise for keeping purity A static exercise, referring to either stabilizing emotion; or caring less of self-idea; or eliminating distracting thought. Bao Puzi is a monograph about traditional Chinese medicine, Qigong and life cultivation entitled *Acme Purity and Perfection*.

抱朴子胎息法【bào pǔ zǐ tāi xī fǎ】 为静功。作法为,初学行气,鼻中引气而闭之,默数至一百二十,乃以口微吐之,可以延年,可治百病。《抱朴子》为医学、气功学和养生学专著。

Bao Puzi's method for fetal respiration A static exercise, marked by inhaling Qi through the nose and closing the nose at the beginning of moving Qi, silently counting to one hundred and twenty, and finally exhaling slowly through the mouth. Such a way of practicing Qigong can prolong life and treat various diseases. Bao Puzi is a monograph about traditional Chinese medicine, Qigong and life cultivation entitled *Acme Purity and Perfection*

抱朴子胎息诀【bào pǔ zǐ tāi xī jué】 为静功,从调节呼吸开始,逐步安定精神。《抱朴子》为医学、气功学和养生学专著。

Bao Puzi's exercise for fetal respiration A static exercise, referring to gradually stabilizing the essence and the spirit through regulation of respiration. Bao Puzi is a monograph about traditional Chinese medicine, Qigong and life cultivation entitled *Acme Purity and Perfection*

抱琴居士【bào qín jū shì】 明代文人,对气功养生颇有研究,著有专著,对指导习练气功、推广运用气功治病起到了积极作用。

Baoqin Jushi A great literati in the Ming Dynasty (1368 AD - 1644 AD) who also well studied Qigong and life cultivation and wrote a monograph of Qigong to contribute a great deal to the practice and development of Qigong.

抱一函三【bào yī hán sān】 抱一为精神意识集中统一,函三乃天、地、人,指人与天地相应,三者协调统一。

embracing one and maintaining three Refers to correspondence of human beings with the sky and the earth, which should be coordinated and unified. In this term, keeping one means combination and unification of the spirit and consciousness while maintaining three refers to the sky, the earth and the human beings.

抱一函三秘诀【bào yī hán sān mì jué】 《抱一函三秘诀》为气功学专著,讲述人体受胎之后与受胎始的各种变异。作者不详。

Baoyi Hansan Mijue (*Recipe of Embracing One and Maintaining Three*) A monograph of Qigong entitled *Recipe of Embracing One and Maintaining Three*, mainly describing various changes at the beginning of pregnancy and after pregnancy. The author was unknown.

抱一冥心【bào yī míng xīn】 指气功中,进入无作无为之时,神形含一,意识宁静。

embracing one and tranquilizing the heart Refers to integration of the spirit and the body and tranquilization of the mind and the brain in practicing Qigong.

抱一为天下式【bào yī wéi tiān xià shì】 指事物相互作用,相反相成,分之为二,合之则一,是自然社会的普遍规律。

embracing one is an exercise in the world This is special discussion about the combination of things in this world, in which they are opposite and complementary, separate into two and integrate into one, indicating the general principle in the natural world and social environments.

抱一子三峰老人丹诀【bào yī zǐ sān fēng lǎo rén dān jué】 《抱一子三峰老人丹诀》为气功专著,由元代金月岩所编。书中认为修炼应性命双修,并且认为性、命二字还有真假。

Baoyizi Sanfeng Laoren Danjue [*Old Man's Dan (Pills of Immortality) Formula for Embracing a Baby in the Three Peaks*] A monograph of Qigong entitled *Old Man's Dan (Pills of Immortality) Formula for Embracing a Baby in the Three Peaks*, written by Jin Yueyan in the Yuan Dynasty (1271 AD – 1368 AD), mainly describing the importance of cultivating both the nature and life in practicing Qigong, indicating that the nature and life sometimes are true and sometimes are false.

抱玉怀珠和子室【bào yù huái zhū hé zǐ shì】 指调节阴阳于子室。

embracing jade, taking pearl and quieting the baby's room A celebrated dictum, referring to regulation of Yin and Yang in the baby's room.

抱元守一【bào yuán shǒu yī】 即神气不分离。元指神,气为一。

embracing the origin and keeping the one A term of Qigong, indicating that the spirit and Qi cannot be separated. In this term, the origin refers to the spirit and the one refers to Qi.

卑监【bēi jiān】 为运气术语。土生万物,其位尊,如土气不及则位卑,其临下视察的职能有失。

humble inspection A term of Qi motion. When the earth has produced all things, it is great; if the earth fails to produce anything, it is humble and unable to reflect its functions.

北斗里藏身【běi dǒu lǐ cáng shēn】 指凝神于气穴,或谓凝神于丹田。

hiding the body in the Big Dipper A celebrated dictum, referring to concentrating the spirit in the Qi point or concentrating in Dantian. Dantian is divided into upper Dantian (the region between the eyes), the middle Dantian (the region below the heart) and the lower Dantian (the region below the navel).

北方莫以心缘心【běi fāng mò yǐ xīn yuán xīn】 指气和于中,神正于内,内照清净。

Heart never connects the heart in the north. This is a celebrated dictum, referring to harmonizing Qi in the center and concentrating the spirit in the internal in order to brighten and tranquilize the internal.

北方正气【běi fāng zhèng qì】 指

肾气。

righteous Qi in the north Refers to kidney Qi.

北方正水【běi fāng zhèng shuǐ】 指肾。

righteous water in the north Refers to the kidney.

北七真【běi qī zhēn】 指道家气功全真派首创者王重阳的七大弟子,即马珏、谭处端、刘处玄、丘处机、王处一、郝大通、孙不二。

seven great masters in the north Refers to the seven important disciples of Wang Chongyang, the founder of the genuine school in Qigong. Those seven important disciples include Ma Jue, Tan Chuduan, Liu Chuxuan, Qiu Chuji, Wang Chuyi, Hao Datong and Sun Buer.

北五祖【běi wǔ zǔ】 指道家全真派对王玄甫、钟离权、吕岩、刘操、王重阳的尊称。

five ancestors in the north Refers to the five important masters in the genuine school of Daoism, including Wang Xuanpu, Zhong Liquan, Lǚ Yan, Liu Cao and Wang Chongyang.

北宗内丹【běi zōng nèi dān】 为大家气功流派之一,以养气兼养神为特点。

internal Dan school in the north One of the schools of Qigong in Daoism, characterized by nourishing Qi and the spirit.

备急千金要方【bèi jí qiān jīn yào fāng】《备急千金要方》为中医专著,由唐代药王孙思邈所撰,其中也谈到了气功养生法等重要内容,为医学和气功做出了重要贡献。

Beiji Qianjin Yaofang (*Valuable Prescriptions for Emergencies*) A great monograph of traditional Chinese medicine entitled *Valuable Prescriptions for Emergencies*, written by Sun Simiao, King of Medicine in the Tang Dynasty (618 AD - 907 AD). This great monograph of traditional Chinese medicine also studied and analyzed the theory and practice of Qigong and life cultivation, contributing a great deal to the traditional Chinese medicine and Qigong.

背【bèi】 ① 指项以下,腰以上部位;② 指整个躯干后面;③ 指躯干四肢的后面皆为背面。

back Back refers to ① either the region below the neck and above the waist; ② or the back of the whole torso; ③ or the back of the torso and the four limbs.

背功【bèi gōng】 为动功。其作法为,两手据床,缩身曲背,拱背向上十三举,可去除心肝之邪。

back exercise A dynamic exercise, marked by putting the hands over the bed, shrinking the body and bending the back, raising the back for thirteen times in order to eliminate pathogenic factors in the heart and the liver.

背后三关【bèi hòu sān guān】 ① 即后三三,指下关、中关和上关;② 指尾闾、夹脊和玉枕。

three joints in the back The same as backward three and three, ① refers to either the lower segment, middle segment and upper segment; ② or coccyx, Jiaji point located in the spine and Yuzhen (BL 9).

背痛导引法【bèi tòng dǎo yǐn fǎ】 为动功。其作法为,两手掌擦热交搭于两肩,用力躬身反复数次,静坐片刻,凝神定志,万念扫除,调息,运气从痛处往手指散出滞气,治脊背痛。

exercise of Daoyin for backache A dynamic exercise, marked by rubbing the hands hot and then putting the hands on the shoulders, bending the body for several times, sitting quietly for a while, concentrating the spirit and stabilizing the heart, eliminating any desires, regulating respiration, moving Qi from the ache place to the fingers in order to disperse stagnant Qi and cure backache.

倍拳【bèi quán】 指手足反向屈曲的导引姿势。

opening and bending A term of Qigong, referring to the style of Daoyin for reversely bending the hands and feet.

本宫【běn gōng】 指人体中丹田,为阳神归伏之宫。

original palace Refers to the middle Dantian (the region below the heart) which is the chamber that Yang spirit enters.

本惑【běn huò】 为佛家气功习用语,指受到外界因素引起的烦恼,含有贪、嗔、痴、慢、疑、恶见等意。

ordinary doubt A common term of Qigong in Buddhism, referring to annoyance caused by external factors, such as greed, anger, stupidity, lowness, doubt and wrong view.

本觉【běn jué】 为佛家气功习用语,指本有常住之觉体,即灵性,即精神意识活动。

original consciousness A common term of Qigong in Buddhism, referring to spiritualism and spiritual and conscious activities in ordinary life.

本神【běn shén】 为足少阳胆经的一个穴位,位于前发际0.5寸,头正中线旁开3寸处。这一穴位为气功运行的一个常见部位。

Benshen(BL 13) An acupoint in the gallbladder meridian of foot Shaoyang, located 0.5 Cun before the front hair line and 3 Cun beside the middle line over the head. This acupoint is a region usually used for keeping the essential Qi in practice of Qigong.

本心【běn xīn】 为佛家气功习用语,指神具有的作用,有形的含义,也有用的含义。

genuine heart A common term of Qigong in Buddhism, referring to the effect of the spirit, indicating physical meaning and active meaning.

本有【běn yǒu】 为佛家气功习用语,指人生及人具有的自然本性,如矿中之金,暗中之宝。

original existence A common term of Qigong in Buddhism, referring to natural property of human beings like gold in the cores and treasures in the dark.

本源【běn yuán】 指下丹田。

origin Refers to lower Dantian (the region below the navel).

鼻不闻【bí bù wén】 指守神于内,精神集中,鼻不闻外气。

nose without taste Refers to keeping the spirit inside the body, concentrating the spirit and no smelling of the external Qi in the nose.

鼻疮【bí chuāng】 为气功适应证,指鼻孔内或鼻部发生疮肿,红肿热痛,多因脾、肺二经壅热所致。

nasal sore An indication of Qigong, referring to swollen sores, redness swelling and hot pain in the nostrils or nasal region, usually caused by accumulation of heat in the spleen and lung meridians.

鼻功【bí gōng**】**　为动功。其作法为,两手大指背擦热,揩鼻三十六次,视鼻端,默数出入息,每晚覆身卧,暂去枕,从膝弯反竖两足向上,以鼻吸纳清气四次,又以鼻出气四次,气出极力后,令微气再入鼻中收纳。

nasal exercise A dynamic exercise, marked by rubbing the back hot with thumbs in two hands, wiping the nose for thirty-six times, viewing the nose, silently counting inhalation and exhalation, lying on bed every night, taking off pillow for a while, bending the knees to stand up the feet, inhaling clear Qi through the nose for four times, exhaling Qi through the nose for four times, and inhaling subtle Qi again through the nose after extreme exhalation.

鼻疾治法【bí jí zhì fǎ**】**　为静功,方法多样。向东而坐,闭息三通,手捻鼻两止;踞坐,合两膝,张两足,不息五通;正坐伸腰,缓缓用鼻吸气,用右手捻鼻,闭目,慢慢吐气;向东而坐,不息三通,以手捻鼻两孔。

exercise for curing nasal disease A static exercise with various methods, marked by sitting to the east, stopping respiration for three times, twisting the nose with hands for twice; sitting with squatting, crossing the knees, stretching the feet, and stopping respiration for five times; sitting upright, stretching the waist, slowly breathing in through the nose, twisting the nose with the right hand, closing the eyes and slowly breathing out; sitting to the east, stopping respiration for three

times and twisting the nostrils with the hands.

鼻衄【bí nǜ**】**　为气功适应证,指鼻孔出血。

nosebleed An indication of Qigong, referring to bleeding in the nostrils.

鼻衄治法【bí nǜ zhì fǎ**】**　为静功。凡鼻血不止,圆开两眼,一气连吸三、九口,意送下丹田即止。

exercise for curing nosebleed A static exercise, marked by opening the eyes when there is constant bleeding in the nose, inhaling Qi for three or nine times, and imagining to send it to the lower Dantian (the region below the navel).

鼻生疮候导引法【bí shēng chuāng hòu dǎo yǐn fǎ**】**　为静功。其作法为,臀部及足掌着地而坐,两膝合拢,两足分开,闭气不息,至极限时慢慢呼出,做五遍。清肺热,通鼻窍,治鼻疮。

exercise of Daoyin for nasal sore A static exercise, marked by sitting with the buttocks and soles on the ground, crossing the knees, separating the feet, stopping respiration, slowly breathing out after maximum of stopping respiration. Such a static exercise is practiced for five times for relieving lung heat, dredging the nostrils and curing nasal sore.

鼻齆【bí wèng**】**　为气功适应证,指鼻塞不知香臭,发音不清。多因肺气虚,卫气失固,伤风感冒所致。

nasal congestion An indication of Qigong, referring to obstructed nose without any taste and clear sound, usually caused by deficiency of lung Qi, weakness of defense Qi and common cold.

鼻齆候导引法【bí wèng hòu dǎo yǐn fǎ**】** 为动静相兼功。其作法为，面向东方而坐，闭气不息，至极限时慢慢呼出，做三遍，用手捻两鼻孔。

exercise of Daoyin for nasal congestion An exercise combined with dynamic exercise and static exercise, marked by sitting to the east, stopping respiration, slowly breathing out for three times after maximum of stopping respiration, and twisting the nostrils with both hands.

鼻息肉候导引法【bí xī ròu hòu dǎo yǐn fǎ**】** 为静功。其作法为，正坐，伸直腰，用鼻慢慢吸气后，用右手捏鼻孔，闭眼、慢慢用口吐气。明目聪耳，治视物昏花，流泪，鼻息肉，耳聋，外感头痛。

exercise of Daoyin for nasal polyp A static exercise, marked by sitting upright, stretching the waist, pinching the nostrils with the right hand after slowly breathing out through the nose, closing the eyes and slowly breathing out through the mouth. Such a static exercise can improve the eyesight and hearing, and cure lacrimation, nasal polyp, deafness and headache due to external contraction.

彼此怀真土【bǐ cǐ huái zhēn tǔ**】** 源自气功学专论，主要阐述真土（意）在金丹（龙虎交媾）返还中的重要作用。

together receiving genuine earth Collected from a monograph of Qigong, mainly describing the important effect of genuine earth（consciousness）in the restoration of golden Dan（pills of immortality）which refers to intercourse of Loong and tiger.

必极【bì jí**】** 指极至，为至人之意，即至人调节意识活动的方法。

supremacy Refers to the thought of lofty man, indicating lofty man's way to regulate the activity of consciousness.

必先岁气无伐天和【bì xiān suì qì wú fá tiān hé**】** 为名言，出自《黄帝内经·素问·五常政大论》。

（One）must be aware of（the condition）of Qi in the year, avoiding violation of natural harmony. This is a celebrated dictum from the *Chapter of Discussion on the Administration of Five-Motions* in Huangdi Neijing（entitled *Yellow Emperor's Internal Canon of Medicine*）.

必一其神【bì yī qí shén**】** 指精神意识活动专一。

spiritual concentration Refers to concentrated activity of the spirit and consciousness.

闭藏【bì cáng**】** 封闭潜藏。气功文献里指精气神不外泄，应伏藏于身内。

hidden secret Refers to closing what is hidden. In the literature of Qigong, it indicates that the essence, Qi and the spirit cannot be leaked and should be hidden in the body.

闭聪掩明【bì cōng yǎn míng**】** 义为切断耳目对外的联系以减少干扰，为古代调神的方法之一。

screening the eyes and ears Means to cut off the external connection of the ears and the eyes in order to stop disturbance, which is one of the methods used in ancient times to regulate the spirit.

闭关【bì guān**】** ① 指意识切断呼吸出入之气；② 指闭息。

controlling pass Refers to ① either cutting off Qi that is inhaled and exhaled with the consciousness；② or regulating respiration in practicing Qigong.

闭摩通滞气【bì mó tōng zhì qì**】** 为动功。其作法为，澄心闭息，以左手摩滞四十九遍，右手亦然，复以津涂之。勤行七日，则气血通畅，永无凝滞之患。

eliminating depression for solving stagnation of Qi A dynamic exercise, marked by purifying the heart and controlling respiration, pressing stagnation with the left hand for forty-nine times, pressing it with the right hand for the same time and moistening it with fluid. After practice for seven days, Qi and blood will be unobstructed without any stagnation.

闭气【bì qì**】** ① 指调息；② 指用意识控制呼吸。

controlling Qi Refers to ① either regulating breath; ② or controlling respiration with consciousness.

闭气法【bì qì fǎ**】** 为静功，① 指调身，即叩齿、咽津、搓面等；② 指调气，即引自然之气咽之，意念导引入气海。

exercise for controlling respiration A static exercise, referring to ① either regulation of the body, including clicking the teeth, swallowing fluid and rubbing the face; ② or regulating Qi, including swallowing natural Qi and transmitting Qi to the sea of Qi with consciousness.

闭气歌【bì qì gē**】** 源自专论，主要阐述闭气疗病的方法。

song of controlling respiration Collected from a monograph that describes the methods to control respiration for treating certain disease.

闭气候极【bì qì hòu jí**】** 指意念控制口鼻，不使其气出。

extreme control of respiration Refers to controlling the mouth and the nose with consciousness in order to prevent dispersion of Qi.

闭气治诸病法【bì qì zhì zhū bìng fǎ**】** 动功，欲引头病者，仰头；欲引腰脚病者，仰足十指；欲引胸中病者，挽足十指；引臂病者，掩臂；欲去腹中寒热、诸不快、若中寒身热，皆闭气、张腹；欲息者，徐以鼻息已，复为至愈乃止。

controlling respiration for curing various diseases A dynamic exercise, marked by raising the head for relieving the disease in the head; raising the ten toes for relieving the disease in the waist and foot; holding the ten toes for relieving the disease in the chest; covering the shoulders for relieving the disease in the arm; controlling respiration and extending the abdomen for relieving cold-heat, various displeasures, cold in the chest and heat in the body; controlling breath through the nose for improving respiration and restoring all activities.

闭任开督【bì rèn kāi dū**】** 指习练周天功的方法，闭任脉，意念导引精气过尾闾，沿督脉而上。

closing the conception meridian and opening the governor meridian Refers to the method for refining the celestial circle marked by closing the conception meridian, transmitting the spiritual Qi through the coccygeal end and upward along the governor meridian with consciousness.

闭塞三关【bì sè sān guān**】** 指闭塞精、气、神三关，即固精护气安神，精气不妄施泄，精神不外弥散。

closing three passes Refers to either

closing the essence, Qi and spirit, indicating that the essence should be fixed, Qi should be protected and the spirit should be stabilized; the essence and Qi should not be leaked; and the essence and spirit should not be dispersed.

闭息【bì xī**】** 指行功时调节呼吸,使之相对稳定。

controlling respiration Refers to regulating and stabilizing respiration.

痹证【bì zhèng**】** 为气功适应证,多因正气不足,腠理不密,卫外不固,感受风、寒、温、热之邪所致。

impediment syndrome/pattern An indication of Qigong, usually caused by insufficiency of healthy Qi, looseness of muscular interstices and invasion of pathogenic wind, coldness, warmth and heat.

辟谷【bì gǔ**】** 即不食。练功到一定程度出现不感饥饿,不进饮食而精力不减,身体轻快而无不适。

stopping diet（inedia） Refers to no hunger after practicing Qigong to a certain stage, during which the energy is not reduced and the body is not discomforted without taking food.

蔽【bì**】** ① 指耳屏;② 指遮掩;③ 指概况;④ 指隐藏。

shelter Refers to ① either tragus; ② or hiding; ③ or generality; ④ or occultation.

蔽骨【bì gǔ**】** ① 指胸骨剑突;② 指穴位名,为任脉中的一个穴位,位于腹正中钱,脐上 7 寸。此穴位为气功习练之处。

Bigu Refers to ① either mucronate cartilage; ② or Jiuwei (CV 15), which is an acupoint in the conception meridian, located in the abdominal middle line, 7 Cun above the navel. This acu-

point is a region usually used in practice of Qigong.

壁观【bì guān**】** 即佛教修行法,要求习练气功之时要完全停止对外在世界的认识,甚至要求连自己的呼吸也感受不到。

mahayana's void The exercise of practicing Qigong in Buddhism, suggesting to stop watching the external world and even to avoid experiencing respiration.

避噩梦法【bì è mèng fǎ**】** 为动静相兼功。其作法为,梦醒后,以左手掐人中二七过,叩齿二七通,开口以前齿啄之。功效为避噩梦。

exercise for avoiding nightmare An exercise combined with dynamic exercise and static exercise, marked by pinching Renzhong (philtrum) and clicking the teeth for two to seven times respectively after getting up, and pecking with the teeth before opening the mouth. Such an exercise combined with dynamic exercise and static exercise can prevent nightmare.

避害【bì hài**】** 指"远嫌疑,远小人"以避免精神损伤。

avoiding harm Refers to being aloof from suspicion and small figures in order to avoid damaging the spirit.

髀【bì**】** ① 指大腿;② 指股骨,即大腿骨;③ 指大腿外侧;④ 指习练大周天。

thigh Refers to ① either the big legs; ② or the femur; ③ or the thighbones; or lateral sides of the thighs; ④ or practice of the great circulatory cycle.

髀关【bì guān**】** ① 指髋关节前方;② 指足阳明胃经中的一个穴位;③ 为精气运行的通道。

thigh joint Refers to ① either the front of the hip joint; ② or an acupoint in the stomach meridian of foot Taiyang; ③ or the way for the movement of the essential Qi.

髀枢【bì shū】　指髋关节。

thigh pivot　Refers to the hip joint.

髀厌【bì yàn】　即股骨大转子。

thigh trochanter　Refers to the greater trochanter of femur.

臂臑【bì rú】　为手阳明大肠经中的一个穴位,位于曲池和肩髃的连线上。此穴位为气功习练之处。

Binao（**LI 14**）　An acupoint in the large intestine meridian of hand Taiyang, located above the line between Quchi（LI 11）and Jianyu（LI 15）. This acupoint is a region usually used in practice of Qigong.

扁鹊【biǎn què】　为战国时杰出的医学家,精通气功。

Bian Que　A great doctor of traditional Chinese medicine and a master of Qigong in the Warring States Period （475 BC – 221 BC）.

遍身疼痛治法【biàn shēn téng tòng zhì fǎ】　为动功。其作法为,端坐舒两脚,握固,闭气一口,拜身向前,次立齐向足,低头垂手扳两脚尖,闭气一口,叩齿一遍。

exercise for curing body pain　A dynamic exercise, marked by sitting upright, stretching the feet, holding the body, stopping respiration for a while, turning the body forward, keeping the feet connected each other, lowering the head to pull the tiptoes with both hands, stopping Qi for a while and clicking the teeth for one time.

表色【biǎo sè】　为佛家气功习用语,指形体在意识作用下反映于外的运动状态,如行、住、坐、卧、取、舍、屈、伸等。

external motions　A common term of Qigong in Buddhism, referring to the external manifestations of movement under the influence of consciousness, such as acting, staying, sitting, lying, taking, abandoning, bending and stretching.

冰壶【bīng hú】　指脑,即脑神冷静空无一物。

cold pot　Refers to the brain, indicating that the spirit in the brain is calm and tranquil without anything.

丙火之腑【bǐng huǒ zhī fǔ】　指小肠。

third fire viscus　Refers to the small intestine.

禀气不能无偏秉【bǐng qì bù néng wú piān bǐng】　指人性虽然相同,个性却是千姿百态,习练气功,选择功法,不能没有差别。

Innate Qi is naturally inclined to a certain side.　This is a celebrated dictum, indicating that human nature is the same, but personalities are in different poses and with different expressions. So in practicing Qigong, selections of exercises are certain different from one to another.

病冷【bìng lěng】　为气功适应证,指虚寒类疾病。因寒邪侵入人体,与卫气相搏,如阴寒偏胜,则出现表寒病。

frigid disease　An indication of Qigong, referring to the category of deficiency-cold diseases usually caused by invasion of pathogenic coldness that strikes against defense Qi, leading to exuberance of Yin cold and frigid disease.

病热【bìng rè】　为气功适应证,指因外感风邪而致发热的疾病。

heat disease　An indication of Qigong,

B

referring to heat disease caused by invasion of external pathogenic wind.

病热候导引法【bìng rè hòu dǎo yǐn fǎ】 为动静相兼功。其作法为，仰卧，两脚舒展，两膝靠拢，腰伸直，用口吸气，鼓部，使气充满，连作七次。清热止痛，舒筋活络；治发热，疼痛，两腿行动不便。

exercise of Daoyin for heat disease An exercise combined with dynamic exercise and static exercise, marked by lying on the back, stretching the feet, crossing the knees, unbending the waist, inhaling Qi through the mouth to increase and enrich it for seven times in order to relieving heat, stopping pain, stretching the sinews and activating the collaterals. This way of practicing Qigong can solve the problems of fever, pain and difficulty in walking.

病有三等【bìng yǒu sān děng】 指时病、年病、身病。

three categories of diseases Include seasonal diseases, yearly diseases and physiological diseases.

波罗蜜【bō luó mì】 为佛家气功习用语，指习练气功，增加智慧，达到涅槃境界。

prajnaparamita (**diversileaf artocarpus fruit**) A common term of Qigong in Buddhism, referring to increasing wisdom and reaching the state of nirvana in practicing Qigong.

帛和【bó hé】 为《太平经》的作者或传人。

Bo He The author or exponent of Taiping Jing entitled *Canon of Peace and Tranquility*.

泊然天真【bó rán tiān zhēn】 指顺应自然，适应社会的变化，保持天和之真。

tranquil celestial truth Means to follow natural principles, adapting to social changes and keeping celestial harmony and truth.

脖映【bó yǎng】 ① 指气海穴，为任脉中的一个穴位；② 指脐。

neck and vision Refers to ① either Qihai (CV 6), which is an acupoint in the conception meridian; ② or navel.

膊【bó】 ① 指上臂外侧面；② 指肩臂。

arm Refers to ① either the lateral side of the upper arm; ② or the shoulder and arm.

不但空【bú dàn kōng】 为佛家气功习用语。习练佛家气功时，观一切法悉皆空，见但空而不见不空。

no emptiness A common term of Qigong in Buddhism, referring to observing void and non-void in practicing Qigong in Buddhism.

不但中【bú dàn zhōng】 为佛家气功习用语，指习练佛家气功，应守中抱一，意识思维活动稳定于形体之中。

stabilized mind A common term of Qigong practice in Buddhism, referring to somatic and spiritual balance and tranquilization of the activities of consciousness and thinking in practicing Qigong.

不畏念起，惟畏觉迟【bú wèi niàn qǐ wéi wèi jué chí】 指习练气功，不畏有杂念，而畏觉悟迟，以其觉悟能守神，排除杂念。

no fearing of full ideas, only fearing of tardy consciousness A celebrated dictum, referring to no fearing of distracting thought, but fearing of no consciousness because only consciousness can keep the spirit and eliminate distracting thought.

补胆气法【bǔ dǎn qì fǎ】 为静功。其

作法为,正身端坐,意想北方,吸玄宫之黑气入口九吞之,意念送入丹田,以补嘻之损。

exercise for tonifying gallbladder Qi A static exercise, marked by sitting upright, imagining the north, inhaling black Qi from Xuangong (north) into the mouth for nine times, entering Dantian with consciousness for curing damage caused by giggle. Dantian is divided into the upper Dantian (the region between the eyes), the middle Dantian (the region below the heart) and the lower Dantian (the region below the navel).

补肺气法【bǔ fèi qì fǎ】 为静功。其作法为,面西平坐,鸣天鼓七,饮玉浆三次,瞑目吸兑宫白气,入口吞之以补呬之损。

exercise for tonifying lung Qi A static exercise, marked by sitting towards the west, sounding to the sky (a method of kneading) for seven times, drinking syrup for three times, closing the eyes to inhale white Qi from Duigong (one of the Eight Trigrams), and swallowing it through the mouth to cure damage caused by gasp for breath.

补肝气法【bǔ gān qì fǎ】 为静功。其作法为,清晨面向东,叩齿三通,闭气七息,吸震宫之青气三吞之,以补嘘之损。

exercise for tonifying liver A static exercise, marked by facing the east in the early morning, clicking the teeth for three times, holding respiration for seven times, taking clear Qi from the east for three times in order to cure damage caused by deficiency.

补脑法【bǔ nǎo fǎ】 为静功。其作法为,① 调身,即自然坐或站式;② 调气

调神,姿势定后调节呼吸。

exercise for tonifying the brain A static exercise, referring to ① either regulation of the body with natural sitting or standing; ② or regulation of Qi and spirit in order to regulate respiration.

补脾气法【bǔ pí qì fǎ】 为静功。其作法为,正身端坐,意想中宫,禁气五息,鸣天鼓七次,吸土宫之黄气入口五吞之,补呼之损。

exercise for tonifying spleen Qi Exercise for tonifying spleen Qi is a static exercise, marked by sitting upright, imagining the central palace, stopping respiration for five times, sounding to sky (a method of kneading) for seven times, inhaling yellow Qi from Tugong (a special joint) into the mouth to swallow for five times in order to cure damage caused by respiration.

补肾气法【bǔ shèn qì fǎ】 为静功。其作法为,正坐端身,面向北方,鸣金梁七,饮玉泉三,吸玄宫之黑气入吞之,以意引入丹田,以补吹之损。

exercise for tonifying kidney Qi A static exercise, marked by sitting upright, facing the north, sounding Jinliang (important region related to the teeth) for seven times, drinking Yuquan (CV 3) located 4 Cun below the navel, inhaling black Qi from Xuangong (north) and leading it to Dantian with consciousness for curing damage caused by exhalation. Dantian is divided into the upper Dantian (the region between the eyes), the middle Dantian (the region below the heart) and the lower Dantian (the region below the navel).

补心气法【bǔ xīn qì fǎ】 为静功。其作法为,清晨面向南,自然端坐,或盘膝

B

坐,叩金梁九,漱玄泉三,静思想吸离宫之赤气入口三吞之,以补呵之损。

exercise for tonifying heart Qi A static exercise, marked by facing the south in the early morning, sitting upright, or sitting with crossed legs, clicking the Jinliang (important region related to the teeth) for nine times, rinsing Xuanquan (saliva) and quietly thinking and taking Qi from Ligong (south) for three times for curing damage caused by respiration.

不测为神【bù cè wéi shén】 指神妙变化,阴阳互根作用。

marvelous change of spirit Refers to marvelous change of the spirit and interaction of Yin and Yang.

不出不入【bù chū bù rù】 为身心稳定平和之意。

no going out and no coming in Refers to stability and harmony of the heart and the body.

不得全闭【bù dé quán bì】 指呼吸完全闭息。意为习练气功时,调匀呼吸,使呼吸出入气缓和均匀。

relaxed respiration Refers to regulation of respiration in practicing Qigong in order to make respiration relaxed and uniform.

不动定【bù dòng dìng】 为佛家气功习用语,指静功,神形清静,无为寂定。

silence A common term and a static exercise of Qigong practice in Buddhism, referring to tranquilization of the spirit and the body.

不二法门【bù èr fǎ mén】 指祖窍之异名,佛学用以称直接入道,不可言传的法门。

unspeakable initial approach Refers to either another name of Zuqiao (an acupoint located in the area between the heart and navel), or the initial way to reach Dao without any description according to Buddhism.

不方不圆闭牖窗【bù fāng bù yuán bì yǒu chuāng】 指精神内守,行为中和,指顺应自然。

closing the window without square and round Refers to keeping the spirit inside, balancing all the activities and following the natural principles.

不放逸【bù fàng yì】 为佛家气功术语,指习练佛家气功,意识活动专注,排除杂念。

concentrated tranquilization A common term of Qigong practice in Buddhism, referring to concentration of attention and relief of distracting thoughts in practicing Qigong.

不寒法【bù hán fǎ】 为静功,指闭口行五火之气一千两百遍。

no cold imagination A static exercise, referring to closing the mouth to practice one thousand and two hundred times of Qi from five fires.

不即不离【bù jí bù lí】 为佛家气功习用语,指习练佛家气功,意识思维活动以和平为佳。

no approach and no leaving A term of Qigong practice in Buddhism, referring to peaceful state in practicing Qigong.

不净观【bù jìng guān】 为佛家功法,即观自身及他身之不净,转移精神意识活动,防治贪欲妄想之病。

foul imagination An exercise of Qigong in Buddhism, referring to exchange of the activities of the spirit and consciousness and prevention of greed through observation of impurity in oneself and others.

不觉【bù jué】 佛家气功习用语,指不理解佛家。功法为,行功不能入静。

no meditation A common term of Qigong in Buddhism, referring to disability for meditation due to failure to understand Qigong in Buddhism.

不来不去【bù lái bù qù】 为佛家气功学习用语,指气根本在于保持神形的稳定状态。

no coming and no going A common term of Qigong in Buddhism, referring to stabilized state in practicing Qigong.

不离于伍【bù lí yú wǔ】 即宇宙间的一切事物,都要按照五行生克规律变化。

indispensability to the five elements Refers to the fact that all the things in the universe must move and change according to the principles of promotion and restraint in the five elements (including wood, fire, earth, metal and water).

不立文字【bù lì wén zì】 为佛家气功习用语,指佛家学习义理,不成文见书,只示人领悟意旨。

no use of characters A common term of Qigong in Buddhism, referring to the fact that the theory and methods in Buddhism are not written in books, only guiding people to comprehend the intention.

不寐【bù mèi】 即失眠。多因思虑劳倦损伤心脾,心肾不交,阴虚火旺,肝阳扰动,心胆气虚及胃不和等所致。

no insomnia Refers to difficulty to sleep usually due to failure to tranquilize the mind that damages the heart and spleen, causing incoordination of the heart and kidney, Yin deficiency and fire excess, disturbance of liver Yang, deficiency of heart Qi and gallbladder Qi as well as disharmony of the

stomach.

不热法【bù rè fǎ】 为静功,指立夏日理想玄冰或飞霜。

no heat imagination A static exercise, referring to imagination of abstruse water or frost in the beginning of summer.

不神神【bù shén shén】 指返璞归真,回复自然本性之神为神神。

natural spirit Indicates to return to original purity and simplicity.

不生【bù shēng】 为佛家气功习用语,指精神意识活动的相对稳定状态。

mental stability A term of Qigong practice in Buddhism, referring to tranquility of the activities of the spirit and consciousness.

不生不灭【bù shēng bù miè】 为佛家气功习用语,指稳定、涅槃、中性。

no bearing and no dying A common term of Qigong in Buddhism, referring to stability, nirvana and mutuality.

不时御神【bù shí yù shén】 指不善于驾驭和使用精神,只专求心志的一时之快,妄耗神气,心至早衰。

improper use of spirit Refers to inability of elaborating the spirit, dissipation of the spirit and temporary indulgence that have declined the heart.

不识阴阳莫乱为【bù shí yīn yáng mò luàn wéi】 源自气功专论。主要阐述阴阳消长、升降交媾在练功中的重要作用。

avoidance of disordered application of Yin and Yang Collected from a monograph of Qigong, mainly describing the important effect of wane and wax of Yin and Yang as well as ascent, descent and coition in practicing Qigong.

不思议【bù sī yì】 佛家气功术语,指气功义理殊深,不在思议中,只在觉悟领会。

no contemplation A common term of

B

Qigong in Buddhism, referring to the fact that the theory and practice of Qigong is abstruse and cannot be stored in the mind.

不死浆【bù sǐ jiāng】 即习练气功时口中产生的津液。

saliva Refers to fluid and humor appearing in the mouth when practicing Qigong.

不忘禅【bù wàng chán】 佛家气功习用语,指修炼佛家气功,增强记忆,亦指能增强记忆的气功功法。

no memory of dhyana A common term of Qigong in Buddhism, referring to increasing memory and ability in practicing Qigong.

不妄语戒【bù wàng yǔ jiè】 指学习佛家气功,禁止一切虚妄不实之言。

forbidden avarice Refers to inhibition of false ideas in practicing Qigong according to Buddhism.

不信【bù xìn】 为佛家气功习用语,指习练佛家功法杂念未除,意识思维活动不稳定。

no stability A common term of Qigong practice in Buddhism, referring to failure to relieve distracting thoughts and to tranquilize the activities of consciousness and thinking.

不有中有【bù yǒu zhōng yǒu】 指通过反复习练,全身保持相对平衡状态。

from nonexistence to pass into existence Refers to keeping balanced state through repeated practice of Qigong.

不欲以静【bù yù yǐ jìng】 指根绝欲念,全身各部才能协调稳定。

stabilization without any desire Refers to the fact that only when avarices are eliminated can the whole body be regulated and stabilized.

不远复【bù yuǎn fù】 指调节意识活动中,不符合事情的言行,出未远而即复正,有益神形的稳定。

close recovery Refers to stabilizing the spirit and the body as well as avoiding speaking and doing any improper things in order to stabilize the spirit and the body.

不住【bù zhù】 指脑神无丝毫念头留住,为至静至虚的境界,亦指精神意识思维活动不会凝住不变。

absolute tranquility Refers to no existence of any idea in the brain spirit which is the ideal state of tranquility without any deficiency.

布气【bù qì】 ①指气功中,发放外气治病;②指风、火、燥、湿、寒五气在自然界的运行。

releasing Qi Refers to ① either treatment of disease by providing external Qi in practicing Qiong; ② or wind Qi, fire Qi, dry Qi, damp Qi and cold Qi in the natural movement.

布气攻疾【bù qì gōng jí】 指发放外气攻逐疾病,使之痊愈。

releasing Qi to expel disease Refers to expelling disease by providing external Qi in order to cure disease.

布宇观法【bù yǔ guān fǎ】 为佛家气功功法,即同一真而共一味。

exercise for releasing universal view A method for practicing Qigong in Buddhism, referring to the same genuine Qi with the same pure taste.

C

擦面【cā miàn】　为动功。其作法为，用两手掌从下到上轻搓面部，次数不拘。搓时动作应缓慢，协调，不用重力，精神集中于手心劳宫。

rubbing face A dynamic exercise, marked by kneading the face from the lower to the upper with both fists for several times, slowing kneading for coordination without gravity, and concentrating the spirit in the palms in kneading.

擦肾腧穴法【cā shèn shù xué fǎ】　为动功。其作法为，临卧时，坐于床垂足，解衣闭气，舌柱上腭，目视顶，仍提缩谷道，以手摩擦两肾腧穴，各一百二十次，以多为妙，毕即卧。治肾气虚、尿频。

exercise for rubbing the kidney and acupoint A dynamic exercise, marked by sitting on the bed before sleeping, drooping the feet, disrobing clothes, stopping respiration, sustaining the supramaxilla with the tongue, seeing the top with the eyes, lifting and shrinking the anus, rubbing the acupoints in the kidney regions with both hands for one hundred and twenty times and sleeping after finishing practice of Qigong. Such a dynamic exercise can cure deficiency of kidney Qi and frequent urination.

擦肾腧治频诩法【cā shèn shù zhì pín xǔ fǎ】　为动功。其作法为，每于卧前，坐床垂足，解衣闭气，舌柱上腭，目视顶，提谷道，以手擦两肾腧穴各三十六次。

frequent brag exercise for rubbing kidney acupoint A dynamic exercise, marked by sitting on the bed before sleeping, drooping the feet, disrobing clothes, stopping respiration, sustaining the supramaxilla with the tongue, seeing the top with the eyes, lifting and shrinking the anus, rubbing the acupoints in the kidney regions with both hands for thirty-six times.

擦涌泉穴法【cā yǒng quán xué fǎ】　为动功。其作法为，平时有空即可作，赤两足，更次用一手握趾，一手摩擦足心涌泉穴。此穴位为气功习练之处。

exercise for rubbing Yongquan（KI 1） A dynamic exercise, marked by practicing at leisure, keeping the feet bare, holding toes with one hand and kneading the soles with the other hand. This acupoint is a region usually used in practice of Qigong.

才全【cái quán】　指情性保持平和，不受自然和社会的干扰。

whole harmony Refers to pacifying the temperament and avoiding interference of social factors.

采补还丹【cǎi bǔ hái dān】　指肾中液还于心中，水火相交，合而为一。

collecting and tonifying exercise for returning of Dan（pills of immortality） Refers to humor in the kidney returning to the heart, indicating combination and integration of water and fire.

采补之法【cǎi bǔ zhī fǎ】　① 指练功中采先天一气，因神的作用，炼而为药，贮藏在下丹田；② 指采日月之精华，以补胎息练气之不足。

exercise for collection and supplementation Refers to ① either collecting the innate Qi in practicing Qigong because of the effect of the spirit that can produce medicinal and store it in the lower Dantian (the region below the navel); ② or the essence of the sun and the moon that can tonify fetal respiration and improve refining Qi.

采飞根法【cǎi fēi gēn fǎ】 为动功。其作法为，日初出时，面向东方，自然站立，叩齿九通，然后默念。

exercise for collecting flying root A dynamic exercise, marked by naturally standing up and turning to the east in sunrise, clicking the teeth for nine times and silently reading some important concepts.

采日精法【cǎi rì jīng fǎ】 为静功。其作法为，择风和日丽的日子，寅卯时刻，太阳出后，在庭园、河滨，林木茂盛，日光能照射处，东向坐（或立）定，双肩微耸，身体放松，不可前俯后仰，弯腰驼背，亦不可硬劲强直。

exercise for collecting solar essence A static exercise, marked by sitting (or standing up) towards the east in garden or streamside with flourishing trees to be shined by the sun after sunrise in Yin (the period of the day from 3 a.m. to 5 a.m. in the early morning) and Mao (the period of a day from 5 a.m. to 7 a.m. in the early morning) in the sunny day, shrugging the shoulders, relaxing the body, avoiding to bend forward and backward, refusing stoop and humpback, and preventing hard strength and rigidity.

采日精月华【cǎi rì jīng yuè huá】 日为心，月为肾，指采心之真液，肾之真气。

collecting the sun-essence and moonlight Refers to collecting the genuine humor in the heart and the genuine Qi in the kidney. In this term, the sun refers to the heart and the moon refers to the kidney.

采时用目守泥丸【cǎi shí yòng mù shǒu ní wán】 指习练周天功时，两目意视泥丸，导引精气沿督脉升上泥丸。

protection of the mud bolus (the brain) with the eyes during collection A celebrated dictum, indicating that the eyes observe the brain with consciousness, leading the essence and Qi to flow upwards to the brain through the governor meridian.

采药【cǎi yào】 ① 指行动中形神的稳定状态；② 指午时阴阳平秘，或相交；③ 指习练气功为采药；④ 指气随意动。

selecting medicinal Refers to ① either stable condition of the body and the spirit in practicing of Qigong; ② or balance or coordination of Yin and Yang in Wu period (the period of the day from 11 a.m. to 1 p.m.); ③ or practice of Qigong which is known as selection of medicinal; ④ or movement of Qi following the consciousness.

采药时调火功【cǎi yào shí diào huǒ gōng】 采药时，指身中一阳来复之时，此时当注意调整火候，以运金行。

exercise for regulating fire in collecting medicinal Refers to regulation of duration of heating in order to move golden activity when a Yang has returned during collection of medicinal.

采药与进火【cǎi yào yǔ jìn huǒ】 源自气功学专论，主要阐述采药与进火的关系。

collecting medicinal and entering fire Collected from a monograph of Qigong, mainly describing the relationship between collection of medicinal and entrance of fire.

采药之法【cǎi yào zhī fǎ**】** 指习练气功，咽津握固，控制意识思维活动，蓄炼真气。

exercise for collecting medicinal Refers to swallowing fluid, setting the thumbs in the palms, controlling the activities of consciousness and thought as well as storing and refining the genuine Qi.

参禅【cān chán**】** 佛家气功习用语，指学习佛家义理，亦含有学习并习练气功之意。

practicing dhyana Refers to the Buddhism principles, which also indicates the significance of studying and practicing Qigong.

参同炉火而言内丹【cān tóng lú huǒ ér yán nèi dān**】** 其中的炉指形体，火指神，内丹指气功养生法。

Participate furnace fire and discuss internal Dan (pills of immortality). This is a celebrated dictum, in which furnace refers to the body, fire refers to the spirit and internal Dan (pills of immortality) refers to the exercise for cultivating life in Qigong practice.

苍锦云衣午龙蟠【cāng jǐn yún yī wǔ lóng pán**】** 苍锦指肾之外象，云衣为肾膜之象，午龙蟠为肾之青脉。

green brocade, cloudy cloth and coiled Wu Loog A celebrated dictum, in which green brocade refers to the external manifestation of the kidney, cloudy cloth refers to the external manifestation of kidney membrane and Wu

Loong refers to the green meridian of the kidney. In this term, Wu (the period of a day from 11 a.m. to 1 p.m. in the noon) refers to afternoon.

藏德不止【cáng dé bù zhǐ**】** 指修炼气功时天人相应之理。

constant storage of virtue Constant storage of virtue is a term of Qigong, referring the principle of correspondence between man and the universe in practicing Qigong.

藏伏【cáng fú**】** 指习练气功时，自然太和之气及先天元气深藏归伏于丹田。

hiding and bending Refers to deeply storing the natural and harmonious Qi as well as the innate original Qi in Dantian during the practice of Qigong. Dantian is divided into the upper Dantian (the region between the eyes), the middle Dantian (the region below the heart) and the lower Dantian (the region below the navel).

藏金斗【cáng jīn dòu**】** 同虚危穴，即九灵铁鼓，为精气聚散常在此处，水火发端也在此处，阴阳变化也在此处，有无出入也在此处。

storage of golden iron The same as deficient and anxious point and nine genius-fire drums, refers to the region where the essential Qi concentrates and disperses there, water and fire appear there, Yin and Yang change there, exit and entrance exist there.

操一【cāo yī**】** 习练气功时，意识思维活动集中统一。

concentration Refers to combination and unification of the activities of consciousness and thinking in practicing Qigong.

曹慈山【cáo cí shān**】** 清代乾隆年间

气功养生家,撰写有老年气功养生专著。
Cao Cishan A master of Qigong and life cultivation in the Qing Dynasty (1636 AD – 1912 AD), who wrote a monograph of Qigong and life cultivation for old people.

曹国舅抚云阳板【cáo guó jiù fǔ yún yáng bǎn**】** 为动功。其作法为,身体坐在椅子上,左脚弯膝置于椅上,右腿斜向自然置地上,两手相抱向左右上举,眼向右前方看,运气廿四口。主治瘫痪。
Cap Guojiu's exercise for overlooking the cloud and the sun A dynamic exercise, marked by sitting on the chair, bending the right knee to the chair, slanting the right foot to the ground, holding the hands to raise from the left and right, turning the eyes to the right front, and moving Qi for twenty-four times. Such a dynamic exercise can cure paralysis.

曹国舅脱靴法【cáo guó jiù tuō xuē fǎ**】** 为动功。其作法为,站立定,左手作报墙形,右手垂下,右脚向前虚蹬,运气一十六口,左右同。主治腿脚疼痛。
Cao Guojiu's exercise for taking off shoes A dynamic exercise, marked by standing up, raising the left hand like a wall, drooping the right hand, imagining to stretch the right foot forward, moving Qi for sixteen times from the left to the right and vice versa. Such a dynamic exercise can cure pain in the leg and foot.

曹溪路【cáo xī lù**】** 即虚危穴,精气聚散常在此处,水火发端也在此处,阴阳变化也在此处,有无出入也在此处。
Caoxi road The same as Xuwei acupoint, is the region where the essential Qi concentrates and disperses there, water and fire appear there, Yin and Yang change there, exit and entrance exist there.

曹仙姑胎息诀【cáo xiān gū tāi xī jué**】** 为静功口诀,指习练时神气相须。
Female Immortal Cao's formula for fetal respiration A static exercise, referring to mutual promotion between the spirit and Qi in practicing Qigong.

漕溪路【cáo xī lù**】** 指脊骨,亦指脊髓。
Caoxi road Refers to backbone, or spinal marrow.

差夏【chà xià**】** 指一年中长夏季与秋令季相交之时。
late summer Refers to the period between the late summer and the beginning of autumn.

姹女【chà nǚ**】** ① 指心;② 指水银,炼丹药物之一。
beautiful female Refers to ① either the heart; ② or mercury, one of the medicinal produced by alchemy.

禅【chán**】** ① 指静虑没有杂念,为稳定精神的方法;② 指精神宁静专注于一境。
dhyana Refers to ① either tranquil contemplation without any distracting thought, which is the way to stabilize the spirit; ② or tranquilization and concentration of the spirit in a special state.

禅病【chán bìng**】** 指一切杂念、妄念为禅定的病魔。
dhyana disease Indicates that all distracting thoughts and wild fancy are the serious illnesses.

禅定【chán dìng**】** 即思维修,为佛家气功习用语,指佛家静坐凝神,专注一境的习练方法。
dhyana stability The same as thinking cultivation, is a common term of

Qigong in Buddhism，referring to sitting quietly and concentrating the spirit in practicing Qigong in Buddhism.

禅寂【chán jì】　指寂静思虑，泛指习练气功，导引入静。

dhyana quietness　A common term of Qigong in Buddhism，referring to quiet and silent contemplation，indicating tranquilization in practicing Qigong.

禅那【chán nà】　即思维修，为佛家气功习用语，指佛家静坐凝神，专注一境的习练方法。

dhyana scene　The same as thinking cultivation，is a common term of Qigong in Buddhism，referring to sitting quietly and concentrating the spirit in practicing Qigong in Buddhism.

禅思【chán sī】　指精神意识活动的集中统一。

dhyana thinking　Dhyana thinking is a common term of Qigong in Buddhism，referring to concentration and unification of the activities of the spirit and consciousness.

禅味【chán wèi】　指习练佛家气功，神形合一，有轻安静寂之妙味，神宁形适之安乐。

dhyana taste　A common term of Qigong in Buddhism，referring to integration of the spirit and the body with wonderful taste of natural stability and tranquility as well as peace and happiness of the spirit and the body.

禅坐【chán zuò】　同结跏趺坐，即吉祥座，为佛家气功坐式，方式有二，一为吉祥，二为降魔。

dhyana sitting　The same as sitting with crossed legs，refers to auspicious sitting which is an exercise of sitting for practicing Qigong in Buddhism with two ways，one is to be auspicious，the other is to expel evil.

蟾光【chán guāng】　指一阳生。

toad light　Refers to the formation of Yang.

躔【chán】　指日月星辰运行的度次。

course of stars　Refers to the degrees and times of the movement of the sun，the moon and the stars.

产药【chǎn yào】　指气化作用，阴阳和合而产药。

producing medicinal　Refers to the effect of Qi transformation. Only when Yin and Yang are harmonized can ideal medicinal be produced in the body.

产药川源处【chǎn yào chuān yuán chù】　源自气功专论，主要阐述药产下丹田及采药火候。

source of medicinal production　Collected from a monograph about Qigong，mainly describing that medicinal is produced in the lower Dantian（the region below the navel）under certain duration and degree of heating.

产在坤，种在乾【chǎn zài kūn zhǒng zài qián】　在气功学中，人腹为坤，首为乾；坤居下为炉，乾居上为鼎。

production in the Kun（abdomen）and growing in the Qian（head）　In traditional Chinese culture，Kun refers to the earth while Qian refers to the sky. In Qigong studies，Kun refers to the abdomen while Qian refers to the head. The abdomen is located in the lower part of the body and acts as a stove while the head is located in the upper part of the body and acts as a cauldron.

长城【cháng chéng】　指任、督二脉。

long wall　Refers to the conception

meridian and the governor meridian.

长春观【cháng chūn guān】 在武昌城东门外,为气功家丘处机练功处之一。

Long spring view Refers to the place where Qiu Chuji, a great master of Qigong, practiced Qigong.

长春真人【cháng chūn zhēn rén】 是对宋元时期气功学家丘处机的称赞。

Long Spring Immortal The reputation of Qiu Chuji, a great master of Qigong.

长春子【cháng chūn zǐ】 为宋元时期气功学家长春真人,即丘处机的另外一个称谓。

Long Spring Man Another name of Qiu Chuji also known as Changchun Zhenren, who was a great scholar and master of Qigong in the Song Dynasty (960 AD - 1279 AD) and Yuan Dynasty(1271 AD - 1368 AD).

长存之道因专志【cháng cún zhī dào yīn zhuān zhì】 指健康长寿之道,在于调节精神,意定志专。

the way of longevity depending on great will A celebrated dictum, referring to the fact that regulation of spirit and stabilization of mind are the ways for cultivating health and prolonging life.

长气【cháng qì】 指火气,心火之气。

long Qi Refers to cardiopyretic Qi.

长生久视【cháng shēng jiǔ shì】 即永不衰退。

longevity without senility Refers to never declining.

长生胎元服气法【cháng shēng tāi yuán fú qì fǎ】 为静功。其作法是,习练时,先排除杂念,外绝思虑,内守神真。

fetal inhaling exercise for longevity A static exercise, characterized by elimination of distracting thought, exclusion

of consideration and stabilization of genuine spirit in practicing Qigong.

长生胎元神用经注【cháng shēng tāi yuán shén yòng jīng zhù】 为气功养生专著,作者不详。

Changsheng Taiyuan Shenyong Jingzhu (*Annotation About Cultivation the Mind and Whole Body*) A monograph of Qigong entitled *Annotation About Cultivation the Mind and Whole Body*, the author was unknown.

长生真人【cháng shēng zhēn rén】 对金代气功学家刘处玄的称赞。

Long Life Immortal The celebration of Liu Chuxuan who was a great scholar and master of Qigong in Jin Dynasty (115 AD - 1234 AD).

长生之道,要在神丹【cháng shēng zhī dào yào zài shén dān】 指的是健康长寿之道,关键在于气功养生。

longevity depending on spiritual Dan (**pills of immortality**) A celebrated dictum, referring to the fact the way for cultivating health and prolonging life depends on practice of Qigong.

长生子【cháng shēng zǐ】 金代气功学家刘处玄的另外一个称谓。

Long Life Man Another name of Liu Chuxuan who was a great scholar and master of Qigong in Jin Dynasty (115 AD - 1234 AD).

长息【cháng xī】 指深长的呼吸。

deep breath Refers to breathing in Qi through the nose and breathing out Qi through the mouth.

长息吐气法【cháng xī tǔ qì fǎ】 为静功,指一吸气,六吐气。

long respiration and exhalation technique A static exercise, marked by one inhalation and six exhalations.

长夏【cháng xià**】**　指农历六月。

long summer　Refers to June in traditional Chinese calendar.

长揖诀【cháng yī jué**】**　为动功。其作法为，叉两手，托天当面，揖伏于地者九；叉两手，左右揖伏于地者五。

long bow exercise　A dynamic exercise, marked by clasping both hands, raising both hands upwards and bending both hands over the ground for nine times; or clasping both hands and bending over the ground from the left to the right for five times.

长斋久洁【cháng zhāi jiǔ jié**】**　指习练气功的注意事项，如饮食清淡。

to pay attention to dos and don'ts　Refers to the announcement in practicing Qigong, such as light diet.

长真子【cháng zhēn zǐ**】**　金元时期气功学家谭玉的另外一个称谓。

Long Immortal　Another name of Tan Yu who was a great master in the late Jin Dynasty (115 AD - 1234 AD) and early Yuan Dynasty (1271 AD - 1368 AD).

肠虫腹痛治法【cháng chóng fù tòng zhì fǎ**】**　为动功。其作法为，身体微屈，咽气十口，两掌重叠，掌心正对肚脐，旋转按摩腹部数百次。

treatment of intestinal parasite and abdominal pain　A dynamic exercise, marked by mildly bending the body, inhaling for ten times, overlapping the fists against the navel and rotating and kneading the abdomen for several hundred times.

肠气证治法【cháng qì zhèng zhì fǎ**】**　为动功。其作法为，凡小肠气冷痛，端坐，两手相擦，务令极热，覆向丹田，数息二十九口。

treatment of intestinal Qi disorder　A dynamic exercise, marked by sitting upright if small intestinal Qi is cold and painful, rubbing the hands hot, turning to Dantian and breathing for twenty-nine times. Dantian is divided into the upper Dantian (the region between the eyes), the middle Dantian (the region below the heart) and the lower Dantian (the region below the navel).

尝罚【cháng fá**】**　指调节阴阳，一年之中春阳生谓之尝，秋阴束谓之罚。一日之中，六阳时进火为尝，六阴时退火为罚。

emergence and penalty　Refers to regulation of Yin and Yang. In every year, Yang begins to grow in spring, which is called emergence; while Yin begins to control in autumn, which is called penalty. In every day, fire produced by six kinds of Yang is called emergence while fire dispersed by six kinds of Yin is called penalty.

常合即吉【cháng hé jí jí**】**　指形体与精神合而为一则身体健康，各部功能协调稳定。

constant integration composing health　Indicates that integration of the body and spirit cultivates health and stabilize the functions of all parts of the body.

常念【cháng niàn**】**　① 指佛家气功功法；② 指经习练气功。

constant idea　Refers to ① either the exercises of Qigong in Buddhism; ② or often practice of Qigong.

常念三房相通达【cháng niàn sān fáng xiāng tōng dá**】**　指经常习练气功，调气调神，三房一气通达，全身无障碍身体健康。三房为黄庭、元海、丹田。

constant hope to interlink three chambers

C

A celebrated dictum in Qigong, indicating that constant practice of Qigong can regulate Qi and spi-rit, interlink three chambers and eliminate any obstacle in the body. The so-called three chambers refers to Huang-ting (the region below the navel), Yuanhai (the region below the heart) and Dantian. Dantian is divided into the upper Dantian (the region between the eyes), the middle Dantian (the region below the heart) and the lower Dantian (the region below the navel).

常清净【cháng qīng jìng**】** 即常常保持清静无为。

constant tranquility Refers to keeping quietism.

常人呼吸【cháng rén hū xī**】** 指呼吸之气从咽喉而下，至胸而回，不能与祖气相连，所以不能产生气功效应。

routine respiration Indicates that Qi from respiration flows downwards from the throat to the chest and then returns, and that it cannot be connected with the original Qi. That is why it cannot be effective as that of Qigong.

常在【cháng zài**】** 指脾神名。

constant existence Refers to the spirit in the spleen.

常住心月轮【cháng zhù xīn yuè lún**】** 即是意想心为明静的圆月，通体清凉明洁如朗月，随之身体与月相合为一，身即是月，月即是身。

imagined integration with the moon Indicates that the heart is imagined as the moon to make the whole body cool and refreshing like the moon, enabling the body to integrate with the moon. In this term, the body refers to the moon and the moon refers to the body.

畅外【chàng wài**】** 为动功。其作法为，手掌摩擦生热，慰通经络，逐邪于外，而使身体轻快。

rubbing exercise A dynamic exercise, marked by rubbing the palms warm, promoting movement of the meridians and collaterals, expelling pathogenic factors and relaxing the body.

超三界【chāo sān jiè**】** 指练功过程中要抛弃一切欲望和杂念，忘掉周围环境一切事物，也不有一切幻想，才能做到高度入静，精神进入某种高级境界。

exceeding three states A term of Qigong in Daoism, indicating that eliminating all desires and distracting thought, forgetting all the things in the surrounding environment, and avoiding illusions in practicing Qigong that can tranquilize the body and enable the spirit to reach the ideal state.

巢氏病源补养宣导法【cháo shì bìng yuán bǔ yǎng xuān dǎo fǎ**】** 《巢氏病源补养宣导法》由清代廖平摘编，对巢氏书中的导引法予以整理。

Chaoshi Bingyuan Buyang Xuandao Fa (*Mr. Chao's Publicized Exercise for Tonifying and Nourishing the Sources of Diseases***)** Written by Liao Pingzhai in the Qing Dynasty (1636 AD - 1912 AD), collecting the exercises of Daoyin mentioned in the monographs of traditional Chinese medicine written by Chao Yuanfang in the Sui Dynasty (581 AD - 618 AD).

巢元方【cháo yuán fāng**】** 隋代著名医学家，主张用导引治疗疾病。

Chao Yuanfang A great doctor of traditional Chinese medicine in the Sui Dynasty (581 AD - 618 AD), advocating to treat diseases with Daoyin.

朝华【cháo huá】　指上齿根之唾液。

facial essence　Refers to saliva in the upper dedendum.

朝天岭【cháo tiān lǐng】　即虚危穴，指九灵铁鼓，精气聚散常在此处，水火发端也在此处，阴阳变化也在此处，有无出入也在此处。

celestial mountain　The same as deficient and anxious point and nine genius-fire drums, refers to the region where the essential Qi concentrates and disperses there, water and fire appear there, Yin and Yang change there, exit and entrance exist there.

朝元【cháo yuán】　指练功中根据不同的时间，五脏之气、液朝集于不同的地方。

origin of direction　Indicates that practice of Qigong depends on different times, Qi from the five Zang-organs (including the heart, the liver, the spleen, the lung and the kidney) and humor concentrated in different areas.

嗔【chēn】　指精神活动，为仇恨、仇视之意。

rage　Refers to hatred and hostility in the activity of the spirit.

嗔火【chēn huǒ】　指邪火，损伤情志。

awful fire　Refers to pathogenic fire that damages emotion.

臣火【chén huǒ】　气为臣火，心为君火。

ministerial fire　Traditionally Qi refers to ministerial fire while the heart refers to monarchy fire.

尘世【chén shì】　① 指世间；② 指身体肛门附近。

human society　Refers to ① either the world; ② or the region near the anus.

陈冲用【chén chōng yòng】　唐代气功学家陈朴的另外一个称谓，其撰写了气功专著，生动、切实、深入地介绍和论述了气功的理论、方法和实践。

Chen Chongyong　Another name of Chen Pu, a master of Qigong in the Tang Dynasty (618 AD-907 AD) who wrote a monograph of Qigong, vividly and thoroughly introduced and described the theory, methods and practice of Qigong.

陈翠虚【chén cuì xū】　宋代气功学家陈楠的另外一个称谓，其著有气功专著，颇为深入地分析、研究和总结了气功养生学。

Chen Cuixu　Another name of Chen Nan, a master of Qigong in the Song Dynasty (960 AD - 1279 AD) who wrote a monograph of Qigong with thorough analysis, study and conclusion of Qigong and life cultivation.

陈观吾【chén guān wú】　元代气功学家陈致虚的另外一个称谓，其撰写了多部气功专著，对后世气功学的发展有较大的贡献。

Chen Guanwu　Another name of Chen Zhixu, a great master of Qigong in the Yuan Dynasty (1271 AD - 1368 AD) who wrote several monographs of Qigong, making certain contribution to the development of Qigong in the later generations.

陈南木【chén nán mù】　宋代气功学家陈楠的另外一个称谓，其著有气功专著，颇为深入地分析、研究和总结了气功养生学。

Chen Nanmu　Another name of Chen Nan, a master of Qigong in the Song Dynasty (960 AD - 1279 AD) who wrote a monograph of Qigong with thorough analysis, study and conclusion of Qigong and life cultivation.

陈楠【chén nán】　宋代气功学家,著有气功专著,颇为深入地分析、研究和总结了气功养生学。

Chen Nan　A master of Qigong in the Song Dynasty（960 AD - 1279 AD）who wrote a monograph of Qigong with thorough analysis, study and conclusion of Qigong and life cultivation.

陈泥丸【chén ní wán】　宋代气功学家陈楠的另外一个称谓,其著有气功专著,颇为深入地分析、研究和总结了气功养生学。

Chen Niwan　Another name of Chen Nan, a master of Qigong in the Song Dynasty（960 AD - 1279 AD）who wrote a monograph of Qigong with thorough analysis, study and conclusion of Qigong and life cultivation.

陈朴【chén pǔ】　唐代气功学家,撰写了气功专著,生动、切实、深入地介绍和论述了气功的理论、方法和实践。

Chen Pu　A master of Qigong in the Tang Dynasty（618 AD - 907 AD）who wrote a monograph of Qigong, vividly and thoroughly introduced and described the theory, methods and practice of Qigong.

陈图南【chén tú nán】　唐代气功学家陈抟的另外一个称谓,撰写了多部气功专著,对气功的发展做出了突出的贡献。

Chen Tunan　Another name of Chen Tuan, a master of Qigong in the Tang Dynasty（618 AD - 907 AD）who wrote several monographs of Qigong, making a great contribution to the development of Qigong.

陈抟【chén tuán】　唐代气功学家,撰写了多部气功专著,对气功的发展做出了突出的贡献。

Chen Tuan　A master of Qigong in the Tang Dynasty（618 AD - 907 AD）who wrote several monographs of Qigong, making a great contribution to the development of Qigong.

陈希夷【chén xī yí】　唐代气功学家陈抟的另外一个称谓,撰写了多部气功专著,对气功的发展做出了突出的贡献。

Chen Xiyi　Another name of Chen Tuan, a master of Qigong in the Tang Dynasty（618 AD - 907 AD）who wrote several monographs of Qigong, making a great contribution to the development of Qigong.

陈希夷熟睡华山【chén xī yí shú shuì huà shān】　为静功。其作法为,侧卧,右手枕于头下,左手轻握拳在腹脐上下往来按摩,右腿在下微屈腿,左腿压在右腿上,收气三十二口在腹,如此运气十二口。

Chen Xiyi's soundly sleeping in Huashan Mountain　A static exercise, marked by sitting on one side, keeping the right hand under the pillow, holding the fist with the left hand to kneading the abdomen from the upper to the lower, slowly bending the right leg, pressing the right leg with the left leg, receiving Qi in the abdomen for thirty-two times and moving Qi for twelve times.

陈希夷胎息诀【chén xī yí tāi xī jué】　为静功,本功主要是存精、养神、练气,法参四时自然阴阳变化。

Chen Xiyi's formula of fetal respiration　A static exercise, mainly including the practice of containing the essence, nourishing the spirit and refining Qi according to the natural changes of Yin and Yang in the sour seasons.

陈先生内丹诀【chén xiān shēng nèi

dān jué】《陈先生内丹诀》为气功专著，由宋代陈朴撰，以诗词的形式描述气功。

Chenxiansheng Neidan Jue（*Mr. Chen's Formula for Internal Dan*）　A monograph of Qigong entitled *Mr. Chen's Formula for Internal Dan*（*Pills of Immortality*），written by Chen Pu in the Song Dynasty（960 AD – 1279 AD），describing the theory and practice of Qigong in poetry.

陈虚白先生规中指南【chén xū bái xiān shēng guī zhōng zhǐ nán】《陈虚白先生规中指南》为气功专著，内容涉及止念、采药、入药起火、识鼎炉、坤离交媾、乾坤交媾、忘神合虚等方面。作者不详。

Chenxubai Xiansheng Guizhong Zhinan（*Mr. Chen Xubai's Guidance in the Principles of Qigong Practice*）　A monograph of Qigong entitled *Mr. Chen Xubai's Guidance in the Principles of Qigong Practice*，including the contents of stopping contemplation，collecting medicinal，taking medicinal to break out fire，understanding cauldron，intercourse of Kun（Trigram）and Li（Trigram），intercourse of Qian（Trigram）and Kun（Trigram），forgetting the spirit and combining deficiency. The author was unknown.

陈阴阳【chén yīn yáng】　古代圣人，也指令阴阳相等，各无偏胜，而达阴阳平衡之目的，为气功学基础理论之一。

Chen Yinyang　A sage in ancient China，also referring to quality and balance of Yin and Yang，one of the theories of Qigong.

陈直【chén zhí】　宋代气功养生家，主张老年人应注意四时调摄，避免精神刺激，提倡应用气功防治疾病。

Chen Zhi　A master of Qigong and life cultivation in the Song Dynasty（960 AD – 1279 AD），suggesting that old people should pay attention to the regulation in the four seasons and avoiding stimulation，and advocating that diseases should be prevented and cured by Qigong.

陈致虚【chén zhì xū】　元代气功学家，撰写了多部气功专著，对后世气功学的发展有较大的贡献。

Chen Zhixu　A great master of Qigong in the Yuan Dynasty（1271 AD – 1368 AD）who wrote several monographs of Qigong，making certain contribution to the development of Qigong in the later generations.

晨昏火候【chén hūn huǒ hòu】　源自气功专论，主要阐述产丹时要据身中阴阳消长调整火候。

duration and degree of fire in the early morning　Collected from a monograph of Qigong，mainly describing that production of Dan（pills of immortality）depends on wane and wax of Yin and Yang to regulate duration and degree of fire.

成道宫【chéng dào gōng】　位于陕西宝鸡市东南六十里处，为丘处机修练之处。

Chengdao Temple　About sixty li（a Chinese unit of length）towards Baoji City，Shaanxi Province，located in the southeast，where Qiu Chuji，a great master in the South Song Dynasty（1127 AD – 1279 AD），practiced and studied Qigong.

成和之修【chéng hé zhī xiū】　指完满纯和的意境，是由精练气功而获得。

ideal state Refers to a perfect natural state produced by practicing Qigong.

成基【chéng jī】 指习练气功,精、气、神三宝合炼成一谓之成基。

entirety Refers to integration of the essence, Qi and the spirit in practicing Qigong.

承蝉【chéng chán】 即发挥人的主观能动作用。

supreme concentration Refers to bringing into play the subjective initiative, indicating the special function.

承负【chéng fù】 指身体超负荷运行。

loading Indicating that the body moves beyond the movement of load.

承浆【chéng jiāng】 ① 指人体部位名;② 指任脉中的一个穴位名,位下唇下颏唇沟正中凹陷处。这一穴位为气功运行的一个常见部位。

Chengjiang Refers to ① either mandibular fossa; ② or Chengjiang（CV 24）, an acupoint in the conception meridian, located in the depression at the midpoint of the mentolabial sulcus. This acupoint is a region usually used for keeping the essential Qi in practice of Qigong.

承泣【chéng qì】 为足阳明胃经中的一个穴位,位于眶下缘与眼球之间。这一穴位为气功运行的一个常见部位。

Chengqi（ST 1） An acupoint in the stomach meridian of foot Yangming, located between the infraorbital margin and the eyeball. This acupoint is a region usually used for keeping the essential Qi in practice of Qigong.

承山【chéng shān】 为足太阳膀胱经中的一个穴位,位于腓肠肌肌腹下。这一穴位为气功运行的一个常见部位。

Chengshan（BL 57） An acupoint in the bladder meridian of foot Taiyang, located in the gastrocnemius below the belly. This acupoint is a region usually used for keeping the essential Qi in practice of Qigong.

乘跷【chéng qiāo】 指腾空上升之工具。

lifting up Refers to the instrument for rising to the sky.

澄心【chéng xīn】 即洗心涤虑。

purifying the heart Refers to rinsing the heart and doing away with cares.

鸥顾【chī gù】 指动功之一式,即身体不动,头往后顾,意识随势亦向后。

fixed observation An exercise of Qigong practice, indicating that the body does not move, the head turns to observe the back and the consciousness follows the procedure to turn backwards.

鸥视【chī shì】 指动功之一式,即身体不动,头往后瞧,视力集中不散乱。

fixed vision An exercise of Qigong practice, indicating that the body does not move, the head turns to see the back and the vision is concentrated without any dispersion.

痴【chī】 为佛家气功习用语,指对事理愚昧无知。

dementia A term of Qigong, referring to benightedness about anything.

驰骋呼吸【chí chěng hū xī】 指呼吸急促,不能节制。

galloping respiration Refers to rapid respiration which is difficult to control.

持其志【chí qí zhì】 即调节意识活动。

controlling the will Means to regulate the activity of consciousness.

持息念【chí xī niàn】 为动功。其作法为,引自然清气入身内(吸),然后持息出，即引体内宿气出身（呼），一入一出为一息，意识集中于息，并计数之。每次作功时间根据练功者自己的情况而定，可长亦可短。久行之，增加智慧，提高身体健康水平。

controlling respiration　An exercise of Qigong in Buddhism, marked by natural inhaling clear Qi and then exhaling turbid Qi. Respiration means to inhale one and exhale one for several times. The time of practice can be decided according to the condition of practitioner. After a long time of practice, wisdom will be increased and health will be improved.

持心【chí xīn】　即调节精神意识活动。

controlling the heart　Means to regulate the activities of the spirit and consciousness.

尺泽【chǐ zé】　属手太阴肺经中的一个穴位，位肘横纹中。

Chize（LU 5）　An acupoint in the lung meridian of hand Taiyin, located in the middle of the elbow.

尺宅【chǐ zhái】　即面、脸面。

little residence　Refers to the face and complexion.

齿功【chǐ gōng】　为动功。其作法为，齿三十六遍，以集心神。小便时，闭口紧咬牙齿，可除齿痛。

dental exercise　A dynamic exercise, marked by clicking the teeth for thirty-six times to concentrate the spirit in the heart, closing the mouth and gritting the teeth in order to cure toothache.

齿痛【chǐ tòng】　为气功适应证，可治疗牙痛。

toothache　An indication of Qigong practice.

齿龈肿【chǐ yín zhǒng】　为气功适应

证，多由风邪侵入头面所致。

gingivitis　An indication of Qigong, usually caused by invasion of pathogenic wind into the head and the face.

齿中后养生方【chǐ zhōng hòu yǎng shēng fāng】　为静功。其作法为，面向东而坐，闭气不息四次，叩齿三十六次。治牙痛。

life cultivation exercise for dental syndrome　A static exercise, marked by sitting towards the east, stopping respiration for four times, clicking teeth for thirty-six times for curing toothache.

赤白痢疾治法【chì bái lì jí zhì fǎ】　为动功。其作法为，两手前后如探马状，又前后左右进步行功。凡水泻痢疾，闭目，两脚相交直立，两手直垂，夹紧谷道，用意上提，以至无数。

treatment of multi-coloured dysentery　A dynamic exercise, marked by stretching the hands forward like exploring a horse and then moving forward and backward, and to the left and right sides. If there is dysentery, practitioners should close the eyes, cross the legs to stand up, raise the hands directly upwards, clamp the grain trail（anus）and image to lift it for many times.

赤城童子【chì chéng tóng zǐ】　指心。

baby in red city　Refers to the heart.

赤肚子胎息诀【chì dǔ zi tāi xī jué】　源自气功学专论，对气功锻炼中极为重要的神气相抱做了简明的阐述，对气功学说的发展有较大促进作用。

exercise of fetal respiration in red abdomen　Collected from a monograph of Qigong, concisely describing the important spirit and Qi in practicing Qigong and making great contribution to the development of Qigong.

C

赤凤髓【chì fèng suǐ】《赤凤髓》为气功养生学专著,由明代周履靖所著。全书所论,内容丰富,言简意赅。

Chifeng Sui (*Red Phoenix and Marrow*) A monograph of Qigong and life cultivation entitled *Red Phoenix and Marrow*, written by Zhou Lǚjing in the Ming Dynasty (1368 AD – 1644 AD). The content of this monograph is rich, concise and comprehensive.

赤龙【chì lóng】① 指舌;② 指妇女月经。

red Loong Refers to ① either the tongue; ② or menstruation.

赤龙搅海【chì lóng jiǎo hǎi】 即舌在口腔、齿龈内外转动,为练功前的准备动作之一。赤龙指舌,海指口腔。

red Loong disturbing sea Refers to the tongue that rotates in the mouth and gingiva, which is one of the ways for preparing practice of Qigong. In this term, red Loong refers to the tongue and sea refers to the mouth.

赤水【chì shuǐ】 指心血。

red water Refers to the blood in the heart.

赤松子【chì sōng zǐ】 为古代传说中的仙人,对气功有高深造诣。

Chi Songzi A legendary immortal in ancient China who made great contribution to the study and development of Qigong.

赤松子导引法【chì sōng zǐ dǎo yǐn fǎ】 为动功。其作法为,清旦未起,先啄齿十四次,闭目、握固,漱津,唾三咽气,寻闭息极,乃徐徐顿踵三还,上床叉手顿项上,左右自引掖不息,复三伸两足返手前。当早晚为之,能数尤善。

immortal exercise of Daoyin A dynamic exercise, marked by lying on bed in the early morning, pecking the teeth for fourteen times, closing the eyes, holding the fists, gargling fluid, spiting for three times to inhale air, slowly holding respiration, mildly pausing the heel in three ways, crossing the hands to hold the neck from the left to the right to turn respiration and returning the feet in three ways. To practice in such a way in the morning and night, all the body will be well cultivated.

赤松子干浴法【chì sōng zǐ gàn yù fǎ】 为动功。其作法为,清旦初起,摩手令热以摩身体,从上至下,名干浴法。令人胜风寒时热、头痛等疾病,并皆除也。

immortal exercise for dry bathing A dynamic exercise, marked by getting up in the early morning and rubbing the hands warm to rub the body from the upper to the lower in the dry bathing way in order to expel fever, headache and other diseases.

赤松子摩耳法【chì sōng zǐ mó ěr fǎ】 为动功。其作法为,清旦初起,以两手叉两耳,极上下之十四次,令人耳不聋。

immortal exercise for rubbing ears A dynamic exercise, marked by getting up in the early morning, forking the ears with both hands up and down for fourteen times in order to prevent deafness.

赤松子摩面法【chì sōng zǐ mó miàn fǎ】 为动功。其作法为,清旦初起,摩手令热以摩面,从上而下十四次止,去邪气,令面有光。

immortal exercise for rubbing face A dynamic exercise, marked by getting up in the early morning, rubbing the hands warm, and then rubbing the face with the warm hands up and down for fourteen times in order to expel evil Qi and to spotlight the face.

赤松子坐引法【chì sōng zǐ zuò yǐn fǎ】 为动功。其作法为,长跪,两手向前分开,五指向外为起式,次则两手叉腰,右手曳向后,左手叉于腹前,再次则左右于均曳向前,两手叉腰而收功。

immortal exercise for sitting A dynamic exercise, marked by prostrating on the ground, separating the hands forwards, stretching the five fingers laterally, forking the waist with both hands with the right hand turning backwards and the left hand turning forwards to the abdomen, and again forking the left hand and right hand all forwards. When both hands fork the waist, the practice will be successful.

赤珠【chì zhū】 指胆的外象。

red pearl Refers to the external manifestation of the gallbladder.

赤子【chì zǐ】 指心神。

newborn baby Refers to the spirit in the heart.

冲和【chōng hé】 ① 指阴阳之气的相互协调;② 指机体身、心、意三家相互烹炼熏蒸之和气。

mutual harmony Refers to ① either mutual coordination of Qi in Yin and Yang; ② or the body, the heart and the mind that combine with each other to balance and harmonize the whole body.

冲脉【chōng mài】 为奇经八脉之一,起于小腹内,下出于会阴部,向上行于脊柱之内,与足少阴肾经交会,沿腹部两侧,上达咽喉,环绕口唇。此脉为气功习练之处。

thoroughfare meridian One of the eight extraordinary meridians, starting from the lower abdomen, coming out from the pudendal region, raising up through the spine and connected with the kidney meridian of foot Shaoyin, reaching the throat and lips along the two sides of the abdomen. This meridian is a region usually used in practice of Qigong

冲门【chōng mén】 ① 足少阴脾经的一个穴位,耻骨联合上缘中点旁开 3.5 寸处;② 指精气运行的要冲。

Chongmen Refers to ① either an acupoint called Chongmen (SP 12) in the spleen meridian of foot Shaoyin, located 3.5 Cun lateral to the central region of the pubic bone connected with the upper region; ② or the central region where the essence and Qi circulate. This acupoint is a region usually used for keeping the essential Qi in practice of Qigong.

冲虚观【chōng xū guān】 位于广东惠州,为东晋时期葛洪炼丹之处。

Chongxu temple Located in Huizhou City, Guangzhou Province, where Ge Hong in the East Jin Dynasty (317 AD - 420 AD) studied and practiced alchemy.

冲应真人【chōng yìng zhēn rén】 东晋时期医药学家和气功学家葛洪的赞称。

Chongying Immortal A celebration of Ge Hong, a great doctor and master of Qigong in the East Jin Dynasty (317 AD - 420 AD).

冲用【chōng yòng】 指一气之内,阴阳之间的交合作用。

intercourse Refers to the effect of intercourse in one kind of Qi and the place between Yin and Yang.

重阳宫【chóng yáng gōng**】** 位于陕西户县,为全真派祖师王重阳埋骨处。

Great Yang Palace Located in Huxian County in Shaanxi Province, the mausoleum of Wang Chongyang, the founder of genuine religion and also a great master of Qigong in the Song Dynasty (960 AD - 1279 AD).

重阳立教十五论【chóng yáng lì jiào shí wǔ lùn**】** 《重阳立教十五论》为气功专著,由金代王嚞所著。

Chongyang Lijiao Wushi Lun（*Discussions about Education of Chongyang*） A monograph of Qigong entitled Fifteen *Discussions about Education of Chongyang*, written by Wang Zhe in the Jin Dynasty (1115 AD - 1234 AD).

重阳全真集【chóng yáng quán zhēn jí**】** 《重阳全真集》为气功专著,由金代王嚞所著,内收传道诗词千余首。

Chongyang Quanzhen Ji（*Collection of All Genuine Chongyang*） A monograph of Qigong entitled *Collection of All Genuine Chongyang*, written by Wang Zhe in the Jin Dynasty (1115 AD - 1234 AD). In this monograph there are over one thousand poems about inheritance of Daoism.

重阳之人【chóng yáng zhī rén**】** 指阳气盛,性格急躁之人。

people with vigorous Yang Refers to people with exuberant Yang Qi and irritability.

重阳子【chóng yáng zǐ**】** 为王重阳的另外称谓,其为宋代真教创始者,也为气功的发展做出了特殊贡献。

Chong Yangzi Another name of Wang Chongyang who was the founder of genuine religion and also a great master of Qigong in the Song Dynasty (960

AD - 1279 AD).

抽铅添汞【chōu qiān tiān gǒng**】** 指气功习练功夫。抽由下丹田之真气上升,添汞由铅升至顶上,化为金精,入于脑海。

taking lead and adding mercury A term of Qigong, referring to the effect of Qigong practice. In this term, taking lead refers to raising of genuine Qi from the lower Dantian (the region below the navel) and adding mercury refers to lead raising to the top and transforming into golden essence that enters the sea in the brain.

抽添【chōu tiān**】** ① 指四时寒暑之变化为天地阴阳之抽添;② 指练功中气定神定;③ 指练功中,平秘阴阳。

taking and adding Refers to ① either the changes of cold and heat in the four seasons belonging to the changes of Yin and Yang in the sky and the earth; ② or stability of the spirit and Qi in the practice of Qigong; ③ or stable Yin and compact Yang in practicing Qigong.

抽胁法【chōu xié fǎ**】** 为动功。其作法为,两手抱头,宛转胜上,有理气作用。

exercise for extending the sides A dynamic exercise, marked by holding the head with both hands, mildly turning the body and regulating Qi.

臭乱神明胎气零【chòu luàn shén míng tāi qì líng**】** 指习练气功,辟谷不食,不闻食味。食则损伤精气,耗竭能源。

confusion of the spirit and loss of fetal Qi Referring to the fact that practice of Qigong should stop diet and avoid smelling taste, otherwise essential Qi will be damaged and the source of energy will be dissipated.

臭皮囊【chòu pí náng】　指形体躯壳。
mortal flesh Refers to the human body.

出清入玄【chū qīng rù xuán】　指调节呼吸之气,出入之气变化著明。
clear and supreme Refers to Qi that regulates respiration and change of Qi that goes out and comes in.

出日入月【chū rì rù yuè】　指阴阳之间的往来变化。
interchange of the sun and the moon Refers to the communication and change of Yin and Yang.

出神【chū shén】　指神出于外,而感知事物。
appearance of the spirit Refers to the spirit that appears in the external in order to enable the practitioner to understand everything.

初步凝神处【chū bù níng shén chù】指泥丸两眉中间、心窍一寸三分处是初步凝神守窍地。
preliminary fixation of the spirit region Refers to the region between the mud bolus (the brain) and the eyes or the region located 1 Cun or 3 Fen towards the heart orifice, in which the spirit is concentrated.

初禅【chū chán】　即意念与眼、耳、鼻、舌、身、意之六识相结合,气息调和,神形稳定。
preliminary dhyana A technique of Qigong practice in Buddhism, referring to combination of the eyes, the ears, the nose, the tongue, the body and the consciousness for regulating respiration and stabilizing the spirit and the body.

初服气须知【chū fú qì xū zhī】　源自气功专论,主要阐述初服气的注意事宜。
notice of preliminary analysis of respira- **tion** Collected from a monograph of Qigong, mainly describing the attentions of preliminary analysis of respiration.

初机下手【chū jī xià shǒu】　指初学气功,认识基本知识并实践之。
preliminary study of Qigong A celebrated dictum, referring to understanding the basic knowledge and continuing practice in studying Qigong.

初结胎看本命【chū jié tāi kàn běn mìng】　即练气功中,意守脐部才能结丹。
preliminary connection of fetus for observing life Marked by concentration of consciousness in the navel in practicing Qigong in order to connect with Dan (pills of immortality).

初入道法【chū rù dào fǎ】　为静功,即端身正坐,放松神形,凝神入静。
preliminary entrance of Dao A static exercise, marked by sitting upright, relaxing the spirit and body, concentrating the spirit and tranquilizing the mind in practicing Qigong.

初阳赤辉化生内景【chū yáng chì huī huà shēng nèi jǐng】　为静功。其作法为,于夏历每月初一日寅时在清净的室内坐定,叩齿三十六通。意想自身坐在昆仑山顶上,下为大海,太阳从海底射出灿烂的光芒。
exercise of sunshine imagination A static exercise, marked by sitting in the room in Yin (the period of a day from 3 a.m. to 5 a.m. in the morning) on the first day of every month in summer, clicking teeth for thirty-six times, imagining sitting on the top of Kunlun Mountain and running into the sea to appreciate brightness of the sunshine

from the seafloor.

初真【chū zhēn】 指习练气功获得成效的第一步,形体和精神意识活动相互作用,维持协调。

preliminary truth Referring to the first successful step to practice Qigong that has ensured the mutual effect and coordination of the body with the activities of the essence, the spirit and the consciousness.

除烦恼禅【chú fán nǎo chán】 指入静坐禅,能消除一切烦恼。

eliminating distracting thought Refers to sitting in meditation with tranquility in order to eliminate annoyance.

除秽去累【chú huì qù lèi】 指排除杂念,精神内守而专一,返璞归真而明敏。

eliminating dirt and relieving fatigue A celebrated dictum, referring to eliminating distracting thought, internally concentrating the spirit and recovering the original simplicity and genuineness.

除五谷【chú wǔ gǔ】 指习练气功,除五谷汤水,即不食五谷汤水。

eliminating five grains Refers to eliminating the soup of five grains. That means the practitioners of Qigong should not take the soup of the five grains.

处暑七月中坐功【chǔ shǔ qī yuè zhōng zuò gōng】 为静功。其作法为,每日丑寅时正坐,转头左右举引,正反两手捶背各五、七次,叩齿、吐纳、咽液。

sitting exercise in the middle of July in summer A static exercise, marked by sitting in Chou (the period of a day from 1 a.m. to 3 a.m. in the morning) and Yin (the period of a day from 3 a.m. to 5 a.m. in the morning), turning the head from the left to the right, pressing the back with both hands for five and seven times, clicking the teeth, breathing in and out, and swallowing saliva.

处中【chù zhōng】 即意识活动在身体之中。

central Indicating that the activity of consciousness is in the body.

触【chù】 ① 指接触,眼、耳、鼻、舌、身、意的感触;② 指感觉,即对外界事物的感觉。

touch Referring to ① either contacting with the eyes, the ears, the nose, the tongue and the body; ② or feeling of things in the external world.

传精神【chuán jīng shén】 指圣人习练气功,调节精神意识思维活动。

regulating the essence and the spirit Refers to sages practicing Qigong and regulating the activities of the spirit, consciousness and emotion.

喘证【chuǎn zhèng】 为气功适应证,多因外感风寒之邪壅滞于肺,肺失宣降等所致。

dyspnea syndrome An indication of Qigong, usually caused by stagnation of external pathogenic wind and cold in the lung that makes the lung unable to diffuse and descend.

疮疽治法【chuāng jū zhì fǎ】 为静功。其作法为,凡久生疮疽,端坐,左拳拄右胁,右手按膝,专心存运气到患处,左右各运气六口。

treatment of sore and furuncle A static exercise, marked by sitting upright if there are chronic sore and furuncle, pressing the right rib with the left fist, pressing the knee with the right hand, concentrating Qi to move into the location of sore and furuncle and moving Qi from the left to the right and vice versa for six times respectively.

垂拱无为【chuí gǒng wú wéi**】**　指脑神清净不妄为。

whim-free mind　Refers to tranquility and purity of the spirit in the brain without any wild activity.

垂帘【chuí lián**】**　指双眼轻轻闭合。

closed curtain　Refers to mild closure of eyes.

垂帘运目法【chuí lián yùn mù fǎ**】**　为静功。其作法为，坐时开眼则神不聚，须宜闭之。

exercise for moving closed eyes　A static exercise, marked by sitting with closed eyes for tranquility. If the eyes are not closed, the spirit cannot be concentrated.

春分二月中坐功【chūn fēn èr yuè zhōng zuò gōng**】**　为动功。其作法为，每日丑寅时伸手回头，左右拗引，各六七次，叩齿三十六次，吐纳、漱咽九次。

exercise of sitting in the middle of February　A dynamic exercise, marked by stretching the hands and turning the head in Zi（the period of the day from 11 p.m. to 1 a.m.）and Yin（the period of a day from 3 a.m. to 5 a.m. in the morning），wiping from the left to the right and vice versa for six or seven times respectively, clicking the teeth for thirty-six times, breathing, rinsing and swallowing for nine times.

春令导引法【chūn lìng dǎo yǐn fǎ**】**　为动功。其作法为，用嘘字导引，以两手相重接肩上，徐徐缓缓，身左右转各三遍。又可正坐，两手相叉，翻复向胸引三五遍。

exercise of Daoyin in spring　A dynamic exercise, marked by starting Daoyin with the Chinese character Xu（slow exhalation），holding the shoulders with both hands mildly, turning the body from the left to the right and vice versa for three times respectively, then sitting upright, crossing the hands and repeatedly turning to the chest for three or five times respectively.

纯粹不杂【chún cuì bù zá**】**　指意识思维活动专一，没有杂念，安静自守。

purity without any mixture　Refers to concentrated activity of consciousness and thought with tranquility and without any distracting thought.

纯粹真精【chún cuì zhēn jīng**】**　指脑之气。

pure genuine essence　Refers to Qi in the brain.

纯气之守【chún qì zhī shǒu**】**　指至人具神形合一，有特异功能，是习练气功的结果。

integration of pure Qi　Refers to integration of the spirit and the body in lofty man with peculiar function due to practice of Qigong.

纯乾【chún qián**】**　① 指十五岁的青少年，精满未泄；② 指纯阳，乾为天，为阳。

pure Qian　Refers to ① either youngster of fifteen years with rich essence and without any diarrhea; ② or pure Yang because Qian refers to the sky and Yang.

纯素之道【chún sù zhī dào**】**　指守神于身内，排除杂念，保养精神是纯正朴素之道。

pure Dao　Refers to concentration of the spirit inside the body in order to eliminate distracting thought and to nourish the essence and the spirit.

纯阳【chún yáng**】**　指纯一之阳。

pure Yang Refers to a pure Yang in the human body.

纯阳金耀焕明内景 【chún yáng jīn yào huàn míng nèi jǐng】 为静功。其作法为,于夏历每月二十日清净的室内静坐,排除杂念,意想身在"日宫"中,身体与太阳混为二体,太阳散发九道光芒,整个天空一片赤红色。

pure Yang and golden shine arousing internal scene A static exercise, marked by quietly sitting in a clean room on the twentieth day in every month in summer, eliminating any distracting thought, imagining that the bod is in the celestial palace, integrating the body with the sun to send out the sunshine to nine ways to make all the sky full of redness.

纯阳天宫 【chún yáng tiān gōng】 指脑。

pure Yang in celestial palace Refers to the brain.

纯阳子兜肾功 【chún yáng zǐ dōu shèn gōng】 为动功。其作法为,先以手搓小腹部八十一次,再以一手将阴囊托住,另一手轻搓揉阴囊八十一次,两手交换进行。到了申时,一边吸气一边上提阴囊,收膀胱气于丹田,纳心之气于下腹部。

pure Yang wrapping kidney function A dynamic exercise, marked by rubbing the lower abdomen with both hands for eighty-one times, holding the scrotum with one hand, rubbing the scrotum with the other hand for eighty-one times, both hands interchanging with each other in the same way. In Shen (the period of a day 3 p. m. to 5 p. m. in the afternoon), respiration is started, scrotum is lifted, Qi from the bladder is transmitted into Dantian and Qi is the heart is led to the lower abdomen. Dantian is divided into the upper Dantian (the region between the eyes), the middle Dantian (the region below the heart) and the lower Dantian (the region below the navel).

纯阳祖师任脉诀法 【chún yáng zǔ shī rèn mài jué fǎ】 为动静相兼功。其作法为,用两手按日月两旁穴九次,运气九口。又一法:两手按膝,左右扭肩,运气十四口。预防疾病,健康形体。

exercise of grand master with pure Yang for conception meridian An exercise with dynamic exercise and static exercise, marked by pressing the acupoints located in the right and left sides with both hands for nine times and moving Qi for nine times. Another way of practice is to press the knees with the hands, turning the shoulders from the left to the right and vice versa, and moving Qi for fourteen times. Such a way of practice can prevent any disease and cultivate health.

纯阳祖师五行功 【chún yáng zǔ shī wǔ xíng gōng】 为动功。其作法为,双托一度通三焦,左肝右肺如射雕,调养脾胃须单举,元海华池内顾潮。摇肩摆臂和心气,手扳涌泉理肾腰,每日如此行三次,方才发火边烧身,延年除百病。

five exercises of grand master with pure Yang A static exercise, marked by raising the hands for a period of time to connect with the triple energizer to promote the liver and the lung like shooting eagles, nourishing the spleen and the stomach with single raising, taking care of tide in original sea (bladder) and the mouth, waving the shoulders, posing the arms and harmonizing heart Qi, holding Yongquan and regulating the kidney and the waist with the hands. To practice in such a way of exercise for three times every day will increase fire to heat the body, prolong life and cure all diseases.

纯一迁矣【chún yī qiān yǐ】 指外物干扰,情志失调,精神意识活动不能专一。

disintegration of pure one Refers to disturbance of external factors that causes maladjustment of emotion and disintegration of the essence, the spirit and the consciousness activities.

淳德全道【chún dé quán dào】 指气功养生的涵养道德达到了高深的境界。

pure and perfect Daoism Refers to the highest and deepest state of Qigong and life cultivation.

淳熙观【chún xī guān】 位于浙江仙居,葛玄曾炼丹于此。

Chunxi Temple Located in Xianju County in Zhejiang Province, where Ge Xuan, a Daoist in the East Han Dynasty (25 AD - 220 AD), refined Dan (pills of immortality).

慈悲【cí bēi】 指同情。

pity Refers to sympathy.

慈悲观【cí bēi guān】 为静功。其作法为,向一切有情动物,如牛、马、羊等,意念观想其可怜的形象,发慈悲之心,增加同情。功在调节精神,防治嗔恚。

idea of pity A static exercise, marked by being compassionate to those who are poor and pitiable as benevolent animals like cattle, horse and sheep. Such a static exercise can regulate the spirit, and prevent anger and vexation.

雌火【cí huǒ】 雌为阴,火为阳,即阴

火,为阳中之阴。

female fire (Yin fire) In this term, the so-called female refers to Yin and fire refers to Yang, indicating female fire (Yin fire) is Yin within Yang.

雌雄【cí xióng】 指阴阳两个方面。

female and male Referring to Yin and Yang. In this term, the so-called female refers to Yin while the so-called male refers to Yang.

雌阴黄包【cí yīn huáng bāo】 雌阴为柔阴,黄包即黄芽,为阴极阳生之意。

female Yin and yellow bag In this term, the so-called female Yin refers to soft Yin while the so-called yellow bag refers to yellow bud, indicating that extreme Yin turns into Yang.

此中【cǐ zhōng】 指形体之中,或心之中,或泥丸之中。

somatic center Refers to either the region inside the body; or the center of the heart; or the center of the mud bolus (the brain).

刺风【cì fēng】 为气功适应证,为风邪侵袭人体所致。

wind attack An indication of Qigong, usually caused by invasion of pathogenic wind.

聪耳法【cōng ěr fǎ】 为动功。其作法为,龙导虎引,熊经龟咽,燕飞蛇屈鸟伸,天俛地仰。令自然赤黄之景,不去泥丸,布散于耳,防治耳聋、耳鸣。

exercise for improving ears A dynamic exercise, marked by leading with Loong, guiding with tiger, moving with bear, swallowing with tortoise, flying with swallow, bending with snake, stretching with bird, lowering the sky and raising the earth. Such a dynamic exercise leads red and yellow scene natural to the ears and not to the mud bolus (the brain), quite effective for preventing and curing deafness and tinnitus.

从革【cóng gé】 为运气术语,指金运不及则火化而变革。

obeying reform A term of Qi motion, referring to fire transformation and change due to insufficiency of metal movement.

从四正【cóng sì zhèng】 指言、行、坐、立四正。

obeying the four kinds of righteousness Refers to speech, movement, sitting and standing which are regarded as the four kinds of righteousness.

从阴阳则生,逆之则死 【cóng yīn yáng zé shēng nì zhī zé sǐ】 指顺从阴阳就能生存,违背阴阳就会死亡。

Following the rules of yin and yang is key to life while violation causes death. A celebrated dictum, referring to the fact that following Yin and Yang ensures life while violence of Yin and Yang results in death.

蹙气【cù qì】 即闭气之意。

urgent Qi Means to stop respiration in practicing Qigong.

卒被孙瘀血【cù bèi sūn yū xiě】 气功适应证,因意外伤害,外部被损伤而内有瘀血所致,即"瘀血证"。

abrupt blood stasis An indication of Qigong, usually caused by accidental damage that causes external injury and internal blood stasis. Such a disease is usually called blood stasis syndrome.

卒被损瘀血候导引法【cù bèi sǔn yū xiě hòu dǎo yǐn fǎ】 为动功,方法多样,如正坐,伸直腰,左手上举,手掌向上,右手托右胁,用鼻吸气,至极限时慢慢呼

出,作七息。可理气活血,治瘀血气滞。

exercise of Daoyin for adverse damage and blood stasis A dynamic exercise with various methods, such as sitting upright, stretching the waist, raising the left hand and the palm, supporting the right flank with the right hand, inhaling through the nose and slowly exhaling for seven times in order to regulate Qi and activate the blood as well as to treat blood stasis and Qi stagnation.

卒上气【cù shàng qì】 气功适应证,因气突然上逆所致。

adverse raise of Qi An indication of Qigong, caused by Qi flowing adversely upwards.

卒上气候导引法【cù shàng qì hòu dǎo yǐn fǎ】 为动功。其作法为,两手在下颌下交叉,尽量用力,可降逆止咳,治突然气逆咳嗽。

exercise of Daoyin for adverse raise of Qi A dynamic exercise, marked by forcibly overlapping both hands in mandible, downbearing counterflow of Qi and stopping cough in order to treat sudden counterflow of Qi and cough.

卒魇【cù yǎn】 气功适应证,指患者突然因惊险怪诞之噩梦而惊叫,多因心火炽盛所致。

nightmare An indication of Qigong, referring to scream of patients in nightmare, usually caused by exuberance of fire in the heart.

卒魇导引法【cù yǎn dǎo yǐn fǎ】 为动功。其作法为,弯曲大拇指,用四指握住。养成习惯,睡眠时亦不要松开。

exercise of Daoyin for nightmare A dynamic exercise, marked by bending the thumb held by the four fingers and avoiding relaxation of it even in sleep.

篡【cuàn】 ① 指会阴部；② 指肛；③ 指夺取，相争；④ 指经穴名，即会阴穴；⑤ 指下丹田，为气功意守处。

Cuan Refers to ① either perineum；② or anus；③ or capture and struggle；④ or Huiyin（RN 1），an acupoint in the conception meridian；⑤ or lower Dantian（the region below the navel）which is the region for concentrating consciousness in Qigong practice.

崔公入药镜【cuī gōng rù yào jìng】《崔公入药镜》为气功学专著，为唐代气功家崔希范所著，认为精、气、神为炼丹之药，心火内照，能见五脏六腑，故称为镜。

Cuigong Ruyao Jing（*Mr. Cui Entering Medicinal Mirror*） A monograph of Qigong entitled *Mr. Cui Entering Medicinal Mirror*，written by Cui Xifan, a master of Qigong in the Tang Dynasty（618 AD - 907 AD），suggesting that the essence，Qi and spirit are the medicinals for refining Dan（pills of immortality）and that heart fire shines the internal side of the body and makes it possible to see the five Zang-organs（including the heart，the liver，the spleen，the lung and the kidney）and the six Fu-organs（including the gallbladder，the stomach，the small intestine，the large intestine，the bladder and the triple energizer）. That is why it is called mirror.

崔公入药镜注【cuī gōng rù yào jìng zhù】《崔公入药镜注》为气功专论，由元代王道渊注。该书的主要内容是习练气功要在调节阴阳，入药的基础是形体和精神的协调，入药的方法是习练周天功，习练周天功的关键是神的作用。

Cuigong Ruyao Jingzhu（*Explanation of Mr. Cui's Entering Medicinal Mirror*） A monograph of Qigong entitled *Explanation of Mr. Cui's Entering Medicinal Mirror*，explained by Wang Daoyuan in the Yuan Dynasty（1271 AD - 1368 AD），mainly indicating that regulating Yin and Yang is the main function of Qigong，coordinating the body and spirit is the foundation for producing medicinal，refining circulatory cycle is the way for producing medicinal and the function of the spirit is the key for practicing circulatory cycle exercise.

崔希范【cuī xī fàn】 唐代著名气功家，撰有气功专著。

Cui Xifan A master of Qigong in the Tang Dynasty（618 AD - 907 AD），who wrote an important monograph of Qigong.

翠微宫【cuì wēi gōng】 指脑。

green vacuum palace Refers to the brain.

翠虚篇【cuì xū piān】《翠虚篇》为气功学专著，由陈楠撰，为古代气功名著。

Cuixu Pian（*A Book about Greenness and Vacuum*） A monograph of Qigong entitled *A Book about Greenness and Vacuum*，written by Chen Nan，which was a famous book of Qigong in ancient China.

翠玄子【cuì xuán zǐ】 宋代的一位杰出的气功学家石泰的另外一个称谓，其也是著名的医学家。

Cui Xuanzi Another name of Shi Tai，a great master of Qigong in the Song Dynasty（960 AD - 1279 AD），who was also a doctor of traditional Chinese medicine.

存北方法【cún běi fāng fǎ】 为静功。其作法为，夜半东向平坐，放松形体，然后意想玄宫（玄宫在头准头直上，至发际5寸处），内现肾形，约二十分钟即可收功。

north contemplative exercise A static exercise, marked by sitting at midnight, relaxing the body, contemplating inside the top of the head, internally reflecting the style of the kidney for about twenty minutes.

存觉性【cún jué xìng】　指内存觉悟之性，不使精神意识外散。

keeping awareness Refers to consciousness inside the body that prevents dispersion of the spirit and the mind.

存泥丸【cún ní wán】　为动功。其作法为，两手摩擦热后，从额揉摩到顶，有健脑作用。

keeping mud bolus（the brain） A dynamic exercise, marked by rubbing the hands to be warm, and then rubbing from the forehead to the top of head for cultivating the brain.

存七元法【cún qī yuán fǎ】　为动功。其作法为，坐式，睡眠之前后及食毕，安神定气。

exercise for keeping seven origins A dynamic exercise, marked by sitting, stabilizing the spirit and fixing Qi before and after sleeping as well as after taking food.

存其心【cún qí xīn】　指存神于身内，即精神内守之意。

keeping the heart Refers to existence of the spirit inside the body, indicating internal concentration of the spirit.

存气注病【cún qì zhù bìng】　为气功治病的一种方式，即运气攻击患病部位，疏通经络，流通气血，以治疗疾病。

activating Qi to attack disease A way to treat disease in practicing Qigong, marked by attacking the location of disease, dredging the meridians, collaterals, Qi and blood in order to treat all diseases.

存日月诀【cún rì yuè jué】　为静功。其作法为，每日日落时，仰卧床上，存想日在额上，月在脐下。能辟秽气，延年却病。

formula for keeping the sun and moon A static exercise, marked by lying on the bed after sunset every day, imagining that the sun in the upper of the forehead and the moon in the lower of the navel. Such a way of practicing Qigong can eliminate pathogenic factors, prolong life and prevent any disease.

存神【cún shén】　指气功习练中之意守。

keeping spirit Indicating mental concentration in practicing Qigong.

存神定志入黄宫【cún shén dìng zhì rù huáng gōng】　源自气功专论，主要阐述练功开始，应先存神于中丹田。

keeping the spirit, stabilizing the will and entering the yellow chamber Collected from a monograph about Qigong, mainly describing the importance of keeping the spirit in the middle Dantian (the region below the heart) first when practicing Qigong.

存神固气论【cún shén gù qì lùn】《存神固气论》为气功专著，作者不详，阐述内丹理论。

Cunshen Guqi Lun（*Discussion about Keeping the Spirit and Concentrating Qi*） A monograph of Qigong entitled *Discussion about Keeping the Spirit and Concentrating Qi*, describing the theory of internal Dan (pills of immortality).

The author was unknown.

存神至要【cún shén zhì yào】 指以意引气，意念与呼吸结合，是存神的关键。

importance of keeping the spirit Refers to guiding Qi with thought. The key for keeping the spirit is combination of thought and respiration.

存视五脏【cún shì wǔ zàng】 为静功。其作法为，用意念存想五脏的形状及其颜色，如肝色青，脾色黄，心色赤，肺色白等。

concentration and vision of the five Zang-organs A static exercise, referring to inward contemplation of the style and color of the five Zang-organs, such as greenness of the liver, yellowness of the spleen, redness of the heart and whiteness of the lung.

存守中黄【cún shǒu zhōng huáng】 指内守脾神，中黄指脾神。

keeping central yellowness Refers to internal concentration of the spleen spirit. In this term, the so-called central yellowness refers to the spleen spirit.

存漱青牙法【cún shù qīng yá fǎ】 为动功。其作法为，立春时，鸡鸣时入室（凌晨三至七时），面向东九拜，叩齿九通，意想东方青气，从口中入，直至肝脏。

exercise for washing green teeth Marked by going into the room from the early morning (3 a.m. to 7 a.m.) in spring, making the ceremonial obeisance to the east for nine times, clicking the teeth for nine times, imagining the green Qi from the east entering the mouth and directly flowing to the liver.

存思【cún sī】 指专一思念丹田、五脏、四象、真气、日月、甘露等。

keeping consideration Refers to con-templation of Dantian, five Zang-organs (including the heart, the liver, the spleen, the lung and the kidney), genuine Qi, the sun and the moon, and sweet dew. Dantian is divided into the upper Dantian (the region between the eyes), the middle Dantian (the region below the heart) and the lower Dantian (the region below the navel).

存思火兵【cún sī huǒ bīng】 指意守阳热之气，或意守火热。

inward contemplation of fire soldier Refers to inward contemplation of Qi in Yang heat or inward contemplation of fire heat.

存思识已形【cún sī shí yǐ xíng】 为动功，即练功时专一地想着自己的形象。

exercise for keeping contemplation and differentiating forms A dynamic exercise, referring to specifically thinking about self-styles in practicing Qigong.

存思在心【cún sī zài xīn】 指养神要靠心静，而心静则要闭目以排除外界的干扰。

keeping thought in the heart Refers to the fact that nourishing the spirit depends on tranquilizing the heart and that only closing the eyes can tranquilize the heart and prevent disturbance of outside.

存威明法【cún wēi míng fǎ】 为动功。其作法为，坐式，意念存想胆神而不倦，功在协调神形。

keeping power and clearing formula A dynamic exercise, marked by sitting with the thought to keep the spirit in the gallbladder in order to regulate the spirit and the body.

存胃神承之【cún wèi shén chéng zhī】 为动功，即用意念想象胃腑之神，张口吸吞。

keeping and inheriting the stomach spirit A dynamic exercise, referring to imagining the spirit in the stomach through contemplation with opening the mouth for inhalation.

存想【cún xiǎng】 ① 指意念在身内以存神；② 指思念导引。

keeping thought Refers to ① either contemplation that enables the spirit to exist; ② or thinking of Daoyin.

存想法【cún xiǎng fǎ】 为静功。其作法为，静坐平息，存我之神，想我之心。

keeping ideas A static exercise, marked by quietly sitting, calming down, concentrating the spirit and contemplating the heart.

存想咽气【cún xiǎng yàn qì】 为静功。其作法为，每连咽气速存下丹田，所纳得元气，以意吹之，送之令入下丹田脐下 3 寸后之二六穴，闭目想。

swallowing Qi through contemplation A static exercise, marked by swallowing Qi to the lower Dantian (the region below the navel), inhaling the original Qi to the two acupoints located 3 Cun below the lower Dantian (the region below the navel) through blowing with contemplation, and closing the eyes.

存心绝虑候晶凝【cún xīn jué lǜ hòu jīng níng】 指亥末子初，天地之阳气至则急采药，存想绝虑静候之，晶津玉液自然生成。

Concentration of the heart ensures pure contemplation and life cultivation. This is a celebrated dictum, referring to quickly collecting medicinal when Yang Qi from the sky and earth starts at the end of Hai (the period of the day from 21 a. m. to 23 p. m. at night) and at the beginning of Zi (the period of the day from 11 p. m. to 1 a. m. in the afternoon), deeply contemplating and naturally producing saliva.

存心养性【cún xīn yǎng xìng】 指调神与调气，使之神与气相抱，和合而为一。

keeping the heart and cultivating the mind Refers to regulation of the spirit and Qi in order to integrate the spirit and Qi.

存心中气【cún xīn zhōng qì】 源自气功专论，阐述存心中气可辟邪、延年、益寿。

keeping Qi in the heart Collected from a monograph of Qigong, mainly describing that concentration of Qi in the heart can prevent pathogenic factors, prolong life and cultivate health.

寸白虫病【cùn bái chóng bìng】 为气功适应证，多因食生肉或未熟猪牛肉所致，症见腹痛、腹胀、泄泻或泻出白色节片等。

taenia An indication of Qigong, referring to the disease caused by eating raw meat, characterized by abdominal pain, abdominal distension and diarrhea.

寸关尺【cùn guān chǐ】 寸口脉分为寸脉、关脉、尺脉三部，是医生把脉的三点。

Cun, Guan and Chi Refers to the three points in the place where doctors take pulse in diagnosing diseases, known as Cun pulse, Guan pulse and Chi pulse.

寸田【cùn tián】 即丹田之意，两眉间为上丹田，心为绛宫中丹田，脐下三寸为下丹田。

small Dantian Refers to the feature of Dantian. Traditionally the upper Dantian refers to the region between the eyes, the middle Dantian refers to the heart and the lower Dantian refers to pubic region.

搓涂自美颜【cuō tú zì měi yán】　动静相兼功。其作法为,静坐,闭目凝神,存养神气,冲胆自内外达,以两手搓热,拂面七次,仍以漱津涂面,搓拂数次。行半月,则皮肤光润,容颜悦泽,大过寻常。

rubbing the face for beautification　An exercise combined with dynamic exercise and static exercise, marked by sitting quietly, closing the eyes, concentrating the spirit, protecting and nourishing the spirit and Qi, rushing the gallbladder from the internal side and the external side, rubbing the hands hot to wipe the face for seven times, rinsing fluid to wipe the face for several times. After practice for half a month, the skin is moistened and the face is beautified.

挫锐解纷【cuò ruì jiě fēn】　指挫折其锋芒,和解其纠纷,使之和平安适。喻气功,排除杂念,调节阴阳。

eliminating whims　Refers to eliminating spearhead and compromising dispute in order to make it peaceful, quiet and comfortable. In Qigong, it refers to eliminating distracting thought and regulating Yin and Yang.

D

达摩禅师胎息诀【dá mó chán shī tāi xī jué】 为静功口诀,本法释道结合,以安定身心,平和精神立法。

Dharma master's formula for fetal respiration A static exercise formula, indicating combination of Buddhism and Daoism in Qigong in order to stabilize the body and the heart as well as to balance the essence and the spirit.

达摩祖师胎息经【dá mó zǔ shī tāi xī jīng】 《达摩祖师胎息经》为气功专论,作者不详,简明阐述了神和气在气功中的关系。

Damo Zushi Taixi Jing(*Bodhidharma's Canon of Fetal Respiration*) A monograph of Qigong entitled *Bodhidharma's Canon of Fetal Respiration*, concisely describing the relationship between the spirit and Qi in practicing Qigong. The author was unknown.

达生【dá shēng】 指调节意识思维活动,畅达生命。

promoting life Refers to regulating the activities of consciousness and thought in order to promote life.

打躬势【dǎ gōng shì】 为动功。其作法为,取直立位,两足稍分开,两手抱头,掌心紧贴耳门,弯腰直膝附首,使头接近两腿,再挺身直立。

bending waist A dynamic exercise, marked by standing in a right way with both feet slightly separating aside, both hands burying the head and both palms clinging to the portals of ears. Then the waist is stooped and the knees are lifted to the head in order to reach the head to the legs and to erect the body.

打天钟【dǎ tiān zhōng】 为动功,指叩左齿,有排除杂念和健齿的作用。

beating the celestial clock A dynamic exercise, referring to clicking the left teeth in order to eliminate distracting thought and to cultivate the teeth.

打坐【dǎ zuò】 是练静功的一种基本姿势,以便排除杂念和外界环境的一切干扰和影响。

sitting in meditation Refers to the fact that sitting in meditation is the basic way to practice Qigong with static exercise in order to eliminate distracting thought and interference of external environment.

大【dà】 指自体宽广,指周遍包含,指多与胜之意,指妙之义,指不可思议。

large Refers to the big body, thorough implication, exuberance and inconceivability.

大包【dà bāo】 属于足太阴脾经的穴位,在腋下 6 寸。此穴位为气功习练之处。这一穴位为气功运行的一个常见部位。

Dabao(**SP 21**) An acupoint in the spleen meridian of foot Taiyin, located 6 Cun below the armpit. This acupoint is a region usually used for moving essential Qi in practice of Qigong.

大宝【dà bǎo】 指眼及眼神。

great treasure Refers to the eyes and

the spirit in the eyes.

大便不通候导引法【dà biàn bù tōng hòu dǎo yǐn fǎ】 为静功。其作法为，用衣被盖住全身及口鼻头面，仰卧，闭气不息。治大小便闭塞不通。

exercise of Daoyin for constipation A static exercise, marked by covering the whole body and mouth, nose and face with clothes, sitting on the back and stopping respiration. Such a static exercise can cure constipation.

大便不通引导法【dà biàn bù tōng yǐn dǎo fǎ】 为动功。其作法为，舌顶上腭，津液生，津润大肠，以手掌复脐，意念将五脏推开后，直落大肠。

exercise of Daoyin for constipation A dynamic exercise, marked by raising the tongue to the palate for increasing fluid and humor and moistening the large intestine, pressing the navel with the hands, imagining to activate the five Zang-organs (including the heart, the liver, the spleen, the lung and the kidney) in order to connect with the large intestine.

大便难候导引法【dà biàn nán hòu dǎo yǐn fǎ】 为动功。其作法为，仰卧，伸直双手。可温中散寒，治腹中冷痛，大便难。

exercise of Daoyin for difficulty in defecation A dynamic exercise, marked by lying on the back and strengthening the arms in order to cure difficulty in defecation, abdominal pain and cold.

大怖生狂【dà bù shēng kuáng】 指恐怖惊悸是狂证之因。

serious horror causing mania A celebrated dictum, referring to the fact that horror and pavor have caused mania syndrome.

大肠俞【dà cháng shū】 足太阳膀胱经的穴位，位于第四腰椎棘突下旁开1.5寸处，为气功常用意守部位。

Dachangshu（**BL 25**） An acupoint in the bladder meridian of foot Taiyang, located 1.5 Cun lateral to the spinous process in the fourth cervical vertebra. This acuppint is a region usually used in practice of Qigong.

大槌【dà chuí】 为大椎的别名，是督脉的一个穴位，位于后正中线，第七颈椎棘突下凹陷中。为气功学重要体表标志之一。此穴位为气功习练之处。

Dachui A synonym of Dazhui（GV 14）, an acupoint in the governor meridian, located in the back midline and in the depression of spinous process in the seventh cervical vertebra, which is the important symbol in Qigong. This acupoint is a region usually used in practice of Qigong.

大丹直指【dà dān zhí zhǐ】 《大丹直指》是气功著作，为元代丘处机所著，阐述了内丹的基本原理。

Dadan Zhizhi（*Direct Guidance of Great Dan*） A monograph of Qigong entitled *Direct Guidance of Great Dan*（*Pills of Immortality*）, written by Jiu Chuji in the Yuan Dynasty（1271 AD－1368 AD）, describing the basic principles of internal Dan（pills of immortality）.

大道【dà dào】 ① 即气功学家认为道乃万物生成之母；② 也指自然规律、治天下之理及道路。

great Dao Refers to ① either originator of all things suggested by the masters of Qigong; or natural principles; ② or the rules and roads for governing the world.

大道歌【dà dào gē】 源自气功专论，主要论述精、气、神、行之间的关系及气功有保养精、气、神的作用。

song of great Dao Collected from a monograph of Qigong, referring to the relationship between the essence, Qi and the spirit as well as the function of the essence, Qi and the spirit in cultivating health.

大道无为【dà dào wú wéi】 指人体意识行为不妄为，即习练气功时，意识思维活动处于相对静止状态。

great Dao with nonexistence Refers to the fact that consciousness activity cannot be done indulgingly, indicating that the activities of consciousness and thinking should be tranquilized in practicing Qigong.

大鼎炉【dà dǐng lú】 指人身头为鼎，腹为炉，炼精气神而结丹之意。

great pot and stove Refers to the head and abdomen as cauldron, the abdomen as furnace as well as the construction of Dan (pills of immortality) in practicing the essence, Qi and the spirit.

大定【dà dìng】 ① 指断一切妄惑；② 指脑神安静，形体放松；③ 指神息相依。

great determination Refers to ① either relief from avarice; ② or tranquilization of the brain spirit in order to relax the body; ③ or interdependence between spirit and respiration.

大敦【dà dūn】 足厥阴肝经的一个穴位，位于跱趾外侧，为气功常用意守部位。

Dadun（LR 1） An acupoint in the liver meridian of foot Jueyin, located lateral to the big toe. This acupoint is a region usually used in practice of Qigong.

大法导引法【dà fǎ dǎo yǐn fǎ】 动静相兼功。其作法为，有火者开目，无火者闭目；欲气上行以治耳、目、口、齿之病；欲气下行以通大小便及健足胫，则屈身为之；欲气达于四肢，则侧身为之；欲引头病者，仰头；欲引腰脚病者，仰足十指；欲引胸中病者，挽足十指；欲引臂病者，掩臂；欲去腹中寒热积聚诸痛及中寒身热，皆闭气满腹偃卧亦可为之。

great method of Daoyin exercise An exercise combined with dynamic exercise and static exercise. It indicates that the eyes are open when there is fire and the eyes are closed when there is no fire; or that Qi is completely closed when there is no sweating and Qi is not closed when there is sweating; or that ascent of Qi can treat diseases related to the ears, the eyes, the mouth and the teeth; or that descent of Qi relaxes urination and defecation; or that raising the head relieves headache; or that raising the ten toes cures diseases related to the back and foot; or that Qi flowing to the four limbs ensures sideways; or that protecting the shoulders relieves disorders in the shoulders; or that closing Qi in the abdomen and lying up eliminates accumulation of cold and heat in the body.

大管【dà guǎn】 指气管，亦指重楼。

great tube Fluid is often taken out of this tube and is transferred to the nose.

大还【dà hái】 指的是一种气功现象。

sudden transformation Refers to a manifestation of Qigong practice.

大寒十二月中坐功【dà hán shí èr yuè zhōng zuò gong】 为动功。其作法为，每日子丑时（二十三时至三时）两手向后踞床,跪坐,左右各三五次,叩齿、漱口、吐纳。可治疗百病。

sitting exercise in the middle of December A dynamic exercise, marked by kneeling with both hands to press backwards on the bed in Zi (the period of a day from 11 p. m. to 1 a. m.) and Chou (the period of a day from 1 a. m. to 3 a. m. in the morning) from the left to the right and vice versa for three or five times respectively, clicking the teeth, rinsing the mouth and breathing in and out. Such a dynamic exercise can cure various diseases.

大河车【dà hé chē】　指羊车、鹿车、牛车,或指小河车、大河车、紫河车。

great river cart Refers to either sheep cart, deer cart and cow cart, or small river cart, large river cart and purple cart, or attack cart, thunder cart and broken cart.

大赫【dà hè】　足少阴肾经的穴位,位于横骨上 1 寸,为气功常用意守部位。

Dahe（KI 12） An acupoint in the kidney meridian of foot Shaoyin, located 1 Cun above the transversum. This acupoint is a region usually used in practice of Qigong.

大横【dà héng】　为足太阴脾经中的一个穴位,位于脐中旁开 3.5 寸处,为气功常用意守部位。

Daheng（SP 15） An acupoint in the spleen meridian of foot Taiyin, located 3.5 Cun lateral to the navel. This acupoint is a region usually used in practice of Qigong.

大还丹【dà huán dān】　指龙虎相交而变黄芽,真气方升,下田入上田,上田复下田。

greatly returning to Dan（pills of immor- tality） Refers to interaction of Loong and tiger that changes into cerebral liquid for increasing the genuine Qi and enabling the lower region to ascend and the upper region to descend.

大寂定【dà jì dìng】　为佛家气功法。指和调神形,进入精神思维活动的稳定状态。

great silence Refers to sitting with crossed legs for regulating and harmonizing the activities of the spirit and thinking.

大寂静妙三摩地【dà jì jìng miào sān mó dì】　为静功。其作法为,和调神形,进入精神思维活动的稳定状态。

great silence in Samadhi A static exercise, marked by sitting with crossed legs for regulating and harmonizing the spirit and the body as well as stabilizing the activities of the spirit and thinking.

大寂灭【dà jì miè】　同涅槃。

great nirvana Refers to ideal state of Qigong practice in Buddhism.

大寂室三昧【dà jì shì sān mèi】　为静功。其作法是,和调神形,进入精神思维活动的稳定状态。

great silence A static exercise, marked by sitting with crossed legs for regulating and harmonizing the spirit and body.

大静【dà jìng】　指静笃,为高度入静状态。大静三百日,中静二百日,小静一百日。

deep tranquilization Refers to tranquilization in practicing Qigong which should be maintained for three hundred days or two hundred days or one hundred days.

大空【dà kōng】　指自身思维活动安静,东西南北等方向的实体。

great vacuum Refers to tranquility in consciousness activity or substance in the north, the south, the east and the west.

大麻疯及诸疮癣癞治法【dà má fēng jí zhū chuāng xuǎn lài zhì fǎ】 为动功。其作法为,立地闭气,两手用力如解木状,左右各扯二十,正扯二十,以汗出为度。

dynamic exercise for leprosy and sores A dynamic exercise, marked by standing up and stopping breath, holding the hands forcefully like relieving wood, pulling from the left to the right and vice versa for twenty times, and pulling straightly for twenty times till sweating.

大念【dà niàn】 指口中念"阿弥陀佛",以一念代万念,稳定精神思维活动二觉悟的功法。

silent recitation Refers to reading Amitabha constantly in order to stabilize the activity of the spirit and thinking.

大怒破阴【dà nù pò yīn】 指大怒损伤身体。

flaming rage harming Yin A celebrated dictum, referring to the fact that rage has damaged the body.

大气【dà qì】 指大邪之气,极峻厉的病邪。

severe Qi Refers to serious pathogenic factors.

大千世界【dà qiān shì jiè】 即万变纷繁的自然界和人类社会。

boundless universe Refers to the natural world and human society with various changes.

大清明【dà qīng míng】 指意识思维活动专一而静,静而生慧,知道、体道、行道。

great pureness Refers to concentration and quietness of the activities of consciousness and thinking for the purpose of understanding Dao, experiencing Dao and practicing Dao.

大人【dà ren】 指与自然、社会相适应的人。

great man Refers to an important person who integrates with the natural world and the social world.

大手印【dà shǒu yìn】 ① 指精神思维活动专注于手印,持之以恒,获得禅定; ② 调节手形成印后,精神思维活动专注于呼吸,达到最高境界。

great hand posture Referring to ① either concentrating the activities of the spirit and thinking in the hands in order to tranquilize the heart and mind with meditation; ② or regulating the posture of hands in order to concentrate the activities of the spirit and thinking in respiration and to reach the ideal state.

大暑六月坐功【dà shǔ liù yuè zuò gong】 为动功。其作法为,每日丑寅时,双拳踞地,返首向肩引,作虎视左右,各三五次,叩齿、吐纳、咽液。此功法可治疗各种疾病。

sitting exercise in dog days A dynamic exercise, marked by pressing the fists on the ground in Chou (the period of a day from 1 a.m. to 3 a.m. in the morning) and Yin (the period of a day from 3 a.m. to 5 a.m. in the morning) every day, returning the head to the shoulders, seeing the right and the left like a tiger for three or five times, clicking the teeth, breathing in and out, and swallowing humor. Such a dynamic exercise can treat various diseases.

大顺【dà shùn】　大敦的别称,是足厥阴肝经的一个穴位,位于跗趾外侧,为气功常用意守部位。

Dashun　A synonym of Dadun (LR 1), an acupoint in the liver meridian of foot Jueyin, located lateral to the big toe. This acupoint is a region usually used in practice of Qigong.

大通【dà tōng】　指的是郝大通,金代(1140—1212)气功学家,撰写了多部气功专著。

Da Tong　Refers to Hao Datong, a great master of Qigong in the Jin Dynasty(1140 AD‑1212 AD), who wrote several monographs of Qigong.

大同【dà tóng】　指神、形、气协调统一。

general coordination　Refers to coordination of the essence, Qi and the spirit.

大威仪先生玄素真人要用气诀【dà wēi yí xiān shēng xuán sù zhēn rén yào yòng qì jué】《大威仪先生玄素真人要用气诀》是气功学专著,介绍了气功基本理论与方法,作者不详。

Daweiyi Xiansheng Xuansu Zhenren Yaoyong Qijue（*Application of Qi for Longevity of Immortals*）　A monograph of Qigong entitled *Application of Qi for Longevity of Immortals*, introducing the basic theory and practice of Qigong. The author was unknow.

大喜坠阳【dà xǐ zhuì yáng】　指喜欢过甚,破损形体之阳而使精神不振。

overjoy impairing Yang　Refers to the fact that overjoy destroys Yang in the body, causing lassitude of the spirit.

大仙【dà xiān】　指习练佛家气功而求长生的人。

great immortal　Refers to a person who has practiced Qigong and has prolonged life.

大小便闭治法【dà xiǎo biàn bì zhì fǎ】　为动功。其作法为,凡男人大小便不通者,调节呼吸,使之平定;凡妇人大小便不通,闭气,两手背交叉入颈,左右各二十四遍,汗出止。

treatment of dysuria and constipation　A dynamic exercise, indicating that all men should regulate respiration, close Qi and shake hands if urination and defecation are not difficult; that all women should stop respiration with both hands crossing and pressing the neck for twenty-four times in order to stop sweating if urination and defecation are not difficult.

大小便难候导引法【dà xiǎo biàn nán hòu dǎo yǐn fǎ】　为动功。其作法为,坐正,以两手交叉放于背后。另外,反叉两手放于背上,向上推至正对心的位置,两脚伸直岔开而坐,头身向后反倒九次。可补虚,理气,通便,治大小便困难。

exercise of Daoyin for dysuria and difficult defecation　A dynamic exercise, marked by sitting upright, crossing the hands and putting on the back; crossing the hands again, putting the hands on the back and pushing to the heart, stretching and crossing the feet to sit, and returning the head and body backwards for nine times. Such a dynamic exercise can reinforce deficiency, regulate Qi, and promote defecation and urination.

大小鼎炉【dà xiǎo dǐng lú】　为百脉交会之处。

great and small pots and furnaces　Refers to the region where all meridians communicate through it.

D

大小还丹【dà xiǎo huán dān】　为静功。其作法为，端身正坐，自肾传肝，自肝传心，自心传脾、传肺，周而复始。调节脏腑功能，治疗脏腑之疾。

great and small returning to Dan（pills of immortality）　A static exercise，marked by sitting quietly every day，transmitting the liver from the kidney，transmitting the heart from the liver，transmitting the spleen and lung from the heart constantly in order to regulate the functions of the viscera and to treat the diseases in the viscera.

大凶【dà xiōng】　指人的精神意识与行为，违背自然规律。

severe fierceness　Refers to the activities of the spirit and consciousness that have violated the natural principles.

大学之道【dà xué zhī dào】　指孔子调节精神意识活动，提高智力的方法。

Dao in the Great Learning　Refers to the exercises of Confucius for regulating the activities of the spirit and consciousness as well as increasing wisdom and ability.

大雪十一月节坐功【dà xuě shí yī yuè jié zuò gong】　为动功。其作法为，每日子丑时（二十三时至三时），起身仰膝，各五七次，叩齿、咽液、吐纳。可治疗各种疾病。

sitting exercise in the feast days of November　A dynamic exercise，marked by standing up and raising the knees in Zi（the period of a day from 11 p.m. to 1 a.m.）and Chou（the period of a day from 1 a.m. to 3 a.m. in the morning）for five or seven times，clicking the teeth，swallowing humor and breathing in and out. Such a dynamic exercise can cure various diseases.

大药【dà yào】　指阳精、肾间动气、内丹、心肾相交、炼精气神所生、阴阳交媾而成。

great medicinal　Refers to either Yang essence（cinnabar），or intra-nephric Qi，or internal Dan（pills of immortality），or coordination between the kidney and heart，or interaction between Yin and Yang.

大药不求争得遇【dà yào bù qiú zhēng dé yù】　指不习练气功，怎么能遇明师？不习练气功，怎么能获得水火既济？

no practice and no achievement　Indicates that no practice of Qigong is impossible to meet great masters and that no practice of Qigong is impossible to coordinate water and fire.

大忧内崩【dà yōu nèi bēng】　指忧虑过度，脏腑及其功能损坏而为病。

serious anxiety impairing the viscera　Refers to serious sorrow that damages the viscera and the functions，eventually causing diseases.

大幽【dà yōu】　指大冥，为北方阴极之地，喻身体会阴部。

perineum　Refers to an area in the north with extreme Yin which refers to perineum.

大圆镜智【dà yuán jìng zhì】　指佛家气功所要达到的理想境界。

great wisdom　Refers to the ideal state of the spirit in Buddhism.

大圆镜智观【dà yuán jìng zhì guān】　是静功，具体做法是意想佛身，融为一体。

buddha imagination　A static exercise，marked by imagination of Buddhism and integration with Buddha.

大圆觉【dà yuán jué】　指广大圆满的

感觉与知觉,为精神意识思维活动。

great satisfaction Refers to complete emotion and consciousness which is the activity of the spirit, consciousness and thinking.

大趾【dà zhǐ】 即蹈趾。足厥阴肝经循行线经大趾,气功排肝经毒气常从此出。

large toe The area through which the liver meridian of foot Jueyin moves around and pathogenic factors in the liver meridian are expelled.

大周天【dà zhōu tiān】 为静功。其作法为,自然坐势,或盘膝坐式,调整意识活动,补脑安神,调节脏腑功能。

great circulatory cycle A static exercise, marked by naturally sitting or sitting with crossed knees, regulating consciousness activity, tonifying the brain, stabilizing the spirit and regulating the functions of the five Zang-organs (including the heart, the liver, the spleen, the lung and the kidney) and six Fu-organs (including the gallbladder, the stomach, the small intestine, the large intestine, the bladder and the triple energizer).

大杼【dà zhù】 为足太阳膀胱经中的一个穴位,位于第一胸椎刺突下旁开1.5 寸处。这一穴位为气功运行的常见部位。

Dazhu（BL 11） An acupoint in the bladder meridian of foot Taiyang, located 1.5 Cun below and lateral to the spinous process of the first thoracic vertebra. This acupoint is a region usually used in practice of Qigong.

大椎【dà zhuī】 督脉的一个穴位,位于后正中线,第七颈椎棘突下凹陷中。为气功学重要体表标志之一。此穴位为

气功习练之处。

Dazhui（GV 14） An acupoint in the governor meridian, located in the back midline and in the depression of spinous process in the seventh cervical vertebra, which is the important symbol in Qigong. This acupoint is a region usually used in practice of Qigong.

大眦【dà zì】 即内眼角,为上下眼睑与鼻侧连接部,是足太阳膀胱经的起点。

large canthus Located between the upper and lower eyelids connected with the nasal side, which is the origin of the bladder meridian of foot Taiyang.

代谢【dài xiè】 指阴尽阳生,阳尽阴生的气化规律。

metabolism Refers to Yin decline and Yang growth as well as Yang decline and Yin growth.

带便【dài biàn】 指端正地坐着,两手相交放于背后的练功姿势。

straight sitting Refers to sitting upright with crossed hands putting over the back.

带缚【dài fù】 为动功。其作法为,正坐,以两手交背后,凝神静守之。

binding belt A dynamic exercise, marked by sitting upright with hands crossed behind for tranquilization.

带脉【dài mài】 ① 为足少阳胆经中的一个穴位;② 为奇经八脉之一。这一穴位为气功运行的一个常见部位。

belt meridian Refers to ① either Daimai（GB 26）which is one of the acupoints in the gallbladder meridian of foot Shaoyang; ② or one of the eight extraordinary meridians. This acupoint or extraordinary meridian is a region usually used for keeping the essential Qi in practice of Qigong.

D

带神符【dài shén fú】　指带人习练气功,为教功之意。

belting hierogram　Means to teach others to practice Qigong.

带执性命守虚无【dài zhí xìng mìng shǒu xū wú】　指讲授性命双修功,并带习练者进入高度入静状态。

protecting life and keeping vacuum and nothingness　Refers to teaching how to cultivate life in two ways and leading the practitioners of Qigong into the high and tranquil state.

丹【dān】　指阴阳两种药物在体内合炼而成丹。后称气功为丹。

Dan（pills of immortality）　Refers to the result of Yin and Yang medicinals that have integrated in the body. It also refers to Qigong practice as Dan（pills of immortality）, indicating an important appellation of Qigong.

丹本【dān běn】　指阴阳相互作用而结,阴阳相互作用的枢机在神。

root of Dan（pills of immortality）　Refers to interaction of Yin and Yang that depends on the spirit.

丹池【dān chí】　即下齿根之唾液。

pool of Dan（pills of immortality）　Refers to saliva from the lower teeth.

丹道【dān dào】　指气功的理论及方法。

Dao of Dan（pills of immortality）　Refers to the theory and methods of Qigong.

丹鼎派【dān dǐng pài】　指习练内丹为主的道家流派。

Daoism school of alchemy　Refers to a school of Daoism that paid more attention to refining the internal Dan（pills of immortality）in practicing Qigong.

丹法【dān fǎ】　指气功功法。

Dan（pills of immortality）method　Refers to the commonly used methods in practicing Qigong.

丹法之祖【dān fǎ zhī zǔ】　《丹法之祖》指《周易参同契》,是习练内丹法之宗,为气功学的第一部专著。

ancestor of Qigong　Refers to the classic entitled Can Tong Qi which is the first book about Qigong study.

丹房语录【dān fáng yǔ lù】　《丹房语录》为气功学专著,阐述神凝精气聚,驻息忘念而成金丹的基本道理。

Danfang Yulu（Quotations of Qigong）　A monograph about Qigong entitled Quotations of Qigong, describing the importance of concentrating the spirit, the essence and Qi, which is the basic rule for practicing Qigong and improving Dantian. Dantian is divided into the upper Dantian（the region between the eyes）, the middle Dantian（the region below the heart）and the lower Dantian（the region below the navel）.

丹基【dān jī】　指产丹的基本物及方位。

foundation of Dan（pills of immortality）　Refers to the region between the left kidney and the right kidney which is the root of life.

丹锦飞裳披玉罗【dān jǐn fēi shāng pī yù luó】　指心之外象,肺似华盖,肺之气如玉罗复于心之上。

the lung coverings the heart　Refers to the manifestation of the heart, the canopy of the lung and Qi of the lung like silk.

丹锦云袍【dān jǐn yún páo】　指心肺的外象,云袍为肺的外象。

cardiac and pulmonary manifestation　Refers to the harmony, balance and influence of the heart and lung.

丹经【dān jīng】《丹经》指气功经典著作。

canon of Dan（**pills of immortality**）Refers to the classic or canon of Qigong.

丹经极论【dān jīng jí lùn】《丹经极论》为气功学专著,作者不详。

Danjing Jilun（***Thorough Annotation of Qigong***）A monograph about Qigong entitled *Thorough Annotation of Qigong*. The author was unknown.

丹扃【dān jiōng】即丹田之门,喻丹田。

knocker of Dan（**pills of immortality**）Refers to the way along which Dantian can be well practiced. Dantian is divided into the upper Dantian（the region between the eyes）, the middle Dantian（the region below the heart）and the lower Dantian（the region below the navel）.

丹诀【dān jué】① 指练气功时默念的口诀;② 指气功习练方法。

formula of Dan（**pills of immortality**）Refers to ① either pretermission of such a formula in Qigong practice; ② or rhymes and techniques for practicing Qigong.

丹母【dān mǔ】① 指阴阳交媾之母;② 指心;③ 指气功获得成效。

mother of Dan（**pills of immortality**）Refers to ① coition of Yin and Yang; ② or the heart; ③ or the effect of Qigong.

丹砂可学赋【dān shā kě xué fù】《丹砂可学赋》为气功学专著,指学习气功,重在变化意识思维活动以调节身体的阴阳。

Dansha Kexue Fu（***Essentials About How To Study Qigong***）A monograph of Qigong entitled *Essentials About How To Study Qigong*, describing the fact that the importance of studying Qigong is to change the activities of consciousness and thinking and to regulate Yin and Yang in the body.

丹髓歌【dān suǐ gē】《丹髓歌》为气功专著,宋代薛道光著,内容有炼丹诗词三十四首,论述甚为精辟。

Dansui Ge（***A Monograph of Qigong***）A monograph of Qigong entitled *A Monograph of Qigong*, written by Xue Daoguang in the Song Dynasty（960 AD－1279 AD）, containing thirty-four poems about how to practice Qigong.

丹台【dān tái】指心。

stage of Dan（**pills of immortality**）Refers to the heart.

丹田【dān tián】指炼丹产丹的部位,为人身之本,真气汇聚之处。

Dantian Refers to the region for producing Dan（pill or cinnabar）in alchemy, which is the root of human body where genuine Qi concentrates. Dantian is divided into the upper Dantian（the region between the eyes）, the middle Dantian（the region below the heart）and the lower Dantian（the region below the navel）.

丹田宫【dān tián gōng】在两眉中入骨3寸。

palace of Dantian Refers to the region between the two eyes. Dantian is divided into the upper Dantian（the region between the eyes）, the middle Dantian（the region below the heart）and the lower Dantian（the region below the navel）.

丹田固守【dān tián gù shǒu】为纳气

于丹田之意。

defence of Dantian　Refers to concentration of Qi at Dantian. Dantian is divided into the upper Dantian（the region between the eyes）, the middle Dantian（the region below the heart）and the lower Dantian（the region below the navel）.

丹田暖融融【dān tián nuǎn róng róng】 指功景象，即神形合一的状态。

warmness of Dantian　Refers to state of somatic and spiritual integration. Dantian is divided into the upper Dantian（the region between the eyes）, the middle Dantian（the region below the heart）and the lower Dantian（the region below the navel）.

丹田真人【dān tián zhēn rén】 为金代气功学家马丹阳的另外一个称谓。

immortal of Dantian　Refers to Ma Danyang, a great master of Qigong and acupuncture in the Jin Dynasty（1123 - 1183）. Dantian is divided into the upper Dantian（the region between the eyes）, the middle Dantian（the region below the heart）and the lower Dantian（the region below the navel）.

丹头【dān tóu】 指阴精阳气相感。

head of Dan（pills of immortality）　Refers to combination of Yin essence and Yang Qi.

丹头只是先天气【dān tóu zhǐ shì xiān tiān qì】《丹头只是先天气》源自气功专论，主要阐述先天气是炼内丹的基础物质。

original Qi as the foundation for practicing Qigong　Collected from a monograph of Qigong, mainly describing the fact that the basic foundation for practicing internal Dan（pills of immortality）is original Qi.

丹阳子【dān yáng zǐ】 宋金时期的气功家和针灸学家马钰的另外一个称谓，著有针灸气功专著。

Dan Yangzi　Another name of Ma Yu, who was a great master of Qigong and acupuncture in the Song Dynasty（960 AD - 1279 AD）and Jin Dynasty（1115 AD - 1234 AD）.

丹元【dān yuán】 指心神。

Danyuan　Refers to cardiac spirit.

丹元宫【dān yuán gōng】 指认真呼吸处，为身体中空窍。

palace of Danyuan　Refers to the orifice of the body through which the immortals can breathe.

丹元宫真人【dān yuán gōng zhēn rén】 指肾脏所主神名。

immortal in the palace of Danyuan　Refers to the special name of the kidney.

单思【dān sī】 指单一之思，即意念纯净为一。

concentrated contemplation　Refers to pure thinking without any desires.

耽玄笃志【dān xuán dǔ zhì】 指习练气功养生法，坚定意志，持之以恒。

perseverance　Refers to firming the will and preserving the purpose in practicing Qigong.

胆病导引【dǎn bìng dǎo yǐn】 为动功。其作法为，平坐床上，合两足掌，仰头，两手分别握住两足腕向垂直方向上提，然后来回摇动，做三五次。

Daoyin for gallbladder disease　A dynamic exercise, marked by sitting on the bed, crossing the soles, raising the head, holding the ankles with both hands to raise directly upwards and then shaking back and forth for three to five times.

胆导引法【dǎn dǎo yǐn fǎ】　为动功。其作法为，平坐，令两脚掌昂头，以两手挽脚腕起，摇动为之，三五度。

exercise of Daoyin for the gallbladder　A dynamic exercise, marked by sitting normally, raising the soles, holding the ankles with both hands and shaking for three or five degrees.

胆理脑升玄【dǎn lǐ nǎo shēng xuán】　指以意内观脑室，引精气上行，上下协调，以补脑神。

supremely managing the gallbladder and increasing the brain　Refers to observing the chamber in the brain with consciousness, leading the essential Qi to move upwards, regulating the upper and lower in order to tonify the spirit in the brain.

胆修养法【dǎn xiū yǎng fǎ】　为静功。其作法为，常以冬月、三月端居净思，北吸玄宫之黑气，入口三吞之以补，嘻之损。以尽益胆之津，以食龟蛇之味，饮玉童之浆，然后神冲体和，众邪不能犯。

exercise for cultivating and nourishing the gallbladder　A static exercise, marked by staying quiet and tranquilizing the mind in the months in winter or in March, inhaling black Qi from the north palace, keeping it in the mouth for three times for tonifying the body and avoiding damage caused by giggle, enriching fluid in the gallbladder, absorbing the taste of turtle and snake, and drinking syrup of immortal baby. To practice Qigong in such an exercise will promote the spirit to move in the whole body and prevent invasion of any pathogenic factors.

旦慧【dàn huì】　指患者一般早晨神气清爽，意识明敏。早晨习练气功，有助于神气的生发。

morning consciousness　Refers to the fact that the patients feel fresh in the morning. Practice of Qigong in the morning is helpful for improving the mind.

但思一部【dàn sī yī bù】　指意念存思三部八景神。

contemplation in one region　Refers to thought and meditation in three regions with eight manifestations of the spirit.

淡然无为神气自满【dàn rán wú wéi shén qì zì mǎn】　神是一切活动的主宰，意静则神自充。

Indifference and inaction can perfect the spirit and Qi.　Indicating that the spirit is the dominator of any activity and tranquilized mind can enrich the spirit.

淡食能多补论【dàn shí néng duō bǔ lùn】　源自气功专论，主要阐述气功养生注意，饮食厚味伤人，淡食能补养五脏六腑的道理。

idea about vegetarian diet for tonifying the body　Collected from a monograph of Qigong, mainly describing that delicious diet damages the body while vegetarian diet nourishes the five Zang-organs (including the heart, the liver, the spleen, the lung and the kidney) and the six Fu-organs (including the gallbladder, the stomach, the small intestine, the large intestine, the bladder and the triple energizer).

当时一句师边得，默默垂帘仔细看【dāng shí yī jù shī biān dé mò mò chuí lián zǐ xì kàn】　指出垂帘返视在练功中的重要性。

Silently sit behind a screen and carefully look after obtaining an instruction from the teacher.　Refers to the importance of silently sitting behind the screen and carefully looking in practicing Qigong.

荡秽【dàng huì】 指气机一有壅滞,百节不流通,以致脉络壅塞,或为瘀血,或为痰浊,令人致病。

foul expelling Referring to stagnation of meridians and collaterals, or blood stasis, or turbid sputum due to stagnation of functional activity of Qi, causing various diseases.

刀圭【dāo guī】 ① 指神;② 指神气合一。

elongated tablet Refers to ① either the spirit; ② or integration of the spirit and Qi.

导气令和,引体令柔【dǎo qì lìng hé yǐn tǐ lìng róu】 导气即导引行气,通过导引行气而使体内气调;引体即肢体活动,通过肢体活动而使体内气血流畅、灵活自如。

transmitting Qi to realize harmony and stretching the body to ensure relaxation Transmitting Qi means to circulate Qi through Daoyin in order to regulate Qi in the body, stretching the body means to smooth Qi and blood in the body through moving the limbs.

导养【dǎo yǎng】 指导引养生,即动功练养身体。

exercise of Daoyin for life cultivation Refers to nourishing the body with the dynamic exercise in practicing Qigong.

导引【dǎo yǐn】 即通过运动肢体,以达到形神谐调的健身方法,属古代气功动功的范畴。

Daoyin Refers to regulation of the body and the spirit through moving the limbs for the purpose of fortifying the body, which belongs to the categories of dynamic exercises for practicing Qigong in ancient times.

导引按蹻【dǎo yǐn àn qiāo】 为动功。其作法为,平身正坐,两手交叉抱颈项,抬头仰视,然后左右转动颈项,继而左手抱左脚趾,闭气以取太冲(穴名)之气。右手动作相同。

exercise of Daoyin for pressing and lifting A dynamic exercise, marked by sitting upright, crossing the hands to hold the neck, raising the head to observe, then turning the neck from the left to the right and vice versa, holding the toes on the left foot with the left hand and closing respiration to take Qi from Taichong (LR 3). The right hand is moving with the same way.

导引法【dǎo yǐn fǎ】 为动功。其作法为,当以丑后卯前,天气清和日为之。先解发散,梳四际,上达顶,三百六十五过,面向东,平坐握固,闭目思神,叩齿三百六十过,乃纵体平气,依次为之。

exercise of Daoyin A dynamic exercise, marked by practice after Chou (the period of a day from 1 a. m. to 3 a. m. in the morning) and before Mao (the period of a day from 5 a. m. to 7 a. m. in the morning) when it is a sunny day. Before practicing Qigong, hair should be freed and groomed in the four sides towards the top of the head for three hundred and sixty-five times. Then the practitioner turns the face to the east, sitting with the hands holding the fists, closing the eyes, contemplating the spirit and clicking the teeth for three hundred and sixty times in order to stabilize Qi. Such a way of practice can be continued for several times.

导引气法【dǎo yǐn qì fǎ】 为静功,指练功时动功姿势与呼吸配合的一种方法。

exercise of Daoyin for respiration A static exercise, referring to a method marked by coordination of the dynamic exercise with respiration in practicing Qigong.

导引去五脏风邪积聚法【dǎo yǐn qù wǔ zàng fēng xié jī jù fǎ】为动功。各脏腑导引法为：肺脏，正坐，两手撑地，缩身曲脊上下五次。心脏，正坐，握拳左右手用力相等。脾脏，坐稳，伸一脚屈一脚，两手往后反擊。肝脏，两手抱项，左右旋转。胆腑，平坐，两脚合拢，两手握脚腕摇动。肾脏，握拳挂两肋，摆动两肩，两足前后迈步，能祛除心、脾、肺、肝、胆风邪积聚。

exercise of Daoyin for eliminating pathogenic wind accumulating in the five Zang-organ A dynamic exercise. There are special exercises of Daoyin for each Zang-organs and Fu-organs (including the gallbladder, the stomach, the small intestine, the large intestine, the bladder and the triple energizer). The exercise for the lung is marked by sitting upright, pressing the ground with both hands, shrinking the body and bending the spine for five times. The exercise for the heart is marked by sitting upright, clenching the fists with the right hand and left hand in the same way. The exercise for the spleen is marked by sitting quietly, stretching one foot and bending the other foot, turning both hands to the back. The exercise for the liver is marked by holding the neck with both hands and rotating from the left to the right and vice versa. The exercise for the gallbladder is marked by sitting quietly, closing two feet and holding the ankles to shake with both hands. The exercise for the kidney is marked by holding the fists over the two sides of the chest, moving the two shoulders and running the feet forwards and backwards. Such special exercises of Daoyin can eliminate accumulation of pathogenic wind in the heart, the spleen, the lung, the kidney, the liver and the gallbladder.

导引却病养生法【dǎo yǐn què bìng yǎng shēng fǎ】为动功，方法多样。如低头，以两手抱两足，不息，十二通，令人身轻，益精气，诸邪恶百病不得入。

exercise of Daoyin for curing disease and cultivating life A dynamic exercise with various methods, such as bowing the head, holding the feet with both hands and suspending respiration for twelve times in order to relax the body, to fortify the essential Qi and to prevent occurrence of any serious diseases.

导引思气【dǎo yǐn sī qì】源自气功专论，主要阐述六字气治五脏之病，即呼时念吹、呼、唏、呵、嘘、呬六字。

Daoyin for contemplating Qi Mainly describing practice of Qigong with six Chinese characters to treat diseases in the five Zang-organs (including the heart, the liver, the spleen, the lung and the kidney), during which six Chinese characters must be read, i.e. Chui (blowing), Hu (exhaling), Xi (sighing), Ke (breathing out), Xu (breathing out slowly) and Xi (panting).

导引图【dǎo yǐn tú】《导引图》即《马王堆汉墓导引图》，为气功导引专著，1973 年于湖南长沙马王堆三号汉墓出土。

D

Daoyin Tu (*Daoyin Pictures in the Mawangdui Tomb of the Han Dynasty*) A monograph of Qigong entitled *Daoin Pictures in the Mawangdui Tomb of the Han Dynasty*, discovered in 1973 from the third tomb of the Han Dynasty (202 BC - 263 AD) in Bawangdui area in Changsha City, Hunan Province.

导引吐纳治病法【dǎo yǐn tǔ nà zhì bìng fǎ】 为动功,方法多样。如平坐,伸腰,两臂覆手据地,口徐纳气,以鼻吐之,除胸中肺中痛。

exercise of Daoyin for curing disease through exhaling the old and inhaling the new A dynamic exercise with various methods, such as sitting down, stretching the waist, pressing the ground with both shoulders and hands, mildly inhaling the new, exhaling the old through the nose in order to relieve pain in the chest and the lung.

导引以通百关【dǎo yǐn yǐ tōng bǎi guān】 指导引(动功)调节形体姿势,开通经络,畅通关节。

Daoyin can pass through all joints Refers to the way of Daoyin (dynamic exercise) to regulate the body and to open the meridians, collateral and joints.

到位次坐向外方,所存在心自相当【dào wèi cì zuò xiàng wài fāng suǒ cún zài xīn zì xiāng dāng】 指脑内百神作用向外,从外又收存向内,向外收内的作用自相当,心为精神意识思维活动。

sitting outside when listing the position and keeping the heart in the natural Refers to extending outside the effects of all the spirits in the brain and then concentrating all the spirits inside. The ways of extending outside and concentrating inside are all natural. The heart reflects the activities of the spirit, consciousness and thought.

道【dào】 ① 指事物一分为二,合二而一的对立统一规律;② 指万物生化之源;③ 指万物变化;④ 指事物正在变化之中;⑤ 指以自然为法;⑥ 指道理,基本理论。

Dao Refers to ① either unity of opposites for dividing one into two and two combined into one; ② or the source of all things; ③ or changes of all things; ④ or things in changing; ⑤ or natural principles; ⑥ or basic theory.

道藏【dào cáng】 《道藏》为道经的总汇,明以前道家气功重要文献均收集于其中。

collection of Daoism Refers to aggregation of important Daoism canons before the Ming Dynasty (1368 AD - 1644 AD).

道冲【dào chōng】 指养形安神应清静自处。

Daoist thoroughfare Refers to cultivating the body and stabilizing the spirit based on tranquilization.

道丹还转【dào dān hái zhuǎn】 指气功中精气神的变化作用。

repeated returning of Daoist Dan (pills of immortality) Refers to the change and effect of the essence, Qi and the spirit in Qigong.

道德【dào dé】 ① 指虚无、化育;② 指形神稳定,形神合一,养育生成;③ 指遵守的行为准则。

Daoist morality Refers to ① either nothingness, transformation and rearing; ② or stability of the body and the spirit, integration of the body and the spirit, and success of nourishing and rearing; ③ or following the rules in action.

道德经【dào dé jīng】《道德经》为《老子》的另外一个名称。老子是春秋末年伟大的思想家、哲学家，为道教的创始人，《老子》中也有气功养生的精神。

Dao De Jing（*Canon of the Virtue of Dao*） Another title of the great canon entitled Lao Zi. Lao Zi was also the name of a great thinker, a great philosopher and the founder of the most important Chinese thought known as Dao in the late Spring and Autumn Period (770 BC－476 BC).

道德相抱【dào dé xiāng bào】 指习练气功，阴阳和平，增进健康。

coordination of Daoism and virtue Refers to harmonizing Yin and Yang and increasing health in practicing Qigong.

道典论【dào diǎn lùn】《道典论》为道书，兼述气功养生，说明作法及注意事项。作者不详。

Daodian Lun（*Discussion of Daoism Canons*） A monograph of Daoism with Qigong and life cultivation entitled *Discussion of Daoism Canons*, explaining the exercises and points for attention. The author was unknown.

道法会元【dào fǎ huì yuán】《道法会元》为道书，兼论气功养生，论述气功养生法的基本理论和具体方法。作者不详。

Daofa Huiyuan（*Metropolitan Origin of Daoist Exercises*） A monograph of Daoism with the discussion of Qigong and life cultivation entitled *Metropolitan Origin of Daoist Exercises*, describing the basic theory and methods of Qigong practice and life cultivation. The author was unknown.

道法自然【dào fǎ zì rán】 指事物的发展规律效法于自然。功中用以喻作精气的运行，任其自然之流行。

Daoist Nature Refers to the natural principles and effects in developing anything. In Qigong, it refers to natural movement of the essential Qi.

道观【dào guàn】 ① 指道教神庙；② 指佛家功法。

Daoist Temple Refers to ① either the temple in Daoism; ② or exercise of Qigong in Buddhism.

道贯真源【dào guàn zhēn yuán】《道贯真源》为气功专著，由清代董元真著，载有多部气功养生之法。

Daoguan Zhenyuan（*Genuine Source of Daoist Penetration*） Daoguan Zhenyuan is a monograph of Qigong entitled *Genuine Source of Daoist Penetration*, written by Dong Yuanzhen in the Qing Dynasty (1636 AD－1912 AD), including several sections about how to practice Qigong and life cultivation.

道家【dào jiā】 ① 指哲学流派；② 指崇尚黄老之说的学者；③ 指具有气功养生法研究的人。

Daoist school Refers to ① either schools of philosophy; ② or those who advocate the thoughts of Yellow Emperor and Lao Zi; ③ or those who have studied Qigong and life cultivation.

道家抱一以独善【dào jiā bào yī yǐ dú shàn】 指道家调节精神，使之专一以适应社会的变化。

Concentration in Daoism is the absolute integrity. Indicates that regulation of the spirit in Daoism is concentrated to conform to social changes.

道家功【dào jiā gōng】 指源于道家，以后较长时间一直在道家内流传的功法。

Daoist exercise Originates from Daoism, which circulates in the Daoism for a very long time.

道家之难【dào jiā zhī nán】 指道家气功,难在守神于身内并随时保持意识的稳定。

difficulty in Daoism Means that it is difficult to keep the spirit inside the body and to stabilize consciousness at any time in practicing Qigong in Daoism.

道家之易【dào jiā zhī yì】 指道家气功,易在自然而然,不劳精神,不运思虑,安时处和。

natural change in Daoism Refers to Qigong in Daoism, characterized by natural practice without exhausting the spirit and keeping contemplation in order to harmonize and to balance the body at anytime.

道教【dào jiào】 为中国教派之一,遵老子为祖。

Daoism One of the region schools in China, taking Lao Zi as the ancestor.

道可受兮不可传【dào kě shòu xī bù kě chuán】 指气功养生法神妙的道理,体内的阴阳变化,精气运行,意识作用等,只能意会(悟得或曰觉悟),不可言传。

Daoism can be understood but cannot be talked. Indicates that the marvelous truth of Qigong and life cultivation, changes of Yin and Yang in the human body, movement of the essential Qi and effects of consciousness can only be sensed, but not be said.

道流【dào liú】 ① 指道家;② 指僧道;③ 也泛指气功养生家。

Daoist style Refers to ① either Dao-

ism; ② or monk; ③ or master of Qigong and life cultivation.

道妙【dào miào】 为对金代气功学家刘处玄的赞美,其为全真随山派创始人。

Daoist wonder The celebration of Liu Chuxuan who was a great master of Qigong in the Jin Dynasty (1120 - 1203) and the founder of Suishan Mountain School in Acme Genuine Dao.

道母道父【dào mǔ dào fù】 指身体阴阳两个方面。

Daoist mother and Daoist father Refers to Yin and Yang in the human body.

道人【dào rén】 ① 指有道术之人,泛指掌握气功养生法的人;② 指佛教徒。

Taoist priest Refers to ① either those who have a grasp of Qigong and life cultivation; ② or Buddhists.

道生【dào shēng】 指长寿是习练气功,善于养生的结果。

Daoist life Refers to results of practicing Qigong and life cultivation among those who have prolonged their life.

道生一【dào shēng yī】 指阴阳运动变化而产生事物。

Dao producing one Refers to things produced by changes of Yin and Yang.

道士【dào shì】 ① 指有道术之人,泛指掌握气功养生法的人;② 指佛教徒。

Daoist Refers to ① either to those who have a grasp of Qigong and life cultivation; ② or Buddhists.

道书十二种【dào shū shí èr zhǒng】《道书十二种》为气功专著,由清代刘一明撰,收载了十二部气功专著,为气功的珍贵文物。

Daoshu Shi'er Zhong (*Twelve Kinds of Daoism Books*) A valuable literature of Qigong entitled *Twelve Kinds of*

Daoism Books, compiled by Liu Yiming in the Qing Dynasty (1636 AD - 1912 AD), including twelve monographs of Qigong.

道枢【dào shū】 ① 为宋代道家大型类书,保存有宋以前的大量气功文献;② 指中。

Daoist pivot Refers to ① either large categories of books about Qigong, into which all kinds of the literature of Qigong before the Song Dynasty (960 AD - 1279 AD) were collected; ② or the center.

道术【dào shù】 指导引、吐纳、玄素、仙药、金丹、黄白、禁咒等术,其中部分即气功养生术,如导引、吐纳、玄素等。

Daoism techniques Refers to the techniques of Daoyin, exhaling the old and inhaling the new, metaphysic, golden Dan (pills of immortality), yellow and white, and Forbidden Mantra, parts of which refer to the techniques of Qigong and life cultivation, such as Daoyin, exhaling the old and inhaling the new and metaphysic.

道胎【dào tāi】 ① 即圣胎,指胎息气功;② 指习练佛家气功;③ 指神气凝结而作丹。

Daoist embryo The same as sacred embryo, refers to ① either fetal respiration in practicing Qigong; ② or Qigong practice in Buddhism; ③ or concentration of the spirit and Qi developing into Dan (pills of immortality).

道心【dào xīn】 ① 指道德观念;② 指悟道,泛指认识气功养生法并实践之;③ 有修道之心,多指在家修道。

Daoist heart Refers to ① either moral concept; ② or realizing truth, which refers to understanding and practicing

the exercise of Qigong and life cultivation; ③ or the idea of monasticism, indicating cultivation of oneself according to Daoism at home.

道学【dào xué】 ① 指老庄之学;② 指宋明理学。

Daoism doctrine Refers to ① either the theories of Lao Zi and Zhuang Zi; ② or neo-Confucianism of the Song Dynasty (960 AD - 1279 AD) and Ming Dynasty (1368 AD - 1644 AD).

道言五种【dào yán wǔ zhǒng】 《道言五种》为气功专著,由清代陶素耜所撰,收集了五部气功专著,保存了气功文献。

Daoyan Wuzhong (*Five Kinds of Daoist Language*) A monograph of Qigong entitled *Five Kinds of Daoist Language*, compiled by Tao Susi in the Qing Dynasty (1636 AD - 1912 AD), collected five kinds of monographs in order to preserve the literature of Qigong.

道意【dào yì】 源自气功专论,阐述有无、多少、动静、升降的辩证关系。

Daoist opinion Collected from a monograph of Qigong, describing the differentiation of presence or absence, more or less, activity or tranquility, and ascent or descent.

道引【dào yǐn】 即导引,指通过运动肢体,以达到形神协调的健身方法,属古代气功动功的范畴。

Daoyin Refers to regulation of the body and the spirit through moving the limbs for the purpose of fortifying the body, which belongs to the categories of dynamic exercises for practicing Qigong in ancient times.

道种智【dào zhǒng zhì】 ① 指三智之一智;② 指修习方法,认为有智才能生慧,生慧才能静定。

all wisdoms Refer to ① all kinds of wisdom and all difference of wisdom; ② or methods of practice, indicating that only wisdom can increase intelligence and only intelligence can tranquilize the body.

得道【dé dào】 即得成真道,喻习练气功达到纯一的境界。

obtaining Dao Refers to achieving the genuine Dao. In Qigong, it refers to the pure state.

得类交感【dé lèi jiāo gǎn】 指阴阳相互作用,即二气相感之意。

interaction of categories Refers to mutual action of Yin and Yang, indicating mutual influence of two kinds of Qi.

得神御气法【dé shén yù qì fǎ】 指控制呼吸的方法。控制的方法重点是调节精神。

exercise for obtaining the spirit and moving Qi Refers to controlling respiration, the important method of which is to regulate the essence and the spirit.

得神者昌【dé shén zhě chāng】 指神气充沛,脏腑功能协调,则形体健康。

prosperity after obtaining the spirit Refers to abundance of the spirit and Qi as well as coordination of the five Zang-organs (including the heart, the liver, the spleen, the lung and the kidney) and the six Fu-organs (including the gallbladder, the stomach, the small intestine, the large intestine, the bladder and the triple energizer), ensuring health of the body.

得药【dé yào】 指得后天鼎中所产先天之外药也。

obtaining medicinal Refers to innate medicinal produced in the postnatal cauldron.

得一【dé yī】 指原则,规律,基础,本根。气功中专用以说明达到阴阳协调统一。

keeping one Refers to the principle, rule, foundation and root. In Qigong, it refers to coordination and integration of Yin and Yang.

得真【dé zhēn】 即证真,指气功中神形相互作用,相顾、相并、相入、相抱,逐步进入俱妙、双舍的境界。

obtaining truth The same as proving truth, refers to mutual effect of the spirit and body, including mutual support, mutual combination, mutual entrance and mutual integration, eventually developing into the wonderful and double alms state.

德和【dé hé】 指意识活动的稳定和协调。

moral harmony Refers to stability and coordination of consciousness activity.

德化政令灾变【dé huà zhèng lìng zāi biàn】 为运气术语,德化是五气正常的吉祥之兆,政令是五气的规则和表现形式,变易是产生胜气和复气的纲纪,灾祸是万物损伤的开始。

De (function), Hua (transformation), Zheng (administration), Ling (order), Zai (harm) and Bian (change) A term of direct Qi, indicating that De (function) and Hua (transformation) are auspicious omen of the five kinds of Qi; Zheng (administration) and Ling (order) are the rules and manifestations of the five kinds of Qi; Bian (change) is the order and law for producing exuberant Qi and renewed Qi; and Zai (harm) is the beginning of damaging all things.

D

德全不危【dé quán bù wēi】　指对气功等养性修身之道有领会，并掌握其方法的人，身体不会受内外病邪的危害。

moral acme ensuring safety Moral acme ensuring safety means that those who are clear about the exercises for nourishing the mind and cultivating life in Qigong practice will not be harmed by external and internal pathogenic factors.

登山采药【dēng shān cǎi yào】　指练功时高度入静后，阴阳协调，和合而成丹。

climbing mountain to collect medicinal Refers to perfect tranquilization and coordination and concordance of Yin and Yang in practicing Qigong，which as formed Dan（pills of immortality）.

登虚【dēng xū】　即练功时的高度入静。

reaching vacuum Refers to perfect tranquilization in practicing Qigong.

堤防【dī fáng】　指专心一意，排除杂念。

dike Refers to concentrating consciousness and tranquilizing the mind to eliminate any distracting thought.

涤除玄览【dí chú xuán lǎn】　即少视少听，排除杂念，导引入静。

eliminating abstruse cognition Refers to visiting less and listening less in order to eliminate distracting thought and to tranquilize the mind.

地【dì】　指行功过程中的阶段次位。

ground Refers to the states in practicing Qigong.

地仓【dì cāng】　为足阳明胃经中的一个穴位，位于口角外侧。这一穴位为气功运行的一个常见部位。

Dicang（ST 4）　An acupoint in the stomach meridian of foot Yangming，located in the outward to the corner of the mouth. This acupoint is a region usually used for keeping the essential Qi in practice of Qigong.

地道不通【dì dao bù tōng】　指月经绝止。

unobstructed earthly way Refers to amenorrhea.

地户【dì hù】　指七孔中的鼻子。

earthly household Refers to the nose in the seven orifices.

地户禁门【dì hù jìn mén】　指九灵铁鼓，精气聚散常在此处，水火发端也在此处，阴阳变化也在此处，有无出入也在此处。

blocked earthly household Refers to nine genius-fire drums，the region where the essential Qi concentrates and disperses there，water and fire appear there，Yin and Yang change there，exit and entrance exist there.

地机【dì jī】　为足太阴脾经中的一个穴位，位于阴陵泉直下 3 寸。这一穴位为气功运行的一个常见部位。

Diji（SP 8）　An acupoint in the spleen meridian of foot Taiyin，located 3 Cun directly below Yinlingquan（SP 9）. This acupoint is a region usually used for keeping the essential Qi in practice of Qigong.

地交于天【dì jiāo yú tiān】　指通过伏羲创建的八卦解读阴阳。

communication of the sky with the earth Refers to explanation of Yin and Yang through exposition of the Eight Trigrams created by Fu Xi，the ancestor of Chinese civilization.

地门【dì mén】　指七门中的尾闾。

earthly gate Refers to coccyx known

as earthly gate in the seven kinds of gates.

地魄【dì pò】 为铅之异名。

earthly ethereal soul A synonym of lead.

地窍【dì qiào】 指腹部丹田。

earthly orifice Refers to Dantian in the abdomen. Dantian is divided into the upper Dantian (the region between the eyes), the middle Dantian (the region below the heart) and the lower Dantian (the region below the navel).

地天泰【dì tiān tài】 指坤卦、乾卦和泰卦,即天地合而成泰卦。在气功学文献中,坤阴乾阳相互作用而平秘身体,故曰泰。

Di Tian Tai Refers to Qian Trigram (sky), Kun Trigram (earth) and Tai Trigram, in which the combination of the sky and the earth have formed Tai Trigram. In the literature of Qigong, interaction of Yin (the earth) and Yang (the sky) balances the body, known as peace.

地轴【dì zhóu】 指九灵铁鼓,精气聚散常在此处,水火发端也在此处,阴阳变化也在此处,有无出入也在此处。

earthly axis Refers to nine genius-fire drums, the region where the essential Qi concentrates and disperses there, water and fire appear there, Yin and Yang change there, exit and entrance exist there.

帝乡【dì xiāng】 指脑。

Emperor's village Refers to the brain.

第一义天【dì yī yì tiān】 即意识活动,不前不后,不上不下,不左不右,身体神形维持协调稳定之义。

the first righteous sky Indicates that the activity of consciousness is neither forward nor backward, neither upward nor downward, neither for the left side and nor for the right side, ensuring to coordinate and stabilize the spirit and body.

颠倒【diān dǎo】 指河车逆转运行,元精坎水性沉,元神离火性浮,顺则成人。

reversion Refers to counter movement of river cart (lead), deepening of the original essence and floating of the original spirit. If the river cart (lead), the original essence and the original spirit are normalized in movement, life will be cultivated.

颠倒由离坎【diān dǎo yóu lí kǎn】 源自气功专论,主要阐述离降坎升,逆行成丹。

reversion with Li (Trigram) and Kan (Trigram) Collected from a monograph of Qigong, mainly describing descent of Li (Trigram) and ascent of Kan (Trigram), converse movement of which will produce Dan (pills of immortality).

癫狂【diān kuáng】 为气功适应证,指精神失常的疾病。

Mania An indication of Qigong, referring to disease caused by lunacy.

点化【diǎn huà】 指点睛。

pointing out Refers to clinching point.

调伏【diào fú】 指调节意识活动,排除神形不稳定的因素。

mental regulation Refers to regulating the activity of consciousness and eliminating pathogenic factors responsible for imbalance of the spirit and the body.

调五事【diào wǔ shì】 为佛家气功习练中应注意的五件事,即调心不沉不浮,调身不缓不急,调息不涩不滑,调眠不节不恣,调食不饥不饿。

regulating five affairs　Refers to paying attention to five affairs in practicing Qigong, including regulating the heart without any sinking and floating, regulating the body without any lentitude and urgency, regulating respiration without any astringency and slipperiness, regulating sleep without any division and indulgency, and regulating diet without any hunger.

掉散【diào sàn】　为佛家气功习用语,指神形不调,意识行为紊乱。

drop and dispersion　A common term of Qigong in Buddhism, referring to imbalance of the spirit and body as well as disorder of consciousness activity.

跌坐【diē zuò】　指盘腿而坐的练功姿势。

sudden sitting　Refers to sitting with crossed legs in practicing Qigong.

叠手【dié shǒu】　为导引姿势,指两手重叠放在一起。

hands-piled posture　The style of Daoyin, referring to overlapped hands at the same place.

丁火之脏【dīng huǒ zhī zàng】　指心脏。

exercise of Dinghuo viscus　Refers to the heart.

顶性脐命喻【dǐng xìng qí mìng yù】源自气功专论,阐述顶性、脐命之喻名,说明身体含阴阳两个方面。

comparison of the property on the top and the life in the navel　Collected from a monograph of Qigong, mainly describing the metaphor of the property in the top the life related to the navel, indicating that the human body contains two sides, i.e. Yin and Yang.

鼎【dǐng】　① 指头;② 指阳气;③ 指烹炼之器;④ 指丹田。

cauldron　Refers to ① either the head; ② or Yang Qi; ③ or cooking cauldron; ④ or Dantian which is divided into the upper Dantian (the region between the eyes), the middle Dantian (the region below the heart) and the lower Dantian (the region below the navel).

定【dìng】　① 指精神思维活动专注一境而不散乱;② 指生定,即与生俱有的"心一境性";③ 指修定,即修习气功后获得的精神稳定。

concentration　Refers to ① either concentrated state of the activities of the spirit and thought; ② or tranquility of life that depends on the pure state of the heart; ③ or cultivation, which indicates stability of the spirit after practice of Qigong.

定而能静【dìng ér néng jìng】　指神形和调安定,才能意识活动保持安静。

stabilization ensuring tranquilization　Refers to the fact that only when the spirit and body are harmonized and stabilized can the activity of consciousness be tranquilized.

定庚甲【dìng gēng jiǎ】　意即定为金木和合而稳定。庚即西方金,甲即东方木。

stabilizing Geng (Trigram) and Jia (Trigram)　Refers to harmonization and stability of metal and wood. In this term, Geng (Trigram) refers to the west and metal while Jia (Trigram) refers to the east and wood according to the five elements (including wood, fire, earth, metal and water) that match the five directions.

定观鉴形【dìng guān jiàn xíng】 指入静后反观自己的形体。

stabilizing vision and scrutinizing form Refers to observing self-body after being tranquilized.

定光清冷玉光结璘内景【dìng guāng qīng lěng yù guāng jié lín nèi jǐng】 为静功。其作法为,于夏历每月二十日,在室内坐定,入静,意想自己与太阴(月亮)混而为一,似乎已感觉不到自身的存在,只觉一片清朗。叩齿咽津,良久收功。

internal state of stabilized chilly light and the jade light with the moon spirit A static exercise, marked by sitting quietly in the room on the twentieth day of every month in summer, tranquilizing the mind and imagining to integrate with Taiyin (the moon). Under the imagined integration with Taiyin (the moon), the practitioner will feel clear and bright without any sense of self-existence. After clicking the teeth and swallowing saliva for a long time, the practice of Qigong will be successful.

定里见丹成【dìng lǐ jiàn dān chéng】 指意识思维活动寂然定静而后丹成。

Stabilizing the internal can achieve Dan (pills of immortality). Indicates that the tranquilized activities of consciousness and thought can produce Dan (pills of immortality).

定力【dìng lì】 指通过气功获得的神形稳定力。

stabilizing power Refers to stability of the spirit and the body after practice of Qigong.

定息【dìng xī】 指通过习练气功稳定和谐之意。

stabilizing respiration Means to stabilize and to harmonize all parts in the body after practice of Qigong.

定息之法【dìng xī zhī fǎ】 指调节呼吸的方法,即使呼吸之气匀、细、深、长。

exercise for regulating respiration Refers to the way for regulating respiration, enabling the respiration to be even, thin, deep and long.

定心【dìng xīn】 指通过习练佛家气功,获得意识思维活动的集中统一。

stabilizing the heart Refers to concentration and unification of the activities of consciousness and thinking after practice of Qigong in Buddhism.

定学【dìng xué】 指学习佛家气功,定神而治散乱的意识活动。

dhyana cognition Refers to stabilizing the spirit and controlling dispersion of consciousness activity after practice of Qigong in Buddhism.

定意【dìng yì】 即稳定精神意识活动。

stabilizing thinking Means to stabilize the activities of the spirit and consciousness.

东方朔置帻官舍【dōng fāng shuò zhì zé guān shě】 为动功。其作法为,以两手抱耳及后枕部,运气十二次,按摩风池、风府、哑门穴十二次。

grand summit in the east A dynamic exercise, marked by holding the ears and the back of pillow with double hands, transporting Qi for twelve times and pressing Fengchi (GB 20), Fengfu (GV 16) and Yamen GV 15) for twelve times.

东华帝君倚杖【dōng huá dì jūn yǐ zhàng】 为动功。其作法为,端立,以手挂杖,项、腰左右运转,运气十八口,一气运三遍,用膝拂地摆。

exercise for moving waist A dynamic exercise, marked by standing up, hold-

D

ing sticks with the hands, moving the neck and waist from the left to the right and vice versa, transporting Qi through the mouth for eighteen times, transporting Qi once for three times and pressing the ground with the knees.

东坡居士【dōng pō jū shì】 为宋代诗人、文学家苏轼的另外一个称谓。苏轼精于气功研究,注重气功实践,善于静功。

Dongpo Jushi Another name of Su Shi, a great poet and litterateur in the Song Dynasty (960 AD – 1279 AD) who also was a master of Qigong study, paying great attention to Qigong practice and adept at static exercise.

东岳真人【dōng yuè zhēn rén】 为宋代大道教创始人、气功学家刘德仁的另外一个称谓。

Liuyue Zhenren Another name of Liu Deren, the founder of Daoism and a greater master of Qigong.

冬令导引法【dōng lìng dǎo yǐn fǎ】为动功。其作法为,可正坐,以两手耸托,左右引胁三五度,能去腰肾风邪积聚。

exercise of Daoyin in winter A dynamic exercise, marked by sitting right, raising up the hands, turning the flanks to the right and left for three and five degrees in order to eliminate accumulation of pathogenic wind in the waist and kidney.

冬十月节坐功【dōng shí yuè jié zuò gōng】 为动功。其作法为,每日丑寅时,正坐,一手按膝,一手挽肘,两手左右托三五次,吐纳、叩齿、咽液。

sitting exercise in the feast days in October in winter A dynamic exercise, marked by sitting right in Chou (the period of a day from 1 a.m. to 3 a.m. in the morning) and Yin (the period of a day from 3 a.m. to 5 a.m. in the morning), pressing the knee with one hand, holding the elbow with the other hand, both hands holding and pressing for three and five times, breathing in and out, clicking the teeth and swallowing saliva.

冬至十一月中坐功【dōng zhì shí yī yuè zhōng zuò gōng】 为动功。其作法为,每日子丑时,平坐,伸两足、两手按两膝,左右极力三五次,吐纳、叩齿、咽液。

sitting exercise in the middle of November in winter A dynamic exercise, marked by sitting right in Zi (the period of the day from 11 p.m. to 1 a.m.) and Chou (the period of a day from 1 a.m. to 3 a.m. in the morning), stretching the feet and pressing the knees from the left to the right with both hands for three and five times, breathing in and out, clicking the teeth and swallowing saliva.

董仲舒养气法【dǒng zhòng shū yǎng qì fǎ】 为静功。其作法为,将欲无念,固守一德,神形合调;闲欲止恶,平意静神,外泰内充;和悦劝善,慎小防微,行为中正平和;见利不诱,见害不惧,稳定精神意识思维活动。

Dong Zhongshu's exercise for nourishing Qi A static exercise, marked by eliminating any desires, keeping virtue and regulating the spirit and body; eliminating any wickedness, stabilizing consciousness, tranquilizing the spirit, pacifying the external and enriching the internal; kindly exhorting the

D

mind, being careful about minute details, harmonizing and pacifying; avoiding allure with profit and fear with harm for stabilizing the activities of the spirit, consciousness and thinking.

动而生昏【dòng ér shēng hūn**】** 指精神躁动不安，意识昏沉迷乱。

dynamic activity with dizziness Refers to restlessness of the spirit that causes dizziness of the mind.

动功【dòng gōng**】** 指行功时躯体外形运动的功法，古称导引。

dynamic exercise Refers to the techniques used to promote external movement, known as Daoyin in antiquity.

动功按摩秘诀【dòng gōng àn mó mì jué**】**《动功按摩秘诀》是气功专著，为清代王启贤、汪启圣所辑，主要阐述气功、按摩对疾病的治疗。

Donggong Anmo Mijue（*Secret of Dynamic Kneading***）** A monograph of Qigong entitled *Secret of Dynamic Kneading*, compiled by Wang Qixian and Wang Qisheng in the Qing Dynasty (1636 AD – 1912 AD), mainly describing the effect of Qigong and kneading for treating diseases.

动合无形【dòng hé wú xíng**】** 指精神专一，动静变化无形迹，为协调之意。

invisibility of dynamic and integrative activities Refers to concentration of the spirit and invisibility of dynamic and static changes, indicating the effect of regulation.

动极而静，静极而动【dòng jí ér jìng jìng jí ér dòng**】** 指动静是相互依存的两种状态，两者对立统一。

Extreme dynamic activity finally transforms into static state and static activity finally transforms into dynamicity. Indicating combination and integration of dynamic activity and static activity.

动静【dòng jìng**】** 动为运动，静为静止，动静交相以成阴阳互根，阴阳交媾之用。

dynamics and statics Dynamics refers to movement and statics means motionlessness. Only when movement and motionlessness combine with each other can Yin and Yang integrate with each other.

动静观【dòng jìng guān**】** 源自气功学专论，主要阐述气功动静之间的辩证关系。

dynamic and static view Collected from a monograph of Qigong, mainly describing the dialectical relationship between dynamic activity and static activity.

动静交相养赋【dòng jìng jiāo xiāng yǎng fù**】**《动静交相养赋》为气功专论，由唐代白居易所作，以动静立论，专述气功气化作用。

Dongjing Jiaoxiang Yangfu（*Combination of Dynamic and Static Activities for Cultivating Life***）** A monograph of Qigong entitled *Combination of Dynamic and Static Activities for Cultivating Life* written by Bai Juyi, a great poet and master of Qigong in the Tang Dynasty (618 AD – 907 AD), mainly describing the effect of Qigong and Qi transformation.

动静双忘【dòng jìng shuāng wàng**】** 指保持形体和精神平静。

neglecting both dynamicity and static state Refers to tranquility of the body and the spirit.

动静说【dòng jìng shuō**】** 源自气功学

专论,阐述动静的含义及其相互关系。

discussion about dynamic and static activities Collected from a monograph about Qigong, mainly describing the meaning and correlation of the dynamic and static activities.

动静一源【dòng jìng yī yuán】　指动静之间的对立统一。

origin of both dynamics and statics Refers to unity of opposites of dynamics and statics.

动脉摇筋,血气布泽【dòng mài yáo jīn xuè qì bù zé】　指动功使筋骨活动自如,血气流畅敷布,且能滋润全身。

artery activating sinews and blood Qi moistening the body Refers to the fact that dynamic practice can activate the sinews and the bones, promote the flow of the blood and Qi, and moisten the whole body.

动起于静【dòng qǐ yú jìng】　指动起于静,而又归于静,是事物变化规律。

dynamicity starting from static state Refers to the fact that dynamics starts from statics, but also returns to the statics, which is the principle for the changes of all things.

动情【dòng qíng】　指躁动情感。情感躁动,引起精神损伤。

emotional activity Refers to emotional manifestation caused by distracting thought and damaging the spirit.

动心【dòng xīn】　指意识思维躁动,躁扰,疑惑丛生。

restlessness Refers to distracting thought that causes dysphoria and anxiety.

洞房【dòng fáng】　指脑中洞房宫。

nuptial chamber Refers to the chamber in the brain.

洞房紫极灵明户【dòng fáng zǐ jí líng míng hù】　指脑神为灵明之户。

Nuptial chamber is purple, clever and bright. Indicates that the brain spirit is the nuptial chamber.

洞观【dòng guān】　指能观察细微变化。

subtle observation A term of Qigong, referring to observing subtle changes.

洞视起居安眠法【dòng shì qǐ jū ān mián fǎ】　为动功。其作法为,闭目,叩齿九次,咽津九次;以手按鼻之左右,上下十次;再咽津九次,按摩面目令小热,每晚睡前做一次。

exercise for thorough observation, daily life and sleep A dynamic exercise, marked by closing the eyes, clicking the teeth for nine times, swallowing fluid for nine times; pressing the lateral sides of the nose upwards and downwards for ten times; swallowing fluid again for nine times and rubbing the face warm before sleep at every night.

洞虚观【dòng xū guàn】　位于江西安福,为南岳魏夫人修炼之处。

Dongxu Temple Located in Anfu County in Jiangxi Province. It was said in ancient China that Ms. Wei in the North Song Dynasty (960 AD – 1127 AD) practiced Qigong in this temple.

洞玄金玉集【dòng xuán jīn yù jí】《洞玄金玉集》为气功专著,为金代马丹阳所著,主张练功要脱离俗尘,清静以修炼性命。

Dongxuan Jinyu Ji (*A Collection of Supreme Golden and Jade Exercises*) A monograph of Qigong entitled *A Collection of Supreme Golden and Jade Exercises*, written by Ma Danyang in the Jin Dynasty (1115 AD – 1234 AD), suggesting to break away from the social world and to tranquilize the mind for cultivating life.

洞玄灵宝自然九天生神玉章经解

【dòng xuán líng bǎo zì rán jiǔ tiān shēng shén yù zhāng jīng jiě】《洞玄灵宝自然九天生神玉章经解》为气功专著,由宋代王希巢撰,主要论述气功药调神、调息、调身,重视保护元气。

Dongxuan Lingbao Ziran Jiutian Sheng-shen Yuzhang Jingjie(*Classical Explanation of Important Chapters about Natural Production of the Spirits in Nine Celestial Ways in the Supreme Cave and the Treasured Temple*) Written by Wang Xichao in the Song Dynasty (960 AD - 1279 AD), mainly describing the regulation of the spirit, respiration and body in Qigong practice; paying great attention to the protection of the original Qi.

洞阳火龙奔飞内景

【dòng yáng huǒ long bēn fēi nèi jǐng】 为静功。其作法为,于夏历每月十二日在清净的室内静坐,排除杂念,叩齿三十六次,意想高空中从太阳上降下一团火红色的云,逐渐形成一座桥。

fire Loong in the nuptial chamber running and flying to the internal scene A static exercise, marked by sitting quietly in a clear room on the twelfth day in every month in summer, eliminating distracting thought, clicking the teeth for thirty-six times, and imagining that hot cloud from the sun descends and gradually forms a bridge.

洞元子内丹诀

【dòng yuán zǐ nèi dān jué】《洞元子内丹诀》为气功专著,应用八卦的基本精神,说明人体的生理功能、阴阳变化,论述气功状态下人体的气化作用。作者不详。

Dongyuanzi Neidan Jue(*Dong Yuanzi's Formula for Internal Dan*) A monograph of Qigong entitled *Dong Yuanzi's Formula for Internal Dan*(*Pills of Immortality*), explaining the physiological functions and Yin and Yang changes in the human body according to the basic spirit of the Eight Trigrams, discussing the effects of Qi transformation under the practice of Qigong. The author was unknown.

兜礼治伤寒法

【dōu lǐ zhì shāng hán fǎ】 为动静相兼功。其作法为,端坐盘足,以两手托起阴囊,闭口缄息,存想真气自尾闾升,过夹脊,透泥丸,逐其邪气,低头屈仰如礼拜状,不拘数,以汗出为度。治元气亏弱,腠理不密,感受风寒之证。

exercise for curing cold damage with scrotum An exercise combined with dynamic exercise and static exercise, marked by sitting with crossed legs, holding up scrotum with both hands, closing the mouth to stop respiration, imagining that the genuine Qi raises from the coccyx along the Jiaji acupoints located on both sides of the spine and through the mud bolus (the brain), expelling pathogenic Qi, lowering the head like religious service, caring less about times, and just taking sweating as the degree. Such an exercise combined with dynamic exercise and static exercise can improve weakness of original Qi and cure syndromes of closure of muscular interstices and wind-coldness.

斗日月

【dòu rì yuè】 指调节阴阳,使其平秘。即日月合璧之意。

fighting against the sun and the moon

Refers to regulating and balancing Yin and Yang, indicating that Yin and Yang coordinate with each other.

督脉【dū mài】 为奇经八脉之一,为习练大小周天功精气运行的通道。此经脉为气功习练之处。

governor meridian One of the eight extraordinary meridians, is the way along which the essential Qi moves in practicing the exercises of large and small celestial cycles. This meridian is a region usually used in practice of Qigong.

督脉络脉【dū mài luò mài】 为十五络脉之一,从尾骨尖下的长强穴分出,沿脊柱两旁上循颈项,散布头上,下行的络脉,延至肩胛部,向左右别走足太阳膀胱经,入内贯脊柱两旁的肌肉。此脉络为气功习练之处。

governor meridian with its collateral One of the fifteen collaterals, starts from Changqiang (GV 1) below the coccyx, moving along the lateral sides of the spine to the head, descending along the scapula, moving along the left side and the right side of the bladder meridian of foot Taiyang and entering the muscles at lateral sides of the spine. This meridian and collateral are the regions usually used in practice of Qigong.

毒气【dú qì】 指贪、嗔、痴三毒之习气,可使精神失调。

toxic Qi Refers to Qi from three toxins (greediness, annoyance and stupidity), causing imbalance and disorder of the spirit.

独立守神【dú lì shǒu shén】 指自我控制精神,超然独处,脱离世俗干扰,把注意力集中于体内而不外驰,以颐养形神。属气功"调神"方法之一。

independent protection of the spirit Refers to self-control of the spirit, aloofly living alone, breaking away from the disturbance of the secular world, concentrating consciousness inside the body in order to nourish the body and spirit. This is one of the methods for regulating the spirit in practicing Qigong.

独头心,重缘心【dú tóu xīn zhòng yuán xīn】 指忽然意念生起,并想善恶等事,谓之独头心。更相续独头心之意识活动,称之为重缘心。均为杂念,妨碍导引入静。

starting daydream and continuing daydream In this term, starting daydream means to suddenly think about some good things and some bad things; continuing daydream means to continuously think about good things and bad things. Such a daydream is distracting thought, impeding tranquilization in practicing Daoyin.

杜胜真阴阳复媾法【dù shèng zhēn yīn yáng fù gòu fǎ】 为静功。其作法为,右侧卧式,意识活动内守丹田,导引入静,主治失眠,多眠,梦游。

Du Shengzhen's exercise for intercourse of Yin and Yang A static exercise, marked by lying on the right side, concentrating the activity of consciousness in Dantian and tranquilizing the mind with Daoyin in order to cure insomnia, somnia and sleepwalking. Dantian is divided into the upper Dantian (the region between the eyes), the middle Dantian (the region below the heart) and the lower Dantian (the region below the navel).

度【dù】 即度过生命的方法。

pass Refers to the method for passing

through life.

度度咽纳【dù dù yān nà】 即动作与咽液配合。

coordinated swallowing and inhaling Refers to coordination of actions and swallowing humor.

断谷法【duàn gǔ fǎ】 为动功。其作法为,食十二时气,从夜半子时开始,服十二时气;春、夏、秋、冬四时服气;食六戊之精;意想脾神黄裳子;但合口食内气。

exercise for stopping diet A dynamic exercise, marked by eating Qi in the twelve periods from midnight, and taking Qi in the twelve periods; taking Qi in the four seasons, i. e. spring, summer, autumn and winter; eating the essence from six kinds of Wu (Trigram); imagining that the spleen spirit is yellow; closing the mouth to eat internal Qi.

断圆【duàn yuán】 指断除一切疑惑。

elimination cycle Refers to eliminating all doubts.

断缘【duàn yuán】 指练功者应摆脱过多的社会交往和名利富贵思想,才能做到心神入静。

elimination of predestined affinity Indicates that only when social association and the idea of fame and wealth are shaken off can the heart spirit be tranquilized.

锻炼【duàn liàn】 指不断调节阴阳,反复锤炼的功夫。

taking exercise Refers to repeatedly regulating Yin and Yang and repeatedly tempering the body in practicing Qigong.

对境无心【duì jìng wú xīn】 指面对自然、社会环境及其变化,不起意念。

free of desire Refers to paying no at-

tention to the natural, social and environmental changes.

对修常居【duì xiū cháng jū】 为动功。常以两手按眉后小穴中十八次,坚持锻炼一年,能夜间看书、写字。

normal residence for life cultivation A dynamic exercise, marked by pressing the small acupoints behind the eyes for eighteen times, persevering practice for a year, reading and writing at night.

兑【duì】 ① 指卦名,为泽;② 指取象比类,为口舌;③ 指人与自然社会相适应;④ 对待人态度和蔼。

Dui ① Refers to either Dui Trigram, related to pool; ② or analogy, related to the mouth and tongue; ③ or suitability of human beings with the natural world and social environment; ④ or kind attitude to human beings.

兑宫白气【duì gōng bái qì】 指西方自然生发之气。

white Qi in Dui palace Refers to the natural Qi in the west regions.

兑虎【duì hǔ】 即白虎,① 指二十八宿中西方的七宿;② 内丹书中指"心中元神谓之龙,肾中元精谓之虎"。

dui tiger The same of white tiger, ① refers to either the seven constellations in the west among the twenty-eight constellations; ② or "the original spirit in the heart called Loong and the original essence in the kidney called tiger" mentioned in the books about internal Dan (pills of immortality).

敦艮【dūn gèn】 为静功。其作法为,意念于头部,稳定意识思维活动,从而全身吉,悦而无忧。

celebral concentration A static exercise, marked by consciousness in the head and stabilizing the activities of consciousness and thinking in order to save the whole body without any annoyance.

顿法【dùn fǎ】　练功过程中,直修上关炼神还虚,到虚极静笃时,精自化气(初关),气自化神(中关)。

transformation exercise　Refers to directly cultivating the upper joint and refining the spirit in practicing Qigong. At the tranquility stage, essence will transform into Qi (the first joint) and Qi will transform into the spirit (the middle joint).

多睡目盲【duō shuì mù máng】　指多睡伤气,五脏精气不能上达于目,可导致目盲。

dim sight due to oversleep　Refers to oversleep injuring Qi, making it difficult to transmit the essential Qi in the five Zang-organs (including the heart, the liver, the spleen, the lung and the kidney) to the eyes and causing blindness.

多唾心烦【duō tuò xīn fán】　气功学认为唾液是人体的宝贵津液,练功时常吞咽津液以润五脏,不可轻易唾出。

restlessness due to excessive spitting　According to Qigong, saliva is a valuable fluid and humor in the human body. In practicing Qigong, fluid and humor should be swallowed to moisten the five Zang-organs (including the heart, the liver, the spleen, the lung and the kidney) and cannot be exhaled.

D

E

额【é】　指眉上发下之处。

forehead　Refers to the lowering part of the eyebrow.

峨眉山【é méi shān】　在四川峨眉，为我国佛教四大名山之一。

Emi Mountain　Located in Emi County in Sichuan Province, is one of the four important mountains in Buddhism.

呃逆【è nì】　为气功适应证，多因脾胃虚寒所致。

hiccup　An indication of Qigong, usually caused by deficiency and cold of the spleen and the stomach.

恶眉【è méi】　为气功适应证，指眉毛枯萎无泽，为气血虚损之象。

dry brows　Refers to withered eyes due to deficiency of Qi and blood.

嶤锋【è fēng】　为齿神名。

mountain sword　Refers to the dental spirit.

頞【è】　指鼻根。

nasal bridge　Refers to the root of the nose.

儿产母【ér chǎn mǔ】　练功者以后天之水火（子）添先天之元精（金）、元神（木），称为儿产母。

reverse generation　Refers to increasing innate original essence (known as metal) and original spirit (known as wood) with postnatal fire (known as child).

耳病导引法【ěr bìng dǎo yǐn fǎ】　为动功。其作法为，凡两耳起疮流脓，用两手掩耳门，闭气正身，前后点头二十四，左右横点头十二，待耳热响止，少停再行。

exercise of Daoyin for auricular disease　A dynamic exercise, marked by covering the ears with both hands when there is ear ulceration and suppurative otorrhea, suspending respiration to rectify the body, nodding the head forwards and backwards for twenty-four times as well as the left and the right for twelve times, which is stopped when there is no heat and noise in the ears.

耳功【ěr gōng】　为动功。其作法为，耳宜按抑左右多数，谓以两手按两耳轮，一上一下摩擦之。平坐伸一足，屈一足，横伸两手，直竖两掌，向前若推门状，扭头左右各顾七次。

ear exercise　A dynamic exercise, marked by pressing the ears upwards and downwards for several times, sitting with one foot stretching and the other foot bending, horizontally stretching the hands and standing up the fists like pushing the gate and turning the head to the left and the right for seven times.

耳疾治法【ěr jí zhì fǎ】　为动功。其作法为，坐地交叉两脚，两手从脚弯中伸入，低头将手交叉放在项上。

exercise for auricular disease　Dynamic exercise, marked by sitting with crossed feet, stretching the hands from behind the feet, lowering the head to cross the hands over the neck.

耳廓【ěr kuò】 指耳道以外的全部可见部分,与脏腑经络有密切的关系。
auricle The external part of the internal acoustic meatus, closely related to the meridians and collaterals of the viscera.

耳聋【ěr lóng】 为气功适应证,指听力障碍,可由先天或外感内伤所致。
deafness An indication of Qigong caused by prenatal or external contraction.

耳聋候导引法【ěr lóng hòu dǎo yǐn fǎ】 为动功。其作法为,坐在地上,交叉两脚,手从脚弯中入,低头,两手交叉放在顶上。
exercise of Daoyin for deafness A dynamic exercise, marked by sitting on the ground, crossing the feet, stretching the hands from behind the feet, lowering the head to cross the hands over the neck.

耳鸣【ěr míng】 为气功适应证,常伴有心烦不眠、手足心热、耳赤、口舌生疮等。
tinnitus An indication of Qigong, marked by vexation, insomnia, feverish palms and soles, redness of ears and orolingual sore.

耳目内通【ěr mù nèi tōng】 指耳内听,目返视,意识活动向内。
inward clearing of the ears and eyes Refers to internal hearing of the ears, opposite seeing of the eyes and activity of consciousness inside.

耳视目听【ěr shì mù tīng】 指习练气功,能产生视听不用耳和目的功能。
auricular seeing and ophthalmic hearing Refers to the miracle that vision and hearing formed in practicing Qigong do not need the function of the ears and the eyes.

耳行气法【ěr xíng qì fǎ】 为静功。其作法为,凡初行气小不调久行,易耳行气还至胃中,咽气自觉至胃中。治头眩、耳聋。
auricular regulation of Qi A static exercise, marked by slowly regulating Qi at first, transmitting Qi to the stomach and swallowing saliva to the stomach in order to relieve dizziness and deafness.

二便不通功法【èr biàn bù tōng gōng fǎ】 为动静相兼功。其作法为,正坐,两手交叉在背,将手向上推,至心上下,两脚伸直岔开而坐,头身向后反倒九次。
double blockage maneuver An exercise combined with dynamic exercise and static exercise, marked by sitting upright with the hands crossed on the back, shoving the hands from the heart to the upper and the lower, sitting by stretching and branching off the feet, and turning the head backwards for nine times.

二采【èr cǎi】 指采药应辨老嫩,采之嫩,则气微而不和调;采之老,则气以久而虚散。二采均不能获气功之成及得药之真。
double collections The term of double collections refers to differentiation of tender and withered medicinal in collection. Collection of tender herbs will make Qi weak and collection of withered medicinal will make Qi scattered, making it difficult to practice Qigong and to take medicinal for nourishing health.

二道【èr dào】 ① 指前后二阴;② 指两种练功的方法,即无间道、解脱道。
double ways A common term of Qigong in Buddhism, referring to ① ei-

ther anus and genital; ② or infernal affairs and liberation path, which are the two ways for practicing Qigong.

二分【èr fēn】 指一年中的春分、秋分。

double equinox Refers to the spring equinox and autumn equinox.

二观【èr guān】 ① 指事观,观因缘所生之事相;② 指理观,观万法之实性。

double observation A common term of Qigong in Buddhism, referring to ① either observation of the cause related to anything; ② or observation of the reason of various reality.

二火【èr huǒ】 指体内的君火、相火。

double fire Refers to monarch fire and ministerial fire.

二惑【èr huò】 指引起神形失调的两种意识思维活动。

double disintegrations Refer to disintegration of the body and spirit that affects the activities of consciousness and thinking.

二极【èr jí】 指南极、北极。

double poles Refer to south pole and north pole.

二纪【èr jì】 指日、月。

double sorts Refer to the sun and the moon.

二景【èr jǐng】 指心、肾两脏之象。

double views Refer to the heart and the kidney.

二景相随【èr jǐng xiāng suí】 指泥丸与命门相通,精气上下运行,贯通一身。

double views linkage Refers to communication of mud bolus (the brain) and life gate which enables the essential Qi to flow upwards and downwards all through the body.

二觉【èr jué】 指本觉和始觉。本觉指众生之心体,始觉指众生本觉之心源。

double senses Refer to original awakening and primary consciousness in all the people.

二六时【èr liù shí】 为时间概念,指一日十二时,即二六为十二。

two-six time A concept of time, referring to twelve periods in a day. The so-called two-six means twelve. In traditionally Chinese calendar, one day is divided into twelve periods and one period contains two hours.

二漏【èr lòu】 ① 指有漏,有烦恼;② 无漏,无烦恼。无漏又指无烦恼的清静法和不引起烦恼的方法。

double leakages Refer to ① either leakage, which means annoyance; ② or no leakage, which means no annoyance. No leakage also refers to the methods for tranquilization and elimination of annoyance.

二门【èr mén】 指净土门、圣道门。

double gate Refers to the pure gate and holy gate.

二气【èr qì】 指阴气、阳气,指先天元气与后天呼吸之气,亦指母气与子气。

double Qi Refers to Yin Qi and Yang Qi, indicating the innate primordial Qi and postnatal Qi in breath. It also refers to mother Qi and child Qi.

二入【èr rù】 包含理入、行入二义。理入,指认识基本知识,用功体验。行入,不断深化气功实践。

double entrance Indicates theoretical entrance and practical entrance. Theoretical entrance means to study the basic knowledge for practicing Qigong while practical entrance means to constantly intensify the practice of Qigong.

二身【èr shēn】 ① 指法身和真身;② 指真身和应身。

double bodies Refers to ① eithers dharmakaya and real body; ② or real body and Nirmanakaya.

二生三【èr shēng sān】　指合二而一，对立的阴阳双方作用后，产生新的第三者。泛指气功将人之阴精、阳气和合成丹。

two producing three Refers to two integrating into one. When the opposite Yin and Yang coordinate with each other, the third element will appear, indicating that Qigong integrates Yin essence and Yang Qi in the human body to produce Dan (pills of immortality).

二十八脉【èr shí bā mài】　指手、足三阴三阳十二经，有十二脉，左右两侧共二十四脉，加阴跷、阳跷、任脉、督脉各一，共二十八脉。

twenty-eight meridians Refer to the combination of the twelve meridians of three Yin and three Yang connected with the hand and foot on both sides of the body (altogether 24 meridians), and Yinyao meridian, Yangyao meridian, conception meridian and governor meridian.

二十八宿【èr shí bā xiù】　指二十八颗星，即东方的角、亢、氐、房、心、尾、箕，南方的井、鬼、柳、星、张、翼、轸，西方的奎、娄、胃、昴、毕、觜、参，北方的斗、牛、女、虚、危、室、壁。

twenty-eight constellations Refer to seven constellations in the east, including Jiao, Kang, Di, Fang, Xin, Wei and Ji; seven constellations in the south, including Jing, Gui, Liu, Xing, Zhang, Yi and Zhen; seven constellations in the west, including Kui, Lou, Wei, Mao, Bi, Zi and Can; and seven constellations in the north, including

Dou, Niu, Xu, Wei, Shi and Bi.

二十四节气斗纲【èr shí sì jié qì dòu gāng】　与我国古代历法相关，把一年划分为二十四个节气。根据天人相应的理念，练功中要根据不同的节气，而采用相应的练功方法。

practice in twenty-four solar terms Related to traditional Chinese calendar that divides a year into twenty-four solar terms. In practicing Qigong, different solar term should be selected for different exercise of Qigong according to correspondence between man and the universe.

二十四时【èr shí sì shí】　一日分为子、丑、寅、卯、辰、巳、午、未、申、酉、戌、亥十二时，每时二分为初时和正时，共为二十四时。

twenty-four hours Refer to the division of a whole day into twenty-four hours. Traditionally one day is divided into twelve periods, i. e. Zi, Chou, Yin, Mao, Chen, Si, Wu, Wei, Shen, You, Xu and Hai. Each period contains two hours and all together there are twenty-four hours.

二十四真【èr shí sì zhēn】　指上、中、下三部八景，合为二十四真。

twenty-four essences Refer to twenty-four spirits in the upper, middle and lower regions of the body.

二时【èr shí】　气功文献中的含义有二：道家指子、午二时；佛家指晨、昏二时。

double times Means two things in the literature of Qigong: or Zi (the period of the day from 11 p. m. to 1 a. m.) and Wu (the period of the day from 11 a. m. to 1 p. m.) in Daoism; or early morning and dusk in Buddhism.

E

二守【èr shǒu】 指服药和调养。

double care Refers to taking medicinal and recuperation.

二竖【èr shù】 指病魔。

double verticals A term of Qigong, referring to disease.

二物归黄道【èr wù guī huáng dào】 二物归黄道源自气功专论,主要阐述阴阳交媾,就能产丹。

two things leading to yellow Dao Collected from a monograph of Qigong, mainly describing the fact that Yin and Yang are combined to create Dan (pills of immortality).

二象【èr xiàng】 指乾、坤,即阴、阳二气之象。

double shapes Refer to the sky and earth, indicating Yin and Yang.

二心【èr xīn】 ①指有异心;②指散乱之心,意识思维纷繁散乱不定,佛家气功习用;③指修定善之心。

double minds Refer to ① either abnormal mind; ② or scattered heart and disorder of consciousness and thinking, which is a common term of Qigong in Buddhism; ③ or benevolent heart mind. In this term, the heart also refers to the mind.

二仪【èr yí】 指人体中的阴阳。

double genres Refer to Yin and Yang in the human body.

二月节后导引法【èr yuè jié hòu dǎo yǐn fǎ】 为动功。其作法为,二月节后,每日丑寅时,自然坐式或盘膝坐式,选择空气清新地,呼吸清新空气一刻(古代计时,十五分为一刻),两手取握固式,转颈项五六次,以意引气向上,口中唾液在口腔中作漱咽二三次,然后以意引咽下之唾液、气到两肾间,慢慢呼气。其功效为强肺肾,身健行动轻便。

exercise of late February Daoyin A dynamic exercise, marked by sitting naturally or sitting with crossed knees in Chou (from 1 a. m. to 3 a. m. in the morning) and Yin (the period of a day from 3 a. m. to 5 a. m. in the morning) after February, selecting a place with fresh air, breathing in fresh air for a quarter, tightly grasping the hands, turning the necks from the left to the right and vice versa for five to six times respectively, promoting Qi to flow upwards with consciousness, rinsing and swallowing saliva in the mouth for two or three times, then mentally leading swallowed saliva and Qi to the region between the kidneys, and slowly breathing out. Such a dynamic exercise can strengthen the lung and kidney, nourish and relax the body.

二月中导引法【èr yuè zhōng dǎo yǐn fǎ】 为动功。其作法为,二月中每日丑寅时,取坐式,调息一刻,两手指交叉向左右上方屈伸各六七次,引下腹部气到口,慢慢吸气三次,以意引气回下腹部。功效为除胸腹胀满。

exercise of Daoyin in the middle of February A dynamic exercise, marked by sitting during the period of Chou (the period of a day from 1 a. m. to 3 a. m. in the morning) and Yin (the period of a day from 3 a. m. to 5 a. m. in the morning), crossing the hands for raising and bending at the left and right for six or seven times in order to lead Qi in the lower abdominal to the mouth, slowly breathing in for three times, turning Qi to the lower abdomen with consciousness. Such a dynamic exercise can relieve abdominal and thoracic distension.

二障【èr zhàng**】**　指烦恼障,能障涅槃。

double obstacles　Refer to annoyance and Nirvana.

二真【èr zhēn**】**　指真水、真气,喻身体内阴阳两方面。

double essences　Refer to true water and genuine Qi，indicating Yin and Yang in the human body.

二至【èr zhì**】**　指一年中的冬至、夏至。

double solstices　Refer to winter solstice and summer solstice.

二至启闭【èr zhì qǐ bì**】**　二至即冬至、夏至。冬至一阳生,夏至一阴生。

start and stop in two solstices　Refers to winter solstice during which Yang begins to grow and summer solstice during which Yin begins to grow.

二中【èr zhōng**】**　指北方之中,内产阳而物始动于下,得东方之和而生,即中春。南方之中,内萌阴而物始养于上,得西方之和而成,即中秋。

double middle　Refers to the middle in the north and south. In the middle of the north，Yang exists inside and materials appear in the lower that begin to develop in the mid-spring. In the middle of south，Yin exists inside and materials grow in the upper that succeed to develop in the mid-autumn.

E

F

发汗法【fā hàn fǎ】 为动功。其作法为，两手握拳，足趾亦缩紧，调息而卧，自然汗出周身，有发汗功效。

sweating exercise A dynamic exercise, marked by clenching the fists, tightening the toes, regulating breath for lying and sweating all over the body.

法轮【fǎ lún】 指气功中，阴阳交替变化，有如车轮转运，故称为法轮。

cyclic alteration Refers to mutual changes of Yin and Yang in Qigong practice, like transportation of a cart. That is why it is called cyclic alteration.

法轮自转法【fǎ lún zì zhuàn fǎ】 为静功。其作法为，取坐势，排除杂念之后，意守下腹部，随之以意引气旋转，由中而达外，由小而至大。

exercise for cyclic alternation A static exercise, marked by sitting, eliminating distracting thought, concentrating mentality in the abdomen, leading Qi to rotate from the middle to the external and from the small state to the large state.

法乾坤【fǎ qián kūn】 乾为天，坤为地，人身之中，乾为首，坤为腹。练功者亦宜效法，令头中元神下降，腹内元精上升，两者相交。

following Qian (Trigram) and Kun (Trigram) Qian (Trigram) refers to the sky and Kun (Trigram) refers to the earth. In the human body, Qian (Trigram) refers to the head and Kun (Trigram) refers to the abdomen. In practicing Qigong, the original spirit in the head should descend and the original essence in the abdomen should ascend in order to intersect them.

法术【fǎ shù】 指各种各样的道术，其中也包含气功养生术。

basic technique Refers to various important techniques, including the technique for cultivating life in Qigong.

法水【fǎ shuǐ】 指运气攻逐治病的方法，适用于治疗轻病或初病，亦可用于养生预防。

focal inhalation Refers to expelling disease and curing disease with movement of Qi, adapting to treatment of minor disease and primary disease, or cultivating life and preventing disease.

法天地【fǎ tiān dì】 即以天地为法，顺应自然。

following the sky and the earth Refers to complying with the natural principles.

法象会一于丹田【fǎ xiàng huì yī yú dān tián】 指习练气功，意守专一，精气神会聚于丹田。

concentration of basic image in Dantian Refers to tranquility of mentality in practicing Qigong and concentration of the essence, Qi and the spirit in Dantian. Dantian is divided into the upper Dantian (the region between the eyes), the middle Dantian (the region below the heart) and the lower Dantian （the region below the navel）.

法性【fǎ xìng】　指气功基本知识和习练方法。

basic nature Refers to the basic knowledge and exercise in Qigong.

法眼圆通【fǎ yǎn yuán tōng】　法为功法，眼即练功者的认识，圆通指气功的效验。说明习练气功，提高认识能力。

cognitive enlightenment Refers to the knowledge about Qigong practice and the experience in practicing Qigong, indicating definition of Qigong practice and improvement of ability.

法药【fǎ yào】　即气功，气功养身法是治疗神形疾病之药。

basic medicinal Refers to Qigong, indicating that the method of life cultivation in Qigong is the medicinal for treating diseases related to the spirit and the body.

法于阴阳，和于术数【fǎ yú yīn yáng hé yú shù shù】　指效法于天地自然变化的规律，运用气功、导引、按跷等手段，以达养生益寿的目的。

following the rules of Yin and Yang and adjusting the ways to cultivate health Refers to following the natural principles to practice Qigong, Daoyin and Anqiao（techniques for life cultivation and treatment of diseases）in order to cultivate health and to prolong life.

髪际【fà jì】　① 指头发的边缘；② 指经外穴位。

hair margin Refers to ① either edge of hair；② or a nomenclature of extra-point.

髪神【fà shén】　为身神之一，位于头上之中。

hair spirit Refers to one of the spirits in the human body, which is usually in the brain.

髪为星辰【fà wéi xīng chén】　指发为星辰，数在万余。

hair as stars Hair refers to the stars, indicating that there are about millions of stars over the head.

翻江倒海法【fān jiāng dǎo hǎi fǎ】　为静功。其作法为，闭口，用脐下转气，左七右八，各为翻江倒海，如此不计遍数，自然暖气。主治伤食过饱，消化不良。

exercise for overturning river and sea A static exercise, marked by closing the mouth, returning Qi below the navel for seven times at the left side and eight times at the right side like overturning rivers and seas without any counting, and warming Qi naturally. Such a static exercise can cure dyspepsia and indigestion.

凡人呼吸与圣人殊【fán rén hū xī yǔ shèng rén shū】　源自气功专著，主要阐述练功者神气长存于气海，与常人出入于咽喉不同。作者不详。

differentiation of ordinary people's respiration from that of Shengren（sage） Collected from a monograph of Qigong, mainly describing the fact that the spirit and Qi in those who have practiced Qigong are stored in the sea of Qi and that those who have practiced Qigong are different from others in respiration.

烦恼【fán nǎo】　指烦躁恼怒，是损伤情志之因。

annoyance Refers to upset and anger that damage emotion.

烦恼病【fán nǎo bìng】　指烦恼引起精神损伤，神形失调而为病。

annoyance disease Refers to annoyance

damaging the spirit and causing imbalance of the spirit and the body.

反济【fǎn jì】 指养形调神，必先去欲，为内省功夫。

eliminating desires Refers to introspection in order to nourish the body, to regulate the spirit and to tranquilize the mind.

反舌塞喉法【fǎn shé sāi hóu fǎ】 为动功。其作法为，先使精神集中，意守不适处，将舌抵上腭，反舌塞喉，待唾液满口咽之，反复数次，不宁之处即感舒适，如仍不宁，重复为之。

tongue rolling exercise A dynamic exercise, marked by concentrating the spirit first, stabilizing consciousness, keeping the tongue over the mandible, turning the tongue to cover the throat, swallowing saliva repeatedly for several times after it is enriched in the whole mouth. After several times of such practice, discomfort will be relieved. If discomfort is not relieved, practice should be continued.

反诸己【fǎn zhū jǐ】 指调节精神意识思维活动，顺应自然的变化。

following natural changes Refers to regulating the activities of the spirit and consciousness in order to follow the natural way.

返老还童【fǎn lǎo huán tóng】 指习练气功后，人虽年老，但容颜如孩童。

rejuvenation Refers to the facial appearance of old men like that of children after practice of Qigong.

返内存三【fǎn nèi cún sān】 返内为精神内守之意，存三为精、气、神内存三丹田。

inward concentration maintaining three A term of Qigong, in which inward concentration means to internally concentrate the essence and the spirit and maintaining three means to internally concentrate the essence, Qi and the spirit in three kinds of Dantian. Dantian is divided into the upper Dantian (the region between the eyes), the middle Dantian (the region below the heart) and the lower Dantian (the region below the navel).

返璞【fǎn pǔ】 即返回其初时本来的面目。

returning to original nature Refers to tranquilizing the mind, coordinating the organs and balancing essence, Qi and spirit in practicing Qigong.

范长生【fàn cháng shēng】 晋代气功学家，精于炼神养形。

Fan Changsheng A master of Qigong in the Jin Dynasty (226 AD - 420 AD), skillful in refining the spirit to nourish the body.

范重九【fàn chóng jiǔ】 晋代气功学家范长生的另外一个称谓，其精于炼神养形。

Fan Chongjiu Another of Fan Changsheng, a master of Qigong in the Jin Dynasty (226 AD - 420 AD), skillful in refining the spirit to nourish the body.

范名文【fàn míng wén】 晋代气功学家范长生的另外一个称谓，其精于炼神养形。

Fan Mingwen Another of Fan Changsheng, a master of Qigong in the Jin Dynasty (226 AD - 420 AD), skillful in refining the spirit to nourish the body.

范希文【fàn xī wén】 北宋杰出的思想家和文学家范仲淹的另外一个称谓，其对气功研究也有造诣，其专著中也论及气功理论和实践。

F

Fan Xiwen　Another name of Fan Zhongyan, great political thinker and litterateur in the North Song Dynasty (960 AD - 1127 AD), also quite familiar with Qigong. In his monographs, he well described the theory and practice of Qigong.

范延九【fàn yán jiǔ】　晋代气功学家范长生的另外一个称谓,其精于炼神养形。

Fan Yanjiu　Another of Fan Changsheng, a master of Qigong in the Jin Dynasty (226 AD - 420 AD), skillful in refining the spirit to nourish the body.

范仲淹【fàn zhòng yān】　北宋杰出的思想家和文学家,对气功研究也有造诣,其专著中也论及气功理论和实践。

Fan Zhongyan　Great political thinker and litterateur in the North Song Dynasty (960 AD - 1127 AD), also quite familiar with Qigong. In his monographs, he well described the theory and practice of Qigong.

范字元【fàn zì yuán】　晋代气功学家范长生的另外一个称谓,其精于炼神养形。

Fan Ziyuan　Another of Fan Changsheng, a master of Qigong in the Jin Dynasty (226 AD - 420 AD), skillful in refining the spirit to nourish the body.

梵【fàn】　指寂静、清净、清洁、离欲等。

sanskrit　Refers to quietness, lustration, cleanness and elimination of greediness.

梵轮【fàn lún】　同法轮,为佛家气功学习用语,指气功中,阴阳交替变化,有如车轮转运,故称为法轮。

pure wheel　The same as cyclic alteration, is a common term of Qigong in Buddhism, referring to mutual changes of Yin and Yang in Qigong practice, like transportation of a cart. That is why it is called cyclic alteration.

梵天【fàn tiān】　指远离世俗世界、清净之地。

pure sky　Refers to leaving the vulgar world in order to find the quiet and clean place.

梵行【fàn xíng】　指修炼要节制性欲。

pure activity　Refers to controlling sexuality in practicing Qigong.

梵音【fàn yīn】　指五中清净之音声。

pure sound　Refers to five kinds of clear sound.

方便【fāng biàn】　指使人觉悟的方法,泛指气功。

applied method　Refers to Qigong and the method that enables people to understand anything.

方寸【fāng cùn】　指心。

square Cun　Refers to the heart.

方寸之中念深长【fāng cùn zhī zhōng niàn shēn cháng】　源自气功专论,方寸为关元穴,谓意守丹田。

contemplating deep and long in sqare Cun　Collected from a monograph of Qigong. In this term, the so-called square Cun refers to Guanyuan (CV 4), indicating to keep consciousness in Dantian. Dantian is divided into the upper Dantian (the region between the eyes), the middle Dantian (the region below the heart) and the lower Dantian (the region below the navel).

方上【fāng shàng】　指鼻准头的两旁处。《黄帝内经》说:"方上者,胃也。"

upper side　Refers to double sides of the nose. In Huangdi Neijing (entitled *Yellow Emperor's Internal Canon of Medicine*), it says that "the upper side

F

refers to the stomach".

方士【fāng shì】 指古代掌握气功诸术的学人。

alchemist Refers to the great master of Qigong in ancient China.

方外【fāng wài】 指方域之外,喻气功家安时处顺。

external region Refers to the region far away from the ordinary area where masters of Qigong practiced and lived smoothly.

方圆一寸【fāng yuán yī cùn】 指泥丸九宫,方圆在一寸。

one Cun circumference Refers to nine chambers in the mud bolus (the brain), circumference of which is just one Cun.

方诸【fāng zhū】 指经练功而感化相通。

big mussel Refers to influence and communication after practice of Qigong.

防危【fáng wēi】 指习练气功应掌握火候。

preventing danger Refers to control duration of heating in practicing Qigong.

房劳【fáng láo】 指性生活不节,纵欲过度。

room act Refers to sexual intercourse with fleshliness.

房门【fáng mén】 指绛宫。

house gate Refers to precordium.

房中术【fáng zhōng shù】 古代研究性生活与健康的一门学问。

coition A course of study about sexuality and health in ancient China.

仿龟蛇行气【fǎng guī shé xíng qì】为静功。其作法为,每旦引首东望,吸初日之光咽之,遂不复饥,身轻力强。

imitating tortoise and snake to move

Qi A static exercise, marked by seeing the east when the sun is raising, and inhaling the sunlight in the early morning which makes practitioners light and strong without any hunger.

仿仙经闭气法【fǎng xiān jīng bì qì fǎ】 为静功。其作法为,以鼻纳气后便闭之于内,久极乃开口微吐之。

exercise of imitating immortal's way of suspending breath A static exercise, marked by keeping Qi inside the body after inhaling it with the nose, and mildly exhaling it after maintaining it for a long time.

放神【fàng shén】 指无思无虑,神意自在的意境。

free spirit Refers to no contemplation and consideration as well as the natural state of the spirit and consciousness.

放心【fàng xīn】 指专心于修养神形,不为外物所牵。

concentrating the heart Means to attentively cultivate and to nourish the spirit and the body, avoiding invasion of anything from the external world.

飞门【fēi mén】 指叩唇。

flying gate Refers to the lips.

非行非坐三昧法【fēi háng fēi zuò sān mèi fǎ】 其作法为,不拘行住坐卧,意起即修三昧,稳定精神,专注一境即可。

samadhi exercise without activity and sitting Marked by natural walking, staying, sitting and lying in order to cultivate Samadhi, to stabilize the spirit and to concentrate attention in one state.

非礼勿动【fēi lǐ wù dòng】 即无礼仪(道理)的事不做。

no rite no action Indicates that anything opposite to the rite (the truth of

Qigong) cannot be done.

非礼勿视【fēi lǐ wù shì**】**　即不符合礼仪的事不看。

no rite no vision　Indicates that anything opposite to the rite cannot be observed.

非礼勿听【fēi lǐ wù tīng**】**　即无礼仪（道理）的事不听。

no rite no listening　Indicates that anything opposite to the rite (the truth of Qigong) cannot be noticed.

非礼勿言【fēi lǐ wù yán**】**　即没有礼仪的话不说。

no rite no speaking　Indicates that anything opposite to the rite cannot be said.

非有非空【fēi yǒu fēi kōng**】**　指中，用以说明意念活动的状态，为守中之意。

neither existence nor vacuum　Refers to the center, indicating concentration of thought activity in the center.

匪人【fěi rén**】**　原指非亲信人，后指行为不正之人。气功文献中讲气功不要向行为不正的人传授。

bandit　Originally refers to those who were not close and trustful, later on referring to those who behaved badly. In the literature of Qigong, it indicates that the practice of Qigong should not be taught to those who behave badly.

肺【fèi**】**　为人体五脏之一，功能为司呼吸，主一身之气，助心行血而贯通百脉，通调水道，主皮毛，开窍于鼻，与大肠相表里。

lung　One of the five Zang-organs (including the heart, the liver, the spleen, the lung and the kidney). Its function is to control respiration and Qi in the human body, to help the heart circulate the blood in all the meridians and vessels, to promote the movement of water passage, to control the skin and hair, to open the nose and to be related internally and externally with the large intestine.

肺痹【fèi bì**】**　为气功适应证，由皮痹日久不愈，复感外邪，或感寒受热，或悲哀过度，使肺气受损所致。

lung impediment　An indication of Qigong, usually caused by damage of lung Qi due to chronic skin impediment, invasion of external pathogenic factors, or attack of cold and heat, or sorrow.

肺病【fèi bìng**】**　为气功适应证，泛指肺脏发生的各种疾病。

lung disease　An indication of Qigong, referring to various diseases related to the lung.

肺病候导引法【fèi bìng hòu dǎo yǐn fǎ**】**　为动功。其作法为，无声用嘘字出气，宣肺理气，治肺病胸脊痛满，四肢烦闷；或用两手撑地，伏身向下，口吸气，鼻呼气，宣肺理气，治胸中及肺部病变。

exercise of Daoyin for lung disease　A dynamic exercise, marked by breathing silently, diffusing the lung and regulating Qi in order to treat lung disease with pain in the chest and spine and irritancy of the four limbs; or pressing the ground with both hands, prostrating over the ground, inhaling through the mouth, exhaling through the nose, diffusing the lung and regulating Qi in order to treat disease in the chest and the lung.

肺经导引法【fèi jīng dǎo yǐn fǎ**】**　为静功。其作法为，先行调息，令息微微，似从心起，导引入静，安定精神，放松身体，导气从身体各处毛孔中出，通畅无障,息息归根,清金养肺。

exercise of Daoyin for the lung meridian A static exercise, marked by mild respiration with regulation from the heart, tranquilization in practice of Daoyin, stabilization of the spirit, relaxation of the body, and leading Qi to flow without any hindrance and naturally entering the root in order to clearing and nourishing the lung.

肺痨【fèi láo】 为气功适应证,因肺脏虚损所致。

pulmonary tuberculosis An indication of Qigong, caused by deficiency and damage of the lung.

肺气【fèi qì】 ① 指肺的功能;② 指肺所吸入的自然界的清气。

lung Qi Refers to ① either the function of the lung; ② or the clear air in the natural world inhaled by the lung.

肺神【fèi shén】 为肺的物质精微结构和功能作用。

lung spirit Refers to the microscopic structure and function of the lung.

肺神去【fèi shén qù】 指肺神损伤于魄,不在身,鼻不通。

loss of lung spirit Refers to the fact that the spirit in the lung is damaged by dispersion of the corporeal soul and obstructed nose.

肺俞【fèi shū】 为足太阳膀胱经中的一个穴位,位于第三胸椎棘突下旁开1.5寸。这一穴位为气功运行的一个常见部位。

Feishu（BL 13） An acupoint in the bladder meridian of foot Taiyang, located 1.5 Cun laterally below the spinous process of the third thoracic vertebra. This acupoint is a region usually used for keeping the essential Qi in practice of Qigong.

肺痿【fèi wěi】 为气功适应证,指肺叶痿弱不用的慢性虚损性疾患。

consumptive lung disease An indication of Qigong, referring to a chronic and asthenic disease caused by weakness and flaccidity of the lung.

肺系【fèi xì】 指喉咙。

lung system Refers to the throat.

肺脏导引法【fèi zàng dǎo yǐn fǎ】 为动功。其作法为,正坐,以手据地,缩身曲脊,向上三举,去肺家风邪积劳,反拳捶脊上,左右各十五度,去胸臆间风毒,闭气为之良久,闭目咽液,三叩齿为止。

exercise of Daoyin for the lung A dynamic exercise, marked by sitting upright, pressing the ground with hands, shrinking the body and bending the spine, raising up for three times, eliminating pathogenic factors in the lung, turning the fists to pound the spine from the left to the right and vice versa for fifteen times, expelling wind toxin in the chest, stopping breath for a while, closing the eyes, swallowing humor and clicking the teeth in three ways.

肺脏修养法【fèi zàng xiū yǎng fǎ】 为动静相兼功。其作法为,常以秋三月朔望旭旦,西面平坐,鸣天鼓七次,饮玉泉三次,然后瞑目正心,思吸兑宫白气入口,吞七次,闭气七十息。盖所以调补神气,安息灵魄之所致也。

exercise for cultivating the lung An exercise combined with dynamic exercise and static exercise, marked by sitting upright after sunrise on the first day and fifteenth day in every month in autumn, pressing the back of the brain for seven times, swallowing saliva for three times, closing the eyes to straighten the heart, inhaling white Qi in to the mouth for seven times, closing respiration for seventy times in order to regulate and nourish the spirit and Qi as well as to stabilize the ethereal soul and corporeal soul.

肺中空洞【fèi zhōng kōng dòng】 指肺的结构。

alveolus in the lung Refers to the structure of the lung.

费长房【fèi zhǎng fáng】 为东汉方士，精通气功。

Fei Changfang An alchemist in the East Han Dynasty (25 AD - 220 AD), who was quite familiar with Qigong.

分而为二【fēn ér wéi èr】 指世间一切事物，都可以分而为二。这是个普遍现象，这就是辩证法。从无限大到无暇小的事物，均有阴阳对立的双方，一分为二，乃至于无穷。人体也不例外，含阴含阳，阴阳双方对立而存在于一体。一体中的任何一个部分，都可分而为二。

division of one into two Means that all the things in this world can be divided into two, which is an ordinary phenomenon and dialectics. From the infinitely largest things to the infinitely smallest things, all things contain two different sides like Yin and Yang, and thus dividing into two in infinity. The human body is the same, containing Yin and Yang in the whole body. Thus any part in the human body all can be divided into two like Yin and Yang.

分肉【fēn ròu】 指肌肉纹理，十二经脉，均伏行分肉之间。

skin texture Refers to the fact that all the twelve meridians are moving through the muscles.

分形【fēn xíng】 指太极生两仪而为阴阳之象。

separation of sides Refers to Taiji (Supreme Pole) that produces Liangyi (the sky and the earth).

分至【fēn zhì】 分者，半也；至者，极也。分至意指自然界的节气、时辰和人体阴阳交接或阴阳多寡的分界。

half and extreme Refers to the fact that Fen is half and Zhi is extreme, indicating combination and separation of Yin and Yang in the human body.

焚身【fén shēn】 指练功中以意念使身体有热感。

burning the body Means that in practicing Qigong thought heats the body.

忿【fèn】 ① 指精神活动，为愤怒、恼怒；② 指烦恼，为佛家气功习用语。

anger Refers to ① either resentment in the activity of essence and spirit; ② or annoyance, which is a common term of Qigong in Buddhism.

忿怒陨身【fèn nù yǔn shēn】 指过分的发怒能使阴阳失调，气血运行紊乱而损害人体的健康。

Anger damages the body. This is a celebrated dictum, indicating that excessive anger imbalances Yin and Yang, causing disorder of Qi and the blood movement, and injuring human health.

风痹【fēng bì】 为气功适应证，指肌肉麻木疼痛之证。痹证是因风、寒、温三气合而伤人所致，可通过习练气功治疗。

wind arthralgia An indication of Qigong, referring to numbness or pain of the muscles caused by pathogenic wind, pathogenic cold and pathogenic Qi. It can be treated by practice of Qigong.

风痹候导引法【fēng bì hòu dǎo yǐn

fǎ】为动功,方法多样。如用右脚跟勾住左脚蹈趾,去风痹;用左脚跟勾住右脚蹈趾,去厥痹;用两手交替拉两足背于膝上,去体痹;还有其他一些方法。

exercise of Daoyin for wind impediment（arthralgia） A dynamic exercise of Qiong with various methods, such as catching the thumb on the left foot with the right foot in order to cure wind impediment; holding the first toe in the right foot with the left heel in order to cure reversal impediment; crossing the hands to pull the acrotarsiums of two feet over the knees in order to cure body impediment. There are still some other methods for practicing Qigong in such a way.

风不仁候导引法【fēng bù rén hòu dǎo yǐn fǎ】为动功。其作法为,仰卧,舒展手脚,足跟向外,足趾相对,鼻吸气至极后慢慢呼出,连续七次。能温经散寒,活血通络。

exercise of Daoyin for wind attack A dynamic exercise of Qigong, marked by lying supine, relaxing and stretching the hands and feet, turning the heels laterally, crossing the toes from two feet, breathing in deeply and breathing out slowly through the nose for seven times in order to warm the meridians, to expel cold, to activate the blood and to unobstruct the meridians.

风池【fēng chí】足少阳胆经中的一个穴位,位于项部。这一穴位为气功运行的一个常见部位。

Fengchi（GB 20） An acupoint in the gallbladder meridian of foot Shaoyang, located in the neck. This acupoint is a region usually used for keeping essential Qi in practice of Qigong.

风齿【fēng chǐ】为气功适应证,多因手阳明经脉虚,风邪袭入头面所致。可通过习练气功治疗。

wind tooth An indication of Qigong, referring to gingivitis caused by deficiency of large intestine meridian of hand Yangming and invasion of wind evil into the head and complexion. It can be treated by Qigong practice. It can be treated by practice of Qigong.

风齿候导引法【fēng chǐ hòu dǎo yǐn fǎ】为动功。其作法为,仰面,抬肩向上,以治疗外感寒热,脊腰颈项痛,风痹,口内生疮,牙齿痛,头眩晕。

exercise of Daoyin for wind tooth（gingivitis） A dynamic exercise of Qigong, marked by raising the shoulders and face in practicing Qigong in order to treat disease caused by wind-heat, pain of the waist and neck, wind impediment, oral ulcer, toothache and dizziness.

风癫【fēng diān】为气功适应证,由血气虚,邪入于阴经所致。其发作原因是心气不足,复受风邪侵袭所致。可通过习练气功治疗。

wind epilepsy An indication of Qigong, is caused by deficiency of blood and Qi and invasion of pathogenic factors in the Yin meridians due to insufficiency of heart Qi and invasion of pathogenic wind. It can be treated by practice of Qigong.

风癫候导引法【fēng diān hòu dǎo yǐn fǎ】为动功。其作法为,自然站立,回头向后看,闭气不息,至极限时慢慢吐出,作七次,两手抓住单杠,身体侧立,或坐在地上能祛风活络,治头晕目眩,风邪癫疾。

exercise of Daoyin for wind epilepsy A

dynamic exercise, marked by naturally standing up, turning the head to see backward, stopping respiration, slowly breathing out for seven times after stopping respiration to the extreme, grasping horizontal bar with the hands, standing up to one side, or sitting on the ground. Such a dynamic exercise can expel wind, activate collaterals, treat dizziness and madness due to pathogenic wind.

风府【fēng fǔ】 为督脉中的一个穴位，位于后正中线。这一穴位为气功运行的一个常见部位。

Fengfu（GV 16） An acupoint in the governor meridian, located in the middle line on the back. This acupoint is a region usually used for keeping essential Qi in practice of Qigong.

风惊【fēng jīng】 为气功适应证，由体虚，心气不足，为风邪所乘而致。可通过习练气功治疗。

wind convulsion An indication of Qigong, referring to the disease caused by insufficiency of heart Qi and attack of exogenous pathogenic wind. It can be treated by practice of Qigong.

风冷【fēng lěng】 为气功适应证，由脏腑虚弱，气血不足，感受风冷之邪所致。可通过习练气功治疗。

wind cold An indication of Qigong, referring to the disease caused by deficiency of the viscera, insufficiency of Qi and the blood and attack of wind cold. It can be treated by practice of Qigong.

风冷候导引法【fēng lěng hòu dǎo yǐn fǎ】 为动功。其作法为，通过站立、蹲坐、正坐、俯卧、侧卧、正仰卧、俯卧等方式习练气功。

exercise of Daoyin for wind cold（frigidity） A dynamic exercise of Qigong, marked by standing up, sitting upright, lying prostrate, lying on the side and lying supine for practicing Qigong.

风轮【fēng lún】 眼之五轮之一，包括角膜和虹膜。

wind wheel Refers to one of the five wheels in the eyes, including cornea and iris.

风门【fēng mén】 足太阳膀胱经中的一个穴位，位于第二胸椎刺突下旁开1.5寸。这一穴位为气功运行的一个常见部位。

Fengmen（BL 12） An acupoint in the bladder meridian of foot Taiyang, located 1.5 Cun below the thoracic vertebra. This acupoint is a region usually used for keeping essential Qi in practice of Qigong.

风木之脏【fēng mù zhī zàng】 指肝脏。肝在五行属木，在五气属风，故称。

wind-wood viscus Refers to the liver because the liver pertains to wood in the five elements（including wood, fire, earth, metal and water）and wind in the five kinds of Qi.

风逆【fēng nì】 气功适应证，指外感风邪厥气内逆的病证。可通过习练气功治疗。

wind converse An indication of Qigong, referring to the disease caused by exogenous pathogenic wind. It can be treated by practice of Qigong.

风偏枯【fēng piān kū】 气功适应证，血气偏虚，则腠理开，受于风湿致病，风湿客于半身所致。可通过习练气功治疗。

wind paralysis Refers to the disease caused by deficiency of Qi and blood,

F

F

invasion of wind and dampness, and existence of pathogenic factors in half of the body. It can be treated by practice of Qigong.

风偏枯候导引法【fēng piān kū hòu dǎo yǐn fǎ】 为静功,方法多样。如端正靠墙站立,放松;站立,两足趾上仰,呼吸五次;背靠墙,端正地站立,舒展两脚和足趾,入静;背靠墙站立,闭气不息,至极限时慢慢吐出。

exercise of Daoyin for wind paralysis A static exercise with various methods, such as standing upright against the wall, standing up with the toes of the feet to raise up and breathing for five times; then standing up with the back against the wall for comforting the feet and toes, and tranquilizing the mind; then standing up with the back against the wall with no respiration for a while and slowly spitting later on, etc.

风气【fēng qì】 气功适应证,指肺气虚而感受风邪所引起的病证。

wind Qi An indication of Qigong, referring to the disease caused by pathogenic wind due to deficiency of lung Qi.

风气候导引法【fēng qì hòu dǎo yǐn fǎ】 为动功。其作法为,自然站立,一手尽力向前伸展,另一手从乳房向后快速拉开,松散自如,不用大力。舒肝理气,开郁畅怀,两手各交替二十一次。然后,臀部及足掌着地,两手抱膝头,随身向后,尽力作二十一次。通过理气通络,治烦恼闷痛。

exercise of Daoyin for wind Qi A dynamic exercise of Qigong, marked by standing up naturally, stretching forward one hand, quickly pulling the other hand from the breast backward, re-laxing the body without forcefulness; smoothing the liver and regulating Qi, opening stagnation and smoothing the chest, and alternating both hands for twenty-one times respectively; then touching the ground with the buttocks and the soles, holding the knees with both hands and turning the body backwards forcefully for twenty-one times. Such a dynamic exercise can relieve annoyance and pain through regulating Qi and the collaterals.

风湿【fēng shī】 气功适应证,指脚病的类证,与一般的风湿证不通。可通过习练气功治疗。

wind dampness An indication of Qigong, referring to rheumatism related to beriberi, different from other kinds of rheumatism. It can be treated by practice of Qigong.

风湿痹候导引法【fēng shī bì hòu dǎo yǐn fǎ】 方法多样。如任意放松两臂,闭气不息,至极限时慢慢吐出,连作十二次;正卧,用手自下而上摩腹。

exercise of Daoyin for wind dampness and impediment A dynamic exercise of Qigong with various methods, such as naturally relaxing the shoulders, suspending respiration and slowly exhaling for twelve times; or lying supine with both hands rubbing the abdomen from the lower to the upper.

风水【fēng shuǐ】 气功适应证,指水肿病之一种。可通过习练气功治疗。

wind water An indication of Qigong, referring to a kind of edema. It can be treated by practice of Qigong.

风头眩【fēng tóu xuàn】 气功适应证,由血气虚,风邪入脑而引目系所致。

wind dizziness An indication of

Qigong, referring to vertigo caused by weakness of the body and invasion of pathogenic wind into the brain. It can be treated by practice of Qigong.

风头眩候导引法【fēng tóu xuàn hòu dǎo yǐn fǎ】 为动功,方法多样。如用两手抱右膝靠近胸部,用两手抓住单杠,身体侧立,一手长伸,手掌向上,正坐,仰卧,低头等。

exercise of Daoyin for wind dizziness A dynamic exercise of Qigong with various methods, such as holding the right knee with both hands to the chest, grasping the horizontal bar with both hands, stretching up one hand and grasping the lower jaw with the other hand, sitting upright and lowering the head, etc.

风邪候导引法【fēng xié hòu dǎo yǐn fǎ】 为动功。其作法为,先使两脚温暖,然后用手按摩脐上下和气海穴,次数不限,越多越好。可温中散寒,宽中理气,治腹中气胀。

exercise of Daoyin for wind evil A dynamic exercise of Qigong, marked by warming the feet, kneading the upper and the lower of the navel and Qihai (CV 6) for more times. Such a dynamic exercise can warm the middle, eliminate cold, stabilize the middle, regulate Qi, and relieve flatulence of Qi in the abdomen.

风虚劳【fēng xū láo】 为气功适应证,因血气虚弱,其肤腠虚疏,风邪易侵所致。可通过习练气功治疗。

wind asthenic disease An indication of Qigong, referring to a disease caused by overexertion, deficiency of Qi and blood, weakness of muscles and invasion of pathogenic wind. It can be trea-

ted by practice of Qigong.

风虚劳候导引法【fēng xū láo hòu dǎo yǐn fǎ】 为动功,方法多样。如正坐,一脚屈膝,趾向地,一手握住足腕部向上提,另一手按在地上,尽力作二十一次,使腰、脚、踝关节有骨松气散之感。

exercise of Daoyin for wind asthenic disease A dynamic exercise, marked by sitting upright, bending the knee with one foot, turning the toes to the ground, holding one ankle with one hand to raise upwards, pressing the ground with the other hand for twenty-one times respectively. Such a dynamic exercise can relax the waist, the feet and ankles and disperse Qi stagnated in these regions.

风注候导引法【fēng zhù hòu dǎo yǐn fǎ】 为动功。其作法为,两手相交按于肩上,两肘尽力上抬,头仰身正,肘头上下摇动二十一次。可祛风通络,治肩肘风邪,咽项拘急,血脉不通。

exercise of Daoyin for wind focus A dynamic exercise of Qiong, marked by crossing the hands to press the shoulders, raising the elbows, rising up the head and keeping the body upright, shaking the elbows upward and downward for twenty-one times. Such a dynamic exercise can expel exogenous pathogenic wind to open the collaterals, relieve pathogenic wind invading the shoulders, and cure spasm of the neck and obstruction of vessels.

封固火候法【fēng gù huǒ hòu fǎ】 为静功。其作法为,正坐安神,意引真气朝元(脑),阴阳反复,交媾一番。久行之,自觉身体风平浪静,恬适安和。

exercise for closing fire A static exercise, marked by sitting upright, stabilizing the spirit, leading genuine Qi to the brain with consciousness, returning Yin and Yang to intercourse with each other. After a long time of such a practice, the body will be relaxed, tranquilized, balanced and harmonized.

封固牢藏法【fēng gù láo cáng fǎ】为静功。其作法为，坐静端身，精神放松，莫昏睡，要清醒，凝神于神室，伏气于气根，照时心中湛然，虽照也忘，忘时性光朗彻。

exercise for closing, fixing and storing A static exercise, marked by sitting quietly and upright, relaxing the spirit, avoiding lethargy, concentrating the spirit in the spiritual chamber, bending Qi to the root of Qi, lighting the heart serenely without memory but with sincerity and purity.

封君达存日月法【fēng jūn dá cún rì yuè fǎ】 为静功。其作法为，偃卧，酉时作，意念日在额上，月在脐上，调节阴阳，有安神之功。

Solar and lunar exercise for closure and existence A static exercise, marked by lying supine in You（the period of a day from 5 p.m. to 7 p.m. in the afternoon）and keeping the sun in the forehead and the moon in the navel with consciousness in order to regulate Yin and Yang and stabilize the spirit.

封炉【fēng lú】 指精神意识内守，目内视，使之达到静谧状态。

closing furnace Refers to internal concentration of the spirit and consciousness, and internal observation with the eyes in order to tranquilize the body.

冯晴川【féng qíng chuān】 清代养生学家和气功学家冯曦的另外一个称谓，其撰有气功专著，推崇气功调息、服气、叩齿、咽津、胎息等多方面养生延命。

Feng Qingchuan Another name of Feng Xi, a great doctor for nourishing life and a great master of Qigong in the Qing Dynasty（1636 AD - 1912 AD），who wrote a monograph of Qigong, emphasizing the exercises of Qigong practice for regulating respiration, taking Qi, clicking the teeth, swallowing fluid and protecting fetal respiration, which can nourish health and prolong life.

冯曦【féng xī】 清代养生学家和气功学家，撰有气功专著，推崇气功调息、服气、叩齿、咽津、胎息等多方面养生延命。

Feng Xi A great doctor for nourishing life and a great master of Qigong in the Qing Dynasty（1636 AD - 1912 AD），who wrote a monograph of Qigong, emphasizing the exercises of Qigong practice for regulating respiration, taking Qi, clicking the teeth, swallowing fluid and protecting fetal respiration, which can nourish health and prolong life.

凤池【fèng chí】 指心、肺之间。

phoenix pool Refers to the region between the heart and the lung.

凤刚阙病发【fèng gāng què bìng fā】为静功。其作法为，闭目内视，心使生火以烧身。

metal burning exercise A static exercise, marked by closing the eyes to observe the internal environment of the body in order to produce fire for heating the body.

凤凰观【fèng huáng guàn】 现在山西代州凤山，为古代名师所居之处。

Phoenix Temple Refers to the mountain in Shanxi Province where great masters in ancient China lived.

凤阙【fèng què】　指心、肺之间。

phoenix watchtower　Refers to the region between the heart and the lung.

佛【fó】　指觉或智，如觉悟、觉察、觉知诸法之事理，而了了分明。

Buddhism　Refers to sense or wisdom，such as consciousness，detection and awareness.

佛法【fó fǎ】　指佛家气功。

Buddhist exercise　Refers to special methods for practicing Qigong in Buddhism.

佛教以无念为宗【fó jiào yǐ wú niàn wéi zōng】　指释家气功，以维持意识活动的静止状态为正宗。

Buddhism takes non-contemplation as authenticity.　This is a celebrated dictum，indicating that Qigong practice in Buddhism regards the exercise for tranquilizing the activity of consciousness as authenticity.

佛心【fó xīn】　指觉悟之心。

Buddhist heart　A term of Qigong，referring to the sense of consciousness or awareness.

佛性【fó xìng】　指觉悟之性。

Buddhist nature　A common term of Qigong in Buddhism，referring to the nature of consciousness or awareness.

跌坐【fū zuò】　跌坐同结跏趺坐，即吉祥座，为佛家气功坐式，方式有二，一为吉祥，二为降魔。

sitting with crossed legs　Refers to auspicious sitting which is an exercise of sitting for practicing Qigong in Buddhism with two ways，one is to be auspicious，the other is to expel evil.

跗【fū】　人体部位名，即足背。

instep　Refers to acrotarsium.

跗阳【fū yáng】　足太阳膀胱经中的一个穴位，位小腿后外侧，为气功中常用的意守部位。

Fuyang（**BL 59**）　An acupoint in the bladder meridian of foot Taiyang，located in the lateral side of the shank，which is the region for concentrating consciousness in practicing Qigong.

敷和【fū hé】　指木象春气，其平气有散布温和的作用，使万物得以生长发育。

goodwill and harmony　Indicates that wood is like spring Qi which spreads warmth and harmony in order to promote the growth of all things.

伏藏【fú cáng】　指巧拙之人，皆可藏神明于脑。

hidden secret　Refers to the fact that no matter ingenious people or clumsy people all hide the spirit in the brain.

伏姹女【fú chà nǚ】　指降心火，或谓肾水上承于心。

hidden beautiful woman　Refers to either descent of heart fire；or kidney water entering the heart.

伏虎【fú hǔ】　① 指制除纷繁的杂念；② 指持心，即调节精神意识活动。

hidden tiger　Refers to ① either elimination of various distracting thoughts；② or concentrating the heart，which means regulating the activities of the spirit and consciousness.

伏明【fú míng】　为运气术语，指阳热光明之气，伏藏不用。

hidden fire　A term about Qi motion，referring to Qi of heat and brightness that is hidden and not used.

伏牛幽阙【fú niú yōu què】　指肾和肾的外象。

hidden secret cattle　Refers to the kidney and the outward expression of the kidney.

伏气【fú qì】 ①指呼吸之气还复归于气海而成不呼不吸的状态；②指滞塞于体内经脉不行而郁结之气；③即胎息；④指结成圣胎之因。

hidden Qi Refers to ① either Qi in respiration returning to the sea of Qi, indicating no inhalation and no exhalation; ② or stagnation of Qi due to obstruction of the meridians inside the body; ③ or fetal respiration; ④ or the reason of holy embryo.

伏尸候导引法【fú shī hòu dǎo yǐn fǎ】为静功。其作法为，叩齿十四次，咽气十四次，如此做三百次止，练百日，大病除，各种病邪皆去。

hidden exercise of Daoyin A static exercise, marked by clicking the teeth for fourteen times and inhaling for fourteen times. After three hundred times of practice, severe disease will be cured and all diseases will be prevented.

伏兔【fú tù】 为足阳明胃经的一个穴位，位于髌骨外上缘6寸处。这一穴位为气功运行的一个常见部位。

Futu（ST 32） An acupoint in the stomach meridian of foot Yangming, located 6 Cun above the outer and upper margin of the kneecap. This acupoint is a region usually used for keeping the essential Qi in practice of Qigong.

伏羲【fú xī】 中国神话中人类的始祖。

Fu Xi In traditional Chinese myth, Fu Xi was the primogenitor of human beings.

伏阳【fú yáng】 ①指阳热之邪潜伏于体内；②气功文献里指阳伏于阴内。

hidden Yang Refers to ① either evil heat in Yang concealing in the body;

② or Yang existing in Yin according to the literature of Qigong.

凫浴【fú yù】 指气功功法之一，姿势如凫之浴。一谓意想全身从头至足放松。

wild duck bathing Refers to one of the methods used in practicing Qigong like a wild duck bathing. It also means to imagine that the whole body from the head to the feet should be relaxed.

扶桑【fú sāng】 指青龙，喻元神。气功文献为性之代名词。

mulberry Refers to Green Loong which refers to the original spirit. In the literature of Qigong, it is the synonym of property.

扶摇子【fú yáo zǐ】 为唐末宋初著名气功学家陈抟的另外一个称谓。

Fu Yaozi Another name of Chen Tuan, a great master of Qigong in the late Tang Dynasty（618 AD - 907 AD）and early Song Dynasty（960 AD - 1279 AD）.

孚祐帝君拔剑法【fú yòu dì jūn bá jiàn fǎ】 为动功。其作法为，站立，足呈"丁"字，以右手扬起视左，运气九口，再以左手扬起视右，运气九口。主治一切胸腹部疼痛。

drawing sword exercise for sincerely supporting monarch A dynamic exercise, marked by standing up with the feet stretching like T-shaped, raising the right hand to see the left side and circulate Qi for nine times, and raising the left hand to see the right side and to circulate Qi for nine times in order to cure thoracic and abdominal pain.

服丹【fú dān】 为阴丹，即口中唾液。指习练气功，吞津咽液。

absorbing Dan（pills of immortality）

Means Yin Dan（pills of immortality），referring to saliva in the mouth. It means to swallow saliva in practicing Qigong.

服闾瞑目【fú lú míng mù**】**　为静功。其作法为，身体盘膝端坐，两手抱脐下，行功运气四十九口。主治腹痛。

absorbing dhyana and closing eyes　A static exercise，marked by sitting with crossed legs，holding the region below the navel with both hands，moving Qi for forty-nine times for treating abdominal pain.

服气【fú qì**】**　气功养生法之一，即吐纳法。

respiration　One of the methods for cultivation of life in Qigong，referring to the method for inhalation and exhalation.

服气并导引咽津法【fú qì bìng dǎo yǐn yān jīn fǎ**】**　为静功。其作法为，先导引，继后服气，每日咽得津液三五十次，胜服诸药。

exercise of Daoyin for absorbing Qi and swallowing fluid　A static exercise，marked by practicing Daoyin first，then absorbing Qi，and swallowing fluid and humor for thirty or fifty times every day，which is more effective than any medicinals.

服气不长生，长生须伏气【fú qì bù cháng shēng cháng shēng xū fú qì**】**　习练气功，关键是归藏气于气海，不能归藏气于气海者，服气不一定有好效果。能伏气丹田，定息于中，神息相依，才能获得成功。

Absorbing Qi cannot prolong life while controlling respiration can prolong life.　This is a celebrated dictum. The key point for practicing Qigong is to store Qi in the sea of Qi. If Qi is not stored in the sea of Qi，absorbing Qi is ineffective. Only when Qi is stored in Dantian，respiration is concentrated in the center，and the spirit and respiration are interdependent，can the ideal results be achieved. Dantian is divided into the upper Dantian（the region between the eyes），the middle Dantian（the region below the heart）and the lower Dantian（the region below the navel）.

服气导引法【fú qì dǎo yǐn fǎ**】**　为动静相兼功。其作法为，取日中子、午、卯、酉时服气。但冬天子时气属寒，不可服。夏午时气属热，不可眠。

exercise of Daoyin for absorbing Qi　An exercise combined with dynamic exercise and static exercise，marked by absorbing Qi in Zi（the period of the day from 11 p.m. to 1 a.m.），Wu（the period of the day from 11 a.m. to 1 p.m. in the noon），Mao（the period of the day from 5 a.m. to 7 a.m. in the early morning）and You（the period of the day from 5 p.m. to 7 p.m. in the dusk）. Zi（the period of the day from 11 p.m. to 1 a.m.）in winter is cold，practitioners cannot absorb Qi. Zi（the period of the day from 11 p.m. to 1 a.m.）in summer is very hot，practitioners cannot sleep.

服气精义论【fú qì jīng yì lùn**】**　《服气精义论》为气功专著，由唐代司马承祯著，是气功养生的重要文献。

Fuqi Jingyi Lun（*Discussion about Absorbing Qi with Succinct Principles***）**　A monograph of Qigong entitled *Discussion about Absorbing Qi with Succinct Principles*，written by Sima Chengzhen in the Tang Dynasty（618 AD – 907 AD），an important literature of Qigong and life cultivation.

服气疗病法【fú qì liáo bìng fǎ**】** 为静功，主要为调身、调气、调神。

exercise for absorbing Qi to treat disease A static exercise for regulating the body, Qi and the spirit.

服气面肿【fú qì miàn zhǒng**】** 源自气功学专著，主要阐述服气面肿的机制和现象。

absorbing Qi for facial swelling Collected from a monograph of Qigong, mainly describing the manifestations and causes of facial swelling during absorbing Qi.

服气吞霞【fú qì tūn xiá**】** 指习练气功的一种方法，服气为食气，吞霞为意引霞光吞入口内。

absorbing Qi and inhaling sunlight A term of Qigong, which is one of the methods to practice Qigong. In this term, absorbing Qi means to take Qi while inhaling sunlight means to enable the sunlight to enter the mouth with consciousness.

服日光芒法【fú rì guāng máng fǎ**】** 为静功。其作法为，日行三次，即日出时，上午十时左右，中午十二时左右，以便调身、调气、调神。

exercise for absorbing sunlight A static exercise, marked by absorbing sunlight for three times every day in 10 o'clock in the morning or the 12 o'clock in the noon for regulating the body, Qi and the spirit.

服日气法【fú rì qì fǎ**】** 为静功。其作法为调身、调气、调神。

exercise for absorbing solar Qi A static exercise, referring to regulation of the body, Qi and the spirit.

服日月法【fú rì yuè fǎ**】** 为静功。习功者于夏历每月朔日（初一），当太阳初出时面向东正坐，调息，令心入静，然后吸气咽下，共咽九次。

exercise for absorbing the sun and the moon A static exercise, marked by sitting to the east in the sunrise on the first day of any month in summer, regulating respiration, tranquilizing the heart, inhaling air and swallowing saliva for nine times.

服三气法【fú sān qì fǎ**】** 为静功。常存青、白、赤三气如綖，从东方日下来，直入口中，挹之九十过，自饱便止。

exercise for absorbing three kinds of Qi A static exercise, marked by normally storing green, white and red Qi, leading it directly into the mouth from the sunrise for ninety times and stopping its movement till feeling full up.

服三五七九法【fú sān wǔ qī jiǔ fǎ**】** 为静功。其作法为，自然站势，或坐势，站（坐）定后，徐徐以鼻引气（吸气）三次，以口吐气；次后鼻引气五次，以口吐气；次后鼻引气七次，以口吐气；次后鼻引气九次，以口吐气。依次三五七九连作，鼻引气二十四次，口吐浊气二十四次。

exercise for absorbing three-five-seven-nine A static exercise, marked by naturally standing or sitting, then inhaling Qi through the nose for three times, exhaling Qi through the mouth; then inhaling Qi for five times through the nose and exhaling Qi through the mouth; then inhaling Qi through the nose for seven times and exhaling Qi through the mouth; then inhaling Qi through the nose for nine times and exhaling Qi through the mouth. After practice for three or five or seven or nine times, the nose should inhale Qi for twenty-four times and the mouth should exhale Qi for twenty-four times.

服食灵药法【fú shí líng yào fǎ】 为静功。其作法为,内视心,想心火烧身及病患痛苦之处,以意火攻疗之,则疾易愈。

exercise for taking food and spiritual medicinal A static exercise, marked by internally observing the heart and imagining that the fire burns the body and the location of disease in order to cure disease.

服四时气法【fú sì shí qì fǎ】 为静功。其作法为,站势或坐势。春向东食岁星青气,入肝;夏服荧惑赤气,使入心;四季之月食镇星黄气,使入脾;秋食太白白气,使入肺;冬服辰星黑气,使入肾。久行之,调节五脏功能,强身延年。

exercise for absorbing Qi in the four seasons A static exercise, marked by standing or sitting, absorbing green Qi in the spring into the liver, absorbing red Qi in the summer into the heart, absorbing yellow Qi in the four seasons into the spleen; absorbing white Qi into the lung in autumn and absorbing black Qi into the kidney in winter. The effect of a long period of practice is to regulate the function of the five Zang-organs (including the heart, the liver, the spleen, the lung and the kidney), to strengthen the body and to prolong life.

服天顺地【fú tiān shùn dì】 为气功学术语,指与自然相应。

absorbing the sky and following the earth Refers to corresponding to all fields naturally.

服雾法【fú wù fǎ】 为静功。其作法为,当以平旦,于寝静之中,坐卧任己,先闭目内视,仿佛使入见五脏,口呼出气二十四过,使自见五色之气,引五色之气入口五十过,咽液六十过。

exercise for absorbing dew A static exercise, marked by sitting or lying quietly at dawn, closing the eyes to imagine seeing the five Zang-organs (including the heart, the liver, the spleen, the lung and the kidney), exhaling through the mouth for twenty-four times in order to observe Qi with five colors and to lead it to the mouth for fifty times, and swallowing humor for sixty times.

服玄根法【fú xuán gēn fǎ】 为动功。其作法为,意念存想胃中,然后仰吸五方太和之气,漱液连气、液咽之入胃中,连做五次。

exercise for absorbing supreme root A dynamic exercise, marked by concentrating consciousness in the stomach, raising the head to inhaling supreme harmonious Qi from five directions, rinsing humor and Qi, and swallowing humor into the stomach for five times.

服药行气【fú yào xíng qì】 指服用药物与气功相结合。行气即气功。

taking medicinal and moving Qi Refers to combination of taking medicinal and Qigong. In this term, moving Qi refers to Qigong.

服阴丹以补脑【fú yīn dān yǐ bǔ nǎo】 指习练气功,吞津咽液,能补脑安神。

Only when Yin Dan (pills of immortality) is absorbed can the brain be tonified. This is a celebrated dictum, referring to swallowing fluid and humor in order to tonify the brain and to stabilize the spirit in practicing Qigong.

F

服玉泉【fú yù quán】　即口服玉泉，为习练气功的一种方法。其中的玉泉指的是口中的唾液。

absorbing jade spring Means to swallow saliva in the mouth, which is one of the methods for practicing Qigong. In this term, jade spring refers to the saliva in the mouth.

服玉泉法【fú yù quán fǎ】　为静功。其作法为，每日子后，正坐端身，鼻内微微吸取清气数口，用舌舐上颚存息。

exercise for absorbing jade spring A static exercise, marked by sitting upright in Zi period (the period of the day from 11 p.m. to 1 a.m.), mildly inhaling clear air through the nose for several times and licking the upper jaw with the tongue.

服元和法【fú yuán hé fǎ】　为静功。其作法为，阳春三月，净理一室，著几案，设以厚暖床席，案上常焚名香。夜半一气初生之时，静虑宁神，叩齿三十六通，两手握固，仰卧瞑目，候常喘息出时，便合口鼓满咽气，以咽入为度，渐渐咽入。

exercise for absorbing the origin and harmony A static exercise, marked by staying in a quiet room with warm bed and spice lighting on the table, tranquilizing the mind and spirit at midnight when Qi begins to appear, clicking the teeth for thirty-six times, holding the hands, lying on the back, closing the eyes, inhaling Qi through the mouth and gradually leading it into the whole body during respiration.

服元气法【fú yuán qì fǎ】　为静功。其作法为，端身正坐，咽气，合口作意，如咽食一般，咽液咽气，皆如咽食。存想入肾，再入命门穴，循脊流上，际入脑宫。又既脐下至五星，五脏相逢，内外相应，各有元气，管系连带。

exercise for absorbing original Qi A static exercise, marked by sitting upright, inhaling Qi, combining the mouth with consciousness like taking food, swallowing humor and Qi all like taking food, imagining to enter the kidney and to reach Mingmen (GV 4) (an acupoint in the governor meridian), circulating along the spine into the brain, flowing it below the navel to the five stars and connecting with the five Zang-organs (including the heart, the liver, the spleen, the lung and the kidney), corresponding to the internal and the external with original Qi in both sides, and coordinating all systems and lines.

服月光芒法【fú yuè guāng máng fǎ】为静功。其作法为，夜间子时左右行功，日一次，以便调身、调气、调神。

exercise for absorbing moonlight A static exercise, marked by absorbing moonlight once a day in Zi period (the period of the day from 11 p.m. to 1 a.m.) for regulating the body, Qi and the spirit.

服月气法【fú yuè qì fǎ】　为静功，以调身、调气、调神为主。

exercise for taking absorbing Qi from the moon A static exercise for regulating the body, Qi and the spirit.

服紫霄法【fú zǐ xiāo fǎ】　为静功。其作法为，坐忘握固，意念从头而出，钻屋直上，直到天边。引紫霄而来，直下穿屋，而从头上入内于腹中。久行此法，补脑安神，益气壮阳，轻身延年。

exercise for absorbing celestial light A static exercise, marked by sitting quietly without holding any part, leading the

F

consciousness out of the brain that rises up from the room and directly to the sky，drawing the celestial light directly into the room and from the head into the abdomen. Such a way of practicing Qigong can tonify the brain and stabilize the spirit， enriching Qi and strengthening Yang，relaxing the body and prolonging life.

浮沉【fú chén**】** 指练功者，使沉者升，浮者降，而令水火交而结丹。

floating and sinking Indicates that in practicing Qigong the sinking should be raised while the floating should be lowered in order to coordinate water and fire and produce Dan（pills of immortality）.

浮游【fú yóu**】** 同优游，为气功学术语，指习练气功，意守景物。

swimming The same as leisurely travel，is a term of Qigong，referring to concentrating mind on photographic field in practicing Qigong.

呋吸宝华【fú xī bǎo huá**】** 源自气功专论，叙述习练气功的方法及入静可神形合一的状态。

significance of respiration Collected from a monograph，mainly describing the methods for practicing Qigong and the integrating condition of the spirit and the body after tranquilization.

府舍【fú shě**】** 为足太阴脾经中的一个穴位，位于耻骨联合上缘 0.7 寸，腹正中线旁开 3.5 寸处。这一穴位为气功运行的一个常见部位。

Fushe（SP 13**）** An acupoint in the spleen meridian of foot Taiyin，located 0.7 Cun to the upper part of pubic symphysis and 3.5 Cun lateral to the middle line of the abdomen. This acupoint

is a region usually used for keeping the essential Qi in practice of Qigong.

胕【fǔ**】** ① 音义同"腐"，古代指腐臭的食物；② 音义同"浮"，即浮肿；③ 音义同"跗"，即足背。

Fu ① The same as the Chinese character decay，referring to putrid food；② the same as the Chinese character dropsy，referring to edema of the body；③ the same as the Chinese character instep，referring to the back of the foot known as acrotarsium.

俯按山源【fǔ àn shān yuán**】** 为动功。其作法为，用第二和第三指端，分别伸入两鼻孔，挟住鼻中隔，轻轻捏按、揉摩，然后以手按鼻片刻。山源指鼻中隔。

bending to press mountain source A dynamic exercise，marked by putting the second and the third fingers into the nostrils to hold nasal septum，mildly pinching and kneading，then rubbing the nose with hands for a while. In this term，mountain source refers to nasal septum.

父曰混丸母雌一【fù yuē hún wán mǔ cí yī**】** 指元阴、元阳，又可指阴神、阳神。

father's brain and mother's oocyte Refers to original Yin and original Yang，or Yin spirit and Yang spirit.

父曰泥丸母雌一【fù yuē ní wán mǔ cí yī**】** 指元阴、元阳，又可指阴神、阳神。

father's mud bolus（the brain）and mother's one Refers to original Yin and original Yang，or spiritual Yin and spiritual Yang.

负局先生磨镜【fù jú xiān shēng mó jìng**】** 为动功。其作法为，身体端坐，两腿平放，两手轻握拳，身手向前如磨镜样，运气十二口，治遍身疼痛。

Mr. Fuju wearing mirror A dynamic exercise, marked by sitting upright, stretching the legs flat, mildly holding the fists, the body and hands turning forwards like wearing mirrors and circulating Qi for twelve times in order to relieve pain in the whole body.

负日之暄【fù rì zhī xuān】 ① 指端坐，意想日光照身，身体温暖舒适；② 指日光照身，脊背得暖，遍体和畅。

warming sunshine Refers to ① either sitting upright, imagining that the sunshine is shining the body and makes the body warm and comfortable; ② or the sunshine that shines over the body, making the back and spine warm and the whole body comfortable.

负阴抱阳【fù yīn bào yáng】 指事物含有对立的阴阳两个方面。气功文献中，为阴中有阳，阳中有阴，阴平阳秘之意。

Yin backward and Yang forward Refers to the fact that everything contains Yin and Yang that are antagonized. In the literature of Qigong, it suggests that there is Yin within Yang, Yang within Yin, and stable Yin and compact Yang.

复骨【fù gǔ】 指第六颈椎以上之颈椎。

renewed bone Refers to the cervical vertebra above the sixth cervical vertebra.

复命关【fù mìng guān】 指下丹田。

renewed life joint Refers to the lower Dantian (the region below the navel).

复性之初【fù xìng zhī chū】 指返璞归真，回复意识活动的自然本性。

natural state of returning Refers to returning to the original purity and simplicity in order to return to the natural principle of consciousness activity.

傅仁宇动功六字延寿法【fù rén yǔ dòng gōng liù zì yán shòu fǎ】 为动功，方法多样。如举手则呵，反手则吸，呵则通于心，去心家一切热气或上攻眼目，或面色红，舌上疮或口疮。冬日省盐增苦，以养其心。

Fu Renyu's dynamic exercise for longevity with six Chinese characters A dynamic exercise with various methods, such as raising the hands to breathe out and turning the hands to breathe in; communicating with the heart through breathing out in order to eliminate heat Qi in the heart, or invasion of the eyes, or reddish face, or lingual sore, or mouth sore. Saving salt in winter can nourish the heart.

傅元虚抱顶形【fù yuán xū bào dǐng xíng】 为动静相兼功。其作法为，端坐，将两手搓热，按抱顶门，闭目凝神，吹呵鼓气，升腾顶上，复行功运气十七口。主治头昏头晕。

exercise for assisting origin deficiency and embracing the top An exercise combined with dynamic exercise and static exercise, marked by sitting upright, rubbing both hands hot, pressing and embracing the top, closing the eyes, concentrating the spirit, bowing and breathing out Qi to raise it to the top, moving Qi again for seventeen times. Such an exercise combined with dynamic exercise and static exercise can cure dizziness and vertigo.

腹【fù】 为人体的一个部位，膈以下，左、右腹股沟韧带、耻骨联合（相当于毛际）以上称腹。

abdomen Refers to the region below

the diaphragm and above the left and right sides of inguinal ligament and pubic symphysis.

腹哀【fù āi】 为足太阴脾经中的一个穴位,位于脐上 3 寸,为气功中常用的意守部位。

Fu'ai（**SP 16**） An acupoint in the spleen meridian of foot Taiyin, located 3 Cun above the navel, which is the region for concentrating consciousness in practicing Qigong.

腹功【fù gōng】 为动功。其作法为,两手摩腹,移行百步,闭息,存想丹田火,自下而上,遍烧其体。

abdominal exercise A dynamic exercise, marked by kneading the abdomen, moving for hundred steps, stopping respiration, imagining Dantian fire from the lower to the upper to heat the whole body. Dantian is divided into the upper Dantian (the region between the eyes), the middle Dantian (the region below the heart) and the lower Dantian (the region below the navel).

腹神去【fù shén qù】 指腹神损伤于胃肠而神散。

loss of abdominal spirit Indicates that the spirit in the abdomen is damaged by dispersion of the spirit in the stomach and the intestines.

腹痛【fù tòng】 为气功适应证,由寒热、饮食不调、寄生虫感染、情志不调等因素引起气血受阻而导致腹部发生疼痛。

abdominal pain An indication of Qigong, usually caused by cold-heat, irregular food intake, parasitic infection and abnormal emotion.

腹痛候导引法【fù tòng hòu dǎo yǐn fǎ】 为静功,方法多样。如正身仰卧,弯曲疼痛的腿和臂,口鼻闭气,待觉腹痛

时,以意念于痛处推动气行,使气行处有热感,温经通络。治四肢疼痛。

exercise of Daoyin for abdominal pain A static exercise with various methods, such as lying on the back, bending painful legs and arms, stopping respiration with the mouth and nose, moving Qi in the tender spot with consciousness when the abdominal is painful in order to make the region with Qi movement hot, warming the meridians and dredging the collaterals. Such a static exercise can cure pain in the four limbs.

腹胀【fù zhàng】 为气功适应证,由消化不良、情志不舒、湿热、寒湿等原因所致。

abdominal distension An indication of Qigong, usually caused by indigestion, discomforting emotion, dampness-heat and cold-dampness.

腹胀候导引法【fù zhàng hòu dǎo yǐn fǎ】 动静相兼功,方法多样。如蹲坐,静心存想,用两手从心向下按摩,摇动左右手臂,使身体左右侧倾,两肩尽量用力,低头向肚,两手沿冲脉按摩至脐下二十一次。温中理气,消食化积,治腹胀闷,食不消化。

exercise of Daoyin for abdominal distension An exercise combined with dynamic exercise and static exercise with various methods, such as squatting, tranquilizing the heart with inward contemplation, pressing from the heart downwards with both hands, shaking the left and right arms, rolling the body from the left to the right and vice versa with forceful shoulders, lowering the head to the abdomen, kneading from the thoroughfare meridian to the navel with both hands for twenty-one

F

times. Such an exercise combined with dynamic exercise and static exercise can warm the center，regulate Qi，digest food and transform accumulations as well as cure abdominal distension and indigestion.

腹之一【fù zhī yī】 指脐。

one part in the abdomen　Refers to the navel.

腹中泪泪【fù zhōng gǔ gǔ】 指气功服气时，腹中发出的声音。

gurgle in the abdomen　Refers to sound in the abdomen in taking Qi during practicing Qigong.

G

干浴【gān yù】　为动功。其作法为，摩手令热以摩面，从上至下，去邪气，令人面上有光彩。摩手令热，摩身体，从上至下，名曰干浴。可预防和治疗感冒。

dry bathing　A dynamic exercise, marked by rubbing the face hot for rubbing the face, relieving pathogenic factors and lustering the face; or rubbing the hands hot for rubbing the body from the upper to the lower, known as heating the body. It can prevent and treat common cold.

甘露【gān lù】　为静功，指服炼口中津液。

sweet dew　A static exercise, referring to fluid and humor swallowed in the mouth.

肝【gān】　为人体五脏之一，与精神活动有关，助脾胃运化。

liver　One of the five Zang-organs, is related to the activity of the essence and the spirit that support the transportation and transformation of the spleen and the stomach.

肝痹【gān bì】　气功适应证，由于筋痹日久不愈，复感外邪，或恼怒伤肝，肝气瘀滞所致。

liver impediment　An indication of Qigong, caused by sinew impediment that has failed to heal for a long time, invasion of external pathogenic factors, or annoyance that has injured the liver, and stagnation of liver Qi.

肝病【gān bìng】　为气功适应证，泛指肝脏发生的多种病证。

liver disease　An indication of Qigong, can be treated by Qigong. It refers to all maladies located in the liver.

肝病导引【gān bìng dǎo yǐn】　为动功。其作法为，正面坐好，两手用力按在两肋部位，然后左转身，再右转身，三至五次。

Daoyin for liver disease　A dynamic exercise, marked by sitting upright, pressing the libs with both hands and turning the body from the left to the right and vice versa for three or five times respectively.

肝病候导引法【gān bìng hòu dǎo yǐn fǎ】　为静功。其作法为，无声读呵字出气。疏肝解郁，治肝愁忧不乐，悲思嗔怒，头旋眼痛。

exercise of Daoyin for liver disease　A static exercise, usually marked by reading the Chinese character He (respiration) without any voice for improving breath, soothing the liver to relieve stagnation in order to eliminate annoyance and unhappiness and to cure dizziness and ophthalmalgia.

肝神【gān shén】　为肝的精微物质和功能作用的总称。

liver spirit　The general appellation of the essential substance and function of the liver.

肝神去【gān shén qù】　即七神去，指损伤五脏六腑的情况。肝神损伤于魂散失目不明，心神损伤于神散失唇见青白，肺神损伤于魄不在身鼻不通,肾神损伤于意出身外食不甘味,头神损伤于神出泥丸头目眩晕,腹神损伤于胃肠神散,四肢神损伤于骨关节重滞不动。

loss of liver spirit　The same as loss of seven spirits, referring to different ways to damage the spirit from the five Zang-organs (including the heart, the liver, the spleen, the lung and the kidney) and six Fu-organs (including the gallbladder, the stomach, the small intestine, the large intestine, the bladder and the triple energizer). The spirit in the liver is damaged by dispersion of the ethereal soul, the spirit in the heart is damaged by loss of the spirit and change of the lips, the spirit in the lung is damaged by dispersion of the corporeal soul and the obstructed nose, the spirit in the kidney is damaged by no pure emotion and no good food, the spirit in the brain is damaged by dispersion of the spirit from the mud bolus (the brain) and dizziness, the spirit in the abdomen is damaged by dispersion of the spirit in the stomach and the intestines, the spirit in the four limbs is damaged by stagnation of the joints.

肝俞【gān shū】　为足太阳膀胱经中的一个穴位,位于第九胸椎刺突下旁开1.5寸处。这一穴位为气功运行的一个常见部位。

Ganshu（BL 18）　An acupoint in the bladder meridian of foot Taiyang, located 1.5 Cun below the spinous process of the ninth thoracic vertebra. This acupoint is a region usually used for keeping the essential Qi in practice of Qigong.

肝脏修养法【gān zàng xiū yǎng fǎ】

为静功。其作法为,常以正月、二月、三月朔旦,东面平坐,叩齿三通,闭气九十息,努力养精。

exercise for nourishing the liver　A static exercise, usually marked by sitting toward the east at the beginning of January, February and March, clicking the teeth for opening up in three ways and holding respiration for ninety times in order to nourish the essence.

感冒【gǎn mào】　为气功适应证,即感受触冒风寒、风热之邪而引起的一系列症状。

common cold　An indication of Qigong, usually caused by invasion of pathogenic wind-cold and wind-heat.

感应【gǎn yìng】　指阴阳二气交相感应。

interaction　Refers to mutual interaction of Qi from Yin and Yang.

刚风【gāng fēng】　即高处之风。在气功文献中,刚风指损伤人体的猛烈致病因素。

strong wind　Refers to wind in the highlands or mountains. In the literature of Qigong, it refers to the serious pathogenic factors that have damaged human body.

刚柔【gāng róu】　指阴阳两个方面,阳刚而阴柔。

firm and soft form　Refers to Yin and Yang, in which Yang is firm and Yin is soft.

刚柔相推【gāng róu xiāng tuī】　指动静的相互作用是事物变化的基础。

mutual effect of firmness and softness Refers to the mutual effect of dynamics and statics that is the foundation of changes for all things.

高拱无为魂魄安【gāo gǒng wú wéi

hún pò ān】 指诸神内存泥丸,高高在上,端拱无为,寂静安谧,则魂魄安和,阴阳平秘。

supreme tranquility of ethereal soul and corporeal soul Refers to storage of all the spirits in the mud bolus (the brain) with height, tranquility and stability, ensuring balance of the ethereal soul and the corporeal soul as well as peace and compactness of Yin and Yang.

高濂【gāo lián】 为明代养生家,对气功有研究,其专著介绍了气功养生法。

Gao Lian A master of life cultivation in the Ming Dynasty (1368 AD - 1644 AD), who also studied Qigong. In his monograph, he introduced the exercises for practicing Qigong.

高攀龙【gāo pān lóng】 为明代气功家,其专著介绍了气功的历史、发展与功效。

Gao Panlong A master of Qigong in the Ming Dynasty (1368 AD - 1644 AD), who introduced the history, development and effects of Qigong.

高瑞南【gāo ruì nán】 为明代养生家高濂的另外一个称谓,其对气功有研究,其专著介绍了气功养生法。

Gao Ruinan Another name of Gao Lian, a master of life cultivation in the Ming Dynasty (1368 AD - 1644 AD), who also studied Qigong. In his monograph, he introduced the exercises for practicing Qigong.

高上玉皇心印妙经【gāo shàng yù huáng xīn yìn miào jīng】 《高上玉皇心印妙经》为气功专著,论述内丹修炼中精气神之关系。作者不详。

Gaoshang Yuhuang Xinyin Miaojing (*Magical Canon of Great Jade Emperor and Heart Scene*) A monograph of Qigong entitled *Magical Canon of Great Jade Emperor and Heart Scene*, describing the relation of the essence, Qi and spirit in practicing the internal Dan (pills of immortality). The author was unknown.

高深甫【gāo shēn fǔ】 为明代养生家高濂的另外一个称谓,其对气功有研究,其专著介绍了气功养生法。

Gao Shenfu Another name of Gao Lian, a master of life cultivation in the Ming Dynasty (1368 AD - 1644 AD), who also studied Qigong. In his monograph, he introduced the exercises for practicing Qigong.

高象先凤张法【gāo xiàng xiān fèng zhāng fǎ】 为动功。其作法为,以身蹲下,曲拳弯腰,起手上顶,口鼻微出清气六口,左脚向前,右脚尖顶左脚跟,仍运气六口。主治腰腿疼痛。

exercise with high scene and ancestral phoenix A dynamic exercise, marked by squatting, bending the fists, curving the waist, raising over the top of the head, mildly breathing out clear Qi through the mouth and nose for six times, walking up with the left foot, pushing the left heel with the toes at the right foot and moving Qi for six times for relieving pain in the waist and legs.

高子怡养立成【gāo zǐ yí yǎng lì chéng】 源自气功专论,主要阐述一日间的修养及气功方法。

very happy success in cultivating health Collected from a monograph of Qigong, mainly describing life cultivation and exercise of Qigong practice.

高子游说【gāo zǐ yóu shuì】 源自气功专论,主要阐述在四时不同季节,到环境幽美的大好河山中,呼吸新鲜空气,运动身作,使体内气血流畅,阴阳平衡,情绪稳定,心旷神怡,有益于健康长寿。

highly canvassing Collected from a monograph of Qigong, mainly describing breathing fresh air in the beautiful great rivers and mountain in the four seasons, moving the body to smooth the flow of Qi and blood, balancing Yin and Yang, stabilizing emotion, freeing the heart and relaxing the spirit in order to cultivate health and to prolong life.

膏肓【gāo huāng】 ① 指病重;② 指疾病位置;③ 指穴位,此穴位为气功习练之处。

Gaohuang(**the region below the heart and above the diaphragm**) Refers to ① either a severe disease; ② or the location of a disease; ③ or Gaohuang(BL 43), an acupoint. This acupoint is a region usually used in practice of Qigong.

膏淋【gāo lín】 为气功适应证,多因湿热下注,肾虚不能制约脂液所致。

chyloid stranguria An indication of Qigong, usually caused by downward pouring of dampness heat and deficiency of the kidney that fails to control blood lipid.

歌咏所以养性情【gē yǒng suǒ yǐ yǎng xìng qíng】 说明唱歌可以欢娱心性,陶冶情操。

Singing nourishes disposition. This is a celebrated dictum, indicating that singing song can excite disposition and cultivate temperament.

葛长庚【gě cháng gēng】 宋代气功学家白玉蟾(1194—1229)的另外一个称谓。

Ge Changgeng Another name of Bai Yuchan, a great master of Qigong in the Song Dynasty (960 AD - 1279 AD).

葛洪【gě hóng】 晋代医药学家及气功养生家。

Ge Hong A great doctor of traditional Chinese medicine and master of Qigong and life cultivation in the Jin Dynasty (266 AD - 420 AD).

葛洪摄生法【gě hóng shè shēng fǎ】源自气功专论,阐述摄生之要,在于综合气功与药物治疗之长。

Ge Hong's exercise for regimen Collected from a monograph of Qigong, mainly describing the importance of regimen and treatment with combination of Qigong and medicinal.

葛仙公【gě xiān gōng】 东汉时期的炼丹家葛玄的另外一个称谓。

Ge Xiangong Another name of Ge Xuan, a great master of alchemy in the East Han Dynasty (25 AD - 220 AD).

葛仙翁开胸法【gě xiān wēng kāi xiōng fǎ】 为动功。其作法为,正站立,脚呈八字,将两手相叉,向胸前往来擦摩,运气二十四口。又一法以左手用力向左,右手也用力随之,头侧向右,目右视,运气九口。治胸痞闷,呼吸不利。

Ge Xianwong's exercise for opening the chest A dynamic exercise, marked by standing up, emerging eight Chinese characters in the feet, crossing the hands to rub the chest and moving Qi for twenty-four times; then turning the left hand to the left side, turning the right hand to the right side, turning the head to the right side, seeing the right side and moving Qi for nine times. Such a dynamic exercise can cure gastric fullness and oppression as well as difficulty in breath.

葛孝先【gě xiào xiān】 东汉时期的炼丹家葛玄的另外一个称谓。

Ge Xiaoxian Another name of Ge Xuan, a great master of alchemy in the East Han Dynasty (25 AD - 220 AD).

葛玄【gě xuán】 东汉时期的炼丹家。

Ge Xuan A great master of alchemy in the East Han Dynasty (25 AD - 220 AD).

葛稚川【gě zhì chuān】 晋代医药学家及气功养生家葛洪的另外一个称谓。

Ge Zhichuan Another name of Ge Hong, a great doctor of traditional Chinese medicine and master of Qigong and life cultivation in the Jin Dynasty (266 AD - 420 AD).

根【gēn】 指能产生精神活动的根本。

root A common term of Qigong in Buddhism, referring to the foundation for spirit activity.

根本【gēn běn】 ① 指太极;② 指生命之本。

foundation Refers to ① either Taiji (Supreme Pole); ② or the root of life.

根尘【gēn chén】 指引起情志损伤,精神失调的六尘。

dirty root Refers to the six blemishes that damage the emotion and imbalance the spirit.

根心【gēn xīn】 即意识思维活动之根在心,实际为脑神。

root of the heart Indicates that the root of the activities of consciousness and thinking is the heart, actually referring to the spirit in the brain.

根源【gēn yuán】 指存精炼神而达到"身心不动"的境地。

original source Refers to storing the essence and refining the spirit in order

to reach the state marked by tranquilization of the body and the heart.

艮【gèn】 ① 指卦名,即集中注意(视力);② 指意识活动的相对稳定;③ 指去类比象;④ 指方向;⑤ 指山。

Gen Refers to ① either the name of Trigram in Bagua (Eight Trigrams), indicating focus of concentration (vision); ② or relative stabilization of the consciousness activity; ③ or analogy; ④ or direction; ⑤ or mountain.

艮背【gèn bèi】 为静功,意念集中于背,忘其周围的人和事,神形和调,自然无咎,身体健康。

back concentration A static exercise, referring to concentration of the consciousness on the back in order to neglect all the men and things around and regulate the spirit and body, which will naturally avoid any blame and well cultivate health.

艮背法【gèn bèi fǎ】 为静功,初学之人,开始时静坐片刻,将万念扫除,凝神定志于水火之中,口念太乙救苦,而渐归于心,渐归于背。

exercise of back concentration A static exercise. Those who first study Qigong should sit quietly for a while to eliminate any ideas and thoughts, concentrating the spirit and stabilizing the will in the water and fire, reading Taiyi (Daoism) in the mouth to relieve any sufferings and gradually turning it to the heart and the back.

艮腓【gèn féi】 为静功,意念集中腿肚。行功时注意精神放松,形体(腿肚)亦相应放松。

calf concentration A static exercise, referring to concentration of the consciousness on the calf. In walking or practicing Qigong, the spirit and the body (legs and abdomen) should be relaxed.

艮辅【gèn fǔ】 为静功,意念集中于额面部,平素注意言语有伦序,或言之有规律,思维就平和。如不注意言语,其言不正,或妄言妄语,则思维紊乱,悔且至矣。

forehead concentration A static exercise, referring to concentration of the consciousness on the forehead. Only when speech is sequent and regular can thinking be gentle and mild. If speech is not cared and or even rubbish, thinking will certainly be chaotic and nonsense.

艮三田【gèn sān tián】 即意念集中于三丹田。

concentration of triple Dantian Refers to concentration of the consciousness on the three kinds of Dantian, i. e. the upper Dantian (the region between the eyes), the middle Dantian (the region below the heart) and the lower Dantian (the region below the navel).

艮身【gèn shēn】 为静功,即意念集中于腹部(丹田),有益于身体健康。

abdominal concentration A static exercise, referring to concentration of the consciousness on the abdomen (Dantian) which is effective for cultivating health. Dantian is divided into the upper Dantian (the region between the eyes), the middle Dantian (the region below the heart) and the lower Dantian (the region below the navel).

艮限【gèn xiàn】 为静功,即意念集中于腰部,行功时注意协调各部。

lumbar concentration A static exercise, referring to concentration of the consciousness on the waist. In practicing Qigong, attention should be paid to the regulation of all aspects.

艮趾【gèn zhǐ】 为静功,指意念集中于趾,和调形神。

toes concentration Static exercise, referring to concentration of the consciousness on the toes in order to regulate the body and spirit.

庚金之腑【gēng jīn zhī fǔ】 指大肠,为六腑之一。

Gengjin Fu-organ Refers to the large intestine which is one of the six Fu-organs (including the gallbladder, stomach, small intestine, large intestine, bladder and triple energizer).

工倕达生法【gōng chuí dá shēng fǎ】 为功法。其作法为,调节意识思维活动,内养精神,外与事象相适应。

internal nourishment and external adaptation A static exercise, marked by regulating the activities of consciousness and thinking in order to internally nourish the spirit and externally adapt to the environment.

功德【gōng dé】 道家积善派的一个概念,认为行善者积德累功为功德。

merits and virtues A concept in the Moral School of Daoism, referring to accumulation of merits and virtues in following the law of Daoism.

功夫【gōng fu】 指习练气功的时间、时机,致力于气功的程度、造诣之浅深,均谓之功夫。

Gongfu (skill) Refers to the time and opportunity for practicing Qigong, during which measures should be taken to reach the level and the state of Qigong.

肱骨【gōng gǔ】 又称为臑骨,是上肢最粗壮的骨。

humerus Also called forelimb, referring to the strongest bone in the upper limbs.

龔居中【gōng jū zhōng】　明代中医学家,对气功养生有研究,其专著中介绍了气功养生。

Gong Juzhong　A doctor of traditional Chinese medicine and a master of Qigong in the Ming Dynasty（1368 AD‐1644 AD）. In his monograph of traditional Chinese medicine，he also introduced the theory and practice of Qigong with life cultivation.

龔廷贤【gōng tíng xián】　明代太医院医师,著有中医专著,对呼吸静功和用六字(吹、呼、唏、呵、嘘、呬)气诀治五脏六腑疾患有专门论述。

Gong Tingxian　A doctor of traditional Chinese medicine in the Imperial Hospital in the Ming Dynasty（1368 AD‐1644 AD）. He wrote a monograph of traditional Chinese medicine，also describing static exercises for respiration and the formula with six Chinese characters to treat diseases in the five Zang-organs（including the heart，the liver，the spleen，the lung and the kidney）and the six Fu-organs（including the gallbladder，the stomach，the small intestine，the large intestine，the bladder and the triple energizer）. The six Chinese characters include Chui（blowing），Hu（exhaling），Xi（sighing），Ke（breathing out），Xu（breathing out slowly）and Xi（panting）.

龔云林【gōng yún lín】　明代太医院医师龚廷贤的另外一个称谓,著有中医专著,对呼吸静功和用六字(吹、呼、唏、呵、嘘、呬)气诀治五脏六腑疾患有专门论述。

Gong Yunlin　Another name of Gong Tingxian，a doctor of traditional Chinese medicine in the Imperial Hospital in the Ming Dynasty（1368 AD‐1644 AD）. He wrote a monograph of traditional Chinese medicine，also describing static exercises for respiration and the formula with six Chinese characters to treat diseases in the five Zang-organs（including the heart，the liver，the spleen，the lung and the kidney）and the six Fu-organs（including the gallbladder，the stomach，the small intestine，the large intestine，the bladder and the triple energizer）. The six Chinese characters include Chui（blowing），Hu（exhaling），Xi（sighing），Ke（breathing out），Xu（breathing out slowly）and Xi（panting）.

G

龔子才【gōng zǐ cái】　明代太医院医师龚廷贤的另外一个称谓,著有中医专著,对呼吸静功和用六字(吹、呼、唏、呵、嘘、呬)气诀治五脏六腑疾患有专门论述。

Gong Zicai　Another name of Gong Tingxian，a doctor of traditional Chinese medicine in the Imperial Hospital in the Ming Dynasty（1368 AD‐1644 AD）. He wrote a monograph of traditional Chinese medicine，also describing static exercises for respiration and the formula with six Chinese characters to treat diseases in the five Zang-organs（including the heart，the liver，the spleen，the lung and the kidney）and the six Fu-organs（including the gallbladder，the stomach，the small intestine，the large intestine，the bladder and the triple energizer）. The six Chinese characters include Chui（blowing），Hu（exhaling），Xi（sighing），

Ke（breathing out），Xu（breathing out slowly）and Xi（panting）.

汞投铅【gǒng tóu qiān】 即神与气，为气功学术语，指身体内阴阳两个方面。

mercury putting into lead A term of Qigong, the same as the term of the spirit and Qi, referring to Yin and Yang in the body.

垢腻【gòu nì】 指习练气功，目明心宽，不受外界困扰，排除污秽及壅滞。

deposits of sweat A term of Qigong, referring to brightening the eyes, relaxing the heart, avoiding disturbance of the external world and eliminating filthiness and stagnation.

媾精【gòu jīng】 即男女阴阳相感，合其精则人体化生。

sexual intercourse Refers to copulation of man and woman, intercourse of which can produce embryo.

古今医统大全【gǔ jīn yī tǒng dà quán】《古今医统大全》为中医学综合性类书，为明代徐春圃所编，其中收藏了许多气功养生资料。

Gujin Yitong Daquan A series of books about traditional Chinese medicine, compiled by Xu Chunpu in the Ming Dynasty（1368 AD - 1644 AD），which has also collected many documents about Qigong.

古龙虎歌【gǔ lóng hǔ gē】 源自气功专论，说明习练精液血以还丹的道理。

song about ancient Loong and tiger Collected from a monograph about Qigong, referring to the principle for refining the essence, humor and the blood in order to enrich Dan（pills of immortality）.

古圣强言为火药，不离神气相随【gǔ shèng qiáng yán wéi huǒ yào bù lí shén qì xiāng suí】 练功就是以神御气，神是火，气是药。分而言之是火、是药，合而言之即神气。

Eloquent words of ancient immortals are gunpowder and only when the spirit and Qi be maintained can the gunpowder be followed. This is a celebrated dictum, referring to controlling Qi with the spirit in practicing Qigong, in which the spirit is fire and Qi is medicinal. In separate explanation, it refers to fire and medicinal; in combined explanation, it refers to the spirit and Qi.

古文龙虎经注疏【gǔ wén lóng hǔ jīng zhù shū】《古文龙虎经注疏》为气功学著作。作者不详。

Guwen Longhu Jing Zhushu（*Notes about Passages of Loong and Tiger in Ancient China*） A monograph of Qigong entitled *Notes about Passages of Loong and Tiger in Ancient China*. The author was unknown.

古文龙虎上经注【gǔ wén lóng hǔ shàng jīng zhù】《古文龙虎上经注》为气功学专著，为保义朗王道注。

Guwen Longhu Shangjing Zhu（*Explanation about Upper Passages of Loong and Tiger in Ancient China*） Written by Wang Dao in the Song Dynasty（960 AD - 1279 AD）.

古仙导引按摩法【gǔ xiān dǎo yǐn àn mó fǎ】《古仙导引按摩法》为气功专著。作者不详。

Guxian Daoyin Anmo Fa（*Methods of Ancient Immortals about Daoyin and Kneading*） The author was unknown.

谷春坐县门【gǔ chūn zuò xiàn mén】 为静功。其作法为，盘膝端坐，两手按膝，左右扭身运气十四口。主治一切杂病。

sitting at gate in spring A static exercise, marked by sitting with crossed legs, pressing the knees with both hands, turning the body from the left to the right and vice versa, moving Qi for fourteen times in order to cure various miscellaneous diseases.

谷道【gǔ dào】 ① 指气功养生术之一,即辟谷不食的方法;② 指肛门。

grain trail Refers to ① either one of the methods used to cultivate life in Qigong, i. e. the way to practice inedia (stopping diet); ② or the anus.

谷神【gǔ shén】 ① 指虚空之山谷,谷为山谷,神为神妙;② 指腹中消谷之神。

mountain spirit Refers to ① either vacant mountain, in which the spirit means marvelous; ② or the spirit in the abdomen that digests food.

谷神歌【gǔ shén gē】 《谷神歌》为气功专论,作者为吕岩,为唐代的八仙之一,即吕洞宾。

Gushen Ge(*Song of Grain Spirit*) A monograph of Qigong entitled *Song of Grain Spirit*, written by Lǔ Yan who was one of the eight immortals in the Tang Dynasty (618 AD – 907 AD), also called Lǔ Dongbin.

谷神篇【gǔ shén piān】 《谷神篇》为气功专论,论述了气功理论,介绍了功法并抒发了练功感受,作者为元代林辕述。

Gusshen Pian(*Chapter of Grain Spirit*) A monograph of Qigong entitled *Chapter of Grain Spirit*, written by Lin Yuanshu in the Yuan Dynasty (1271 AD – 1368 AD), describing the theory of Qigong and the experience of practicing Qigong.

谷神是动念处【gǔ shén shì dòng niàn chù】 指谷神调节呼吸,为呼之根,吸之蒂。

Grain spirit is the region for dynamic contemplation. This is a celebrated dictum, referring to regulation of inhalation and exhalation, in which exhalation is the root of respiration and inhalation is the result of respiration.

谷药【gǔ yào】 指导引后要慢慢散步,吃不冷不热、清洁卫生的食物,细嚼慢咽,饭后不要立即睡觉等养生方法。

grain medicinal Refers to the way for cultivating health made by slowly walking after practice of Qigong, eating tepid and good food, chewing carefully and swallowing slowly, and avoiding immediate sleep after taking food.

谷雨三月中坐功【gǔ yǔ sān yuè zhōng zuò gōng】 为动功。即每日丑寅时平坐,换手左右,举托移臂,左右掩乳,各五七次,叩齿、吐纳、漱咽。

middle March dhyana A dynamic exercise, marked by quietly sitting in Chou (the period of a day from 1 a.m. to 3 a.m. in the morning) and Yin (the period of a day from 3 a.m. to 5 a.m. in the morning), changing the hand from the left to the right, raising the hands to change the shoulders, covering the breasts with the left and the right hands for five or seven times respectively, clicking the teeth with exhaling and inhaling as well as rinsing and swallowing.

股【gǔ】 指大腿。

thigh Refers to the big leg in the human body.

股阳【gǔ yáng】 指大腿外侧。

thigh Yang Refers to the lateral side of the thigh.

股阴【gǔ yīn】 指大腿内侧。

thigh Yin Refers to the interior side of the thigh.

骨痹【gǔ bì】 为气功适应证,指以骨节证候为突出表现的痹证。

bone impediment An indication of Qigong, usually referring to the obvious manifestation of bone syndromes.

骨髓【gǔ suǐ】 指藏于骨腔内的精髓。

bone marrow Refers to the marrow in the bone cavity.

骨蒸【gǔ zhēng】 气功适应证,多由阴虚所致。

steaming bone An indication of Qigong, usually caused by Yin deficiency.

骨之一【gǔ zhī yī】 指脊。

one of the bones Refers to the spine.

蛊毒候导引法【gǔ dú hòu dǎo yǐn fǎ】 为动功,方法多样。如两手交叉放头上,坐在地上,慢慢伸展下肢,用两手从外抱住膝部,低头进入两膝间,两手交叉放头十二次。杀虫,治蛊毒,三尸毒。

exercise of Daoyin for parasitic disease A dynamic exercise with various methods, such as overlapping the hands to put on the head, sitting on the ground, slowly stretching the legs, holding the knees from the lateral sides with both hands, lowering the head to reach the region between the knees, overlapping the hands to put on the head for twelve times. Such a dynamic exercise can kill worms, cure parasitic disease and expel triple corpse toxin.

鼓腹淘气【gǔ fù táo qì】 为动功。其作法为,闭目仰面,腰脊伸直,将气海中气鼓荡起来,令气内外流转。将浊气吐出,出气时以两耳听不到出气声为好,鼓腹淘气连做九次或十八次均可。

promoting the abdomen and cleaning out Qi A dynamic exercise, marked by closing the eyes, raising the face, stretching the waist and spine, instigating Qi from Qi sea in order to flow Qi internally and externally, breathing out turbid Qi without any sound in the ears, and promoting the abdomen and cleaning out Qi for nine or eighteen times respectively.

鼓呵消积聚法【gǔ hē xiāo jī jù fǎ】 为动静相兼功。其作法为,正身端坐,闭目凝神,鼓动胸腹,待其气满时缓缓呵出,如此行五或七次。

exercise for abdominal mass with deep inhaling and slow exhaling An exercise combined with dynamic exercise and static exercise, marked by sitting upright, closing the eyes, concentrating the spirit, instigating the abdomen, and slowly breathing out for five or seven times when Qi is enriched.

瞽听聋视【gǔ tīng lóng shì】 即眼睛失明的人,听力特别好;耳朵失聪的人,视力特别好。

blind person listening well and deaf person seeing well Indicates that those with blindness can listen well while those with deafness can see clearly.

固济【gù jì】 指水火既济,养心益肾,并温养团固。

strict harmonization Refers to coordination of water and fire, nourishing the heart, fortifying the kidney, and warmly cultivating the whole body.

固瘕【gù jiǎ】 为气功适应证,即大便先硬后溏,由肠胃虚寒所致。

chronic diarrhea An indication of Qigong, also referring to dry feces followed by sloppy stool caused by deficiency and coldness of the intestines and the stomach.

固守虚无【gù shǒu xū wú】 指习练气功时，保持精神意识活动相对静止状态。

defending nihility Refers to relatively tranquilizing the activities of the essence, the spirit and the consciousness in practicing Qigong.

固元气【gù yuán qì】 即固守虚无以补养元气。

reinforcing original Qi Refers to defending nihility and nourishing original Qi.

故妪泣拜文宾【gù yù qì bài wén bīn】 为动功。其作法为，自然站立，两脚分开同肩宽，左脚向前半步，右脚跟提起，弯腰低头如鞠躬状。

trying to be an apprentice of the master A dynamic exercise, marked by standing naturally and separating the feet with the same width of the shoulders with the left foot running forward for half a step, lifting the right heel, stooping the waist and lowering the head like bowing.

卦气【guà qì】 ① 坎、离、震、兑为四时卦；② 复、临、泰、大壮、夬、乾、姤、遁、否、观、剥、坤为十二消息卦，谓之卦气；③ 将八卦配洛书数，以奇偶分阴阳，亦谓之卦气；④ 分卦爻值日，一爻主一日，六十卦每卦六爻为三百六十日，余震、离、坎、兑四卦，分主春分、秋分、夏至、冬至。

Trigram Qi Refers to ① either Kan Trigram, Li Trigram, Zhen Trigram and Dui Trigram in the four seasons as well as Fu Trigram, Lin Trigram, Tai Trigram, Dazhuang Trigram, Guai Trigram, Qian Trigram, Gou Trigram, Dun Trigram, Pi Trigram, Guan Trigram, Bo Trigram and Kun Trigram in the twelve periods, which all refer to Trigram Qi; ② or combination of the Eight Trigrams with Luo Shu (the ancient Chinese mythological fiction) that have divided the odd number and even number into Yin and Yang, also known as Trigram Qi; ③ or six levels in each Trigram that pertain to six days, indicating that one level in a Trigram refers to one day and all the levels in sixty Trigrams belong to three hundred and sixty days; ④ Besides, Kan Trigram, Li Trigram, Zhen Trigram and Dui Trigram represent the spring, summer, autumn and winter, the four seasons in a year.

卦气方隅论【guà qì fāng yú lùn】 源自气功专论《类经图翼》，述先天、后天八卦的秩序方位，认为先天为易之体，后天为易之用。

discussion about the procedure of Trigram Qi Collected from a monograph entitled Leijing Tuyi or *The Illustrated Wings of the Classified Canon*, describing the procedure and positions of the innate Eight Trigrams and the postnatal Eight Trigrams, indicating that the innate is the origin of Yijing or *Simplification, Change and No Change* and the postnatal is the foundation of the Yijing or *Simplification, Change and No Change*.

卦脏时论【guà zàng shí lùn】 源自气功专论《至游子》，阐述八卦、五脏、四时的关系。

discussion about Trigrams and viscera Collected from a monograph of Qigong entitled Zhi Youzi or *Sincere Traveller*, describing the relationship between the Eight Trigrams, five Zang-organs (including the heart, the liver, the spleen, the lung and the kidney) and four seasons (including spring, summer, autumn and winter).

挂金索【guà jīn suǒ】 源自气功专论,以五更练功为喻,简明地论述了练功的不同阶段。

hanging golden rope Collected from a monograph of Qigong, a metaphor of practicing Qigong at midnight, describing different stages of Qigong practice.

关冲【guān chōng】 手少阳三焦经中的一个穴位,位于无名指尺侧。这一穴位为气功运行的一个常见部位。

Guanchong (TE 1) An acupoint in the triple energizer meridian of hand Shaoyang, located in the ulnar side of the fourth finger. This acupoint is a region usually used for keeping the essential Qi in practice of Qigong.

关门【guān mén】 指玄关。玄关有二门,左为玄门,右为牝门。左通呼气,右通吸气。

pass gate Refers to abstruse pass which is composed of two gates, i. e. abstruse gate in the left for exhalation and female gate in the right for inhalation.

关尹子【guān yǐn zǐ】 古代气功学家,著有气功专论,年代不详。

Guan Yinzi A great master of Qigong in ancient China and wrote a monograph about Qigong. The related dynasty was unknown.

关元【guān yuán】 ① 指任脉中的一个穴位,位于前正中线,脐下 3 寸;② 指气功中常用的意守部位,即下丹田。

Guanyuan Refers to ① either an acupoint called Guanyuan (CV 4) in the conception meridian, located 3 Cun be-low the navel in the front middle line; ② or the region for concentrating consciousness in practicing Qigong known as the lower Dantian (the region below the navel).

观【guān】 为佛家气功习用语,① 指观察思维;② 指智慧;③ 指神形活动开朗、大观。

vision A common term of Qigong in Buddhism, ① referring to either observation and thinking; ② or wisdom; ③ or sparky activity of the spirit and the body.

观鼻法【guān bí fǎ】 为静功,指通过调身调气,补脑安神、益气养形、和调阴阳。

exercise for observing the nose A static exercise, referring to regulating the body and Qi in order to tonify the brain, to stabilize the spirit, to fortify Qi, to nourish the body and to regulate Yin and Yang.

观世音【guān shì yīn】 指听音声,以转移意识活动注意力,而去除妄念,获得解脱。

observation of world voice Refers to listening voice in order to transfer the attention of consciousness activity, to eliminate distracting thought and to free from worldly worries.

观想【guān xiǎng】 指意识活动,为意想之意。

observation of thought Refers to the activity of consciousness and imagination of idea.

观心【guān xīn】 指观察意识活动。

observation of the heart Refers to observation of consciousness activity.

观心法【guān xīn fǎ】 为静功,指排除外界干扰,神志安宁清静。

exercise for observing the heart　A static exercise, referring to eliminating disturbance of the external world and making the consciousness stable and quiet.

观一切空法【guān yí qiè kōng fǎ】佛家气功习用语,其作法为,趺坐观空,维持意识活动的稳定。

exercise for inspecting vacuum　A common term of Qigong in Buddhism, referring to observing nothingness in sitting and stabilizing consciousness activity.

观照【guān zhào】　指用美好意识温煦体内。

observation of idea　Refers to warming the internal of the body with fine consciousness.

观止【guān zhǐ】　观指目光真意,止指意识停留在此,即意识着于一个美好的念头。

observation and stop　Indicates that the consciousness must be a fine idea. In this term, observation refers to genuine intendment of the eyes and stop refers to keeping the consciousness on this genuine intendment.

观志【guān zhì】　指观察意识思维活动,测其神思所游。

observation of will　Refers to observation of consciousness and thinking activities and application of the spiritual idea.

管敬仲【guǎn jìng zhòng】　春秋初期杰出的政治家管子的另外一个称谓,其对气功学的发展有一定的贡献。其经典著作《管子》也介绍了气功学,论述了人体的精气,并提出了一些行之有效的功法。

Guan Jingzhong　Another name of

Guan Zi, a great politician in the initial stage of Spring and Autumn Period (770 BC－476 BC), who made certain contribution to the development of Qigong. In his great canon entitled *Guan Zi*, Qigong was introduced, essential Qi in the human body was described and the effective exercises were suggested.

管夷吾【guǎn yí wú】　春秋初期杰出的政治家管子的另外一个称谓,其对气功学的发展有一定的贡献。其经典著作《管子》也介绍了气功学,论述了人体的精气,并提出了一些行之有效的功法。

Guan Yiwu　Another name of Guan Zi, a great politician in the initial stage of Spring and Autumn Period (770 BC－476 BC), who made certain contribution to the development of Qigong. In his great canon entitled *Guan Zi*, Qigong was introduced, essential Qi in the human body was described and the effective exercises were suggested.

管仲【guǎn zhòng】　春秋初期杰出的政治家管子的另外一个称谓,其对气功学的发展有一定的贡献。其经典著作《管子》也介绍了气功学,论述了人体的精气,并提出了一些行之有效的功法。

Guan Zhong　Another name of Guan Zi, a great politician in the initial stage of Spring and Autumn Period (770 BC－476 BC), who made certain contribution to the development of Qigong. In his great canon entitled *Guan Zi*, Qigong was introduced, essential Qi in the human body was described and the effective exercises were suggested.

管子【guǎn zǐ】　春秋初期杰出的政治家,对气功学的发展有一定的贡献。其经典著作《管子》也介绍了气功学,论述了人体的精气,并提出了一些行之有效的功法。

Guan Zi A great politician in the initial stage of Spring and Autumn Period (770 BC – 476 BC), who made certain contribution to the development of Qigong. In his great canon entitled *Guan Zi*, Qigong was introduced, essential Qi in the human body was described and the effective exercises were suggested.

管子平正法【guǎn zǐ píng zhèng fǎ】为静功。其作法为,止怒用诗,去忧用乐,节乐用礼,守礼用敬,守敬用静。根据不同情性变化,应用不同的方法调节意识思维活动和行为。

Guan Zi's exercise for peace and calm A static exercise, marked by stopping rage with poems, eliminating anxiety with music, controlling joy with rite, keeping rite with esteem and keeping esteem with tranquility. Such a static can regulate the activities of consciousness and thinking with different ways according to the changes of temperament.

管子养生法【guǎn zǐ yǎng shēng fǎ】为静功。其作法为,存精养精,养气以和,守中抱一,效在安养形体,内守精神。

Guan Zi's exercise for nourishing life A static exercise, marked by keeping the essence and nourishing the essence, nourishing Qi for harmonization, keeping somatic and spiritual balance. Such a static exercise can nourish the body and keep the spirit inside.

灌溉中岳【guàn gài zhōng yuè】为动功。其作法为,用手指摩擦鼻部两旁至发热,有润肺,防治伤风感冒,去鼻疾的作用。

irrigation of the central mountain A dynamic exercise, marked by kneading and rubbing the lateral sides of the nose hot for moistening the lung. Such a dynamic exercise can prevent and cure common cold and nasal disease.

灌溉中州【guàn gài zhōng zhōu】为动功。其作法为,用手指摩擦鼻部两旁至发热,有润肺,防治伤风感冒,去鼻疾的作用。

irrigation of the central plains A dynamic exercise, marked by kneading and rubbing the lateral sides of the nose hot for moistening the lung. Such a dynamic exercise can prevent and cure common cold and nasal disease.

光明【guāng míng】足少阳胆经的一个穴位,位于外踝尖上 5 寸。这一穴位为气功运行的一个常见部位。

Guangming（SP 11） An acupoint in the gallbladder meridian of foot Shaoyang, located 5 Cun above the lateral malleolus. This acupoint is a region usually used for keeping the essential Qi in practice of Qigong.

光若玄【guāng ruò xuán】指发色黑而光亮,为脑中华。

supreme brightness Refers to the hair that is black but also bright, indicating the prosperity of the brain.

广成宫【guǎng chéng gōng】在河南汝州的山上,为气功学家广成子隐居处。

Guang Cheng Temple Located in a mountain in Ruzhou city in Henan Province, where Guang Chenzi, a great master of Qigong, lived in seclusion.

广成先生【guǎng chéng xiān shēng】唐代气功学家刘元靖的另外一个称谓,主要通过辟谷练气。

Mr. Guang Cheng Another name of Liu Yuanqing, who was a great master of Qigong in the Tang Dynasty（618 AD－907 AD）. He refined Qi only with inedibility.

广成子【guǎng chéng zǐ】 气功学家，据说是轩辕黄帝时期之人，重视养生之道。

Guang Chengzi A great master of Qigong who devoted much attention to the ways for cultivating life. According to the legendary story, he lived together with Yellow Emperor.

广成子解【guǎng chéng zǐ jiě】 《广成子解》是气功养身学专著，为北宋苏轼所撰，阐述修身、养生之道。

Guang Chen Zi Jie（*Explanation of Guang Chengzi*） Written by Su Shi, a great scholar and poet in the North Song Dynasty（960 AD－1279 AD）, mainly describing the ways for cultivating the body and nourishing the life.

广成子至道法【guǎng chéng zǐ zhì dào fǎ】 为功法，指认识气功的基本知识、调节意识思维活动、行功时的注意事项、功能作用。

Guang Chengzi's perfect method An exercise of Qigong practice, referring to the basic knowledge for practicing Qigong, regulating the activities of consciousness and thinking, paying attention to the practice of Qigong and the function of Qigong.

广寒【guǎng hán】 指月宫。气功文献说习练气功到一定时候，脑神清净无杂念，而延年益寿。

moon temple Refers to the palace of the moon. It is described in the literature of Qigong that the brain spirit is tranquilized and the life is prolonged

after practicing Qigong for a certain period of time.

广宁真人【guǎng níng zhēn rén】 金代气功学家郝大通的另外一个称谓，其撰写了多部气功专著。

famous immortal The celebration of Hao Datong, a great master of Qigong in the Jin Dynasty（1115 AD－1234 AD）, who wrote several monographs of Qigong.

广宁子【guǎng níng zǐ】 金代气功学家郝大通的另外一个称谓，其撰写了多部气功专著。

Guang Ningzi Another name of Hao Datong, a master of Qigong in the Jin Dynasty（1115 AD－1234 AD）, who wrote several monographs of Qigong.

归伏【guī fú】 指真人呼吸，神气蛰藏气穴而不散。

quiet entrance Refers to immortal respiration and entrance of spiritual Qi in the Qi point without any dispersion.

归复变化【guī fù biàn huà】 指精气神归藏于丹田之中，反复锤炼，化育为丹。

multiple purification Refers to returning the essence, Qi and spirit to Dantian and transforming into Dan（pills of immortality）after repeated practice. Dantian is divided into upper Dantian（the region between the eyes）, the middle Dantian（the region below the heart）and the lower Dantian（the region below the navel）.

归根复命【guī gēn fù mìng】 即神归神宅脑，气归气海膻中，亦说气归丹田。

returning to the original life Refers to the spirit returning to the brain and Qi returning to Tanzhong（CV 17）or Dantian. Dantian is divided into upper

Dantian (the region between the eyes), the middle Dantian (the region below the heart) and the lower Dantian (the region below the navel).

归根窍【guī gēn qiào】 ① 指"祖窍"的异名;② 指"下丹田"的异名。

root returning orifice Refers to ① either another synonym of Zuqiao which is an acupoint located in the area between the heart and the navel; ② or another synonym of the middle Dantian (the region below the navel).

归命于身中【guī mìng yú shēn zhōng】 指气功状态下,神运精气于身中。

distribution of life inside the body Refers to the fact that the spirit leads essence and Qi to the body in practicing Qigong.

归心寂静【guī xīn jì jìng】 指心静神守,弃除妄想杂念,则可以长寿。

tranquilized heart Refers to tranquilizing the heart and stabilizing the spirit, eliminating delusion and distracting thought in order to prolong life.

归一【guī yī】 指意识活动集中于一。

concentration Refers to concentration of consciousness activity.

归婴至道【guī yīng zhì dào】 指以手心或指按摩目下颧上,是返老还童之道。

the way for renewing youth Refers to pressing the cheekbone with palms or fingers in order to renew youth.

归正论【guī zhèng lùn】 源自气功专论,主要阐述真种与还丹,并提出归正的具体方法。

discussion about returning to the right way Collected from a monograph about Qigong, mainly describing truth and Huandan (mercury or immortality) and suggesting the method for returning to the right way.

归中【guī zhōng】 指丹田,亦指气穴。

centralization Refers to Dantian or Qi point. Dantian is divided into upper Dantian (the region between the eyes), the middle Dantian (the region below the heart) and the lower Dantian (the region below the navel).

龟鳖行气法【guī biē xíng qì fǎ】 为动功,方法多样。如坐地直舒两脚,以两手叉,挽两足自极。

turtle exercise for moving Qi A dynamic exercise with various methods, such as sitting on the ground, stretching the feet, crossing the hands and turning the feet naturally.

龟行气【guī xíng qì】 为静功,如龟一样呼吸。其作法为,藏身衣被之中,遮盖头面口鼻,正卧位,闭气不息九次,以鼻微缓出气,治大便不通。

turtle breath A static exercise, referring to respiration like that of a turtle, marked by lying on the right way, covering the body, head and face with quilt, stopping respiration for nine times and exhaling mildly through the nose in order to cure constipation.

龟蛇相缠【guī shé xiāng chán】 即神气相抱。龟指命,指气;蛇指神,指性。

combination of turtle and snake Refers to combination of the spirit and Qi. In this term turtle refers to life and Qi while snake refers to the spirit and nature.

龟息记【guī xī jì】 为气功故事,通过龟的方式说明自然运动的规律。

record of turtle respiration A story about Qigong, describing the natural ways to practice Qigong.

规中【guī zhōng】 指脐。

umbilical region　Refers to navel.

规中守一说【guī zhōng shǒu yī shuō】
源自气功专论《了三得一经》,主要阐述
上药三品,神于气精和合为一之说,即神
凝精气聚而作丹的道理。

idea about protecting navel in umbilical region　Collected from a monograph of Qigong entitled Liaosan Deyi Jing or *Canon of Understanding Three and Obtaining One*, mainly describing three grades of medicinal, indicating combination of the spirit with Qi and spirit, referring to the principle for coagulating the spirit with the essence and Qi in order to produce Dan (pills of immortality).

规中直指元关说【guī zhōng zhí zhǐ yuán guān shuō】　源自气功专论《了三得一经》,主要阐述调身体阴阳以保持神形稳定的道理。

idea about umbilical region directly aiming at the original joint　Collected from a monograph of Qigong entitled Liaosan Deyi Jing or *Canon of Understanding Three and Obtaining One*, mainly describing and regulating the body and Yin and Yang in order to stabilize the spirit and the body.

闺房【guī fáng】　指脑。

boudoir　Refers to the brain.

鬼谷子胎息诀【guǐ gǔ zi tāi xī jué】
为静功口诀,即"故炼心为神,炼精为形,炼气为命,此是阴阳升降之气也"。

Gui Guzi's formula for fetal respiration
A static exercise, marked by "refining the heart for nourishing the spirit, refining the essence for nourishing the body, refining Qi for nourishing life", indicating the condition of Qi during the ascent and descent of Yin and Yang".

鬼井【guǐ jǐng】　为人中的异名。

ghost well　The synonym of Renzhong (the region below the nose and above the lip).

鬼神之情【guǐ shén zhī qíng】　指阴阳两方面的变化情况。

affection of the ghost and spirit　Refers to two ways of changes in Yin and Yang.

癸水之脏【guǐ shuǐ zhī zàng】　指肾脏,五行中肾属水,故称癸水。

viscus of Gui water　Refers to the kidney. In the five elements (including wood, fire, earth, metal and water) the kidney pertains to water. That is why the kidney is called Gui water. The so-called Gui is the tenth Heavenly Stem.

贵生【guì shēng】　指以生命为贵,亦养生。气功中讲究耳目鼻口,不得擅行,必有所制,返朴归真,顺应自然。

treasuring life　Refers to the importance of life, also referring to cultivation of life. In Qigong practice, great attention must be paid to the ears, eyes, nose and mouth which cannot be moved arbitrarily. Practitioners must return to nature and follow the natural principles.

贵一【guì yī】　指以一为贵。因一生二,一中含阴阳两个方面,是万物生发之母。

treasuring one　Refers to the importance of one because one produces two and one contains both Yin and Yang. Thus one is the mother all the things in the universe.

跪坐【guì zuò】　为导引坐势之一,指两膝着地,臀部放在脚跟上。

sitting on knees One of the sitting styles in practicing Qigong, referring to kneeling on the ground and pressing the heels with the buttocks.

郭真人胎息诀【guō zhēn rén tāi xī jué】 为静功口诀，重在定心养神，以高度集中精神意识思维活动为修养大法。

immortal Guo's formula for fetal respiration A static exercise, paying great attention to the tranquilization of the heart and cultivation of the spirit, regarding concentration of the activities of the spirit, consciousness and thought as the great exercise for cultivating life.

腘【guó】 指膝关节的后方。

popliteal space Popliteal space refers to the posterior side of the knee-joint.

果园【guǒ yuán】 即达到理想境界。

result cycle Refers to the ideal state.

过三关说【guò sān guān shuō】 源自气功专论，主要阐述习练气功时大要发生，气动三关时的感受和意念导引过三关的方法。

discussion about crossing the triple pass Connected from a monograph of Qigong, mainly describing production of medicinal in practicing Qigong, experience of Qi crossing the triple pass and the method of mental Daoyin through the triple pass.

H

海蟾真人胎息诀【hǎi chán zhēn rén tāi xī jué】 为静功,以守神于丹田,调气微微出入,使心与神气相合。

immortal Hai Chan's formula for fetal respiration A static exercise, referring to keeping the spirit in Dantian, mildly regulating inhalation and exhalation in order to balance the heart with the spirit and Qi. Dantian is divided into the upper Dantian (the region between the eyes), the middle Dantian (the region below the heart) and the lower Dantian (the region below the navel).

海蟾子【hǎi chán zǐ】 宋代气功实践家,常将自己进行气功锻炼的体会和练功方法写成诗文。

Hai Chanzi An important practitioner of Qigong in the Song Dynasty (960 AD‐1279 AD), who summarized his experiences of Qigong practice in poems.

海琼传道集【hǎi qióng chuán dào jí】 《海琼传道集》为气功学专著,由宋代洪知常集,主张凝气、聚神、绝念。

Haiqiong Chuandao Ji (*Collection of Propagating Daoism in the South Sea*) A monograph of Qigong entitled *Collection of Propagating Daoism in the South Sea*, written by Hong Zhichang in the Song Dynasty (960 AD‐1279 AD), emphasizing concentration of Qi, accumulation of the spirit and elimination of desires.

海琼子【hǎi qióng zǐ】 宋代气功学家

白玉蟾(1194—1229)的另外一个称谓。

Hai Qigongzi Another name of Bai Yuchan, a great master of Qigong in the Song Dynasty (960 AD‐1279 AD).

海源【hǎi yuán】 指肾,肾主水,为水之源。

sea source Refers to the kidney which controls water and is the source of water.

亥子中间【hài zǐ zhōng jiān】 指天人合发之机。亥为阴尽,子为阳生,即阴尽阳生之际。

center of Hai and Zi Center of Hai (the period of a day from 21 p. m. to 23 p. m. in the evening) and Zi (the period of a day from 11 p. m. to 1 a. m. at night) is a term of Qigong, referring to the time that the sky and human beings are combined with each other. In this term, Hai (the period of a day from 21 p. m. to 23 p. m. in the vening) refers to exhaustion of Yin and Zi (the period of a day from 11 p. m. to 1 a. m. at night) refers to production of Yang.

含光【hán guāng】 指精神内守,神形清静。

containing brightness Means to internally concentrate the spirit and to tranquilize the spirit and the body.

含精养神【hán jīng yǎng shén】 指人体内精与神互依,精盈而神足,精神内藏,则充养一身。

enriching the essence and nourishing the spirit A term of Qigong, referring to coordination of the essence and the spirit that ensures sufficiency of the essence and the spirit, and internal storage of the essence and the spirit that enriches and nourishes the whole body.

含气养精口如朱【hán qì yǎng jīng kǒu rú zhū】 指习练气功,含气养精,形体康健。

To enrich Qi and nourish essence will make the mouth bright red. This is a celebrated dictum, referring to enriching Qi, nourishing essence and cultivating health in practicing Qigong.

函三【hán sān】 指调节三丹田之气合而为一。

three cases A term of Qigong, referring to integration of Qi from three ways of Dantian. Dantian is divided into the upper Dantian (the region between the eyes), the middle Dantian (the region below the heart) and the lower Dantian (the region below the navel).

涵养本原【hán yǎng běn yuán】 指精神出而收之于内,荣养脑神。

origin of self-restraint A term of Qigong, indicating that the spirit produced is kept inside the body to nourish the brain spirit.

涵养本源法【hán yǎng běn yuán fǎ】 为静功,可通过调身、调气、调神以补脑安神,协调形神,调节五脏六腑功能,疏通经络,培补元阴元阳。

exercise for nourishing the origin A static exercise, indicating that regulation of the body, Qi and the spirit can tonify the brain, stabilize the spirit, coordinate the body and spirit, regulate the functions of the five Zang-organs (including the heart, the liver, the spleen, the lung and the kidney) and the six Fu-organs (including the gallbladder, the stomach, the small intestine, the large intestine, the bladder and the triple energizer), dredging the meridians and collaterals, cultivating and tonifying the original Yin and original Yang.

韩湘子存气【hán xiāng zǐ cún qì】 为动功。其作法为,身体盘膝端坐,先以两手擦两眼,然两手拄两胁,行功运气,引气上升,运气二十四口。

Han Xiangzi's exercise for keeping Qi A dynamic exercise, marked by sitting with crossed legs, rubbing the eyes with both hands, pressing the rib-sides with both hands, raising Qi and moving Qi for twenty-four times.

寒痹【hán bì】 即痛痹,为气功适应证,由风寒湿邪侵袭肢节、经络所致。

cold impediment The same as pain impediment, is an indication of Qigong, referring to cold impediment caused by invasion of pathogenic cold and dampness into the limb joints, meridians and collaterals.

寒劲子【hán jìn zǐ】 清代气功家、养生家田绵淮的另外一个称谓。

Han Jinzi Another name of Tian Jinhuai, a great master of Qigong and life cultivation in the Qing Dynasty (1636 AD - 1912 AD).

寒露九月节座功【hán lù jiǔ yuè jié zuò gōng】 为动功。其作法为,每日丑寅时(一至五时)正坐,举两臂,踊身上托,左右各三五次,叩齿、吐纳、咽液。治风寒湿邪所致百病。

sitting exercise in September for cold dew

A dynamic exercise, marked by sitting in Chou (the period of a day from 1 a.m. to 3 a.m. in the early morning) and Yin (the period of a day from 3 a.m. to 5 a.m. in the early morning), raising both shoulders, jumping up the body from the left to the right for three to five times respectively, clicking the teeth, exhaling the old, inhaling the new and swallowing humor. Such a dynamic exercise can cure various diseases caused by pathogenic wind, cold and dampness.

寒热厥候导引法【hán rè jué hòu dǎo yǐn fǎ】 为静功。其作法为,正身仰卧,伸展两脚,吸气至极,然后慢慢呼出,两脚左右摇动三十次,通经络,和阴阳,治脚寒厥逆。

exercise of Daoyin for cold-heat syncope A static exercise, marked by lying on the back, stretching the feet, breathing in to the utmost point, slowly breathing out, shaking the feet from the left to the right and vice versa for thirty times respectively. Such a static exercise can dredge the meridians and collaterals, harmonize Yin and Yang, and cure foot cold and reversal cold.

寒疝【hán shàn】 为气功适应证,多因下焦元气不足,风冷寒邪客于肝肾经脉,阴寒凝聚,气滞血瘀所致。

cold hernia An indication of Qigong, usually caused by insufficiency of original Qi in the lower energizer, invasion of pathogenic wind and cold into the liver and kidney meridians, agglomeration of Yin coldness, Qi stagnation and blood stasis.

寒疝候导引法【hán shàn hòu dǎo yǐn fǎ】 为动功。其作法为,屈膝如坐,两

手抬脚,两腿尽量向两侧展开。理气止痛,治气冲部位肿痛、寒疝。

exercise of Daoyin for cold hernia A dynamic exercise, marked by sitting with bent knees, lifting the feet and trying to spread at both sides with both hands. Such a dynamic exercise can regulate Qi to stop pain and cure swelling pain and cold hernia in Qichong (LR 14).

汉钟离【hàn zhōng lí】 为唐代气功学家,传说为八仙之一。

Han Zhongli A great master of Qigong in the Tang Dynasty (618 AD – 907 AD) and one of the eight immortals according to the legendary story.

颔【hàn】 ① 指下颔以下,喉结以上之颈的前上部;② 指点头;③ 指静功调身姿势,颔宜内向。

chin Refers to ① either the region below the lower jaw and above the Adam's apple; ② or nodding; ③ or the way to regulate the body with static exercise.

颔厌【hàn yàn】 为足少阳胆经中的一个穴位,位于鬓发中,为气功中常用的意守部位。

Hanyan (GB 4) An acupoint in the gallbladder meridian of foot Shaoyang, located in earlock, which is the region for concentrating consciousness in practicing Qigong.

沆瀣【hàng xiè】 冬日夜半,水气方凝,清露时刻。

coagulation of water Refers to congealing water with clear dew at midnight in winter.

郝大通【hǎo dà tōng】 金代气功学家,撰写了多部气功专著。

Hao Datong A master of Qigong in the

Jin Dynasty （1115 AD – 1234 AD），who wrote several monographs of Qigong.

浩然得意【hào rán dé yì】　为古代调神的方法之一,任情志放逸而不滞郁。

overwhelming and complacency　One of the ways to regulate the spirit in ancient China，referring to natural emotion without any stagnation.

浩然之气【hào rán zhī qì】　指正气,喻作气功,调呼吸,炼真气。

healthy Qi　Means to regulate respiration and to refine genuine Qi in practicing Qigong.

皓华【hào huá】　即肺神之称。

luminous magnitude　Refers to the lung spirit.

灏气门【hào qì mén】　即下丹田。

boundless Qi gate　Refers to the lower Dantian（the region below the navel）.

合背坐【hé bèi zuò】　为气功治法之一,即气功医师与患者对背而坐,应用导引法治疗,合坐四十九夜而愈。

back to back sitting　One of the treatment method in Qigong，marked by doctor and patient sitting back to back to treat consumptive disease through practicing Qigong. Only sitting together in the same way for forty-nine nights can the disease be finally cured.

合二而一【hé èr ér yī】　指世间一切事物都由阴阳双方和合而成。气功文献中,常用以说明神运精气合而成丹。

integration of two　Refers to all things in this world produced by integration of Yin and Yang. In the literature of Qigong, it usually emphasizes that spiritual transmission of the essence and Qi has formed Dan（pills of immortality）.

合谷【hé gǔ】　为手阳明大肠经中的一个穴位,位于第一与第二掌骨之间。这一穴位为气功运行的一个常见部位。

Hegu（LI 4）　An acupoint in the large intestine meridian of hand Yangming，located in the region between the first metacarpusand the second metacarpus. This acupoint is a region usually used for keeping the essential Qi in practice of Qigong.

合眸固关【hé móu gù guān】　为气功的一种调神方法。

combination of eyes and consolidation of joints　A term of Qigong，referring to the method of regulating the spirit in practicing Qigong.

合三以一【hé sān yǐ yī】　① 指三丹田之气合二为一;② 指精气神合二为一。

integration of three　Refers to ① either integration of Qi from three kinds of Dantian；② or integration of the essence，Qi and the spirit. Dantian is divided into the upper Dantian（the region between the eyes），the middle Dantian（the region below the heart）and the lower Dantian（the region below the navel）.

合十【hé shí】　即合掌,为佛家敬礼之一。习练气功时,常出现此动作。

integration of ten　Refers to clasping the hands which is one of the salutes in Buddhism，usually occurring in practicing Qigong.

合一成基【hé yī chéng jī】　指精、气、神三者合而为一,筑固根基。

integrated base　Refers to integration of the essence，Qi and the spirit in order to consolidate the foundation.

合一大药【hé yī dà yào】　指身体神形合一,阴平阳秘。

integration of one large medicinal　Refers to integration of the spirit and body in practicing Qigong in order to make Yin stable and yang compact.

合阴阳顺道法【hé yīn yáng shùn dào fǎ】 为静功。其作法为，① 旦时著席，仰卧；② 指鼻吸鼻呼（通风），呼吸出入之气，温润绵绵；③ 指闭目，意想自己彬彬有礼的形貌。

exercise of following the way of Yin and Yang A static exercise, referring to ① either lying on the back over the bed in the morning; ② or inhaling and exhaling through the nose to moisten the body; ③ or closing the eyes to imagine ceremonious style.

合掌【hé zhǎng】 为佛家敬礼之一。习练气功时，常出现此动作。

clasping hands Refers to one of the salutes in Buddhism, usually occurring in practicing Qigong.

合真【hé zhēn】 指气功中，神形相互作用，相顾、相并、相入、相抱，逐步进入俱妙、双舍的境界。

combination of truth Mutual effect of the spirit and the body in practicing Qigong, indicating mutual support, mutual combination, mutual entrance and mutual embrace, eventually leading to wonderful and dedicated state.

何仙姑【hé xiān gū】 为八仙之一，唐代特殊人物，其胎息诀颇有影响。

He Xiangu One of the eight immortals, a special immortal in the Tang Dynasty (618 AD－907 AD) whose fetal respiration exercise greatly influenced many people.

何仙姑胎息诀【hé xiān gū tāi xī jué】 为静口诀，强调练功以精气神为主，息气本源以清净真气为主。

He Xiangu's formula for fetal respiration A static exercise, emphasizing the importance of essence, Qi and spirit in practicing Qigong and the tranquil genuine Qi as the foundation of respiration.

何仙姑簪花【hé xiān gū zān huā】 为静功。其作法为，身体端坐，两手抱头行功运气十七口。

He Xiangus' flower arrangement A static exercise, marked by sitting upright and holding the head with both hands to circulate Qi for seventeen times.

和合聚集【hé hé jù jí】 指神气和合，凝聚而为一。

Harmonic concentration Refers to integration of the spirit and Qi.

和合四象【hé hé sì xiàng】 四象即青龙、白虎、朱雀、玄武。青龙于脏为肝，开窍于目、藏魂；白虎于脏为肺，开窍于鼻，藏魄；朱雀于脏为心，开窍于舌，藏神；玄武于脏为肾，开窍于耳，藏精。和合指精、神、魂、魄谐调于中央。

coordination of four images A term of Qigong, in which the four images refer to Qinglong, Baihu, Zhuque and Xuanwu. Qinglong refers to the liver, opening the eyes and storing the ethereal soul; Baihu refers to the lung, opening the nose and storing the corporeal soul; Zhuque refers to the heart, opening the tongue and storing the spirit; Xuanwu refers to the kidney, opening the ears and storing the essence. In this term, coordination refers to concentration of the essence, the spirit, the ethereal soul and the corporeal soul into the center of the body.

和髎【hé liáo】 为手少阳三焦经中的一个穴位，即耳和髎，位于耳门前上方。这一穴位为气功运行的一个常见部位。

Heliao（TE 22） An acupoint in the tri-

H

ple energizer meridian of hand Shao-yang, also called Erheliao (TE 22), located in the upper part of the ear portal. This acupoint is a region usually used for keeping the essential Qi in practice of Qigong.

和乃无一和【hé nǎi wú yī hé】 指和一则全身各部皆和。

Harmony means complete integration. This is a celebrated dictum, indicating that integration of one part will enable all the parts in the body to be integrated.

和气【hé qì】 指自然阴阳调和之气。

harmonic Qi Refers to natural regulation of Qi in Yin and Yang.

和气汤【hé qì tāng】 为静功。作法为先"忍",后"忘",治一切怒气、客气和抑郁不平。

harmonious decoction A static exercise, marked by tolerating first and forgetting later in practicing Qigong in order to relieve annoyance, pathogenic factors and depression.

和三气法【hé sān qì fǎ】 为静功。其作法为,意想中和之道,调节太阴、太阳,合三归一,阴阳相得。久行之,太平中和,养性延年。

exercise for harmonizing three Qi A static exercise, marked by imagining harmony, regulating Taiyin and Taiyang, integrating three into one and coordinating Yin and Yang. Long time of practicing Qigong in such a way can pacify and harmonize the body, cultivate health and prolong life.

和神导气法【hé shén dǎo qì fǎ】 为静功。其作法为,在一间安静舒适的室内,关好门,安置床铺寒温适中,枕高二寸半,身体平正地仰卧于床上,轻轻闭上眼,吸入的气停于胸脯,约三百次呼吸的时间,耳听不到声音,眼看不到东西,心内安宁无思念。

exercise for harmonizing the spirit and regulating Qi A static exercise, marked by closing the gate of the clean and quiet room, normally warming the bed, selecting a pillow of two and half Cun, lying on the back, mildly closing the eyes and inhaling Qi into the chest for about three hundred times. In such a way of practicing Qigong, the ears will not listen to any sound and the eyes will not see anything and the heart will be tranquilized without any thinking.

和谐【hé xié】 指习练气功,在脾意的作用下,心肾相交,水合既济,一身协调稳定。

harmony A term of Qigong, referring to combination of the heart and the spirit, balance of water, and regulation and stability of the body under the influence of the spleen function in practicing Qigong.

和制魂魄【hé zhì hún pò】 指和合肝肺之神,使之协调平秘。

harmonic control of the ethereal soul and corporeal soul Refers to integration of the spirit from the liver and the lung.

河车【hé chē】 ① 指正气、肾气;② 指任脉、督脉。

river cart Refers to ① either healthy Qi and kidney Qi; ② or conception meridian and governor meridian.

河车初动【hé chē chū dòng】 为静功。其作法为,每日先静一时,待身心都安定,气息都和平,始将双目微闭,垂帘观照心下肾上一寸三分之间,不即不离,勿忘勿助,万念俱泯,一灵独存,谓之正念。

primary movement of river cart　A static exercise, marked by tranquilizing for a whole every day, stabilizing the heart, balancing respiration, mildly closing the eyes, lowering the head to observe the 1 Cun and 3 Fen region between the heart and the kidney, keeping tranquility, sincerity and and purity.

河车路【hé chē lù】　指督脉。

way of river cart　Refers to the governor meridian.

河车真动法【hé chē zhēn dòng fǎ】为静功。其作法为, 微微凝照, 守于中宫, 自有无尽生机, 行之一月、二月, 神益静, 静久则气益生。

exercise for real movement of river cart　A static exercise, marked by mildly concentrating mentality in the middle chamber, moving for one or two months with unrestrained vitality, and tranquilizing the spirit to promote Qi.

河上公养神八法【hé shàng gōng yǎng shén bā fǎ】　为静功。其作法为, 行无为、少言语、守五性、内照视、顺天时、专一志、却液昧、去情欲。

He Shanggong's eight methods for cultivating the spirit　A static exercise, marked by performing inactivity, speaking less, keeping five properties (keeping Qi from the five Zang-organs, including the heart, the liver, the spleen, the lung and the kidney), observing the internal organs, following the celestial principles, concentrating the will, eliminating abnormal humor and expelling passion. He Shanggong was the real recluse in ancient China.

河上公治身八法【hé shàng gōng zhì shēn bā fǎ】　为静功。其作法为, 爱气、调气、定静、归神、养德、行无为、去欲、固精。

He Shanggong's eight methods for curing the body　A static exercise, marked by loving Qi, regulating Qi, tranquilizing mind, returning to the spirit, cultivating morality, performing inactivity, eliminating desires and stabilizing the essence. He Shanggong was the real recluse in ancient China.

河图洛书【hé tú luò shū】　为华夏文化的源头。气功文献常引用河图洛书论述五行生克。

Hetu and Luoshu (the ancient Chinese mythological fiction)　The origins of the traditional Chinese civilization and culture. In the literature of Qigong, the mutual promotion and restriction among the five elements (including wood, fire, earth, metal and water) are often analyzed according to Hetu and Luoshu (the ancient Chinese mythological fiction).

核骨【hé gǔ】　① 指足外踝;② 指第一跖趾关节内侧圆形突起。

kernel bone　Refers to ① either lateral malleolus; ② or prominence of the interior circular form of the metatarsal bone and phalanx.

颔【hé】　指耳下骨, 即颔骨支。

jaw　Refers to the bone below the ears, indicating ramus of jaw.

阖辟【hé pì】　① 指呼吸的开合作用;② 指阴阳及其相互作用;③ 指乾坤。

closing and opening　Refers to ① either harmonization of inhalation and exhalation; ② or mutual effects of Yin and Yang; ③ or Qian Trigram and Kun

H

Trigram.

赫赤内景【hè chì nèi jǐng**】** 为静功。其作法为,于夏历每月九日在清净的室内静坐,排除一切杂念,叩齿三十六通,意想从太阳上降下火红色的云,慢慢形成座桥。

imagining internal state A static exercise, marked by sitting in a quiet and clear room on ninth in every month in summer, eliminating all distracting thought, clicking the teeth for thirty-six times, imagining to descend red and hot cloud from the sun to slowly form a bridge.

黑白【hēi bái**】** 指阴阳两个方面。气功中常指金水相生而成丹。

black and white A term of Qigong, referring to Yin and Yang. In Qigong, it refers to mutual promotion of metal and water that produces Dan（pills of immortality）.

黑肠【hēi cháng**】** 为膀胱。

black intestine Refers to the bladder.

黑汞红铅【hēi gǒng hóng qiān**】** 指真阴真阳交相会合,结为一体。

black mercury and red lead Refers to combination and integration of genuine Yin and genuine Yang.

黑龟【hēi guī**】** ① 即白虎,指二十八宿中西方的七宿;② 内丹书中指"心中元神谓之龙,肾中元精谓之虎"。

black tortoise The same as white tiger, refers to ① either the seven constellations in the west among the twenty-eight constellations; ② or "the original spirit in the heart called Loong and the original essence in the kidney called tiger" mentioned in the books about internal Dan（pills of immortality）.

黑虎【hēi hǔ**】** 即白虎,① 指二十八宿

中西方的七宿;② 内丹书中指"心中元神谓之龙,肾中元精谓之虎"。

black tiger The same as white tiger, refers to ① either the seven constellations in the west among the twenty-eight constellations; ② or "the original spirit in the heart called Loong and the original essence in the kidney called tiger" mentioned in the books about internal Dan（pills of immortality）.

黑铅【hēi qiān**】** 即白虎,① 指二十八宿中西方的七宿;② 内丹书中指"心中元神谓之龙,肾中元精谓之虎"。

black lead The same as white tiger, refers to ① either the seven constellations in the west among the twenty-eight constellations; ② or "the original spirit in the heart called Loong and the original essence in the kidney called tiger" mentioned in the books about internal Dan（pills of immortality）.

黑中有白【hēi zhōng yǒu bái**】** 指肾阴中有真阳。

white within black Refers to genuine Yang within kidney Yin.

恒山【héng shān**】** 在河北曲阳,古代传说中的八仙之一张果老曾在此修道。

Hengshan Mountain Located in the Quyang County in Hebei Province. It was said in ancient China that Zhang Guolao, one of the eight immortals, studied and developed Daoism in this mountain.

横骨【héng gǔ**】** ① 指耻骨上支、耻骨联合;② 指舌骨;③ 指经穴名,属足少阴肾经,位于耻骨联合上旁开 0.5 寸处。

transverse bone Refers to ① either the upper part of the pubic bone and pubic symphysis; ② or the hyoid bone; ③ or Henggu（KI 11）, which is an acupoint in the kidney meridian of foot Shaoyin, located 0.5 Cun lateral to the upper part of pubic symphysis.

横理【héng lǐ】 指脾。脾横在身体中，故叫横理。

transverse texture Refers to the spleen because the spleen is located transversely in the body.

骱骨【héng gǔ】 小腿胫、腓骨之统称。

tibia The general designation of the shank of the calf and fibula.

衡山【héng shān】 湖南衡山，为唐代初司马承祯修道之处。

Hengshan Mountain Located in the Hengshan County in Hunan Province, where Sima Chengzhen in the Tang Dynasty studied and practiced Daoism.

红炉点雪【hóng lú diǎn xuě】《红炉点雪》为中医学专著，为明代龚居中著，主要论述痰火病防治及阐述养生之法，强调守丹田对延年却病的重要性。

Honglu Dianxue（*Putting Snow into Hot Stove*） A traditional Chinese medicine monograph entitled *Putting Snow into Hot Stove*, written by Gong Juzhong in the Ming Dynasty（1368 AD – 1644 AD）. It mainly describes prevention and treatment of phlegm fire disease and cultivation of health, emphasizing concentration of Dantian and importance of preventing disease for prolonging life. Dantian is divided into the upper Dantian（the region between the eyes）, the middle Dantian（the region below the heart）and the lower Dantian（the region below the navel）.

洪炉上一点雪【hóng lú shàng yì diǎn xuě】 为静功。其作法为，卷舌以舐悬雍垂，但行之数日间，舌下筋微急痛，当以渐训至。

a little snow in the firing stove A static exercise, marked by rolling the tongue to lap the uvula gradually for several days if the sinews below the tongue are painful.

洪元先生【hóng yuán xiān shēng】 指的是唐代气功学家王玄览，其撰写了多部气功专著，深入研究了气功的理论和方法。

Mr. Hong Yuan Refers to Wang Xuanlan, a great master of Qigong in the Tang Dynasty（618 AD - 907 AD）. He wrote several monographs of Qigong, thoroughly studying and analyzing the theory and methods of Qigong.

鸿蒙养心法【hóng méng yǎng xīn fǎ】 为动功，指调节精神意识思维活动，处无为之道；行功时注意"无问其名，无窥其情，物固自生气"。

exercise of primordial state for nourishing the heart A dynamic exercise, referring to either regulating the activities of the spirit, consciousness and thinking without any desires; or "avoiding the name and emotion of oneself and clearing the natural formation of Qi in all the things" in practicing Qigong.

侯道玄望空设拜【hóu dào xuán wàng kōng shè bài】 为动静相兼功。其作法为，八字站立，低头于胸前，两手相抱子腹下，用功行气十七口。主治前后心疼。

Hou Daoxuan's exercise for bending and embracing An exercise combined with dynamic exercise and static exercise, marked by standing like the form of the Chinese character eight, lowering the head to the chest, holding the abdomen with both hands and moving Qi with the exercise of Qigong for seventeen times. Such an exercise combined with dynamic exercise and static exercise can cure heartache.

喉痹【hóu bì】 为气功学适应证,多因外感风热或阴亏火旺,虚火上炎所致。

throat impediment An indication of Qigong, usually caused by external contraction of wind heat, or blazing fire due to depletion of Yin, or flaming up of deficiency fire.

喉痹候导引法【hóu bì hòu dǎo yǐn fǎ】为动功,方法多样。如两手托两颊而不动,两肘紧靠身体,腰部用力伸直,然后两肘向外抬,使两肋向外,疏散肘肩腰部之气,至极限时止,反复作七遍。利咽喉,治喉痹。

exercise of Daoyin for throat impediment A dynamic exercise with various methods, such as pulling the cheeks with both hands in the stationary way, adjoining the elbows at the body, stretching the waist; then raising the elbows laterally, ultimately scattering Qi from the elbows, shoulders and waist for seven times. Such a dynamic exercise can profit the throat and treat throat impediment.

喉舌治法【hóu shé zhì fǎ】 为动功,方法多样。如一手长伸,手掌向上;一手握住下颌向外拉,连续尽力作十四次,左右相同。然后手不动,头向左右两侧尽量转侧,作快速牵拉动作十四次。

exercise for curing throat and tongue A dynamic exercise with various methods, such as stretching out one hand, raising the palm and holding the mandible with the other hand to haul down and vice versa for fourteen times respectively; then stopping moving the hands and quickly turning the head to the left and the right for fourteen times respective-ly.

喉息【hóu xī】 为较浅的呼吸。

throat breath Refers to shallow breath.

后门【hòu mén】 即七门,指身有七门,即泥丸为天门,尾闾为地门,夹脊为中门,明堂为前门,玉枕为后门,重楼为楼门,绛宫为房门。

back gate The same of seven gates, referring to the mud bolus (the brain) known as celestial gate, coccyx known as earthly gate, back and waist known as middle gate, nose known as front gate, posterior hairline known as back gate, trachea as building gate and precordium known as house gate.

后曲【hòu qǔ】 为足少阳胆经穴位瞳子髎的另外一个称谓,位于目外眦外侧0.5寸。

Houqu A synonym of Tongziliao (GB 1) which is an acupoint in the gallbladder meridian of foot Shaoyang, located 0.5 Cun lateral to the outer canthus.

后三骨【hòu sān gǔ】 ① 指枕外隆凸;② 指玉枕关,属于足太阳膀胱经,位于后发际正中直上2.5寸,此穴位为气功习练之处。

three backward bones Refers to ① either external occipital protuberance; ② or Yuzhen (BL 9), which is an acupoint in the bladder meridian of foot Taiayng, located 2.5 Cun directly above the midline in the hairline. This acupoint is a region usually used in practice of Qigong.

后三三【hòu sān sān】 ① 指下关、中关和上关;② 指尾闾、夹脊和玉枕。

backward three and three Refers to ① either the lower segment, the middle segment and the upper segment;

② or coccyx，Jiaji point located in the spine and Yuzhen（BL 9）.

后天【hòu tiān**】** 指太极，分阴分阳之时际。

previous sky Refers to the supreme pole during which Yin and Yang were separated.

后天气【hòu tiān qì**】** 指呼吸自然之气。

late weather Refers to respiration with natural air.

后弦【hòu xián**】** 即下弦，为二十三日月象，此时阳中阴半。

backward quarter Refers to last quarter，indicating the manifestations of the moon in twenty-three days during which half of Yang is Yin.

厚重【hòu zhòng**】** 指稳定、稳重。

messiness Refers to stability and steadiness.

候【hòu**】** ① 指五日；② 指时候。

Hou Hou refers to ① either a period of five days；② or the time.

候真人胎息诀【hòu zhēn rén tāi xī jué**】** 为静功口诀。"本源者，则是心也。不动不行，心则是源；不停不住，源则是心。其心清净，则成大药；其心惑乱，则成大贼。"

Immortal Hou's formula for fetal respiration A static exercise. "The origin of the body is the heart. No movement and immobility and inactivity indicate that the heart is the origin while continuous movement and activity indicate that the origin is the heart. When the heart is tranquilized，large medicinal is produced；when the heart is confused，large thief is produced."

呼吸出入【hū xī chū rù**】** 指气功中呼浊吸清，吐故纳新，平秘阴阳，和调脏腑

的功能。

inhibition and exhalation A term of Qigong，referring to exhaling turbid Qi and inhaling clear Qi，exhaling the old and inhaling the new，balancing Yin and Yang，and harmonizing the functions of the five Zang-organs（including the heart，the liver，the spleen，the lung and the kidney）and the six Fu-organs（including the gallbladder，the stomach，the small intestine，the large intestine，the bladder and the triple energizer）.

呼吸导引【hū xī dǎo yǐn**】** 指气功调气、调身，为呼吸与动作配合的功法。

exercise of Daoyin for respiration A term of Qigong，referring to regulation of Qi and the body in practicing Qigong，which is the way for combination of respiration and activity.

呼吸精气【hū xī jīng qì**】** 指选择幽静的环境，调节呼吸，吸收最精纯的洁气，以达益气养生之目的。

respiration of essential Qi A term of Qigong，referring to selecting a quiet environment， regulating respiration and inhaling the purest clear Qi to enrich Qi and nourish the body in practicing Qigong.

呼吸卢间【hū xī lú jiān**】** 指意识作用下神气相合，呼吸之气以归黄庭。

respiration in chamber A term of Qigong，referring to combination of the spirit and Qi and Qi from respiration entering Huangting（the region below the navel）.

呼吸微徐【hū xī wēi xú**】** 指气息均匀，不粗不疾。

mild respiration Refers to normal breath without any changes.

H

呼吸元气【hū xī yuán qì】 指呼吸天地阴阳四时五行之气。

inhaling original Qi A term of Qigong, referring to Qi related to inhalation and exhalation, the sky and the earth, Yin and Yang, the four seasons and the five elements (including wood, fire, earth, metal and water).

呼吸元气以求仙法【hū xī yuán qì yǐ qiú xiān fǎ】 即封固牢藏法。

respiration of original Qi in order to receive immortal exercise Refers to the way to protect the body, to solidify the essence, to straighten Qi and to store the spirit.

胡德文【hú dé wén】 为明代文人胡文焕的另外一个称谓,其对气功养生颇有研究,著有专著,对指导习练气功、推广运用气功治病起到了积极作用。

Hu Dewen Another name of Hu Wenhuan, a great literati in the Ming Dynasty (1368 AD - 1644 AD) who also well studied Qigong and life cultivation and wrote a monograph of Qigong to contribute a great deal to the practice and development of Qigong.

胡东邻运化阴阳【hú dōng lín yùn huà yīn yáng】 为静功口诀。本口诀为右侧卧式睡功口诀。按此口诀习练治疗失眠、多梦、梦游等症。

Hu Donglin's regulation of Yin and Yang A static formula marked by lying on the right side for curing insomnia, dreaminess and sleepwalking.

胡跪【hú guì】 指膝跪地的练功姿势。

kneeling posture A term of Qigong, referring to kneeling on the ground to practice Qigong.

胡全庵【hú quán ān】 明代文人胡文焕的另外一个称谓,其对气功养生颇有研究,著有专著,对指导习练气功、推广运用气功治病起到了积极作用。

Hu Quan'an Another name of Hu Wenhuan, a great literati in the Ming Dynasty (1368 AD - 1644 AD) who also well studied Qigong and life cultivation and wrote a monograph of Qigong to contribute a great deal to the practice and development of Qigong.

胡文焕【hú wén huàn】 明代文人,对气功养生颇有研究,著有专著,对指导习练气功、推广运用气功治病起到了积极作用。

Hu Wenhuan A great literati in the Ming Dynasty (1368 AD - 1644 AD) who also well studied Qigong and life cultivation and wrote a monograph of Qigong to contribute a great deal to the practice and development of Qigong.

胡愔【hú yīn】 为唐代女气功学家,撰写了气功专著,对后世气功学的发展有一定的影响。

Hu Yin A female master of Qigong in the Tang Dynasty (618 AD - 907 AD) who wrote a monograph of Qigong, influencing the development of Qigong in the later generations.

虎视法【hǔ shì fǎ】 为动功。其作法为,两手据地左右回顾,如同老虎回视状。

tiger watching exercise A dynamic exercise, marked by pressing the hands over the ground, watching the left side and right side, just like a tiger watching forwards and backwards.

虎戏【hǔ xì】 为华佗五禽戏之一。

tiger boxing One of the five ways of animal boxing.

虎向水中生【hǔ xiàng shuǐ zhōng shēng】 为静功。其作法为,常卷舌上

舐悬雍(一般舐上腭),玉液咽下口,直送至丹田,久则为精。

tiger living in water A static exercise, marked by rolling up the tongue to the upper palate, swallowing saliva through the mouth into Dantian and finally transforming into essence. Dantian is divided into the upper Dantian (the region between the eyes), the middle Dantian (the region below the heart) and the lower Dantian (the region below the navel).

户门【hù mén】 指牙齿。

house gate Refers to the teeth.

护持【hù chí】 即反复习练,以固秘发展。

protection and persistence Refers to repeatedly practicing Qigong in order to protect and to develop the body.

华池【huá chí】 ① 指口;② 指舌下;③ 指肾中液;④ 指华池,在黄庭之下。

magnificent pool Refers to ① either the mouth; ② or the area below the tongue; ③ or humor in the kidney; ④ or Huachi, below the yellow chamber (the region below the navel).

华盖【huá gài】 ① 指脑之象;② 指眉。

canopy Refers to ① either the manifestations of the brain; ② or the brows.

华阳隐居【huá yáng yǐn jū】 指梁代著名医药学家和气功学家陶弘景的生活方式。

living in seclusion in Huayang Refers to the way that Tao Hongjing lived. Tao Hongjing was a great doctor and master of Qigong in the Liang Dynasty (502 AD - 557 AD).

华阳真人【huá yáng zhēn rén】 为唐代著名气功学家施肩吾的另外一个称谓,其著有多部气功著作,提倡习练气功应明四时、阴阳、五行。

Huayang Immortal Another name of Shi Jianwu, a great master of Qigong in the Tang Dynasty (618 AD - 907 AD). He wrote several monographs of Qigong, suggesting to pay attention to the four seasons, Yin and Yang, and five elements in practicing Qigong.

华阳子【huá yáng zǐ】 金代气功学家王处一的另外一个称谓,其为全真道嵛山派的创始人。

Hua Yangzi Another name of Wang Chuyi, a great master of Qigong in the Jin Dynasty (1142 AD - 1217 AD), who was the founder of Yushan school in Acme Genuine Dao.

华阳子论内观【huá yáng zǐ lùn nèi guān】 源自气功专论,阐述内观可以消除佛家气功练而入定。

Hua Yangzi's discussion about internal vision Collected from a monograph of Qigong, describing about how to tranquilize the mind and body through practicing Qigong in Buddhism.

华岳【huá yuè】 为五岳中之西岳,为著名道家和气功家修炼之处。

Huayue Mountain A synonym of Huashan Mountain, is a mountain located in the Shaanxi Province, one of the five important mountains in China. In this great mountain, some of the Daoists stayed there to study and develop Daoism and some of the masters of Qigong stayed there to study and practice Qigong.

华座观【huá zuò guān】 为静功,为佛家气功功法。其作法为,趺坐,意想阿弥陀佛之象,并使意识活动集中于像而不分散。

sitting vision A static exercise, referring to exercise of Qigong in Buddhism, marked by sitting quietly, imagining Amitabha and concentrating consciousness activity without any dispersion.

华座想【huá zuò xiǎng**】** 为静功,为佛家气功功法。其作法为,趺坐,意想阿弥陀佛之象,并使意识活动集中于像而不分散。

sitting contemplation A static exercise, referring to exercise of Qigong in Buddhism, marked by sitting quietly, imagining Amitabha and concentrating consciousness activity without any dispersion.

滑心【huá xīn**】** 指精神意识活动散乱而浮躁。

slippery heart Refers to disordered and fickle activities of the spirit and consciousness.

化身坐忘法【huà shēn zuò wàng fǎ**】** 动静相兼法。每夜入定后,偃卧闭目,然后安神定魄,忘想。

vacuum contemplation exercise An exercise combined with dynamic exercise and static exercise, marked by lying on the back with eyes closed, spirit stabilized, corporeal soul maintained and ideas forgot every night.

华山【huà shān**】** 五岳中之西岳,为著名道家和气功家修炼之处。

Huashan Mountain Located in the Shaanxi Province, one of the five important mountains in China. In this great mountain, some of the Daoists stayed there to study and develop Daoism and some of the masters of Qigong stayed there to study and practice Qigong.

华山睡功法【huà shān shuì gōng fǎ**】** 为静功。其作法为,于日间或夜静,或一阳来之时,端身正坐,叩齿三十六通,逐一唤集身中诸神,然后松宽衣带而侧卧之。可强身明目、交通心肾、安神补脑。

lying exercise in Huashan Mountain A static exercise, marked by tranquilization in the noon or at midnight, or sitting right when one Yang comes, clicking the teeth for thirty-six times, eventually concentrating all kinds of the spirit, then loosening the belt and lying on the side. Such a way of practice can strengthen the body, improve eyesight, stabilize the spirit and tonify the brain.

淮南子【huái nán zǐ**】** 《淮南子》为道家论著,兼述气功。作者为汉代刘安及其同门客苏非、李尚、伍被等。

Huai Nanzi A monograph of Daoism, including the discussion and analysis of Qigong. This monograph of Daoism was written by Liu An in the Han Dynasty(202 BC – 263 AD)with his followers like Su Fei, Li Shang and Wu Bei.

踝【huái**】** ① 指踝关节内、外侧隆起处;② 指手掌后的高骨。

ankle Refers to ① either the internal and external bump pad in anklebone; ② or bone prominence behind the palm.

还丹【huán dān**】** ① 指调节意识思维活动;② 指真气出而复还本处;③ 指习练气功。

returning Dan（pills of immortality） Refers to ① either the activities of consciousness and thinking; ② or the genuine Qi returning the original place;

③ or practice of Qigong.

还丹复命篇【huán dān fù mìng piān】《还丹复命篇》为气功专著,由宋代薛道光撰,全文以诗歌形式论述锻炼内丹之法。

Huandan Fuming Pian(*Monograph of Returning to Dan for Reviving Life*)A monograph of Qigong entitled *Monograph of Returning to Dan*(*Pills of Immortality*)*for Reviving Life*, written by Xue Daoguang in the Song Dynasty(960 AD－1279 AD). This monograph was written in the ways of poetry to discuss the methods for refining internal Dan(pills of immortality).

还丹歌【huán dān gē】《还丹歌》为气功专论,由汉代学者钟离权所撰,主要阐述阴阳、五行在炼丹中的作用。

Huandan Ge(*Song for Returning to Dan*)A monograph of Qigong entitled *Song for Returning to Dan*(*Pills of Immortality*), written by Zhong Liquan, a great scholar in the Han Dynasty(202 BC－263 AD), mainly describing the effect of Yin and Yang as well as the five elements(including wood, fire, earth, metal and water)in making pills of immorality.

还丹金液【huán dān jīn yè】 指气功金液还丹。

returning golden humor to Dan(**pills of immorality**)Refers to the fact that golden humor in the body will return to Dan(pills of immorality)in practicing Qigong.

还丹六法口诀【huán dān liù fǎ kǒu jué】 为静口诀。其作法为,① 九转还丹诀,即以五脏真气、三田真气和合神水而下丹田;② 指七返还丹诀,即以三阴三阳三返,昼夜一循环,三田都过;③ 指

大还丹诀,即以三田反复循环一次;④ 指小还丹诀,即以五脏循环一次;⑤ 指金液还丹诀,即以肺金气,合顶中神水,下还丹田;⑥ 指玉液还丹诀,即肾间真气,合心中神水,而曰玉液,下还丹田。

formula of six ways to return Dan A static formula. ① The first formula is nine transformations, indicating that the genuine Qi from the five Zang-organs(including the heart, the liver, the spleen, the lung and the kidney)and the genuine Qi from the triple energizer combine with spiritual water and enter the Dantian; ② the second formula is seven returns, indicating that three Yin and three Yang return three times at night and in the daytime to pass the triple energizer; ③ the third formula is greatly returning to Dan(pills of immortality), indicating circulation once in the triple energizer; ④ the fourth formula is small turning to Dan(pills of immortality), indicating circulation once in the five Zang-organs(including the heart, the liver, the spleen, the lung and the kidney); ⑤ the fifth formula is golden humor returning to Dan(pills of immortality); ⑥ the sixth formula is combination of Qi in the lung metal with the spiritual water that returns to Dan(pills of immortality); the seventh formula is jade humor returning to Dan(pills of immortality), indicating that combination of the genuine Qi in the kidney with the spiritual water in the heart to return to Dantian. In this term, Dan(pills of immortality)mainly refers to the pills of immortality and

and Dantian. Dantian is divided into upper Dantian (the region between the eyes), the middle Dantian (the region below the heart) and the lower Dantian (the region below the navel).

还丹秘诀养赤子神方【huán dān mì jué yǎng chì zǐ shén fāng】《还丹秘诀养赤子神方》为气功专著,由宋代许明道著,详细论述了习练气功的时节、要领、以及功成出现的境界及特异功能。

Huandan Mijue Yang Chizi Shenfang (*Secret Formula for Returning Dan and Immortal Formula for Nourishing Babies*) A monograph of Qigong entitled *Secret Formula for Returning Dan and Immortal Formula for Nourishing Babies*, written by Xu Mingdao in the Song Dynasty (960 AD - 1279 AD), particularly describing the time and essentials for practicing Qigong as well as the state and special functions after successful practice.

还丹破迷歌【huán dān pò mí gē】《还丹破迷歌》为气功专论,由五代时期的刘海蟾所著,主要阐述单纯行气、闭气、叩齿等法不能成丹。只有抽铅添汞、龙虎交媾才能成丹。所谓五代指的是后梁、后唐、后晋、后汉、后周。

Huandan Pomi Ge (*Songs for Returning Dan and Relieving Confusion*) A monograph of Qigong entitled *Songs for Returning Dan and Relieving Confusion*, written by Liu Haichan in the period of five Dynasties (907 AD - 960 AD), mainly describing that simple ways to move Qi, to close respiration and to click teeth cannot produce Dan (pills of immortality) and that only taking out lead (Qi) and increasing mercury (spirit) as well as intercourse of Loong (original spirit) and tiger (original essence) can produce Dan (pills of immortality). The so-called five Dynasties (907 AD - 960 AD) include the Later Liang Dynasty (907 - 923), the Later Tang Dynasty (923 - 936), the Later Jin Dynasty (936 - 947), the Later Han Dynasty (947 - 950), and the Later Zhou Dynasty (951 - 960).

还丹院【huán dān yuàn】 在陕西宝鸡南二十五里,为纯阳真人炼丹处。

college for returning Dan Located twenty-five Li in the south of Baoji City, Shaanxi Province, where the pure Yang immortals refined Dan (pills of immortality).

还晶入泥丸【huán jīng rù ní wán】其中的晶指精气神合而为一,泥丸为大脑。

returning crystal to enter the mud bolus (the brain) A celebrated dictum, in which crystal refers to the integration of the essence, Qi and the spirit which eventually enters the brain.

还精补脑【huán jīng bǔ nǎo】 指练功中,炼精化气,炼气化神的过程。

returning essence to tonify the brain A term of Qigong, referring to refining essence to train Qi and refining Qi to train the spirit.

还精法【huán jīng fǎ】 为静功。其作法为,意想肾精正赤白,从脐中到背,复上头,入脑中藏之。

exercise for returning to essence A static exercise, marked by imagining the kidney essence as red and white that moves from the navel to the back, from the back to the head and from the head to the brain.

还念两目【huán niàn liǎng mù】 为动功,指精神集中于目。

consciousness in the two eyes A dynamic exercise, referring to concentrating the essence and the spirit on the eyes.

还神摄气【huán shén shè qì】 指还归神于泥丸,摄归气于气穴(丹田)。

returning spirit and absorbing Qi A term of Qigong, referring to returning the spirit to the mud bolus (the brain) and absorbing Qi to Qixue (KI 13) which is similar to Dantian. Dantian is divided into the upper Dantian (the region between the eyes), the middle Dantian (the region below the heart) and the lower Dantian (the region below the navel).

还源篇【huán yuán piān】 《还源篇》为气功专著,由宋代石泰撰,指出积精化气,神合先天真元之气以成内丹。

Huanyuan Pian (*Monograph of Returning to the Origin*) A monograph of Qigong entitled *Monograph of Returning to the Origin*, written by Shi Tai, a great scholar in the Song Dynasty (960 AD – 1279 AD). This monograph mainly describes the ideas about accumulation of the essence and promotion of Qi as well as integration of the spirit with Qi of the innate genuine origin in order to produce internal Dan (pills of immortality).

还真集【huán zhēn jí】 《还真集》为气功专著,内容论心、论元、论中,有一定的参考价值。作者不详。

Haizhen Ji (*Collection of Returning to Genuineness*) A monograph of Qigong entitled *Collection of Returning to Genuineness*, mainly discussing the heart, the origin and the center with certain

reference value. The author was unknown.

环跳【huán tiào】 足少阳胆经中的一个穴位,位于股骨大转子最高点与髓管裂孔连线的中、外交点处。在气功状态下,是精气运行的通道。

Huantiao (**GB 30**) An acupoint in the gallbladder meridian of foot Shaoyang, located in between the middle and lateral sides on the top of the greater trochanter of femur and the medullary canal hole. It is the way to move the essence and Qi in practicing Qigong.

环中【huán zhōng】 指意识活动平和、稳定,在不左不右,不前不后,不上不下之中。

balance Refers to peacefulness and stability of the consciousness activity which is not just in the left or the right, the front or the back, the upper or the lower.

幻丹【huàn dān】 指思虑之神与呼吸之气所结的丹。

phantom Dan (**pills of immortality**) Refers to Dan (pills of immortality) formed by the spirit in consideration and Qi in respiration.

幻丹说【huàn dān shuō】 源自气功专论,主要阐述幻丹由于神识尚未入静,而急于采药所致。

fluctuation of Dan (**pills of immortality**) Collected from a monograph about Qigong. It mainly describes that fluctuating Dan (pills of immortality) is not tranquilized and is anxious to collect medicinal.

幻化【huàn huà】 指玄妙、静漠的变化。

fluctuation A term of Qigong, referring to changes of mysterious and static conditions.

幻心【huàn xīn】 指禅家所认为的忽然而生，忽然而灭的念头。

fluctuating the heart Refers to the idea about sudden existence and sudden loss in Zen Buddhism.

幻真先生【huàn zhēn xiān shēng】 唐代气功家，生卒不详。

Mr. Huanzhen A great master of Qigong in the Tang Dynasty (618 AD – 907 AD), whose life was unclear.

幻真先生服内元气诀【huàn zhēn xiān shēng fú nèi yuán qì jué】《幻真先生服内元气诀》为气功养生专著，论述其作法、功效、应用。作者姓名、成书年代不详。

Huanzhen Xiansheng Funei Yuanqi Jue (***Mr. Huanzhen's Formula for Internally Absorbing Original Qi***) A monograph of Qigong entitled *Mr. Huanzhen's Formula for Internally Absorbing Original Qi*, describing the methods, effects and application of Qigong. The author was unknown.

幻真先生胎息法【huàn zhēn xiān shēng tāi xī fǎ】 为静功。谓人之元神，藏于气穴，犹万物藏于坤土。神入地中，犹天气降而至于地。

Mr. Huanzhen's method about fetal respiration A static exercise, referring to the original spirit in the human body that stays in the Qi point, just like all the things in the world that stay in the earth. The way that the spirit enters the earth is just like that of the celestial Qi that descends into the earth.

幻真行气法【huàn zhēn xíng qì fǎ】 为静功，指调身、调神、调气。其作法为，取仰卧式或自然坐式均可，闭目塞兑，身体自然舒适。坐或卧定后，叩齿三十六

通。平定精神，搓面、搓手，令热后熨目，捏目内眦，按摩迎香穴附近。津生后咽之，导引入胃，存胃中。

Huanzhen's method for regulating Qi A static exercise for regulating the body, the spirit and Qi, marked by lying on the back or sitting naturally, closing the eyes for relaxing the body, clicking the teeth for thirty-six times after sitting or lying naturally, stabilizing the essence and the spirit, kneading the face and hands, pressing the eyes when the hands are kneaded hot, pinching the inner canthus, kneading the region near Yingxiang (LI 20), and entering fluid into the stomach after swallowing fluid.

幻真注解胎息经【huàn zhēn zhù jiě tāi xī jīng】 源自气功专论，主要阐述神、气、形的关系及对人体的重要性。

Huanzhen's canon about fetal respiration Collected from a monograph about Qigong, mainly describing the relationship and importance of the spirit, Qi and the body.

肓俞【huāng shū】 足少阴肾经中的一个穴位，在脐中旁开 0.5 寸。这一穴位为气功运行的一个常见部位。

Huangshu (KI 16) An acupoint in the kidney meridian of foot Shaoyin, located 0.5 Cun lateral to the navel. This acupoint is a region usually used for keeping the essential Qi in practice of Qigong.

黄白【huáng bái】 ① 指黄芽、白雪，为纯粹、清素之意；② 指烧炼丹药，化为金银；③ 同黄芽白雪。

yellow and white Refers to ① either yellow bud and white snow, indicating pure and sincere consciousness; ② or refining Dan（pills of immortality）medicinal and transforming into gold and silver；③ or the same of yellow bud and white snow.

黄白术【huáng bái zhú】 指古代之冶金术。

yellow and white technique Refers to metallurgy in ancient China.

黄道【huáng dào】 指太阳运行的轨道。气功文献中指中宫金丹凝结生成之处。

yellow Dao Refers to the way along which the sun moves. In the literature of Qigong, it refers to the region for the production and concentration of golden Dan（pills of immortality）in the middle palace.

黄帝【huáng dì】 黄帝(公元前2717—公元前2599年)为古华夏部落联盟首领,中国远古时代华夏民族的共主。五帝之首。被尊为中华"人文初祖"。

Yellow Emperor Yellow Emperor（2717 BC–2599 BC）was the leader of Chinese tribal confederacy and Chinese nation in the ancient times, the first of five emperors in ancient China and the father of Chinese culture.

黄帝八十一难经纂图句解【huáng dì bā shí yī nàn jīng zuǎn tú jù jiě】 《黄帝八十一难经纂图句解》为中医学专著,由宋代李駉所撰,除阐述中医基本理论外,对人体五脏六腑、奇经八胁、百骸众窍在练功中出现的效应做了切实记述,对习练气功有较大的指导作用。

Huangdi Bashiyi Nanjing Zuantu Jujie（Compilation and Explanation of Yellow Emperor's Eighty-one Issues） A monograph of traditional Chinese medicine with discussion of Qigong entitled *Compilation and Explanation of Yellow Emperor's Eighty-one Issues*, written by Li Dong in the Song Dynasty（960 AD–1279 AD）, mainly describing the theory of traditional Chinese medicine, recording the effects of the five Zang-organs（including the heart, the liver, the spleen, the lung and the kidney）, the six Fu-organs（including the gallbladder, the stomach, the small intestine, the large intestine, the bladder and the triple energizer）, the eight extraordinary meridians, all the skeletons and orifices in practicing Qigong.

黄帝九鼎神丹经诀【huáng dì jiǔ dǐng shén dān jīng jué】 《黄帝九鼎神丹经诀》为外丹专著,为古代研究外丹的重要文献,作者不详。

Huangdi Jiuding Shendan Jingjue（Yellow Emperor's Classic Formula for Nine Cauldrons and Spiritual Dan） A monograph about external Dan（pills of immortality）entitled *Yellow Emperor's Classic Formula for Nine Cauldrons and Spiritual Dan（Pills of Immortality）*, which is an important literature about external Dan（pills of immortality）in ancient China. The author was unknown.

黄帝内经【huáng dì nèi jīng】 《黄帝内经》为我国现存最早的较为系统和完整的医学典籍,大约成书于战国至秦汉时期。

Huangdi Neijing（Yellow Emperor's Internal Canon of Medicine） The earliest canon of traditional Chinese medicine entitled *Yellow Emperor's Internal Canon of Medicine*, which is the systematic and complete cannon of traditional Chinese medicine, compiled from the Warring States Period（475 BC - 221 BC）to the Qin Dynasty（221 BC - 207 BC）.

黄帝内视法【huáng dì nèi shì fǎ】 为静功。其作法为，端身正坐，存想思念，令见五脏如悬磬，五色了了分明，勿辍也。

Yellow Emperor's exercise for internal inspection A static exercise, marked by sitting upright, imagining consciousness, observing the five Zang-organs（including the heart，the liver，the spleen，the lung and the kidney）like chime stones with bright colors and without any dispersion.

黄帝胎息诀【huáng dì tāi xī jué】 为静功口诀，主要为内守精神，避免精神刺激。

Yellow Emperor's formula for fetal respiration A static exercise, referring to internally concentrating the spirit in order to prevent stimulation of the spirit.

黄帝阴符经【huáng dì yīn fú jīng】 《黄帝阴符经》为古代文化专著，涉及气功，作者不详。

Huangdi Yinfu Jing（*Yellow Emperor's Yin Conception Canon*） A monograph of traditional Chinese culture with Qigong entitled *Yellow Emperor's Yin Conception Canon*. The author was unknown.

黄帝阴符经集解【huáng dì yīn fú jīng jí jiě】 《黄帝阴符经集解》为唐宋时期多位学者所解注，本书论述长生守一大旨、静心存神之道、御气内修之术。

Huangdi Yinfu Jingji Jie（*Collection and Explanation of Yellow Emperor's Yin Conception Canon*） The analysis and explanation made by several scholars in the Tang Dynasty（618 AD - 907 AD）and Song Dynasty（960 AD - 1127 AD）entitled *Collection and Explanation of Yellow Emperor's Yin Conception Canon*，mainly describing the gist for prolonging life and concentrating the mind，the way for tranquilizing the heart and storing the spirit，and the technique for controlling Qi and cultivating the internal.

黄帝阴符经注【huáng dì yīn fú jīng zhù】 《黄帝阴符经注》为气功专著，由宋代唐淳所注.

Huangdi Yinfu Jingzhu（*Explanation of Yellow Emperor's Yin Conception Canon*） A monograph of Qiong, also entitled *Explanation of Yellow Emperor's Yin Conception Canon*，analyzed by Tang Chun, a great scholar and master of Qigong in the Song Dynasty（960 AD - 1279 AD）.

黄房【huáng fáng】 ① 指玄关，玄关指入道之门，泛指气功基础；② 指丹田。

yellow house The same as supreme pass，refers to ① either the gate of Daoism，indicating the function of Qigong；② or Dantian which is divided into the upper Dantian（the region between the eyes），the middle Dantian（the region below the heart）and the lower Dantian（the region below the navel）.

黄宫【huáng gōng】 指脾，为五脏之一。

yellow palace Refers to the spleen which is one of the five Zang-organs（including the heart，the liver，the spleen，the lung and the kidney）.

黄河【huáng hé】 指脊髓。

yellow river Refers to marrow.

黄河水逆流【huáng hé shuǐ nì liú】

指神运精气沿督脉逆上泥丸。

reverse running of water in the yellow river　A term of Qigong, indicating that the spirit moves the essence and Qi along the governor meridian to the mud bolus (the brain).

黄家【huáng jiā】　指气海,指下丹田。

yellow place　A term of Qigong, referring to Qi sea and the lower Dantian (the region below the navel).

黄精【huáng jīng】　指阴气,亦为药名。

yellow essence　Refers to either Yin Qi, or the name of a medicinal.

黄男玄女【huáng nán xuán nǚ】　指肾中之一阳及心中之一阴。黄男指肾阳,玄女指心阴。

yellow man and profound woman　Refers to Yang in the kidney and Yin in the heart. In this term, yellow man refers to Yang in the kidney while profound woman refers to Yin in the heart.

黄宁【huáng níng】　指人身内胃脘之神。

yellow tranquility　Refers to spirit of gastric cavity.

黄婆【huáng pó】　指中央戊己土。

yellow grandmother　A term of Qigong, referring to Wu (the fifth of the ten Heavenly Stems), Ji (the sixth of the ten Heavenly Stems) and earth in the center.

黄婆舍【huáng pó shè】　指中宫意土,亦指祖窍,指位于心与脐之正中。

yellow grandmother's room　A term of Qigong, referring to the imaged earth in the central palace, or the ancestral orifice which refers to the central region between the heart and the navel.

黄泉【huáng quán】　指口中唾液。

yellow spring　Refers to saliva in the mouth.

黄阙【huáng què】　指头面两眉间。

yellow gate　Refers to the head, face and the region between the eyes.

黄阙紫户【huáng què zǐ hù】　在右眉外侧角入骨三分处。

yellow gate and purple household　Located 3 Fen to the bone from the lateral side of the right eyebrow.

黄石公受履【huáng shí gōng shòu lǚ】　为动功。其作法为,身子坐于席上,两腿自然放伸,两手按两大脚跟,边按边移动两手,由脚跟直按至膝。

Huang Shigong's exercise for wearing shoes　A dynamic exercise, marked by sitting on the bed, naturally stretching the feet, pressing the heels with the hands and also moving the hands, then pressing the knees with the heels.

黄庭【huáng tíng】　① 指中;② 指身体内的中虚空窍;③ 指五脏之中;④ 指脐之后;⑤ 指有名无所;⑥ 指黄八极;⑦ 指黄庭在二肾之中;⑧ 指黄庭在心之下。

Yellow hall　Refers to ① either the center; ② or the middle deficiency and empty orifice in the center of the body; ③ or the center of the five Zang-organs (including the heart, the liver, the spleen, the lung and the kidney); ④ or the region below the navel; ⑤ or a person or something with name but without position; ⑥ or eight yellow extremities; ⑦ or Huangting (yellow hall) located in the region between the kidneys; ⑧ or Huangting (yellow hall) located in the region below the heart.

黄庭宫真人【huáng tíng gōng zhēn

rén】 指脾脏所主神名。

immortal in Yellow Palace Refers to the spirit in the spleen.

黄庭观【huáng tíng guàn】 在湖南衡阳,为晋代女道士魏华存修炼处。

Yellow Hall Temple Located in Hengyang City in Hunan Province, where Wei Huacun, a great female Daoist in the Jin Dynasty (266 AD – 420 AD) practiced and developed Qigong.

黄庭经【huáng tíng jīng】 《黄庭经》为气功学经典著作,指《上清黄庭外景经》和《上清黄庭内景经》。《上清黄庭外景经》为气功学专著,世传为东晋魏华存所传。《上清黄庭内景经》为气功学专著,相传为太上老君所作。

Huangting Jing (*Yellow Hall Canon*) A classic monograph of Qigong entitled *Yellow Hall Canon*, referring to Shangqing Huangting Waijing Jing entitled *External Scene About the Root of Body in Qigong Practice* written by Wei Huacun in the East Jin Dynasty (217 AD – 420 AD) and Shangqing Huangting Neijing Jing entitled *Canon About Upper Clearity and Internal Essence of Imperial Palace* compiled by legendarily the Lord Lao Jun.

黄庭内景五脏六腑补泻图【huáng tíng nèi jǐng wǔ zàng liù fǔ bǔ xiè tú】《黄庭内景五脏六腑补泻图》为气功养生专著,由唐代胡愔所撰,是研究气功养生法的专著。

Huangting Neijing Wuzang Liufu Buxie Tu (*Pictures about Supplementation and Draining of the Internal Scene, Five Zang-organs and Six Fu-organs*) A monograph of Qigong and life cultivation entitled *Pictures about Supplementation and Draining of the Internal Scene, Five Zang-organs and Six Fu-organs*, written by Hu Yi in the Tang Dynasty (618 AD – 907 AD), mainly analyzing the exercises for practicing Qigong and cultivating life described in other monographs. The five Zang-organs include the heart, the liver, the spleen, the lung and the kidney; the six Fu-organs include the gallbladder, the stomach, the small intestine, the large intestine, the bladder and the triple energizer.

黄庭内人【huáng tíng nèi rén】 指五脏之阴气。

man in the yellow hall A term of Qigong, referring to Yin Qi in the five Zang-organs (including the heart, the liver, the spleen, the lung and the kidney).

黄庭真人【huáng tíng zhēn rén】 指五脏之阳气。

immoral in the yellow hall A term of Qigong, referring to Yang Qi in the five Zang-organs (including the heart, the liver, the spleen, the lung and the kidney).

黄庭中景经【huáng tíng zhōng jǐng jīng】《黄庭中景经》为气功学专著,主要论述脑及五脏的生理功能,认为脑为一身之主,是精神意识活动的枢纽。

Huangting Zhongjing Jing (*Canon about Yellow Hall and Central Scene*) A monograph of Qigong entitled *Canon about Yellow Hall and Central Scene*, mainly describing the physiological functions of the five Zang-organs (including the heart, the liver, the spleen, the lung and the kidney), indicating that the brain is the master of the whole body and the most important region for controlling the activities of the spirit and consciousness.

黄芽【huáng yá】　① 指脾液；② 指脑中涎；③ 指阴阳和合为一；④ 指真龙、真虎，即心液之气，肾中之水；⑤ 指坎中真阳。

yellow bud　Refers to ① either spleen humor；② or brain liquid；③ or integration of Yin and Yang；④ or genuine Loong and genuine tiger，indicating Qi in heart humor and water in the kidney；⑤ genuine Yang in the Kan Trigram.

黄芽白雪【huáng yá bái xuě】　指脾气之初生和肺气之初成。

yellow bud and white snow　A term of Qigong，referring to the primary production of spleen Qi and primary formation of lung Qi.

黄芽白雪不难寻【huáng yá bái xuě bù nán xún】　《黄芽白雪不难寻》为气功专论，主要阐述真一之水为炼丹原质，土为四象和合的关键。

no difficulty in selecting yellow bud and white snow　Collected from a monograph of Qigong，mainly describing that the genuine water is the hypostasis for refining Dan（pills of immortality）and earth is the key for the four scenes to integrate with each other.

黄野【huáng yě】　指黄庭，亦指中央。

yellow region　Refers to yellow hall or the center.

黄衣紫带【huáng yī zǐ dài】　指脾居谓上。

yellow cloth with purple belt　A term of Qigong，indicating that the spleen is located above the stomach.

黄中【huáng zhōng】　为"祖窍"异名，此穴位为气功习练之处。

yellow middle　A synonym of Zuqiao which is an acupoint located in the region between the heart and the navel. This acupoint is a region usually used in practice of Qigong.

黄中正位【huáng zhōng zhèng wèi】　指心肾之间的位置。

right position in the yellow center　A term of Qigong，referring to the region between the heart and the kidney.

恍惚【huǎng hū】　① 指意识思维活动无思无欲，宁谧安静，中和平衡的状态；② 指神形合一出现的状态。

trance　Refers to ① the condition of stability，tranquility and balance related to the activities of consciousness and thinking without contemplation and desire；② condition under the integration of the spirit and the body.

恍惚说【huǎng hū shuō】　源自气功专论，阐述行动中意守出现的景象。

idea about trance　Idea about trance is collected from a monograph of Qigong，describing the scene of concentrating consciousness in practicing Qigong.

恍惚杳冥【huǎng hū yǎo míng】　指气功中阴阳二气和合，静极至虚的状态。

dim trance　A term of Qigong，referring to harmony and tranquility of Yin Qi and Yang Qi in Qigong.

挥斥八极【huī chì bā jí】　喻气功家高度调合神形，情绪稳定。

freedom to visit eight directions　Means that the masters of Qigong have highly regulated and harmonized the spirit and the body so as to stabilize the mood.

回肠【huí cháng】　相当于西医解剖学中的回肠、盲肠、升结肠。

ileum　Refers to ileum，caecum and ascending colon in modern anatomy.

H

回道人【huí dào rén】 为唐代气功学家吕洞宾的另外一个称谓,其撰有多部气功专著,为气功的发展做出了特殊贡献。

Hui Daoren Another name of Lǚ Dongbin, a great master of Qigong in the Tang Dynasty (618 AD – 907 AD), who wrote several monographs of Qigong, contributing a great deal to the development of Qigong.

回光返照【huí guāng fǎn zhào】 ① 指将驰逐于外之神收回身内;② 指神气归根,根即脑;③ 指神归丹田。

returning light Refers to ① either taking back the spirit flowing outside into the body; ② or the root (the brain) of the spirit and Qi; ③ or the spirit entering Dantian. Dantian is divided into the upper Dantian (the region between the eyes), the middle Dantian (the region below the heart) and the lower Dantian (the region below the navel).

回颜填血脑【huí yán tián xuè nǎo】 为气功养生法,可平秘阴阳,有驻颜、益血、补脑、安神的作用。

returning complexion and filling the brain A term of Qigong, referring to the exercise of Qigong and life cultivation, which can regulate Yin and Yang, normalizing complexion, fortifying the blood, tonifying the brain and stabilizing the spirit.

回紫抱黄入丹田【huí zǐ bào huáng rù dān tián】 ① 指紫河车运精气入丹田;② 指目送脾气于丹田。

returning the purple and taking the yellow into Dantian A term of Qigong, referring to ① either placenta hominis moving the essence and Qi into Dantian; ② or the eyes moving spleen Qi into Dantian. Dantian is divided into the upper Dantian (the region between the eyes), the middle Dantian (the region below the heart) and the lower Dantian (the region below the navel).

会三性【huì sān xìng】 指通过气功锻炼,元气、元精、元神三者有机地结合为一体。

integration of three properties Refers to integration of the original Qi, the original essence and the original spirit through practicing Qigong.

会阳【huì yáng】 即虚危穴和九灵铁鼓,精气聚散常在此处,水火发端也在此处,阴阳变化也在此处,有无出入也在此处。

combination of Yang The same as Xu-wei point and nine genius-fire drums, referring to the region where the essential Qi concentrates and disperses there, water and fire appear there, Yin and Yang change there, exit and entrance exist there.

会阴【huì yīn】 ① 为任脉中的一个穴位,男子位于阴囊与肛门之间,女子位于阴唇后联合与肛门之间;② 指人体部位名;③ 指气功常见意守部位。

Huiyin (CV 1) Refers to ① either an acupoint in the conception meridian, located in the region between the scrotum and anus in men, and in the region between the labia and the anus in women; ② or the name of a part in the body; ③ or the region with mental concentration in practicing Qigong.

晦朔弦望【huì shuò xián wàng】 为古人根据月象之盈虚而命名。① 阴历(以下均指阴历)每月月末,月亮纯黑无光,称为晦;② 每月初一,月虽黑,已受阳光,称为朔;③ 初八之月阴阳各半称为上弦；④ 十五之月圆，称为望。在气功文献中，常以月象之盈虚圆缺来表达练功时之阴阳消长。

the ending, beginning and middle of a month with round moon　A term used to describe lunar image in ancient China. According to traditional Chinese calendar，① the ending of every month is called Hui during which there is no manifestation of the moon；② the first day of every month is called Shuo during which there is no manifestation of the moon but slightly bright；③ the eighth in every month is called Xuan during which Yin and Yang are just half and half；④ the fifteenth in every month is called Wang during which the moon is round. In the literature of Qigong, the wane and wax of Yin and Yang are described according to the images of the moon.

慧【huì】　① 指智慧，为分辨事理，决断疑念的精神作用；② 指通达事理。

wisdom　A common term of Qigong in Buddhism, referring to ① either wisdom for differentiating reasons and deciding doubt；② or understanding reasons.

慧根【huì gēn】　指具有智慧的根基。

wisdom root　Refers to the foundation of wisdom.

慧剑【huì jiàn】　指意识作用，即用意排除杂念，如用剑斩去邪恶。

wisdom sword　Refers to the effects of consciousness, indicating to eliminate distracting thought by consciousness, just like executing evils by sword.

慧眼【huì yǎn】　① 指额部正中之眼，又名天目；② 指眼力，能洞察万物。

ocular wisdom　Refers to ① either the

middle point on the forehead known as celestial eye；② or eyesight that can thoroughly examine all things.

慧圆【huì yuán】　指智慧圆通，明达盈固，神形和调。

wisdom circle　Refers to flexibility of wisdom, clarity with exuberance and regulation of the spirit and body.

昏清【hūn qīng】　指习练气功时的黄昏和凌晨时期。

dusk and morning　A term of Qigong, referring to practicing Qigong in the dusk or in the morning.

浑沦【hún lún】　指太极，喻精神内守，视之不见，听之不闻，循之不得。

tranquilization　Refers to Supreme Pole, comparing to internal concentration of the spirit without any vision, hearing and following.

混百灵于天谷【hún bǎi líng yú tiān gǔ】　指脑调节精神意识活动，并使之和平稳定。

coordination of lark in heavenly valley　A celebrated dictum, indicating that the brain regulates the activities of the spirit and consciousness and makes it pacified and stabilized.

混而为一【hún ér wéi yī】　指视、听、搏合而为一，是神形的高度协调统一。

integration　Refers to integration of vision, hearing and beating, indicating great coordination and unification of the spirit and the body.

混性命【hún xìng mìng】　指练气功达到某一阶段，神和气得到高度的结合和统一。

chaos life　A term of Qigong, indicating that the spirit and Qi are highly combined and unified with each other when practice of Qigong has reached to a certain stage.

混元一窍【hún yuán yī qiào】 指玄牝。玄牝为气功学名词，① 指身中一窍；② 指二肾之间；③ 指天地；④ 指任督二脉；⑤ 指体内阴阳；⑥ 指中宫脾。

a chaos orifice The synonym of Xuanpin, which is a term of Qigong, referring to ① either an orifice in the body；② or a region between the two kidneys；③ or the sky and earth；④ or the conception meridian and governor meridian；⑤ or Yin and Yang in the body；⑥ or the spleen.

魂忽魄糜【hún hū pò mí】 指魂魄不调，魂躁魄朽，神形失调。

neglect of the ethereal soul and disorder of the corporeal soul Refers to imbalance between the ethereal soul and the corporeal soul, indicating that the ethereal soul is restless, the corporeal soul is rotten and imbalance of the spirit and the body.

魂精玉室【hún jīng yù shì】 指神所居之室，即脑。

jade chamber of the ethereal soul and the spirit A term of Qigong, referring to the brain, which is the chamber storing the spirit.

魂静魄安【hún jìng pò ān】 指调节精神的方法。

tranquil ethereal soul and stable corporeal soul Refers to the method for regulating the spirit.

魂魄【hún pò】 魂魄与肝、肺相关。① 肝主魂，魂为肝之神；② 肺藏魄，魄为肺之神。又指精神活动。

ethereal soul and corporeal soul Related to the liver and the lung. According to traditional Chinese medicine，① the liver controls the ethereal soul and the ethereal soul is the spirit in the liver；② the lung stores the corporeal soul and the corporeal soul is the spirit in the lung. It also refers to the activity of the spirit.

魂魄相投【hún pò xiāng tóu】 即幻丹，指思虑之神与呼吸之气所结的丹。

congeniality of the ethereal soul and the corporeal soul The same as phantom Dan (pills of immortality), is a term of Qigong, referring to Dan (pills of immortality) formed by the spirit in consideration and Qi in respiration.

魂台【hún tái】 ① 为人中异名，指人中穴在鼻下唇上，鼻唇沟之正中；② 也指身体九窍中，单窍与双窍的分界点。

ethereal soul stage The synonym of Renzhong which refers to ① either an acupoint located in the area between the upper lip and nose；② or the cut-off point between the single orifice and double orifice among the nine orifices. This acupoint is a region usually used in practice of Qigong.

魂欲上天魄入泉【hún yù shàng tiān pò rù quán】 魂欲上天指魂归于脑，魄入泉为肺魄归于肾水。

The ethereal soul wants to fly to the sky and the corporeal soul wants to enter the spring. This is a celebrated dictum, in which the ethereal soul wanting to fly to the sky means to reach the brain, and the corporeal soul wanting to enter the spring means to enter water in the kidney.

混沌【hùn dùn】 指阴阳二气相融，常用于说人体思维活动未萌发的状态。

chaos Refers to mergence between

Yin and Yang, usually referring to non-germinated activity of thinking.

混沌交接【hùn dùn jiāo jiē】　指阴阳相融从无极到有极的最初变化。

coordination of chaos　A term of Qigong, referring to the primary changes of mergence between Yin and Yang from non-polar to polar.

混沌窍【hùn dùn qiào】　指中极，为任脉中的一个穴位。

chaos orifice　Refers to Zhongji (CV 3), which is an acupoint in the conception meridian.

混沌之根【hùn dùn zhī gēn】　为祖窍异名，位于心与脐之正中。

root of chaos　The synonym of ancestral orifice, which is a term of Qigong, referring to the central region between the heart and the navel.

活命慈舟【huó mìng cí zhōu】　《活命慈舟》为清代本草专著，其中记述了气功导引法。作者不详。

Huoming Cizhou (*Saving Life with Charitable Boat*)　A monograph of materia medica with the discussion of Qigong in the Qing Dynasty (1636 AD - 1912 AD) entitled *Saving Life with Charitable Boat*. The author was unknown.

活人心法【huó rén xīn fǎ】　《活人心法》为养生专著，兼论气功，由明代臞仙所著，论述了气功养生之道。

Huoren Xinfa (*Heart Exercise for Saving People*)　A monograph of Qigong entitled *Heart Exercise for Saving People*, written by Qu Xian in the Ming Dynasty (1368 AD - 1644 AD), discussing the principles for practicing Qigong for cultivating life.

活子时【huó zǐ shí】　① 指习练气功中

形神安静；② 指一日之中均可习练气功。

living in Zi (the period of the day from 11 p. m. to 1 a. m.)　Refers to ① either tranquilization of the body and spirit in practicing Qigong; ② or practicing Qigong at any time every day.

火【huǒ】　① 指真气；② 指慧、日、心；③ 指药；④ 指调神。

fire　Refers to ① either genuine Qi; ② or wisdom, the sun and the heart; ③ or medicinal; ④ or regulation of the spirit.

火逼金行【huǒ bī jīn xíng】　为功法。呼吸时以鼻中吸气，借以接先天之气；吸取食物时，以舌上颚迎取甘露；紧摄谷道内中提，明月辉辉顶上飞；塞兑垂廉兼逆咽，久而神水落黄庭。

fire forcing metal movement　A dynamic exercise, marked by receiving original celestial Qi when the nose is inhaling, receiving sweet dew when the tongue is taking food, pinching the grain trail (anus) to enable the bright moon to raise, and concentrating the essence in order to transmit the spiritual water to flow into the yellow chamber (the region below the navel).

火逼药过尾闾穴【huǒ bī yào guò wěi lú xué】　指习练小周天功，意念导引精气，并耐用意，收腹提肛，促使精气冲过尾闾关，逆流直上。

fire forcing coccyx acupoint　A celebrated dictum, referring to practice of the small celestial circle during which emotion guides the essential Qi and tries to draw the abdomen and to lift up the anus in order to promote the essential Qi to run through the coccyx acupoint and to flow up.

H

火朝元【huǒ cháo yuán】　指五脏之气上朝天元。

fire turning to the origin　Refers to Qi from the five Zang-organs（including the heart，the liver，the spleen，the lung and the kidney）flowing up to the celestial origin.

火炽【huǒ chì】　相火妄为之意。

great fire　Refers to abnormal action of the ministerial fire.

火寒【huǒ hán】　指习练气功时，"意不可散，意散则火冷"。

cold fire　Refers to the fact that mentality should not be dispersed in practicing Qigong，otherwise fire will become cold.

火候【huǒ hòu】　指烧炼药石过程中火力的旺、衰调节。

duration of heating　Refers to regulation of exuberance and decline of fire in practicing Qigong.

火候纯正说【huǒ hòu chún zhèng shuō】　源自气功专论，阐述火候的含义，对源流及诸家学说亦有铺陈。

pure explanation about duration of heating　Collected from a monograph of Qigong，describing the meaning，origin，development and masters' ideas about fire procedure.

火候行持绝句【huǒ hòu xíng chí jué jù】　源自气功专论，阐述了习练气功是强身健体的大道。

poems about the way of duration of heating　Collected from a monograph of Qigong，describing the great ways of Qigong practice in strengthening the body and cultivating health.

火候事条【huǒ hòu shì tiáo】　指火候在不同功法及其不同阶段中，说法不同。

problems with duration of heating　Refers to different explanation about practice of Qigong at different times with different methods.

火候诸家说【huǒ hòu zhū jiā shuō】　源自气功专论，阐述火候的含义及其各家学说。

all explanations about duration of heating　Collected from a monograph of Qigong，describing the meaning and all masters' explanations about fire procedure.

火候足，莫伤丹【huǒ hòu zú mò shāng dān】　指练功练得黄芽满鼎，白雪浸天，婴儿之象。此时，只宜沐浴温养，若再妄意进火，则反损伤已成之丹。

insufficiency of duration of heating never damaging Dan（pills of immortality）　A term of Qigong，means great effect of Qigong practice，appearing like white snow soaking the sky and baby growing up. During this period，only taking bath can warmly nourish the body. If measures are still taken to receive fire，Dan（pills of immortality）that is already well produced will be damaged.

火居深海，阳焰透水【huǒ jū shēn hǎi yáng yàn tòu shuǐ】　指阴中有阳，阳中有阴。

fire in the deep sea and Yang flaming through water　Refers to Yin within Yang and Yang within Yin.

火炼法【huǒ liàn fǎ】　为静功。其作法为，存想两肾中间一点真气，补火助阳，治疗阳虚不足之证。

fire practice exercise　A static exercise，marked by keeping genuine Qi in the kidneys in order to improve fire，to support Yang and to treat the disease caused by Yang deficiency.

火铃【huǒ líng】　指胆之外象。

fire bell　Refers to the external manifestation of the gallbladder.

火龙【huǒ lóng】　火龙指神。

fire Loong　Refers to the spirit.

火龙水虎【huǒ lóng shuǐ hǔ】　指五行颠倒、反克而言。

fire Loong and water tiger　A term of Qigong，indicating perversion and disorder of the five elements（including wood，fire，earth，metal and water）.

火起【huǒ qǐ】　指意想真火，从涌泉起而上行。

fire starting　Refers to imagined genuine fire that starts from Yongquan（KI 1）.

火位【huǒ wèi】　运气术语，为君火相火所主之位。

fire position　A term about Qi motion，referring to the place controlled by monarchy fire and ministerial fire.

火性【huǒ xìng】　火为神，指精神意识活动协调柔缓，协调全身各部，即为火性。

fire property　Fire refers to the spirit，indicating that the activities of the spirit and consciousness should be gently to regulate all parts of the body.

火燥【huǒ zào】　指习练气功时，"念不可起，念起则火燥"。

dryness of fire　Refers to the fact that ideas should not be maintained in practicing Qigong，otherwise fire will become dry.

火燥火寒【huǒ zào huǒ hán】　火燥指的是"念不可起，念起则火燥"；火寒指的是"意不可散，意散则火冷"。

dry fire and cold fire　Refers to the fact that ideas should not be maintained in practicing Qigong，otherwise fire will become dry；and that mentality should not be dispersed in practicing Qigong，

otherwise fire will be cold.

火之功效【huǒ zhī gōng xiào】　火助肾气以生真水，肾火上升交心液，而生真气。

effect of fire　A term of Qigong，indicating that fire supports kidney Qi to produce genuine water and kidney fire ascends to heart humor to produce genuine Qi.

惑【huò】　佛家气功习用语，指烦恼。

puzzle　A common term of Qigong in Buddhism，referring to annoyance.

惑业苦【huò yè kǔ】　佛家气功习用语，指身、口、意所致的贪、嗔、痴。

puzzle and bitter　A term of Qigong，referring to greediness，anger and stupidity caused by the body，mouth and consciousness.

惑以丧志【huò yǐ sàng zhì】　指迷惑引起精神意识失调。

puzzle losing ambition　Refers to imbalance of the spirit and consciousness caused by confusion.

霍乱治法【huò luàn zhì fǎ】　为动功。其作法为，转筋不止，男子以手牵引生殖器，女子以手牵拉乳房两边；仰卧，展两腿手，足跟向外分开，鼻吸气尽力行七息；俯卧，侧头看一旁，立两足尖，伸腰，鼻吸气。

exercise for curing cholera　A dynamic exercise，marked by constantly turning the sinews，towing the genitalia with hands for men and towing the breasts at both sides for women；lying on the back，stretching the hands and legs，turning the feet laterally，breathing in through the nose for seven times；lying on one side，turning the head to see one side，raising the tiptoes，stretching the waist and breathing in through the nose.

J

J

击探天鼓【jī tàn tiān gǔ】 为动功。两手掌心掩耳,手指置脑后,用示指压住中指,弹脑后部位,使耳内如有击鼓之声,声音壮盛,连续不散,能使神气内聚不散,防治头、耳疾病。

exploring celestial drum A dynamic exercise, marked by covering the ears with both palms, keeping the fingers on the back of the head, pressing the middle finger with the thumb, touching the back of the head in order to keep the sound of beating the drum in the brain that continues for a long time in order to concentrate the spirit and Qi inside the body. Such a dynamic exercise can prevent diseases in the head and the ears.

饥渴食饮气津法【jī kě shí yǐn qì jīn fǎ】 为动静相兼功。凡服气、静定安坐,瞑目叩齿,闭口鼓腹,令气满口即咽,至九下一息。

exercise with restricted diet An exercise combined with static exercise and dynastic exercise, marked by quiet sitting for respiration with closed eyes, clicking teeth, closing the mouth, instigating the abdomen and swallowing saliva when Qi is full for nine times.

机发于踵【jī fā yú zhǒng】 为气功形象,即勃勃生机。

vitality originating from heel Refers to manifestation of Qigong, indicating fullness of life.

机括【jī kuò】 指机关,意为悟性。

comprehension Refers to ability of understanding.

机在目【jī zài mù】 指目为脑神之先锋,目视而神随之。

vitality in the eyes Refers to the vanguard of the brain spirit which follows when the eyes look at what is necessary.

鸡子去留【jī zǐ qù liú】 指阴阳相对平衡稳定的状态。

going and staying of chicken A term of Qigong, referring to the balance and stability of Yin and Yang.

积精全神【jī jīng quán shén】 指积蓄精气,集中精神,以达延长寿命、强健身体的目的。

accumulating the essence and completing the spirit A celebrated dictum, indicating that accumulation of the essential Qi and concentration of the spirit can prolong life and fortify the body.

积聚【jī jù】 为气功适应证,指腹内结块,或胀或痛的病证。

mass An indication of Qigong, referring to either abdominal mass; or a disease with distension or pain.

积聚候导引法【jī jù hòu dǎo yǐn fǎ】 为动功,方法多样。如正坐,伸直腰,抬头向太阳,用口慢慢吸气,咽下三十次为止。明目,治视物昏花。

exercise of Daoyin for distension and mass A dynamic exercise with various methods, such as sitting upright, stretching the waist, raising the head to see the sun, slowly inhaling Qi and swallowing for thirty times in order to improve eyesight and to cure blurred vision.

积神【jī shén】　为凝神之意,指凝神诊脉,可以知病的既往与现在。

concentration of the spirit　A term of Qigong and life cultivation, referring to gazing the spirit, indicating that gazing the spirit and diagnosing the meridians can clarify the previous and present symptoms of a disease.

积阳生神【jī yáng shēng shén】　指阳之积而生神,神生而出智慧与技巧。

Yang accumulation formulating the spirit　A term of Qigong, indicating that accumulation of Yang can produce the spirit. When the spirit is produced, wisdom and techniques will be improved.

积阴生形【jī yīn shēng xíng】　指阴之积而生形,形生而有身体、脏腑、肢节。

Yin accumulation formulating the body　A term of Qigong, indicating that accumulation of Yin can form the body. When the body is formed, the five Zang-organs (including the heart, the liver, the spleen, the lung and the kidney), the six Fu-organs (including the gallbladder, the stomach, the small intestine, the large intestine, the bladder and the triple energizer), the limbs and the joints will be made.

嵇康【jī kāng】　魏晋时期的文学家、思想家、音乐家、气功养生家,著有气功专著,提出具体的养生方法。

Ji Kang　A litterateur, thinker, musicologist and master of Qigong and life cultivation in the period of Wei Dynasty and Jin Dynasty (220 AD – 420 AD). He wrote a monograph of

Qigong, suggesting several methods for cultivating life.

嵇康养生法【jī kāng yǎng shēng fǎ】　源自气功专论,指出调节精神,守一养和,体妙心玄,是养生之大法。

Ji Kang's exercise for cultivating life　Collected from a monograph of Qigong, indicating that regulating the spirit, protecting integration and maintaining harmony, keeping the body fine and the heart subtle are the ways to cultivate life.

嵇叔夜【jī shū yè】　魏晋时期的文学家、思想家、音乐家、气功养生家嵇康的另外一个称谓,其著有气功专著,提出具体的养生方法。

Ji Shuye　Another name of Ji Kang, a litterateur, thinker, musicologist and master of Qigong and life cultivation in the period of Wei Dynasty and Jin Dynasty (220 AD – 420 AD). He wrote a monograph of Qigong, suggesting several methods for cultivating life.

吉祥止止【jí xiáng zhǐ zhǐ】　指习练气功时,意识活动相对静止,身体各部和谐,协调统一,神灵自然来至。

perfect auspicious exercise　Refers to quietness of consciousness activity and balance of all parts of the body in order to promote natural development of divinities.

吉祥座【jí xiáng zuò】　佛家气功坐式,方式有二,一为吉祥,二为降魔。

auspicious sitting　An exercise of sitting for practicing Qigong in Buddhism with two ways, one is to be auspicious, the other is to expel evil.

极乐国【jí lè guó】　为"祖窍"异名,位于心脐之中的一个穴位。这一穴位为气功运行的一个常见部位。

very happy country　A term of Qigong, referring to either a synonym of Zuqiao which is an acupoint located in the area between the heart and navel. This acupoint is a region usually used for keeping the essential Qi in practice of Qigong.

极泉【jí quán】　手少阴心经中的一个穴位,位于腋窝正中。这一穴位为气功运行的一个常见部位。

Jiquan（HT 1）　An acupoint in the heart meridian of hand Shaoyin, located in the center of armpit. This acupoint is a region usually used for keeping the essential Qi in practice of Qigong.

极势【jí shì】　指按要领全力完成某一导引动作。

full posture　A term of Qigong, referring to completely finishing a certain exercise of Qigong practice according to the essentials.

极言【jí yán】　源自气功专论,阐述气功皆由学习而得,并要意识专一才能成功。

pure words　Collected from a monograph of Qigong, mainly describing that the success of Qigong practice depends on sincere study and that only when consciousness is concentrated can practice of Qigong be succeeded.

亟夺【jí duó】　指机体内阳气不断地向外泄耗。

constant leakage　Refers to constant discharge and leakage of Yang Qi from the body.

急存白元和六气【jí cún bái yuán hé liù qì】　为动功。其作法为,意守白元于脑神,久而久之和调六气,增强肺的卫外作用。久习此法,形体通达而不滞塞。

immediate protection of white origin and six kinds of Qi　A dynamic exercise, marked by imagining to keep the white origin in the brain spirit, balancing and regulating the six kinds of Qi after a long period of practice in order to increase the effect of the lung to defend the external. After a long period of practicing Qigong in such a way, the body is unobstructed without any stagnation.

集义所生【jí yì suǒ shēng】　源自气功专论,主要阐述守命宫,即能一阳初动,萌发生机。

concentrating righteousness for cultivating life　Collected from a monograph of Qigong, mainly describing keeping the life chamber, which means that primary movement of Yang can geminate vitality.

己【jǐ】　为脑中之灵性。

truth　Refers to the intelligence in the brain.

己土之脏【jǐ tǔ zhī zàng】　指脾脏。

earth viscus　Refers to the spleen.

脊【jǐ】　为骨名,指脊椎骨,为气功精气运行之重要部位。

spine　Refers to vertebra which is an important region for the movement of the essence and Qi in practicing Qigong.

脊脉【jǐ mài】　指督脉。

spine meridian　Refers to the governor meridian.

季胁【jì xié】　① 即季肋;② 为章门穴的另外一个称谓;③ 指气滞在胁肋,为气功适应证。

Jixie　Refers to ① either hypochondrium; ② or a synonym of Zhangmen (LR 13); ③ or stagnation of Qi in lateral thorax which is an indication of Qigong.

济一子道书【jì yī zǐ dào shū】 《济一子道书》为气功学专著,由清代傅金铨所著,深入系统地分析介绍了气功学的基本理论和方法。

Jiyizi Daoshu (*A Daoism Book about Supporting Each Other*) A monograph of Qigong entitled *A Daoism Book about Supporting Each Other*, written by Fu Jinquan in the Qing Dynasty (1636 AD – 1912 AD), systematically analyzing and introducing the basic theory and practice of Qigong.

既济【jì jì】 ① 指卦名,为六十四卦之一;② 指调节周既。

balance Refers to ① either the name of a Trigram in Yijing, in which there are altogether sixty-four Trigrams; ② or entire regulation.

寂静【jì jìng】 佛家气功习用语,指身寂静、心寂静。

concentrated tranquilization A common term of Qigong in Buddhism, referring to tranquilization of the body and the heart.

寂静法【jì jìng fǎ】 佛家气功功法,指神形调和、安静之法。

exercise for silence The exercise for practicing Qigong in Buddhism, referring to regulation, balance and tranquilization of the spirit and the body.

寂寥【jì liáo】 指静之极,广远无边际。

extreme vacuum Refers to perfect tranquility and boundless distance.

寂照【jì zhào】 气功学术语,指精、气、神合而为一,温养沐浴机体。

lone illumination A term of Qigong, referring to integration of the essence, Qi and spirit as well as warming, nour-

ishing and bathing the body.

颊车【jiá chē】 指足阳明胃经中的一个穴位,位齿咬紧时,在隆起的咬肌高点处,为气功中常用的意守部位。

Jiache (ST 6) An acupoint in the stomach meridian of foot Yangming, located in the upper of masseter when the teeth are ground, which is the region for concentrating consciousness in practicing Qigong.

假想观【jiǎ xiǎng guān】 为佛家气功习用语,指意想,或意念活动。

imagined contemplation A common term of Qigong in Buddhism, referring to imagination or consciousness activity.

坚齿法【jiān chǐ fǎ】 动静相兼功。其作法为,安精神,养华池,吞津液,清晨叩齿三百次。能坚齿,治齿牙摇动,或脱落。

exercise for strengthening the teeth An exercise combined with dynamic exercise and static exercise, marked by stabilizing the essence and spirit, nourishing essential pool, taking fluid and humor and clicking the teeth for three hundred times in the early morning in order to strengthen the teeth and to cure mobility or loss of teeth.

坚法【jiān fǎ】 佛家气功习用语,指忘生命、弃财宝、去封累,而专修功法,以提高意志,增加活力。

cultivating devotion A common term of Qigong in Buddhism, referring to neglecting life, eliminating treasure, expelling closure, majoring practice methods, improving consciousness and increasing energy.

肩髎【jiān liáo】 手少阳三焦经中的一个穴位,位于锁骨肩峰端与肩胛骨之间凹陷中。这一穴位为气功运行的一个常见部位。

Jianliao（SJ 14） An acupoint located in the triple energizer meridian of hand Shaoyang, located in the depression between the acromion of clavicle and scapula. This acupoint is a region usually used for keeping the essential Qi in practice of Qigong.

坚实心【jiān shí xīn】 佛家气功习用语，指人固有的自然本性。

natural solid heart A common term of Qigong in Buddhism, referring to natural characteristics in human beings.

间关【jiān guān】 指三丹田中间部位。

middle joint Refers to the middle region of the three Dantian. Dantian is divided into the upper Dantian (the region between the eyes), the middle Dantian (the region below the heart) and the lower Dantian (the region below the navel).

肩功【jiān gōng】 为动功。其作法为，两肩连手，左右轮转，各二十四次。调息神思，以左手擦脐十四遍，右手亦然。

shoulder exercise Dynamic exercise, marked by connecting the hands with both shoulders, rotating from the left to the right and vice versa for twenty-four times respectively, regulating respiration, the spirit and thinking, rubbing the navel with the left hand and the right hand for fourteen times respectively.

肩胛【jiān jiǎ】 指肩胛骨。

shoulder joint Refers to scapula.

肩井【jiān jǐng】 为足少阳胆经中的一个穴位，位于肩上。这一穴位为气功

运行的一个常见部位。

Jianjing（GB 21） An acupoint in the bladder meridian of foot Shaoyang, located in the shoulder. This acupoint is a region usually used for keeping the essential Qi in practice of Qigong.

肩髆【jiān pò】 指肩胛骨。

shoulder blade Refers to the scapula.

肩髃【jiān yú】 手阳明大肠经中的一个穴位，位于肩峰前下方。这一穴位为气功运行的一个常见部位。

Jianyu（LI 15） An acupoint in the large intestine meridian of hand Yangming, located below the acromion. This acupoint is a region usually used for keeping the essential Qi in practice of Qigong.

俭视养神【jiǎn shì yǎng shén】 指闭目少视，眼不受外界事物的影响，可以荣养脑神。

closing the eyes to nourish the spirit Means to close the eyes and to avoid influence of anything in the external world in order to nourish the spirit in the brain.

俭听养神【jiǎn tīng yǎng shén】 指减听噪声安语，可以稳定精神意识思维活动。

avoiding noise to nourish the spirit Means that avoiding any noise and nonsense can stabilize the activities of the spirit, consciousness and thinking.

检情摄念【jiǎn qíng shè niàn】 指习练气功，应解除情欲，收摄杂念。

eliminating sexual desire Refers to eliminating sexual passion and distracting thought in practicing Qigong.

检时含景补泻图【jiǎn shí hán jǐng bǔ xiè tú】 为静功，方法多样。如肺用呬为泻，呼为补；立秋日平旦，面正西坐；鸣

天鼓七通,饮玉泉浆三咽;瞑目正思,兑宫白气入口吞之三,则童神安,百邪不能殃,兵刃不能害,延年益寿。谓补泻神气,安息灵魂。

exercise for purging and tonifying modes of respiration A static exercise with various methods, such as eliminating diarrhea and with Xi (breath) in the lung and tonifying through breath, sitting to the west in the early morning in autumn, clicking teeth for seven times, drinking slurry in Yuquan (CV 3) located 4 Cun below the navel for three times, closing the eyes to purify the mind, swallowing white Qi from the east for three times, taking measures to stabilize the fetal spirit, eliminating all evils and avoiding any harm caused by weapons in order to prolong life and cultivate health. Such a static exercise can tonify the spirit and Qi as well as to stabilize the ethereal soul and corporeal soul.

简寂先生【jiǎn jì xiān shēng】　南朝气功学家陆修德的另外一个称谓,其撰写了气功学专著,分析和研究了气功学的理论和方法。

Mr. Jian Ji Another name of Lu Xiude, a great master of Qigong in South Dynasty (420 AD – 589 AD) who wrote a monograph of Qigong to analyze and to study the theory and practice of Qigong.

篯铿【jiǎn kēng】　上古时代气功养生学家彭祖的另外一个称谓。

Jian Keng Another name of Peng Zu, a great master of Qigong and life cultivation in ancient China.

篯篮观井【jiǎn lán guān jǐng】　为动功。其作法为,自然站立,两脚分开与肩宽,两手握拳,腰弯如鞠躬姿势,两手尽量向下,慢慢起身,两拳随身慢慢举起,过顶,整个过程要闭口,两拳过顶时鼻内微微出气三四口。治腰腿疼。

Jian Lan viewing well A dynamic exercise, marked by standing up naturally, separating the feet similar to the distance between both shoulders, holding the fists with both hands, lowering the waist like bowing, stretching the hands downwards, slowly lifting the body, slowly raising the fists to the top of the head, closing the mouth during the whole process, breathing out through the nose for three to four times when the fists are raised to the top of the head. Such a dynamic exercise can cure waist pain and leg pain.

见道【jiàn dào】　佛家气功功法,指应用"空观",稳定情绪,消除烦恼。

perspective of Dao A method of Qigong practice in Buddhism, referring to stabilizing emotion and eliminating annoyance in order to cultivate health.

见思惑【jiàn sī huò】　佛家气功习用语,指精神思维活动,为思惑之意。引起的原因,一是贪欲嗔恚,反思世间事物;二是邪见。

perspective of avaricious temptation A common term of Qigong practice in Buddhism, referring to avaricious temptation that abnormally observe, analyze and decide anything in the world, which should be absolutely eliminated in practicing Qiong.

见素抱朴【jiàn sù bào pǔ】　指外象单纯,内里朴素,喻气功表里如一,神形和调。

perspective of purity and frugality Refers to simplicity of the external and purity of the internal，indicating that the external and the internal of Qigong are the same and that the spirit and the body are regulated.

见素子【jiàn sù zǐ**】** 唐代女气功家胡愔的另一名称。

Jian Zuzi Another name of Hu Yin who was a great master of Qigong in the Tang Dynasty（618 AD - 907 AD）.

见心【jiàn xīn**】** 指透视人心以静其神。

cardiac perspective Refers to sincerely observing the heart with the mind in order to tranquilize the spirit.

建德观【jiàn dé guàn**】** 在南昌城内，相传为古人习练气功之处。

Jiande Temple Located in the Nanchang City，where some important masters of Qigong studied and practiced Qigong in ancient China.

健忘【jiàn wàng**】** 气功适应证，指记忆减退，遇事善忘。

amnesia An indication of Qigong, referring to hypomnesis that makes the sufferers to forget everything when meeting anything.

渐法【jiàn fǎ**】** 指练功过程中，由初关炼精化气到中关炼气化神，再到上关炼神还虚。

gradual practice A term of Qigong, indicating to refine the essence to transform into Qi at the early level and to transform Qi into the spirit at the middle level，and to refine the spirit to be tranquilized at the high level.

渐门【jiàn mén**】** 指习练气功，应循序渐进，逐步深化。

gradual progress Refers to advancing gradually and deepening eventually in practicing Qigong.

渐悟集【jiàn wù jí**】** 《渐悟集》为气功专著，由金代马丹阳所撰，内容主要以诗词形式谈内丹修炼，清心寡欲，炼精化气，炼气化神，炼神还虚，循序渐进。

Jianwu Ji （*Collection of Gradual Awareness*） A monograph of Qigong entitled *Collection of Gradual Awareness*，written by Ma Danyang in the Jin Dynasty（1115 AD - 1234 AD），mainly describing practice of internal Dan（pills of immortality）with poems, suggesting to cleanse one's heart and limit one's desires，to refine the essence for transforming Qi，to refine Qi for transforming the spirit，and to refine the spirit for gradually tranquilizing the mind.

渐有五门【jiàn yǒu wǔ mén**】** ① 指斋戒；② 指安处；③ 指存想；④ 指坐忘；⑤ 指神解。

gradually forming five stages Refers to ① either fast；② or stability；③ or inward contemplation；④ or sitting quietly；⑤ or imagining the spirit.

楗【jiàn**】** 指股骨上段。

bone Refers to the upper part of thighbone.

将摄保命篇【jiāng shè bǎo mìng piān**】** 《将摄保命篇》为气功专著，主要论述道德修养，避免精神刺激，为气功养生延年的重要措施。作者不详。

Jiangshe Baoming Pian（*Important Formulae of Cultivation in Various Categories*） A monograph of Qigong entitled *A Book about Protection and Cultivation of Life*，mainly describing the importance of morality for cultivating life and suggesting avoidance of stimulated spirit，which is the important measure to cultivate health and prolong life.

The author was unknown.

降龙【jiàng lóng】　龙指心,练功中调心神为降龙。

descending Loong　A term of Qigong, referring to regulating the heart spirit. In this term, Loong refers to the heart.

降心【jiàng xīn】　指人的心思容易妄动,常使意念不易集中。

descending the heart　A term of Qigong, indicating that the mind often takes reckless actions, making it difficult for consciousness to be concentrated.

绛宫【jiàng gōng】　气功中心的别称。

crimson palace　A synonym of the heart in Qigong.

绛宫真人【jiàng gōng zhēn rén】　心之元神。绛宫为心,真人指神。

genuine immortal in crimson palace　Refers to the original spirit in the heart. In this term, crimson palace refers to the heart and genuine immortal refers to the spirit.

交感宫【jiāo gǎn gōng】　指泥丸,或指脑。

interaction chamber　Refers to cerebral spirit or the mud bolus (the brain).

交感之精【jiāo gǎn zhī jīng】　指男女交媾,精自泥丸顺脊而下,至膀胱外肾施泄,遂成渣滓,则为交感之精。

essence in intercourse　Refers to coitus of a man and a woman, during which essence in the mud bolus (the brain) descends from the spine to the bladder and the external side of the kidney, eventually discharging and becoming dregs. This is what the essence in sexual intercourse means.

交媾【jiāo gòu】　指阴阳相交之意,又指男女性交。

intercourse　Refers to either combination of Yin and Yang; or copulation between a man and a woman.

交媾龙虎【jiāo gòu lóng hǔ】　指通过精气神的交流和交会,"液中有真气,气中有真水,互相交合,相依而下,名曰交媾龙虎"。

connection of Loong and tiger　Refers to combination and integration of the essence, Qi and the spirit, during which "there is genuine Qi in humor and there is genuine water in Qi. The so-called connection of Loong and tiger means mutual combination and mutual movement of the essence, Qi and the spirit".

交合【jiāo hé】　指习练气功中,阴精阳气的依附作用。

interdependence　A term of Qigong, referring to the interdependence of Yin essence and Yang Qi in practicing Qigong.

交脚踑踞【jiāo jiǎo qí jù】　指两脚交叉,屈膝张腿而坐的导引姿势。

cross-legged exercise　Refers to the style of sitting marked by crossing the feet, bending the knees and stretching the feet.

交梨火枣【jiāo lí huǒ zǎo】　① 指心源和关元;② 指药物;③ 指练功效应;④ 指阴丹。

linking pear and heating jujube　Refers to ① either heart source and Guanyuan (CV 4); ② or medicinal; ③ or effect of Qigong practice; ④ or Yin Dan (pills of immortality).

交信【jiāo xìn】　足少阴肾经的一个穴位,位于内踝尖与跟腱水平连线中点直上 2 寸,向前 0.5 寸。这一穴位为气功运行的一个常见部位。

Jiaoxin（KI 8） An acupoint in the kidney meridian of foot Shaoyin, located 2 Cun above and 0.5 Cun forward the midline between the top of the medial malleolus and Achilles tendon. This acupoint is a region usually used for keeping the essential Qi in practice of Qigong.

娇女【jiāo nǚ】 ① 指目神;② 指耳神。

tender female Refers to ① either the spirit in the eyes; ② or the spirit in the ears.

焦心劳神【jiāo xīn láo shén】 指思虑纷繁复杂,能劳伤精神。气功中通过意守即为排除焦心而养神。

scorching the heart and bothering the spirit Indicates that contemplation is complicated and damages the spirit. In Qigong practice, anxiety in the heart is eliminated for nourishing the spirit.

角孙【jiǎo sūn】 手少阳三焦经中的一个穴位,位于耳尖上方发际处。这一穴位为气功运行的一个常见部位。

Jiaosun（TE 20） An acupoint in the triple energizer meridian of hand Shaoyang, located above the auricle in the hair line. This acupoint is a region usually used for keeping the essential Qi in practice of Qigong.

绞肠痧治法【jiǎo cháng shā zhì fǎ】 为动静相兼功。其作法为,凡绞肠痧腹痛,侧坐,以两手抱膝齐胸,左右足各蹬板九次,数息二十口。

exercise for abdominal angina An exercise combined with dynamic exercise and static exercise, marked by sitting at one side if there is angina, holding the knees and chest with both hands, kicking the board with both feet for nine

times and breathing for twenty times.

脚气缓弱【jiǎo qì huǎn ruò】 为气功适应证,本病多由感受风寒之邪所致。

flaccid beriberi An indication of Qigong, caused by pathogenic cold and wind.

脚气缓弱候导引法【jiǎo qì huǎn ruò hòu dǎo yǐn fǎ】 为动功,方法多样。如俯卧,眼侧视,脚跟向上,伸直腰,用鼻吸气,至极限时慢慢呼出,作七息。通经络,强腰脚,治脚痛转筋,脚痹弱。

exercise of Daoyin for flaccid beriberi A dynamic exercise with various methods, such as lying prostrate, seeing lateral side, lifting heels, stretching the waist, inhaling Qi through the nose, and slowly exhaling Qi for seven times for dredging the meridians and collaterals as well as strengthening the waist and feet. Such a dynamic exercise can cure foot pain, convulsion of sinews and foot impediment.

脚气治法【jiǎo qì zhì fǎ】 为动静相兼功,方法多样。如俯卧,两眼向旁看,脚跟向内,伸腰,用鼻子吸气,尽力七息。

exercise for curing beriberi An exercise combined with dynamic exercise and static exercise with various methods, such as lying prostrate, seeing laterally with both eyes, turning the heel inward, stretching the waist, and inhaling Qi through the nose for seven times.

教修身则全神俱气【jiào xiū shēn zé quán shén jù qì】 指全神养气以修身,提高智力,健康形体。

Only when the body is cultivated can all kinds of spirit contain Qi. This is a celebrated dictum, indicating that only when all kinds of spirit have nourished

Qi can the body be cultivated, the wisdom be increased and the health be promoted.

教修心则虚心守道【jiào xiū xīn zé xū xīn shǒu dào】　指意识活动清静宁谧,守自然之道,以调节精神。

Only when the heart is cultivated can the heart be tranquilized and defend Dao. This is a celebrated dictum, indicating that tranquilized activity of consciousness can defend natural Dao and regulate the spirit.

教圆【jiào yuán】　指入静能灭烦恼。

tranquility cycle Tranquility cycle means to eliminate annoyance after tranquilization.

接舆狂歌【jiē yú kuáng gē】　为动功。其作法为,自然站立,面对墙,右手扶墙,左手自然下垂,右脚蹬墙,力量适中而舒缓,同时运气十八口,然后换左手扶墙,右手下垂,左脚蹬墙,要求同前。

Jie Yu's song singing heartily　A dynamic exercise, marked by standing up naturally toward the wall, sustaining the wall with the right hand, naturally drooping the left hand, kicking the wall with the right foot to a certain level and moving Qi for eighteen times; then sustaining the wall with the left hand, naturally drooping the right hand, and kicking the wall with the left foot just like the previous practice.

节气法【jié qì fǎ】　为静功。其作法为,先闭口,默察外息从鼻入。可调节身之阴阳,协和五脏,通经络。

exercise of solar term　A static exercise, marked by closing the mouth, silently inhaling external air through the nose in order to regulate Yin and Yang, to harmonize the five Zang-or-gans (including the heart, the liver, the spleen, the lung and the kidney) and to unobstruct the meridians and collaterals.

节宣之和【jié xuān zhī hé】　指进行气功养生,应节制性欲。

command and harmony　A term of Qigong, referring to checking sexual desire in practicing Qigong.

劫【jié】　为佛学外来语。气功文献中,指炼内丹成功之后,生命摆脱生死而获得长生。

extraction　A foreign word in Buddhism. In the literature of Qigong, it refers to longevity after successful practice of Qigong.

结【jié】　指束缚,喻人体为烦恼束缚而神形不调。

trammel　Refers to fetter, indicating annoyance and imbalance between the spirit and body.

结丹【jié dān】　指采外来之药,与真气相聚,结而成丹。

formulating Dan（pills of immortality） A term of Qigong, referring to collecting medicinal in the external world that coordinates with the genuine Qi and forms Dan（pills of immortality）.

结丹定位【jié dān dìng wèi】　指结丹在气海,其位在下丹田,与脐相对。

formulation and location of Dan（pills of immortality）　A term of Qigong, referring to formulation of Dan（pills of immortality）in the sea of Qi, located in the lower Dantian（the region below the navel）.

结跏趺坐【jié jiā fū zuò】　即吉祥座,为佛家气功坐式,方式有二,一为吉祥,二为降魔。

sitting with crossed legs　Refers to auspicious sitting which is an exercise of sitting for practicing Qigong in Buddhism with two ways, one is to be auspicious, the other is to expel evil.

结气【jié qì】 为气功适应证,指肝气郁结不舒的病证,常因情志不遂所致。

stagnant Qi An indication of Qigong, referring to Qi stagnation syndrome / pattern caused by emotional frustration.

结气后导引法【jié qì hòu dǎo yǐn fǎ】为动功。其作法为,正坐,伸直腰,左手上举,手掌上仰,右手下垂向后,手掌向下,用鼻吸气至极限时慢慢呼出,作七息。呼吸时,右手稍顿,活气血,通经络。治两臂背痛,结气。

exercise of Daoyin for stagnation of Qi A dynamic exercise, marked by sitting upright, stretching the waist, raising the left hand sand palm, lowering the right hand and palm, inhaling Qi through the nose to the limit and then slowly exhaling Qi for seven times, mildly pausing the right hand in breathing in order to activate Qi and blood and to promote the meridians and collaterals. To practice Daoyin with such a dynamic exercise can relieve pain in the shoulders and back and cure stagnation of Qi

结胎【jié tāi】 指练功到一定的时候,精气与神融为一体,加上阳气的作用,合而成丹,此称结胎。

formulating embryo Refers to integration of the essential Qi and the spirit in practicing Qigong. Integration of the essential Qi and the spirit with the effect of Yang Qi will produce Dan (pills of immortality), which is called formulating embryo.

解脱【jiě tuō】 为佛家气功习用语,指解除系缚,而使神形合调,安适自在。

stopping collapse A common term of Qigong in Buddhism, referring to eliminating fetter in order to regulate and to comfort the spirit and the body.

解脱身形及诸神【jiě tuō shēn xíng jí zhū shén】 指放松形体,安静精神意识活动之意。

freeing from the body and various spirits A celebrated dictum, referring to relaxing the body, stabilizing and tranquilizing the activities of the spirit and consciousness.

介尔阴妄一念【jiè ěr yīn wàng yī niàn】 为佛家气功习用语,指观想阴妄之一念在"即空即假即中"之间。

sudden thinking about confusion A common term of Qigong practice in Buddhism, referring to the fact that confusion is maintained in emptiness, falseness and middle.

戒【jiè】 为佛家气功习用语,指戒规、戒律,防禁错误、过失。有五戒、八戒、十戒等说,意在使行为不出轨。

discipline A common term of Qigong in Buddhism, referring to precepts and commandment for prohibiting errors and faults. There are five sila (morality), eight sila (morality) and ten sila (morality), which are the important ways for preventing derailment.

戒暴怒养性【jiè bào nù yǎng xìng】指调节情志,修养性格,忌暴发脾气,免使气血逆乱伤身。

eliminating rage to nourish the body A celebrated dictum, referring to regulating emotion and cultivating character in order to prevent eruption of temperament and to avoid Qi and blood to dam-

② 指内丹之金丹。

golden Dan（pills of immortality） Refers to ① either golden Dan（pills of immortality）in the external Dan（pills of immortality）；② or golden Dan（pills of immortality）in the internal Dan（pills of immortality）.

金丹大药【jīn dān dà yào】 指内丹，即习练气功。

large medicinal in golden Dan（pills of immortality） A term of Qigong, referring to internal Dan（pills of immortality）, indicating practice of Qigong.

金丹大要【jīn dān dà yào】《金丹大要》为气功专著，由元代陈致虚所著，认为精气神为金丹之上药三品，强调人皆禀受先天真阳之气而生。

Jindan Dayao（*Great Importance of Golden Dan*） A monograph of Qigong entitled *Great Importance of Golden Dan（Pills of Immortality）*, written by Chen Zhixu in the Yuan Dynasty（1271 AD - 1368 AD）, describing that the essence, Qi and the spirit are the three great medicinals in golden Dan（pills of immortality）, emphasizing that the birth of human beings depends on Qi from the innate genuine Yang.

金丹秘法【jīn dān mì fǎ】 为动功。其作法为，每日十九时至二十一时正坐，一手兜外肾，一手护脐下，左右换手，各八十一次。

secret method of golden Dan（pills of immortality） A dynamic exercise, marked by sitting upright in Zi period（the period of the day from 11 p.m. to 1 a.m.）, wrapping the external kidney with one hand and protecting the navel with the other hand and vice versa for eighty-one times respectively.

---

age the body.

戒定会慧【jiè dìng huì huì】 为佛家气功习用语，防非止恶曰戒，息虑静缘曰定，破恶证真曰慧。

discipline deciding wisdom A common term of Qigong in Buddhism, in which discipline means to prevent disorder and to expel evil; deciding means to eliminate contemplation and to tranquilize respiration mind; and wisdom means to break wickedness and rectify truth.

界分别观【jiè fēn bié guān】 为佛家气功功法。其作法为，分别六界、十八界，停止我见之法，以排除精神不稳定的因素。

distinguishing different states An exercise of Qigong in Buddhism, marked by separating six states and eighteen states without any personal idea in order to eliminate the pathogenic factors affecting the stability of the spirit.

疥候导引法【jiè hòu dǎo yǐn fǎ】 为静功。其作法为，坐或站立，低头向下看，闭气不息，至极限时慢慢呼出，作十二遍。可清热解毒，治疗疥疮。

exercise of Daoyin for scabies A static exercise, marked by sitting or standing, lowering the head to see the ground and stopping respiration to a certain degree to slowly exhale for twelve times. To practice Qigong with this static exercise can relieve heat, expel toxin and treat scabies.

巾金巾【jīn jīn jīn】 指肺在心之上，肺为心之华盖。

mulching lung Indicates that the lung is located above the heart and the lung is the canopy of the heart.

金丹【jīn dān】 ① 指外丹之金丹；

金丹心法【jīn dān xīn fǎ】 《金丹心法》为气功专著,作者不详。

Jindan Xinfa(*Mental Cultivation Methods of Celestial Immortals with Golden Dan*) A monograph about Qigong entitled *Mental Cultivation Methods of Celestial Immortals with Golden Dan*(*Pills of Immortality*). The author was unknown.

金丹要诀【jīn dān yào jué】 《金丹要诀》为气功学专著,为明代伍守阳所著,论述了气功的基础理论和方法。

Jindan Yaojue(*Important Formula of Golden Dan*) A monograph of Qigong entitled *Important Formula of Golden Dan*(*Pills of Immortality*), written by Wu Shouyang in the Ming Dynasty (1368 AD – 1644 AD), mainly describing the theory and practice of Qigong.

金丹之道【jīn dān zhī dào】 指习练气功主要是入静。

the way of golden Dan(*pills of immortality*) A term of Qigong, referring to the importance of tranquility in Qigong practice.

金鼎【jīn dǐng】 指头。

golden cauldron A term of Qigong, referring to the head.

金公【jīn gōng】 ① 指外丹,文献中指金属铅;② 指内丹,文献中指元精、坎水。

golden common A term of Qigong, referring to ① either external Dan(pills of immortality) and metallic lead according to the traditional literature; ② or original essence and water related to Kan Trigram according to the literature of internal Dan(pills of immortality).

金关玉楼【jīn guān yù lóu】 同金室,

① 指练功过程中结"金丹"之所;② 指肺;③ 指脑。

golden joint and jade building The same as golden chamber, refers to ① either the place to form golden Dan(pills of immortality) during the procedure of Qigong practice; ② or the lung; ③ or the brain.

金关玉锁坐法【jīn guān yù suǒ zuò fǎ】 为静功。其作法为,跏趺升身,垂帘塞兑,神凝息定,下提上吸,二气交合,熏蒸四大,上十二重楼,真津满口,以气送之,意归元宫,既住吸提,微微开兑。

sitting exercise with golden joint and jade lock A static exercise, marked by sitting with crossed legs and stretching the waist, closing the curtain and stopping any change, concentrating the spirit and quieting respiration, lifting the lower and inhaling in the upper, coordinating the two kinds of Qi, fumigating in the four important regions, rising up to the twelve important tops, enriching genuine fluid in the mouth, delivering with Qi, entering consciousness into the original chamber, staying with increased inhalation and mildly turning from one joint to another.

金光清虚含真内景【jīn guāng qīng xū hán zhēn nèi jǐng】 为静功。其具体作法为,于夏历每月十七日夜晚,在清净的室内坐定,入静后意想自己进入"月宫",朝拜"月中帝君",默默想学气功之愿望。叩齿、咽津各四十九遍,良久收功。

golden light and clear vacuum containing genuine internal image A static exercise, marked by sitting in the clean and quiet room at night on seventeenth in every month in summer, imagining to enter into "the lunar palace" to worship "the lunar King" after tranquilization, silently thinking about the desire to study Qigong, then clicking the teeth and swallowing fluid for forty-nine times and completing the exercise.

金柜【jīn guì】 指肾。

golden cabinet A term of Qigong, referring to the kidney.

金火混融【jīn huǒ hún róng】 即牛女相逢,喻气功真阴、真阳相逢,阴平阳秘,合为一处。

combination of metal and fire A synonym of meeting of cowherd and maid, is a term of Qigong, referring to integration of genuine Yin and genuine Yang in practice of Qigong and harmony between Yin and Yang.

金浆玉醴【jīn jiāng yù lǐ】 即玉醴金浆,指服炼口中津液。

golden syrup and jade wine The same as jade wine and golden syrup, is a term of Qigong, referring to fluid and humor swallowed in the mouth.

金晶【jīn jīng】 指子时所生之肺液并在肾中。

golden brilliance A term of Qigong, indicating that humor produced in the lung in Zi period (the period of the day from 11 p.m. to 1 a.m.) is also in the kidney.

金醴【jīn lǐ】 指口中之津液。

golden wine A term of Qigong, referring to fluid and humor in the mouth.

金梁【jīn liáng】 指上下牙齿。

golden beam A term of Qigong, referring to the upper and lower teeth.

金铃朱带坐婆娑【jīn líng zhū dài zuò pó suō】 指心之内有室如铃内空,心之脉如朱带,心神安静自守为坐婆娑。

sitting to dance with golden bell and red belt A celebrated dictum, indicating that there is a chamber like bell in the heart, the heart meridian moves life as the red belt and the heart spirit is tranquilized like sitting to dance.

金炉【jīn lú】 即白虎,① 白虎指二十八宿中西方的七宿;② 内丹书中指"心中元神谓之龙,肾中元精谓之虎"。

golden furnace A synonym of white tiger, refers to ① either the seven constellations in the west among the twenty-eight constellations; ② or "the original spirit in the heart called Loong and the original essence in the kidney called tiger" mentioned in the books about internal Dan (pills of immortality).

金炉火炽【jīn lú huǒ chì】 指元精经河车搬运入泥丸时的景象。

golden stove with great fire A term of Qigong, referring to the scene of original essence that has entered the mud bolus (the brain) through the river cart.

金蟆【jīn má】 即玉兔。玉兔,气功文献中指代月。

golden toad Refers to jade rabbit. In traditional literature of Qiong, it refers to the moon.

金木交【jīn mù jiāo】 指肝肺之气和合并协调之。

coordination of metal and wood A term of Qigong, referring to integration and coordination of Qi from the liver and the lung.

金木相刑【jīn mù xiāng xíng】 源自气功专论,论述金木相互制约,才能维持五脏之间的稳定。

control of metal and wood Collected from a monograph of Qigong, describing that only when metal and wood control each other can the five Zang-organs（including the heart, the liver, the spleen, the lung and the kidney）be stabilized.

金男【jīn nán】　指元气,亦指肺金之气。

golden man　A term of Qigong, referring to either the original Qi; or Qi from the lung-metal. Lung-metal means that the lung pertains to metal among the five elements（including wood, fire, earth, metal and water）.

金阙帝君三元真一经【jīn què dì jūn sān yuán zhēn yì jīng】　《金阙帝君三元真一经》为气功专著,阐发气功理论,介绍具体方法,有一定的使用价值。作者不详。

Jinque Dijun Sanyuan Zhenyi Jing（*A Genuine Canon of King's Three Origins in Golden Watchtower*）　A monograph of Qigong entitled *A Genuine Canon of King's Three Origins in Golden Watchtower*, describing the basic theory of Qigong, introducing the detailed methods of Qigong practice, quite effectively in studying and practicing Qigong. The author was unknown.

金室【jīn shì】　① 指练功过程中结"金丹"之所;② 指肺;③ 指脑。

golden chamber　Refers to ① either the place to form golden Dan（pills of immortality）during the procedure of Qigong practice; ② or the lung; ③ or the brain.

金水合处【jīn shuǐ hé chù】　指肺肾滋养。其中金指肺,水指肾。

combination of metal and water　A term of Qigong, referring to enriching and nourishing the lung and the kidney. In this term, metal refers to the lung while water refers to the kidney.

金锁关【jīn suǒ guān】　指舌。

golden lockage　A term of Qigong, referring to the tongue.

金翁【jīn wēng】　① 即金公,指外丹,文献中指金属铅;② 指内丹,文献中指元精、坎水。

golden old man　A synonym of golden common, is a term of Qigong, referring to ① either external Dan（pills of immortality）and metallic lead according to the traditional literature; ② or original essence and water related to Kan Trigram according to the literature of internal Dan（pills of immortality）.

金乌搦兔儿【jīn wū nuò tù ér】　金乌即日,气功学中喻元神;兔儿即月,气功学中喻元精。金乌搦兔儿,喻练功中元神制元精。

golden bird holding young rabbit　A term of Qigong, indicating that the original spirit controls the original essence. In this term, golden bird refers to the sun and in Qigong it refers to the original spirit; young rabbit refers to the moon and in Qigong it refers to the original essence.

金乌玉兔【jīn wū yù tù】　指日月。在气功学中,金乌指心,玉兔指肾。金乌玉兔即心肾相交。

golden bird and jade rabbit　Refers to the sun and the moon. In Qigong, golden bird refers to the heart while jade rabbit refers to the kidney. Golden bird and jade rabbit all mean combination of the heart and the kidney.

金仙【jīn xiān】　指气功锻炼中的性命双修。

golden immortal A term of Qigong, referring to double cultivation of life in practicing Qigong.

金仙证论【jīn xiān zhèng lùn】《金仙证论》为气功专著,由清代柳华阳所撰,书中内容以内丹术为主,吸收了佛家的坐禅功法。

Jinxian Zhenglun (*Demonstration of Golden Immortals*) A monograph of Qigong entitled *Demonstration of Golden Immortals*, written by Liu Huayang in the Qing Dynasty (1636 AD – 1912 AD), mainly describing the techniques of internal Dan (pills of immortality) and collecting the exercises of sitting in meditation in Buddhism.

金液【jīn yè】 ① 指肝之液;② 指肺液;③ 指炼丹的药物,即津液、金水、玉液。

golden humor Refers to ① either humor in the liver; ② or humor in the lung; ③ or medicinal in refining Dan (pills of immortality) which refers to fluid and humor, golden water and jade humor.

金液还丹【jīn yè huán dān】 ① 指真铅与真汞相交合而化生之丹;② 指以肺液入下丹田。

golden humor entering Dan (**pills of immortality**) A term of Qigong, referring to ① either combination of genuine lead and genuine mercury producing Dan (pills of immortality); ② or lung humor entering the lower Dantian (the region below the navel).

金液还丹赋【jīn yè huán dān fù】《金液还丹赋》为气功专论,由元代肖廷芝所撰,阐述肺液(金液)还于丹田的习练方法。

Jinye Huandan Fu (*Composition of Golden Humor Entering Dan*) A monograph of Qigong entitled *Composition of Golden Humor Entering Dan* (*Pills of Immortality*), written by Xiao Tingzhi in the Yuan Dynasty (1271 AD – 1368 AD), describing the practice exercise for entering lung humor (golden humor) into Dantian. Dantian is divided into upper Dantian (the region between the eyes), the middle Dantian (the region below the heart) and the lower Dantian (the region below the navel).

金液还丹印证图【jīn yè huán dān yìn zhèng tú】《金液还丹印证图》为气功专著,由宋代龙眉子所撰,记述了外法象及内法象各九章,阐述了气功的微妙道理。

Jinye Huandan Yinzheng Tu (*Certification Chart of Golden Humor Entering Dan*) A monograph of Qigong entitled *Certification Chart of Golden Humor Entering Dan* (*Pills of Immortality*), written by Long Meizi in the Song Dynasty (960 AD – 1279 AD), narrating the external practice image and the internal practice image in nine chapters, and describing the subtle truth of Qigong.

金液之精【jīn yè zhī jīng】 同金液还丹,指真铅与真汞相交合而化生之丹;指以肺液入下丹田。

essence of golden humor The same as golden humor entering Dan (pills of immortality), is a term of Qigong, referring to either combination of genuine lead and genuine mercury producing Dan (pills of immortality); or lung humor entering the lower Dantian (the region below the navel).

金元朝【jīn yuán cháo】 即五气朝元,

指五脏之气上朝天元。

gold and origin vision A term of Qigong, the same as five Qi turning to the origin, refers to Qi from the five Zang-organs (including the heart, the liver, the spleen, the lung and the kidney) that flows up to the celestial origin.

津【jīn】 ① 指体液;② 指唾液;③ 指汗。

fluid Refers to ① either humor; ② or saliva; ③ or sweating.

津脱【jīn tuō】 为气功适应证,指汗大泄而亡阳。

dehydration An indication of Qigong, referring to loss of Yang due to profuse sweating.

津为续命芝【jīn wéi xù mìng zhī】 指气功咽唾可以养津益津。

Fluid is the glossy ganoderma for protecting life. This is a celebrated dictum, indicating that swallowing saliva in practicing Qigong can nourish fluid and enrich fluid.

津液【jīn yè】 ① 指尿液;② 指体液。

fluid-humor Refers to ① either urine; ② or humor.

津液之道【jīn yè zhī dào】 指廉泉、玉英两穴,为玉液生成之处。

the way of fluid-humor Refers to the acupoints of Lianquan(CV 23) and Yuying(CV 18) where jade syrup is produced.

津液之腑【jīn yè zhī fǔ】 指膀胱,为六腑之一。

Fu-organ of fluid-humor Refers to the bladder, which is one of the six Fu-organs (including the gallbladder, the stomach, the small intestine, the large intestine, the bladder and the triple en-

ergizer).

津液之海【jīn yè zhī hǎi】 指玄膺窍。

sea of fluid-humor A term of Qigong, referring to the supreme thoracic orifice.

津液之山源【jīn yè zhī shān yuán】 指脑,为津液之源。

original mountain of fluid-humor A term of Qigong, referring to the brain which is the origin of fluid and humor.

筋痹【jīn bì】 为气功适应证,指筋脉拘挛,关节疼痛,不能行走的病证。

sinew impediment An indication of Qigong, referring to diseases characterized by spasm of sinews and vessels, joint pain and difficulty to walk.

筋急【jīn jí】 为气功适应证,多见于破伤风、痉病、痹证、惊风等疾病过程中。

sinew spasm An indication of Qigong, usually related to tetanus, convulsive disease, impediment syndrome and convulsion.

筋急候导引法【jīn jí hòu dǎo yǐn fǎ】 为动功,方法多样。如两手抱足向面部靠近,头不功,意想使全身骨节松散,做二十一次,用手握住脚,左右侧身,尽力牵引,腰不动。

exercise of Daoyin for spasmodic sinew A dynamic exercise with various methods, such as holding the feet with both hands toward the face without moving the head, imagining to relax all the joints in the body, grasping the feet with both hands from the left side to the right side and vice versa for twenty-one times respectively in order to drag the legs without moving the waist.

筋瘤【jīn liú】 为气功适应证,多因久站致血壅于下,或寒邪侵袭,筋挛血瘀所致。

sinew tumor An indication of Qigong, usually caused by blood stasis in the lower region due to standing for a long time; or invasion of pathogenic cold, sinew spasm and blood stasis.

尽势【jìn shì】 指一时间尽力保持原来的导引姿势。

concentration of feature A term of Qigong, referring to trying the best to keep the original features of Daoyin in a time.

尽心【jìn xīn】 尽思维之意以知其性。气功文献中常用以认识人的情性，观察人与自然的关系。

concentration of the heart Refers to concentration of consciousness in order to understand the property. In the literature of Qigong, it usually refers to understanding temperament and observing the relationship between human beings and the natural world.

尽性了命【jìn xìng liǎo mìng】 性为神，命为气。指习练气功，神气相互作用，和合而为一。性中有命，命中有性。

integration of the spirit and Qi A term of Qigong, in which the so-called property refers to the spirit and the so-called life refers to Qi. It refers to interaction and integration of the spirit and Qi, indicating that there is Qi in the spirit and there is the spirit in Qi.

进德之基【jìn dé zhī jī】 指气功练养形体，通过厚重、静定、宽缓等法来实现。

foundation for increasing morality Refers to cultivation of the body through messiness, tranquility and relaxation.

进火【jìn huǒ】 指调神御气，使归丹田。

entering fire Refers to regulating the spirit and controlling Qi, making it to enter Dantian. Dantian is divided into the upper Dantian (the region between the eyes), the middle Dantian (the region below the heart) and the lower Dantian (the region below the navel).

进退【jìn tuì】 指阴阳相互作用，阳升阴退，阳退阴进，循环不已。

advance and retreat A term of Qigong, referring to interaction of Yin and Yang, Yang raising and Yin declining, Yang declining and Yin advancing with continuous circulation.

禁酒【jìn jiǔ】 酒可伤神，习练气功应禁酒，以免神伤而不入静。

prohibiting alcohol A term of Qigong, indicating that alcohol can damage the spirit. In practicing Qigong, alcohol must be prohibited, otherwise the spirit will be damaged and tranquilization cannot be realized.

禁绝阴阳【jìn jué yīn yáng】 此处阴阳指男女之房事，即行功期间勿行房事，意在保精敛气。

forbidden Yin and Yang A term of Qigong, referring to refusal of sexual intercourse in order to protect the essence and to stabilize Qi. In this term, Yin and Yang refers to sexual intercourse.

禁门【jìn mén】 指虚危穴，精气聚散常在此处，水火发端也在此处，阴阳变化也在此处，有无出入也在此处。

forbidden gate Refers to an acupoint known as Xuwei, referring to the region where the essential Qi concentrates and disperses there, water and fire appear there, Yin and Yang change there, exit and entrance exist there.

禁气【jìn qì】 指闭气、闭息。

J

forbidden Qi Refers to closing Qi and stopping respiration.

禁烟【jìn yān】 指进行气功养生,应禁吸烟,吸烟一是邪火增加上热,二是烟毒损伤身体。

prohibiting smoking Refers to prohibiting smoking in practicing Qigong and life cultivation. Smoking can increase heat like evil fire and damage the body like tobacco toxin.

茎垂【jīng chuí】 指身中之机,阴精之候,津液之道。

penis and testis The important joints in the human body that lead to the movement of the Yin essence, fluid and humor.

京黑先生行气法【jīng hēi xiān shēng xíng qì fǎ】 为静功。其作法为,平卧床上,两手握固成拳,两足间相距四五寸,两臂间亦相距四五寸,去枕,微微呼吸,共三百六十息。

Mr. Jing He's exercise for moving Qi A static exercise, marked by lying on the back over the bed, holding the fists with the hands with 4 to 5 Cun between the feet and the shoulders, removing the pillow and mildly breathing for three hundred and sixty times.

经络【jīng luò】 指人体中运行气血、沟通内外、联系上下的通路,也是气功中行气的途径。

meridians and collaterals The ways for Qi and blood to move and flow all through the body, also the ways for moving Qi in practicing Qigong.

经气【jīng qì】 即经络之气,存于经络之中与人体真气有密切关系。

meridian Qi Refers to Qi in the meridians and collaterals, which is closely related to the genuine Qi in the human body.

惊则气乱【jīng zé qì luàn】 指惊吓使人神乱而心气无所依附,神不内守而紊乱。

terror disordering Qi Means that terror disorders the spirit and destroys the dependence of heart Qi. If the spirit cannot concentrate inside the body, it will be disordered.

惊蛰二月节坐功【jīng zhé èr yuè jié zuò gōng】 为动功。其作法为,每日丑寅时(一时至五时),握固,转颈,反肘后向,顿掣五六次,叩齿三十六次,吐纳,漱咽九次。

sitting exercise in February A dynamic exercise, marked by griping every day in Chou (the period of a day from 1 a.m. to 3 a.m. in the early morning) and Yin (the period of a day from 3 a.m. to 5 a.m. in the early morning), turning the neck, returning the elbows backwards for five to six times, clicking the teeth for thirty-six times, inhaling and exhaling, rinsing and swallowing for nine times.

晶光清明耀华内景【jīng guāng qīng míng yào huá nèi jǐng】 为静功。其作法为,于夏历每月初七日,在清净的室内坐定,入静后,意想自己登上昆仑山顶,仰望升起的月亮,月亮如半规形。默念咒语二十四遍,咽津二十四次,调息良久收功。

internal scene with glittering light, clear brightness and shining magnificence A static exercise, marked by sitting quietly in a clear room on the seventh every month in summer, imagining to reach the peak of the Kunlun Mountain after tranquilization, looking up at the moon with semicircular shape, then silently reading incantation for twenty-four times, swallowing fluid for twenty-four times and constantly regulating respiration.

睛明【jīng míng】　足太阳膀胱经中的一个穴位,位于目内眦的外上方 0.1 寸处,这一穴位为气功运行的一个常见部位。

Jingming（BL 1）　An acupoint in the bladder meridian of foot Taiyang, located 0.1 Cun above the lateral side of the inner canthus. This acupoint is a region usually used for keeping the essential Qi in practice of Qigong.

精【jīng】　① 指构成世界和人体的本源,又称精气;② 指禀受于父母的"先天之精";③ 指来源于摄入的饮食物,通过脾胃的运化及脏腑的生理活动,化为精微;④ 指阴阳;⑤ 指藏于肾。

essence　Refers to ① either the original source of the world and human body, also known as essential Qi; ② or innate essence originated from parents; ③ or diet taken into the body which is transformed into food essence after digestion of the spleen and stomach and physiological activities of the viscera; ④ or Yin and Yang; ⑤ or storage in the kidney.

精诚【jīng chéng】　指专心用意而守一。

sincerity　A term of Qigong, referring to concentration on the intention.

精根【jīng gēn】　指脑神。

essential root　A term of Qigong, referring to the brain spirit.

精归泥丸【jīng guī ní wán】　指精神和精气归藏泥丸宫。

location of essence in the mud bolus（the brain）　A celebrated dictum, referring to storage of the spirit and essential Qi in the mud bolus（the brain）chamber.

精和【jīng hé】　指自然冲和之气。

essential harmony　A term of Qigong, referring to natural flowing Qi.

精滑引气法【jīng huá yǐn qì fǎ】　为静功。其作法为,平和胁腹,缩尾闾,闭光瞑目,头若石压之状,即引气自背后直入泥丸,而后咽归丹田,不计遍数,行住坐卧皆为之。

exercise of Daoyin for emission　A static exercise, marked by stabilizing the upper part of the body and the abdomen, shrinking coccyx, closing the eyes, lowering the head as being pressed by a stone, leading Qi from the back to the mud bolus（the brain）and swallowing it into Dantian for many times. Such a static exercise can be practiced by staying, sitting and lying. Dantian is divided into the upper Dantian（the region between the eyes）, the middle Dantian（the region below the heart）and the lower Dantian（the region below the navel）.

精金【jīng jīn】　指药物中的精纯物质。

essential metal　A term of Qigong, referring to the essential and pure substance in the medicinal.

精进【jīng jìn】　为佛家气功习用语,指练功时,不懈的努力,排除杂念,或指努力断除恶念。

elimination of distraction　A common term of Qigong in Buddhism, referring to eliminating distracting thought or evil intentions in practicing Qigong.

精景按摩法【jīng jǐng àn mó fǎ】　为动功。其作法为,清晨起床时,使呼吸平和,正坐,又两手,掩项后,并仰面视上,举项,使项与两手争,如此三四次止,做毕,又屈动身体,伸手四极,反张侧掣,宣摇百关,为一各三。起床后,以手巾拭项中四面及耳后,使项觉温温然,再顺发摩顶,如梳发无数次,摩擦双手,以手轻摩面及目。做完后,咽液二十次,以导内液。

exercise for morning Tuina A dynamic exercise, marked by getting up in early morning, breathing peacefully, sitting upright, crossing the hands to cover the retrocollic side, looking up, raising the neck against the hands for three or four times; then bending the body, stretching the hands toward the four sides, lifting the neck to open all the joints for one or three times; wiping the four sides in the neck and below the ears with towel to warm the neck; then kneading the top of the head along the hair like combing hair for countless times; then rubbing both hands and mildly kneading the face and eyes with the hands; then swallowing humor for twenty times in order to lead humor flowing inside the body after practicing Qigong.

精门【jīng mén】 即背下腰软处。

essential gate A term of Qigong, referring to the soft region of the waist below the back.

精明【jīng míng】 指眼神。

eye expression A term of Qigong, referring to the spirit in the eyes.

精明五色【jīng míng wǔ sè】 指眼神和面部反映的青、赤、黄、白、黑五种色泽变化。

five colors of essential brightness Refers to changes of green color, red color, yellow color, white color and black color in the eyes and face.

精明之府【jīng míng zhī fǔ】 指头,为精神意识思维活动。

essential mansion A term of Qigong, referring to the head, indicating the activities of the spirit, consciousness and thinking.

精念存想【jīng niàn cún xiǎng】 指精神、意识、思维活动从目、耳、口而反映于外。意念专一,存神于内,即可切断目、耳、口对外的联系。

thinking essence and existing thought A term of Qigong, indicating that the activities of the spirit, consciousness and thinking reflect externally through the eyes, the ears and the mouth. When emotion is concentrated and the spirit is kept inside, contact of the eyes, the ears and the mouth with the external will be eliminated.

精念玉房【jīng niàn yù fáng】 指精神意识(即意念)活动集中于玉房。玉房为脑之象。

thinking essence in jade chamber A term of Qigong, referring to concentrating the activities of the spirit and consciousness in the jade chamber. In this term, the so-called jade chamber refers to the scene of the brain.

精气【jīng qì】 指阴阳二气。

essential Qi A term of Qigong, referring to Yin Qi and Yang Qi.

精气弛坏【jīng qì chí huài】 指由于生活上嗜欲无穷,精神上忧患不止,导致精气毁坏。

impairing essential Qi Refers to constant addiction of life and hardship of the spirit that have damaged essential Qi.

精气夺则虚【jīng qì duó zé xū】 为气功适应证,指病邪过度耗损人体正气,精气损伤,呈现一派虚象。

deficiency due to depletion of essential Qi An indication of Qigong, referring to excessive depletion of healthy Qi and damage of essential Qi caused by pathogenic factors.

精气神【jīng qì shén】 ① 指上药,为练功的基础;② 指感觉、知觉、运动;③ 精气神一体不离,相互作用;④ 指元精、元气、元神;⑤ 指身体纯一通达和平。

essence, Qi and spirit A term of Qigong, referring to ① either important medicinal which is the foundation for practicing Qigong; ② or sensation, consciousness and action; ③ integration of the essence, Qi and spirit without any separation; ④ or original essence, original Qi and original spirit; ⑤ or purification and harmonization of the body.

精舍【jīng shè】 指精的归藏之处。

essential chamber A term of Qigong, referring to the place that stores the essence.

精神【jīng shén】 ① 指意识思维活动;② 指正气活动。

essence and spirit Refers to ① either activities of consciousness and thinking; ② or activity of healthy Qi.

精神第一【jīng shén dì yī】 源自气功专论,阐述神御形,全形先理神,理神在恬和清静。

the essence and the spirit as the first Collected from a monograph of Qigong, mainly describing that the spirit controls the body, the body manages the spirit and management of the spirit ensures harmonization and tranquility.

精神内守病安从来【jīng shén nèi shǒu bìng ān cóng lái】 从养生之道强调意念集中,神不外驰,内养元气,外慎六淫,阴阳平衡,则不生病。

Concentration of essence and spirit inside will prevent occurrence of any disease. This is celebrated dictum, emphasizing the importance of concentrating consciousness for cultivating life. Only when consciousness is concentrated can the spirit be kept inside to nourish original Qi, to prevent six external pathogenic factors and to balance Yin and Yang in order to prevent any disease.

精神相媾【jīng shén xiāng gòu】 指阴阳合璧,结而为一。精为阴,神为阳。

intercourse of the essence and spirit A term of Qigong, referring to integration of Yin and Yang. In this term, the essence refers to Yin while the spirit refers to Yang.

精神专直【jīng shén zhuān zhí】 指精神集中。

straightening the essence and spirit A term of Qigong, referring to concentration of the essence and the spirit.

精思【jīng sī】 指调神。

essential thought A term of Qigong, referring to regulating the spirit.

精玄【jīng xuán】 指元精。

primordial essence A term of Qigong, referring to the original essence.

精一【jīng yī】 指精粹纯一。

essential one A term of Qigong, referring to succinctness and purity.

精应乾坤说【jīng yìng qián kūn shuō】 源自气功专论,说明精应乾坤(八卦),随着年龄的增加,阴阳变化,身体逐渐衰老,出现衰老性疾病。

idea about correspondence of essence to

Qian Trigram and Kun Trigram Collected from a monograph of Qigong, explaining that the essence corresponds to Qian Trigram and Kun Trigram and senile disease is caused by senility and changes of Yin and Yang due to aging. The Qian Trigram and Kun Trigram are in the Eight Trigrams from Yijing (*Canon of Simplification*, *Change and No Change*).

精转为神【jīng zhuǎn wéi shén】 指精生神。

change of the essence into the spirit A term of Qigong, indicating that the essence produces the spirit.

精浊【jīng zhuó】 指尿道中常有白色分泌物溢出，并有少腹、会阴、睾丸部不适感。

turbid urine Refers to constant white secretion overflow from the urethra and uncomfortableness of the lower abdomen, the pudendal region and the testicle.

颈冲【jǐng chōng】 手阳明大肠经穴位臂臑的另外一个称谓，位于曲池和肩髃的连线上。此穴位为气功习练之处。

Jingchong A synonym of Binao (LI 14) which is an acupoint in the large intestine meridian of hand Taiyang, located above the line between Quchi (LI 11) and Jianyu (LI 15). This acupoint is a region usually used in practice of Qigong.

颈脉【jǐng mài】 指体表部位，在人迎脉搏动处。

neck meridian Refers to the pulse located in the side of the neck.

景阳子【jǐng yáng zǐ】 宋代针灸学家和气功学家王惟一的另外一个称谓。

Jiang Yangzi Another name of Wang Weiyi, a great master of acupuncture, moxibustion and Qigong in the Song Dynasty (960 AD - 1279 AD).

净土【jìng tǔ】 佛家气功习用语，指佛所生之地，泛指良好精神意识活动所产生的环境。

sukhavati（pure land） A term of Qigong, referring to the place where Buddhism was developed, indicating the ideal state made by the activities of the spirit and consciousness.

净土门【jìng tǔ mén】 佛家气功习用语，指通过清净境界而消除诸障，获得精神的稳定。

purifying land gate A common term of Qigong in Buddhism, referring to elimination of various obstacles and stabilization of the spirit based on clean and quiet state.

净心【jìng xīn】 ① 指涤虑，排出脑中妄念、妄思；② 指本来具有的清净之心。

tranquilized heart Refers to ① either elimination of anxiety, indicating elimination of selfish desires and distracting thought；② or innate tranquil and clean heart.

净志【jìng zhì】 指涤虑洗心，减少精神刺激之意。

tranquilized will Means to eliminate anxiety and clean the heart in order to reduce stimulation of the spirit and the essence.

胫【jìng】 ① 指小腿；② 指胫骨。

shank Refers to ① either calf；② or tibia.

胫骨【jìng gǔ】 足太阴脾经的上行之处。

tibia The region through which the spleen meridian of foot Taiyin moves upwards.

敬斋先生卧法【jìng zhāi xiān shēng wò fǎ】 为静功,主要为调身、调气、调神。其作法为,仰卧或侧卧,置身安稳自然,调节呼吸,意念存想真气由两踵生长,然后导引真气由两踵自后而上,过腰,合而为一。

Mr. Jing Zhai's exercise for lying A static exercise for regulating the body, Qi and spirit; marked by lying on the back or lying on one side, naturally stabilizing the body, regulating respiration, imagining to increase genuine Qi from the heels, then leading the genuine Qi from the heels to the upper along the waist, and eventually concentrating Qi from different regions of the body.

敬直老人【jìng zhí lǎo rén】 是对元代医学家兼气功学家邹铉的美誉。

great and pure old man A traditional way to respect and to celebrate Zou Xuan, a great doctor and master of Qigong in the Yuan Dynasty(1271 AD -1368 AD).

静而能安【jìng ér néng ān】 指形神和调,意识活动清静,形体才能安康。

Only tranquility can secure the body. This is a celebrated dictum, indicating that only when the body and spirit are regulated and only when the activity of consciousness is tranquilized can the body be well nourished.

静而生慧【jìng ér shēng huì】 指气功中,脑神清静,智慧自生。

tranquility generating wisdom Means that wisdom increases naturally when the brain spirit is tranquilized in practicing Qigong.

静伏【jìng fú】 指神气合一的状态。

tranquility and bending Refers to inte-

gration of the spirit and Qi.

静功【jìng gōng】 与动功相对,指习练气功时肢体不动的功法。

static exercise Opposite to dynamic exercise, referring to inactivity of the limbs in practicing Qigong with such an exercise.

静观【jìng guān】 指意守丹田,即静观窍妙。

tranquilized sight Refers to concentration in Dantian, indicating view of ingenious aperture with tranquility. Dantian is divided into the upper Dantian (the region between the eyes), the middle Dantian (the region below the heart) and the lower Dantian (the region below the navel).

静观脐下【jìng guān qí xià】 指意守丹田。

quiet view of the region below the navel Refers to concentration in Dantian. Dantian is divided into the upper Dantian (the region between the eyes), the middle Dantian (the region below the heart) and the lower Dantian (the region below the navel).

静呼吸功法【jìng hū xī gōng fǎ】 为静功,主要调身、调气、调神。调身时,以子、午、卯、酉四时为调身之时,以子时为好,不拘时亦可,取自然坐或站式;调气与调神是,坐(站)定后,轻闭目,意念使目视脐,绵塞耳,使不闻外声。

exercise for tranquil respiration A static exercise for regulating the body, Qi and the spirit. Regulating the body can be done in Zi (the period of a day from 11 p.m. to 1 a.m.), Wu (the period of a day from 11 a.m. to 1 p.m. in the noon), Mao (the period of a day from 5 a.m. to 7 a.m. in the early morning) and You（the period of a day from 5 p. m. to 7 p. m. in the dusk）or at any time，sitting or standing up naturally. Regulating Qi and the spirit can be done by sitting or standing up，mildly closing the eyes，mentally viewing the navel，covering the ears with silk floss to avoid listening sound in the external world.

静力【jìng lì】　佛家气功习用语，指意识导引之力。

tranquil energy　A common term of Qigong in Buddhism，referring to the power of Daoyin with consciousness.

静虑【jìng lǜ】　即思维修，为佛家气功习用语，指佛家静坐凝神，专注一境的习练方法。

tranquil consideration　The same as thinking cultivation，is a common term of Qigong in Buddhism，referring to sitting quietly and concentrating the spirit in practicing Qigong in Buddhism.

静漠【jìng mò】　指意识活动安静，淡泊无为。

inactive mood　Refers to tranquilized activity of consciousness without any desires.

静寿躁夭【jìng shòu zào yāo】　指静能藏神养形而多寿，躁可伤神损形而早夭。

tranquility prolonging life while impetuousness damaging life　Indicates that tranquility can store the spirit，nourish the body and prolong the life while impetuousness damages the spirit，injures the body and reduce the life.

静顺【jìng shùn】　指平气之年水得平静柔顺。

tranquility and smoothness　Refers to

quiet and unobstructed water in the peaceful year.

静思【jìng sī】　指行功中，意识思维活动的相对静止。

tranquil contemplation　Refers to relative tranquility of the activities of consciousness and thinking in practicing Qigong.

静为动之基【jìng wéi dòng zhī jī】　指动自静生，不静不动。

Tranquility is the foundation of activity.　This is a celebrated dictum，indicating that activity depends on tranquility.

静为躁君【jìng wéi zào jūn】　指静是动的主宰。浮躁、烦躁只有用宁静、安静来协调。

tranquility controlling impetuousness　Means that tranquility is the dominator of action，indicating that only tranquility and quietness can regulate impetuousness and annoyance.

静虚至极【jìng xū zhì jí】　指习练气功时，意识活动处于相对静止的状态。

extreme tranquility　A term of Qigong，referring to relative tranquility of consciousness activity in practicing Qigong.

静则生慧，动则成昏【jìng zé shēng huì dòng zé chéng hūn】　说明心是神的主宰，心静则使人智慧，躁动则使人昏蒙，沉迷于幻境之中，不能收到练功的效果。

Tranquility produces wisdom while activity causes impetuousness.　This is a celebrated dictum，indicating that the heart is the dominator of the spirit and the tranquilized heart can increase wisdom while impetuousness makes people confused，indulging in fantasy and failing in practicing Qigong.

静者静动【jìng zhě jìng dòng】　指气

功运动是永恒的、绝对的，静动是意识形体运动的一种状态。

tranquility combined with action　Means that dynamic state of Qigong is absolute while static condition of consciousness activity is relative.

静中一动【jìng zhōng yī dòng】　指虚极之中，一阳初动。

one movement in tranquility　A term of Qigong, referring to primary action of Yang after extreme deficiency.

静坐时潜心目于海底【jìng zuò shí qián xīn mù yú hǎi dǐ】　指习练静功，两目内视腹脐下丹田。

Quiet sitting devotes the heart and eyes in the seafloor.　This is a celebrated dictum, indicating that the eyes observe the lower Dantian (the region below the navel) and the navel in practicing Qigong.

静坐吟【jìng zuò yín】　《静坐吟》为气功专论，由明代攀龙撰写，阐述气功静坐的方法、景象和境界。

Jingzuo Yin（*Quiet Sitting with Silent Chanting*）　A monograph of Qigong entitled *Quiet Sitting with Silent Chanting*, written by Pan Long in the Ming Dynasty (1368 AD – 1644 AD), describing the methods, scene and state of Qigong practice with quiet sitting.

鸠尾【jiū wěi】　① 指胸骨剑突；② 指穴位名，为任脉中的一个穴位，位于腹正中线，脐上 7 寸。此穴位为气功习练之处。

Jiuwei　Refers to ① either mucronate cartilage; ② or Jiuwei (CV 15), which is an acupoint in the conception meridian, located in the abdominal middle line, 7 Cun above the navel. This acupoint is a region usually used in practice

of Qigong.

究竟觉【jiū jìng jué】　指于妙觉之位，成究竟至极之始觉。

actual awareness　A term of Qigong, referring to a region with wonderful consciousness, which is a manifestation of perfect awareness.

九【jiǔ】　在《易经》中，九为奇数之阳，为老阳。

nine　In *Yijing*, nine refers to the Yang line in Trigrams. In Yijing, the Chinese character Yi means simplification, change and no change, not just change.

九禅【jiǔ chán】　为静功，佛家气功功法。九禅即自性禅、一切禅、难禅、一切门禅、善人禅、一切行禅、除烦恼禅、此世他世乐禅、清净净禅。其具体作法为，意识思维集中于一，或止观双修而静定，意识内守不散，并逐步相对静止；专注于境、一事、一物而静定；解难而入静；一切法从此入静；思善事而静定；行走而入定静；除烦恼后入清净之境；排除杂念，而入理想提界；观虚空明净而达空寂明亮之境。

nine meditations　A static exercise and the method of Qigong practice in Buddhism, marked by personal meditation, referring to either concentrating the activities of consciousness and thought, or thoroughly tranquilizing and stabilizing with double cultivation in order to internally concentrate the consciousness without any dispersion to eventually reach the state of tranquility and stability; or all meditation, referring to paying attention to just one state, one matter and one thing in order to tranquilize the body; difficult meditation, referring to relieving all the problems for reaching the state of tranquility; all entering meditation, referring to reaching the state of tranquility with all the principles and exercises; kind meditation, referring to tranquilizing the body and the mind with virtual thought; active meditation, referring to reaching the state of tranquility in moving; mediation for eliminating annoyance, referring to eliminating all annoyance after reaching the state of tranquility; meditation for eliminating distracting thought, referring to reaching the ideal state after eliminating distracting thought; and tranquil meditation, referring to reaching the state of vacuum, tranquility and brightness after concentrated observation of vacuum, brightness, clarity and brightness.

九疮【jiǔ chuāng】　指九窍,即两眼、两鼻孔、两耳、一口、两便道。

nine sores　Refers to the sores in the eyes, nostrils, ears, mouth and anus.

九丹【jiǔ dān】　指精、气、神合而为一,也指人禀自然之气,阴阳之精而成。

nine kinds of Dan(**pills of immortality**)　Refers to either integration of essence, Qi and spirit; or receiving natural Qi for the formation of essence in Yin and Yang.

九鼎【jiǔ dǐng】　指纯阳,从始至终,自一而丸,为炼就纯阳之意。

nine treasures　Refers to refined Yang. From the beginning to ending, the practice from one to nine purifies Yang.

九鼎炼心【jiǔ dǐng liàn xīn】　指调神炼心的九个层次。

purifying the heart in nine supremacies　Refers to nine states in regulating the spirit and exercising the heart.

九鼎炼神法【jiǔ dǐng liàn shén fǎ】　为静功,即调身、调气及调神。其作法,自然坐势或卧势(仰卧),做好行功前准备,安定形神:坐定(卧定)后,放松形体,排除杂念,鼻引自然之气,舌舐上腭,以意念导引入丹田;然后引气从口出,呼出气时,舌尖自然放下;吸时腹部鼓起,呼时腹部凹下;意识集中于丹田,两目内视丹田,两耳内听丹田,神气精合而为一;然后意引精气流过尾吕,循督脉而上,通夹脊玉枕,而入头脑;复由泥丸下鹊桥,从任脉经膻中,复归丹田,如此者反复九转;良久,意引清气入肾,从左入肝,上升入心,由心升至泥丸,复由泥丸从右而下入肺,至脾,复归于肾,如此反复九还;良久,意引精气从肾上升入心,随即由心归肾,如此反复九通;意引精气归入丹田,意守之,精气神合而养就灵丹。

technique for purifying the spirit in nine supremacies　A static exercise for regulating the body, Qi and the spirit, marked by naturally sitting or lying on the back, preparing well before practice and stabilizing the body and the spirit; after sitting upright or lying on the back, relaxing the body, eliminating distracting thought, breathing in naturally through the nose, raising at the palate with the tongue, leading it to Dantian with consciousness; breathing out through the mouth, naturally putting down the tongue during exhalation; plucking up the abdomen during inhalation and sinking the abdomen during exhalation; concentrating consciousness in Dantian, internally seeing Dantian with both eyes, listening Dantian with both ears in order to integrate the essence, Qi and the spirit; then leading the essential Qi from the coccyx and along the governor meridian upwards through Yuzhen (BL 9)(an acupoint in the bladder meridian of foot Taiyang) to the brain; then leading the essential Qi from the mud bolus (the brain) to the magpie (the tongue), from Tanzhong (CV 17) in the conception meridian to return again to Dantian, which is moved repeatedly in nine ways; leading clear Qi to the kidney with consciousness after a certain period of time, entering it the liver from the left and the heart, raising it to the mud bolus (the brain) from the heart, and lowering it from the mud bolus (the brain) and the right side to the lung, the spleen and the kidney, which is moved repeatedly again for nine times; leading the essential Qi from the kidney to the heart with consciousness after a certain period of time, then returning it from the heart to the kidney, which is moved repeatedly for nine times; leading the essential Qi to Dantian with consciousness, mentally keeping it and integrating the essence, Qi and the spirit for producing Lingdan (panacea). Dantian is divided into the upper Dantian (the region between the eyes), the middle Dantian (the region below the heart) and the lower Dantian (the region below the navel).

九鼎炼心法【jiǔ dǐng liàn xīn fǎ】 为静功,即调身、调气及调神。其作法与"九鼎炼神法"相同。

technique for purifying the heart in nine supremacies A static exercise for regulating the body, Qi and the spirit, which is the same as that of the te-

chiques for purifying the spirit in nine supuremacies.

九二【jiǔ èr】 卦交位,从下数第二爻为阳爻者,称为九二。

nine-two Refers to the second Yang line of Trigrams.

九方【jiǔ fāng】 指八方与中央。

nine directions Refers to the eight directions and the center in the sky.

九宫【jiǔ gōng】 古人认为人脑分为九部;也指天之八方加中央为九宫。

nine palaces Refers to the nine regions in the brain in ancient China; or the eight directions and the center in the sky.

九宫真人【jiǔ gōng zhēn rén】 即九个器官。古人认为人有心、肾、肝、肺、脾、胆、小肠、大肠、膀胱九个器官。

immortals in the nine palaces Refers to the heart, kidney, liver, lung, spleen, gallbladder, small intestine, large intestine and bladder.

九卦论【jiǔ guà lùn】 主要阐述圣人处丘之道:内养正气,稳定情绪,和调神形。

explanation of nine Trigrams Refers to the right way of health cultivation through practice of Qigong, which can internally nourish the original Qi, stabilize the mind and regulate the spirit and body.

九鬼拔马刀【jiǔ guǐ bá mǎ dāo】 为动功。其作法为,直立侧头,一手向上弯至项后,另一手向上弯至腰后,如拔刀之状,两手交替反复上述动作,同时注意调息均匀。

nine spiritual techniques for drawing swords A dynamic exercise, marked by standing up and turning the body for practicing Qigong, during which one

J

hand repeatedly turns upwards to the nape and the other hand repeatedly turns upwards to the back to relieve disorders in the shoulder, neck and back.

九华【jiǔ huá】　指日月之精华。

nine radiances　Refers to the radiances of the sun and the moon.

九还七返【jiǔ huán qī fǎn】　人体经气之升降与天地之气升降相应。

nine restorations and seven returns　A term of Qigong, referring to correspondence between the ascent and descent of Qi in the human body and the universe.

九江【jiǔ jiāng】　指小肠。

nine rivers　A term of Qigong, referring to the small intestine.

九孔【jiǔ kǒng】　指两眼、两耳、两鼻孔、一口、两便道。

nine holes　Refers to nine orifices, indicting two eyes, two nostrils, two ears, one mouth, one urethra and one anus.

九灵铁鼓【jiǔ líng tiě gǔ】　精气聚散常在此处，水火发端也在此处，阴阳变化也在此处，有无出入也在此处。

nine genius-fire drums　Refers to the region where the essential Qi concentrates and disperses there, water and fire appear there, Yin and Yang change there, exit and entrance exist there.

九难【jiǔ nàn】　指习练气功时，干扰气功锻炼的九种因素。

nine obstacles　Refers to the nine factors that interfere the practice of Qigong.

九气【jiǔ qì】　为三丹田之气。

nine kinds of Qi　Refers to three kinds

of Qi in the upper Dantian (the region between the eyes), the middle Dantian (the region below the heart) and the lower Dantian (the region below the navel).

九窍【jiǔ qiào】　指眼、耳、鼻、口及前后二阴。

nine orifices　Refers to the eyes, ears, nostrils, mouth, scrotum and anus.

九色【jiǔ sè】　指青、赤、黄、白、黑、绿、紫、红、绀九色。

nine colors　Refers to green color, red color, yellow color, white color, black color, blue color, purple color and cyanose color.

九神【jiǔ shén】　指九气，为三丹田之气。

nine spirits　Refers to the three kinds of Qi in the upper Dantian (the region between the eyes), the middle Dantian (the region below the heart) and the lower Dantian (the region below the navel).

九神丹【jiǔ shén dān】　即养生长寿的九种神丹式的药物。

nine kinds of immortal Dan (pills of immortality)　Refers to use of some important medicinals in nine ways to cultivate health and to prolong life.

九室【jiǔ shì】　为九宫之宅及九窍之主。

nine chambers　A term of Qigong, referring to either nine chambers; or nine orifices.

九守【jiǔ shǒu】　气功养生的九条守则，即守和、守神、守气、守仁、守简、守清、守盈、守弱。

nine defenses　Refers to defending harmony, spirit, Qi, morality, simplicity, change, emotion, exuberance and deficiency.

九思【jiǔ sī】 指面对社会的九种思维活动，即思明、思聪、思温、思恭、思忠、思敬、思问、思难、思义的九种因素。

nine contemplations A noun of Qigong, referring to contemplation of brightness through vision, intelligence through listening, warmth through complexion, respect through style, loyalty through speech, worship through matter, question through doubt, difficulty through anger and justice through observation.

九天【jiǔ tiān】 指九气，或八方位及中央天，或头上九穴。

nine skies Refers to either nine kinds of Qi; or the eight directions and the center in the sky; or the nine acupoints located in the head, which are usually used in practice of Qigong.

九微【jiǔ wēi】 指的是脑中的幽深之处。

nine kinds of remoteness A term of Qigong, referring to the deep chamber in the brain.

九无为【jiǔ wú wéi】 指的是不妄为、无生灭变化的绝对存在、精神稳定。

nine inactions Refers to nine kinds of inactivity, absolute existence and spiritual stability.

九霄【jiǔ xiāo】 指天目下，鼻柱之上部。

nine skies Refers to the area between the nose and the eyes.

九邪【jiǔ xié】 指九窍之邪，为损害机体的致病因素。

nine evils Refers to the nine pathogenic factors in the nine orifices that damage the body and cause various diseases.

九咽丹成【jiǔ yān dān chéng】 气功中咽口中唾液，反复九次。

nine times of saliva with internal elixir A term of Qigong, referring to swallowing saliva in the mouth for nine times in practicing Qigong.

九阳【jiǔ yáng】 指的是太阳。

nine kinds of Yang Refers to the sun.

九阳离明真气郁仪内景【jiǔ yáng lí míng zhēn qì yù yí nèi jǐng】 为静功。其作法为，于夏历每月二十日、二十五日、三十日在清静的室内静坐，叩齿，咽津。坚持一年可消灾免病，两年神壮体轻。

merging genuine Qi inside in the summer days A static exercise, marked by sitting quietly in a clear and quiet room, clicking the teeth and swallowing fluid in twentieth, twenty-fifth and thirtieth in every month in summer. To continuously practice Qigong with such a static exercise for a whole year can relieve disaster and disease. After two years of practice the spirit and the body will be strengthened and purified.

九曜【jiǔ yào】 指天上有九种曜。

nine kinds of sunlight Refers to nine stars in the sky.

九野【jiǔ yě】 指天的中央和八方。

nine directional scenes Refers to the eight directions and one center in the universe.

九液【jiǔ yè】 指九窍的津液。

nine humors Refers to fluid and humor in the nine orifices.

九幽【jiǔ yōu】 指阴丹，为日月（阴阳）之气相互作用而成。

nine serenities A noun of Qigong, referring to Yin Dan (pills of immortality) made by interaction of the sun

（Yang）and the moon（Yin）.

九隅【jiǔ yú】 指古代的九方。

nine directions Refers to the nine cantons formed in ancient China.

九原之山【jiǔ yuán zhī shān】 指脑，头脑在身之高巅故名。

mountain in the nine highlands Refers to the brain that is located on the top of the body.

九月节导引法【jiǔ yuè jié dǎo yǐn fǎ】为动功。其作法为,九月节每日丑寅时,正坐,两手向上作托天之势,闭气引气到口中。功效为清心火除痰。

exercise of Daoyin in the feast days of September A static exercise, marked by sitting up with both hands to raising up, closing Qi and inhaling Qi in the mouth in Chou（the period of a day from 1 a.m. to 3 a.m. in the morning）and Yin（the period of a day from 3 a.m. to 5 a.m. in the morning）every day in September for the purpose of clearing away heat in the heart and relieving sputum.

九月中导引法【jiǔ yuè zhōng dǎo yǐn fǎ】 为动功。其作法为,九月中每日丑寅时,静坐,两手重叠抱于下丹田。功效为调和阴阳,健身防病。

exercise of Daoyin in the middle of September A dynamic exercise, marked by sitting quietly with both hands pressing on the lower Dantian（the region below the navel）in Chou（the period of a day from 1 a.m. to 3 a.m. in the morning）and Yin（the period of a day from 3 a.m. to 5 a.m. in the morning）every day in September for the purpose of regulating and combining Yin and Yang as well as cultivating health and preventing disease.

九载功【jiǔ zài gōng】 为动功。其作法为,自然坐正,闭目,调气,收心,坚持九年。可使人体气、血、脉、肉、髓、筋、骨、发、形强健,返老还壮。

nine tranquil techniques A dynamic exercise, marked by sitting upright, closing the eyes, regulating Qi, concentrating the heart in practicing Qigong. After conscientiously practicing Qigong for nine years, it will strengthen Qi, blood, meridians, muscles, marrow, sinews, bones, hair and body, and eventually prolonging life.

九真【jiǔ zhēn】 指高真、天真、神真、上真、玄真、仙真、虚真、太真、至真。

nine truths Refers to high truth, celestial truth, spiritual truth, upper truth, abstruse truth, immortal truth, deficient truth, great truth and perfect truth.

九州【jiǔ zhōu】 指冀、兖、青、徐、扬、荆、豫、梁、雍九个州。以九州言之,肾为冀州,膀胱为徐州,肝为青州,胆为兖州,心为扬州,小肠为荆州,脾为豫州,肺为梁州,大肠为雍州。

nine states Refers to nine cantons set up in antiquity in China, including Jizhou symbolizing the kidney, Yanzhou symbolizing the bladder, Qingzhou symbolizing the liver, Xuzhou symbolizing the gallbladder, Yangzhou symbolizing the heart, Jingzhou symbolizing the small intestine, Yuzhou symbolizing the spleen, Liangzhou symbolizing the lung and Yongzhou symbolizing the large intestine.

九转【jiǔ zhuǎn】 指练功纯深产生精气转化。

nine transformations Refers to transformation of essence, Qi and spirit on the foundation of deep and pure practice of Qigong.

九转金丹【jiǔ zhuǎn jīn dān】　九转即九还。一转降丹,二转交媾,三转养阳,四转养阴,五转换骨,六转换肉,七转换五脏六腑,八转育火,九转飞升。

nine refined golden Dan（pills of immortality）　Refers to nine times of repeatedly practicing Dan（pills of immortality）, the practice of which includes descending Dan（pills of immortality）and coitus, nourishing Yang, nourishing Yin, changing bones, changing muscles, changing five Zang-organs（including the heart, the liver, the spleen, the lung and the kidney）and six Fu-organs（the gallbladder, stomach, small intestine, large intestine, bladder and triple energizer）, making fire and flying up.

九转金丸【jiǔ zhuǎn jīn wán】　即九转之丹,指将丹循环反复烧炼九次。古人认为金丹烧炼次数越多效果就越好。

nine refined golden pills　The same as the term of nine kinds of refined Dan（pills of immortality）, refers to nine times of repeatedly heating and refining Dan（pills of immortality）. It was believed in ancient times that constantly heating and refining Dan（pills of immortality）would be better for practicing Qigong and cultivating life.

九转九易【jiǔ zhuǎn jiǔ yì】　即习练气功日久,反复锤炼,阴阳相对平衡,有补益精神,抵抗早衰之功。

nine transformations and nine changes　Refers to repeated practice of Qigong in order to balance Yin and Yang, to nourish essence and spirit and to avoid presenility.

九转之丹【jiǔ zhuǎn zhī dān】　即将丹循环反复烧炼九次。古人认为金丹烧炼次数越多效果就越好。

nine kinds of refined Dan（pills of immortality）　Refers to nine times of repeatedly heating and refining Dan（pills of immortality）. It was believed in ancient times that constantly heating and refining Dan（pills of immortality）would be better for practicing Qigong and cultivating life.

久视三丹田【jiǔ shì sān dān tián】　为静功。其作法为,久视上丹田,即凝神入上丹田,意识内照之;久视中丹田,即凝神入中丹田,意识内照之;久视下丹田,凝神入下丹田,意识内照之。

concentration on the triple Dantian　A static exercise, referring to long time observing the upper Dantian（the region between the eyes）with the spirit concentrated in it and emotion focused on it; or long time observing the middle Dantian（the region below the heart）with the spirit concentrated in it and emotion focused on it; or long time observing the lower Dantian（the region below the navel）with the spirit concentrated in it and emotion focused on it.

酒积治法【jiǔ jī zhì fǎ】　为动功。其作法为,立地闭气,一手前上伸,一手后下伸,转项扭身两次,觉腹内响、身暖止。

exercise for solving intoxication　A dynamic exercise, marked by standing up and stopping respiration, stretching one hand upwards and the other hand downwards, turning the neck and twisting the body for twice, and feeling that the abdomen is active and the body is warm.

J

酒乱其神【jiǔ luàn qí shén】 指饮酒至醉，损失脑神。

alcohol impairing the spirit Means that intoxication damages the brain spirit.

救护命宝【jiù hù mìng bǎo】 指抵抗衰老，采药练己筑基，萌发生机。

exercise for saving life A term of Qigong, referring to resisting senility, collecting medicinal to refine foundation and germinating vitality.

拘魂法【jū hún fǎ】 为静功。作法为，暮卧，静心存想太阳；朝卧，静心存想月亮。

exercise for keeping the ethereal soul A static exercise, referring to either lying in the evening with tranquilization of the heart and contemplation of the sun; or lying in the morning with tranquilization of the heart and contemplation of the moon.

拘魂魄法【jū hún pò fǎ】 为动静相兼功。其作法为，朝暮入室，放松神形，静坐约 10 分钟。

exercise for keeping the ethereal soul and corporeal soul An exercise combined with dynamic exercise and static exercise, marked by entering the room in the daytime or at night, relaxing the spirit and body, quietly sitting for over 10 minutes every time.

拘三魂法【jū sān hún fǎ】 为静功。其作法为，农历每月初三、十二、二十三日夕作功，卧式，去枕伸足，头在两手心之内，瞑目闭气三息，叩齿三通，存心中有赤气如鸡子，从内仰上，出于目中。

exercise for keeping three ethereal souls A static exercise, marked by lying without pillow for practicing Qigong on the third day, twelfth day and twenty-third day in every month in daytime and nighttime, stretching the feet, holding the head with the hands, closing the eyes and stopping respiration for three times, clicking the teeth for three times, keeping red Qi in the heart like a chicken, raising up from the internal side and through the eyes.

拘于鬼神者，不可与言至德【jū yú guǐ shén zhě bù kě yǔ yán zhì dé】 指执迷于鬼神的，不可与言气功养生法。

Do not talk about the great virtue with those who are superstitious. This is a celebrated dictum, referring to avoidance of talking about Qigong with those who are superstitious.

居家宜忌【jū jiā yí jì】 《居家宜忌》为气功养生专著，由明代瞿韦占所著，主要论述一年中生活起居养生所应注意的事项。

Jujia Yiji (*Compatibility and Incompatibility at Home*) A monograph of Qigong entitled *Compatibility and Incompatibility at Home*, written by Qu Weizhan in the Ming Dynasty (1368 AD - 1644 AD), describing the matters needing attention during cultivation of life in a year.

居髎【jū liáo】 为足少阳胆经中的一个穴位，位于髂前上棘与股骨大转子最高点连线的中点处。这一穴位为气功运行的一个常见部位。

Juliao An acupoint in the gallbladder meridian of foot Shaoyang, located on the hip at the midpoint of the line connecting the anteriosuperior iliac spine and the prominence of the great trochanter. This acupoint is a region usually used for keeping the essential Qi in practice of Qigong.

居脑中【jū nǎo zhōng】 指百神皆居

脑中。

locating in the brain A term of Qigong, indicating that hundred spirits are all located in the brain.

居士【jū shì】 ① 指气功高深之士；② 指为做官的士人；③ 指在家奉佛者。

lay Buddhist Refers to ① either a scholar with profound study and practice of Qigong；② or a scholar without official position；③ or the person who sacrificed Buddhism at home.

疽【jū】 为气功适应证，指疮面深恶、范围较大的疮癌。

ulcer An indication of Qigong, referring to severe eczema and cancer.

疽候导引法【jū hòu dǎo yǐn fǎ】 为静功。其作法为，端正地背靠墙壁，闭气不行，至极限时慢慢呼出，然后用意念引气从头至足，同时行气，用鼻吸五次，吐出一次，行气十二遍。

exercise of Daoyin for ulcer A static exercise, marked by leaning upright on the wall, stopping breath, then slowly breathing out, imagining to promote Qi flowing from the head to the feet, then moving Qi, inhaling through the nose for five times, exhaling once and moving Qi for twelve times.

巨窌【jù liáo】 手少阳三焦经中丝竹空穴位的别称，位于眉毛外侧段凹陷处。这一穴位为气功运行的一个常见部位。

Juliao A synonym of Sizhukong（SJ 23）which is an acupoint in the triple energizer meridian of hand Shaoyang, also called Juliao or Muliao, located in the lateral depression of the eyebrow. This acupoint is a region usually used for keeping the essential Qi in practice of Qigong.

巨气【jù qì】 指人体正气。

great Qi Refers to healthy Qi in the body.

据【jù】 导引姿势，指用两手按着、撑着。

prop An exercise of Daoyin, referring to pressing and controlling with both hands.

聚火载金法【jù huǒ zǎi jīn fǎ】 为静功。其作法为，练功产药之后，提肛引气上行，闭任开督，用吸、舐、撮、闭所聚火，令火炽则水沸，水沸则驾动河车，载金上升泥丸，与真汞配合。

exercise for gathering fire and holding metal A static exercise, marked by lifting anus and promoting Qi to move upwards after production of medicinal in practicing Qigong；closing the conception meridian and opening the governor meridian；gathering fire through inhaling, lapping, pinching and closing for boiling water. Only when the water is boiled can the river cart be driven to the mud bolus（the brain）and cooperate with the original spirit. River cart refers to either healthy Qi and kidney Qi；or conception meridian and governor meridian.

聚火之法【jù huǒ zhī fǎ】 即聚火载金法，为静功。其作法为，练功产药之后，提肛引气上行，闭任开督，用吸、舐、撮、闭所聚火，令火炽则水沸，水沸则驾动河车，载金上升泥丸，与真汞配合。

exercise for gathering fire The same as exercise for gathering fire and holding metal, is a static exercise, marked by lifting anus and promoting Qi to move upwards after production of medicinal in practicing Qigong, closing the conception meridian and opening the governor meridian, gathering fire through inhaling, lapping, pinching and closing for boiling water. Only when the water is boiled can the river cart be driven to the mud bolus (the brain) and cooperate with the original spirit. River cart refers to either healthy Qi and kidney Qi; or conception meridian and governor meridian.

聚精论【jù jīng lùn】 源自气功专论,主要阐述保养精血的养生要点。

idea about gathering the spirit Collected from a monograph of Qigong, mainly describing the importance for nourishing life in protecting and nourishing the essence and the blood.

聚散水火【jù sàn shuǐ huǒ】 指调节水火,喻调节身体阴阳,以维持神形的稳定。

gathering and dispersing water and fire Refers to regulation of water and fire, indicating regulation of Yin and Yang in the body for stabilizing the spirit and body.

聚为玉浆【jù wéi yù jiāng】 指鼓漱后滋生的唾液,有流利百脉,溉脏润身之功。

gathering into immortal beverage Refers to breeding saliva after rinsing the mouth, which promotes the movement of all meridians and vessels, cleanses the viscera and moistens the body.

踞坐【jù zuò】 指两足掌及臀部着地,两膝上耸而坐的练功姿势。

squatting A term of Qigong, referring to touchdown of the soles and buttocks and sitting with the knees raised up for practicing Qigong.

涓子【juān zǐ】 齐国气功研究家,著有《天人经》。

Quan Zi A master of Qigong in the Qi State in the Zhou Dynasty (1046 BC – 256 BC). He wrote an important book entitled *Canon of the Sky and Man*.

涓子垂钓荷泽【juān zǐ chuí diào hé zé】 为静功。其作法为,身端坐,左手自然握拳按摩左胁,右手按摩右膝,同时专心存想,运气于患疠处,左六口,右六口。

Juan Zi's exercise for fishing in lotus pond marked by sitting upright, kneading the left rib with the left hand and kneading the right knee with the right hand, concentrating the attention and moving Qi to the region with furuncle for six times on the left and six times on the right.

卷头筑肚【juǎn tóu zhù dù】 指低头向肚的导引姿势。

Bending the head and building the abdomen A term of Qigong, referring to the style of Daoyin marked by lowering the head toward the abdomen.

窅冥【juàn míng】 指动静,动为运动,静为静止,动静交相以成阴阳互根,阴阳交媾之用。

obscurity Refers to dynamics and statics and is a term of Qigong, in which dynamics refers to movement and statics means motionlessness. Only when movement and motionlessness combine with each other can Yin and Yang integrate with each other.

窅冥端【juàn míng duān】 指极深极奥极静。

extreme obscurity A term of Qigong, referring to extreme depth, extreme obscurity and extreme tranquility.

窅冥景象【juàn míng jǐng xiàng】 源自气功专论,阐述气功所产生的窅冥状态。

scene of obscurity Collected from a monograph of Qigong, describing the condition of obscurity after practice of Qigong.

觉海【jué hǎi】　指脑。

innate sea A term of Qigong, referring to the brain.

觉了【jué liǎo】　佛家气功习用语，指觉悟之后而具有分辨事物的能力，气功中指认识功法的性能作用。

cognition A common term of Qigong in Buddhism, referring to the ability of differentiation after awareness. In Qigong, it refers to effect of studying and practicing the exercises in Qigong.

觉灵【jué líng】　指脑神之用，即精神意识思维活动。

realizing intelligence A term of Qigong, referring to the function of the brain spirit, indicating the activities of the spirit, consciousness and thinking.

觉悟【jué wù】　佛家气功习用语，指会得真理，开通真智，提高认识能力。

realizing consciousness A term of Qigong, referring to understanding truth, promting wisdom and increasing knowledge.

觉心【jué xīn】　指禅家能照见其妄（指幻心），而斩断念头。

realization A term of Qigong, indicating that Buddhists can see fantasy and eliminate distracting thought.

觉性【jué xìng】　佛家气功习用语，指省悟之性。

realizing nature A term of Qigong, referring to coming to realize the truth.

觉照【jué zhào】　指反复习练，以固秘发展。

constant practice A term of Qigong,

refers to repeated practice of Qigong in order to protect and develop the body.

绝谷【jué gǔ】　即辟谷，不饮食。练功到一定程度出现不感饥饿，不进饮食而精神不减，身体轻快而无不适。

inedia（stopping diet） Refers to the marvel in practicing Qigong, characterized by no hunger in practicing Qigong to a certain level. Although food is not taken in practicing Qigong, the spirit is still energetic and the body is still brisk.

绝谷行气法【jué gǔ xíng qì fǎ】　为静功。其作法为，每日减食一口，十日以后可不食。可益气，且生津液。

exercise for inedia（stopping diet）and moving Qi A static exercise, marked by reducing meal each day and stopping taking food after ten days. To practice Qigong with such a static exercise can fortify Qi and increase fluid and humor.

绝骨【jué gǔ】　①指腓骨下段，外踝之上；②指足少阳胆经中的一个穴位，位于外踝直上三寸。这一穴位为气功运行的一个常见部位。

extreme bone Refers to ① either the bone below the fibula and above the external malleolus；② or an acupoint in the gallbladder meridian of foot Shaoyang, located 3 Cun directly above the external malleolus. This acupoint is a region usually used for keeping the essential Qi in practice of Qigong.

绝粒【jué lì】　即辟谷不食，为习练气功养生法。

stopping grain Refers to inedia（stopping diet），which is a way in Qigong practice for cultivating life.

绝虑忘情【jué lǜ wàng qíng】　指大脑

完全清静无思。

tranquilized mind and unruffled emotion Means that the brain is tranquilized without any selfish desires.

绝相【jué xiāng】 指习练气功时，眼不外视任何物体。

invisibility Refers to seeing nothing in the external world in practicing Qigong.

橛骨【jué gǔ】 ① 指尾骨；② 指经穴名长强；③ 指尾闾关。此穴位为气功习练之处。

coccyx Refers to ① either coccyx；② or Changqiang （CV 1）；③ or the end of sacrococcyx. This acupoint is a region usually used in practice of Qigong.

君房服气法【jūn fáng fú qì fǎ】 为静功，方法多样。如胎息服气，从夜半后服内气七咽，每一咽即调气六七息，即便咽之。

exercise for respiration in monarchy chamber A static exercise with various methods. One of the method is to breathe in the way of fetal respiration，to breathe in internal Qi at midnight for seven times of swallowing and regulating Qi for six or seven times during each swallowing.

君房服气养生法【jūn fáng fú qì yǎng shēng fǎ】 《君房服气养生法》为气功养生专著，由宋代张君房辑，主要说明习练气功的基本方法，如调节身体姿势，调节身体的呼吸，调节精神意识活动等。

Junfang Fuqi Yangsheng Fa（*Exercise of Respiration and Life Cultivation in Noble Person's Room*） A monograph of Qigong entitled *Exercise of Respiration and Life Cultivation in Noble Person's Room*，written by Zhang Junfang in the Song Dynasty （960 AD - 1279 AD），mainly descriving the basic methods for practicing Qigong，such as regulating body styles，regulating respiration and regulating activities of the spirit and consciousness.

君火【jūn huǒ】 心为君主，故心火为君火。

monarchy fire A term of Qigong，referring to heart fire. In the human body，the heart is the monarch in the body. That is why heart fire is called monarch fire.

君子思不出其位【jūn zǐ sī bù chū qí wèi】 即君子意识思维不超出身体之外。

Noble person's thinking is nerve beyond his state. This is a celebrated dictum，indicating that the consciousness and thought of a noble person never transcends his body.

K

开关法【kāi guān fǎ】　为动功。其作法为,先以左上肢向前圆转九次,次以右上肢向前圆转九次,然后再以双上股向前回转九次。

switching method　A dynamic exercise, marked by turning the left upper limb to the front for nine times first, then turning the right upper limb to the front for nine times, and finally turning the double upper limbs together to the front for nine times.

开胁法【kāi xié fǎ】　为动功。其作法为,两手抱头,宛转上下,除身体昏沉,不通畅。

method for relieving sides　A dynamic exercise, marked by holding the head with both hands to solve dizziness and difficulty in circulation.

开郁法【kāi yù fǎ】　为动功。其作法为,两手挥动向前向后,两足作白鹭行步状。左手搭在右肩上,右足搭左腘窝而行,仰卧运气下行。然后蹲立,两手用力攀起脚后跟,然后起立,两手相交掩两臂扶胸前。治胸腹胀满。

depression relief method　A dynamic exercise, marked by waving both hands to the front and back, walking in the way of egrets, putting the left hand on the right shoulder, keeping the right foot on the left popliteal space for moving, lying on the back to descend Qi, then sitting with hands grasping the heels, and finally standing up with both hands pressing the chest and arms.

Such a dynamic exercise can cure stagnation of the chest and the abdomen.

坎【kǎn】　① 卦名,为伏羲所造之八卦之一,为水;② 指精神意识活动不专一;③ 指取象比类;④ 指方向。

Kan　Refers to ① either the Kan Trigram among the Eight Trigrams created by Fuxi, indicating water; ② or non-concentration of the activities of the essence, the spirit and the consciousness; ③ or analogy; ④ or directions.

坎离【kǎn lí】　伏羲创建的八卦中的两卦,气功中① 指药物,为阴阳两方面的基本物质;② 指方向。

Kan and Li　Refers to the two Trigrams in the Eight Trigrams created by Fuxi, referring to ① either medicinals in Qigong which are the important substances in Yin and Yang; ② or directions.

坎离颠倒【kǎn lí diān dǎo】　坎和离为伏羲所创建的八卦中的两卦。"坎者,肾宫也,离者,心田也。"气功学中指心阴下降于肾,肾阳上升于心,叫坎离颠倒。

overthrow of Kan and Li　A term of Qigong, in which Kan and Li are the two Trigrams among the Eight Trigrams created by Fuxi. Traditionally "Kan refers to the kidney chamber while Li refers to the heart position". In Qigong, it refers to heart Yin that descends to the kidney and kidney Yang that raises to the heart. That is what overthrow of Kan (Trigram) and

Li (Trigram) means.

坎离会合【kǎn lí huì hé】　坎和离为伏羲所创建的八卦中的两卦。坎指肾,离指心。会合即指心肾相交,阴阳含育。

combination of Kan and Li　A term of Qigong, in which Kan and Li are the two Trigrams among the Eight Trigrams created by Fuxi. In this term, Kan refers to the kidney and Li refers to the heart, combination of Kan and Li means to coordination of the heart and the kidney, indicating the connection of Yin and Yang.

坎离交【kǎn lí jiāo】　坎和离为伏羲创建的八卦中的两卦。气功中① 指日月合璧;② 指阴阳和合;③ 指心肾相交。

integration of Kan and Li　A term of Qigong, in which Kan and Li are the two Trigrams among the Eight Trigrams created by Fuxi. In Qigong, integration of Kan and Li refers to ① either integration of the sun and the moon; ② or integration of Yin and Yang; ③ or integration of the heart and the kidney.

坎离交媾【kǎn lí jiāo gòu】　坎和离为伏羲所创建的八卦中的两卦。术语中的离为心中一阴,坎为肾中一阳。心中一阴与肾中一阳结合,即坎离交媾。

intercourse of Kan and Li　A term of Qigong, in which Kan and Li are the two Trigrams among the Eight Trigrams created by Fuxi. In this term, Li refers to one Yin in the heart while Kan refers to one Yang in the kidney. Combination of one Yin in the heart and one Yang in the kidney indicates intercourse of Kan (Trigram) and Li (Trigram).

坎离交媾之乡【kǎn lí jiāo gòu zhī

xiāng】　与黄庭相同,① 指中;② 指身体内的中虚空窍;③ 指五脏之中;④ 指脐之后;⑤ 指有名无所;⑥ 指黄八极;⑦ 指黄庭在二肾之中;⑧ 指黄庭在心之下。

intercourse village for Kan and Li　The same as Huangting (yellow hall), referring to ① either the center; ② or the middle deficiency and empty orifice in the center of the body; ③ or the center of the five Zang-organs (including the heart, the liver, the spleen, the lung and the kidney); ④ or the region below the navel; ⑤ or a person or something with name but without position; ⑥ or eight yellow extremities; ⑦ or Huangting (yellow hall) located in the region between the kidneys; ⑧ or Huangting (yellow hall) located in the region below the heart.

坎离匡郭【kǎn lí kuāng guō】　坎和离为伏羲所创建的八卦中的两卦,匡郭指乾为天在上,坤为地在下,离坎如日月升降其间。

positions of Kan and Li　A term of Qigong, in which Kan and Li are the two Trigrams among the Eight Trigrams created by Fuxi, and positions (匡郭) indicate that Qian Trigram refers to the sky and is in the high position while Kun Trigram refers to the earth and is in the lower position, among which Kan (Trigram) and Li (Trigram) are just like the rise and set of the sun and the moon.

坎男离女【kǎn nán lí nǚ】　即日月,坎和离为伏羲所创建的八卦中的两卦。指阳中含阴,也指乳头下方足少阳胆经的一个穴位。这一穴位为气功运行的一个常见部位。

Kan man Li woman Refers to the sun and moon, a term of Qigong, in which Kan and Li are the two Trigrams among the Eight Trigrams created by Fuxi. This term refers to either Yin within Yang; or an acupoint in the gallbladder meridian of foot Shaoyang located below the breast.

坎内黄男【kǎn nèi huáng nán】 坎为伏羲所创建的八卦之一。指坎中阳爻。坎为水中之一阳,即真阳。

yellow man in Kan A term of Qigong, in which Kan is one Trigram among the Eight Trigrams created by Fuxi, referring to the Yang level in the Kan Trigram. In Qigong, Kan refers to Yang in water, known as the genuine Yang.

坎内中心实【kǎn nèi zhōng xīn shí】 坎卦之中爻为阳爻,故称为"实"。练功中取肾阳(坎中之阳)与心阴(离中之阴)结合而产金丹。

the central level of Kan Trigram A term of Qigong, in which the central level in the Kan Trigram is called Yang level. In practicing Qigong, combination of kidney Yang (Yang in the Kan Trigram) and heart Yin (Yin in the Li Trigram) can produce golden Dan (pills of immortality).

顑【kǎn】 ① 指腮;② 指鬓前俗称"太阳"的部位。

chin Refers to ① either the cheek; ② or the region in front of the temple.

康南岩守炉鼎【kāng nán yán shǒu lú dǐng】 为静功。其作法为,侧卧式,以头为鼎,以腹为炉,心端正后,炉鼎自坚牢。

kang nanyuan's exercise for keeping furnace cauldron A static exercise, marked by lying on one side and imagining the head as cauldron and the abdomen as furnace. When the heart is straightened and purified, the furnace (the abdomen) and the cauldron (the head) are strong and firm.

亢仓子【kàng cāng zǐ】 为气功养生家,春秋时人。

Kang Cangzi A great master of Qigong for cultivating health in the Spring and Autumn Period (770 BC – 476 BC).

亢仓子胎息诀【kàng cāng zǐ tāi xī jué】 静功口诀,说明要练好气功,应在平素下功夫,稳定情绪,避免有害精神刺激。

Kang Cangzi's fetal respiration formula A static exercise, referring to practicing Qigong with quietness and tranquility in order to stabilize emotion and to avoid damage and irritation of the spirit.

颏【kē】 下颌骨体的前面,承浆以下至下颌骨下缘的部位。

chin Refers to region in front of jawbone and below Chengjiang (CV 24) (an acupoint in the conception meridian) and jawbone.

咳红导引法【ké hóng dǎo yǐn fǎ】 为动功。其作法为,坐小凳子上,双手搭项,蹲身,调息闭气。如气急,微微放之,放而又闭,双手往胸前推开,意念足心,运涌泉水上济心火,守脐下丹田。

exercise of Daoyin for haemoptysis A dynamic exercise, marked by sitting on a small stool, putting the hands over the neck, squatting the body, regulating respiration, keeping breath, mildly closing respiration if Qi is flustered, stretching the hands before the chest, concentrating consciousness in the heart, moving water from Yongquan

（KI 1）upwards to assist heart fire，and keeping the lower Dantian（the region below the navel）.

咳逆候导引法【ké nì hòu dǎo yǐn fǎ**】**为动功。其作法为，先用鼻暖气，然后闭口咳嗽，重复进行，止咳嗽。凌晨去枕，正身仰卧，伸展臂腿，合眼闭口，闭气不息，尽力鼓腹，两腿用力，再呼吸。

exercise of Daoyin for hiccup A dynamic exercise，marked by warming Qi through the nose，closing the mouth to cough with the repetition，taking off the pillow，lying on the back，stretching the legs，closing the eyes and mouth，stopping respiration，bulging the abdomen，straightening the feet and breathing again.

咳嗽【ké sòu**】** 为气功适应证，本病多因外感风寒，邪气直侵肺脏所致。

cough An indication of Qigong，usually caused by invasion of external wind，cold and pathogenic factors into the lung.

咳嗽吐血治法【ké sòu tù xiě zhì fǎ**】**为静功。其作法为，坐墩几，两手搭顶上，蹲身闭息二十一口。如气急难忍，轻轻放出，日行三次。

exercise for curing cough and hemoptysis A static exercise，marked by sitting quietly，keeping the hands over the neck，squatting the body and reducing respiration for twenty-one times. If Qi is flustered and difficult to endure，it can be slightly dispersed for three times a day.

克己复礼【kè jǐ fù lǐ**】** 指克制私欲，恢复天理，稳定情绪的方法。

restrain oneself and restore the rites A celebrated dictum of Confucius，referring to restraining selfish desires and stabilizing emotion.

克念【kè niàn**】** 指克服自己之邪念、杂念。

expelling avarice Refers to eliminate wicked idea and distracting thought.

克念而后可以无念，存心而后可以无心【kè niàn ér hòu kě yǐ wú niàn cún xīn ér hòu kě yǐ wú xīn**】** 指习练气功由初级到高级的过程。即首先控制意念，日久才能静而无念；意念专一，日久思维活动才能维持相对静止。

After restraining selfish desires there will be no desires；after keeping the heart there will be no heart. A celebrated dictum，indicating that the practice of Qigong develops from the primary stage to the high stage. That means the practitioners of Qigong first should control consciousness and eventually tranquilize the mind without any desires. Only when consciousness is concentrated can the activity of consciousness tranquilize the mind.

刻漏【kè lòu**】** 原意指时间，此乃出入息之异名。

carving and leaking A term of Qigong，originally referring to time and then referring to respiration.

刻意【kè yì**】** ① 指调节精神意识；② 指专心致志。

concentration Refers to ① either regulation of the essence，spirit and consciousness；② or concentration of mind in practicing Qigong.

客气【kè qì**】** 指非时而至之气，即风、寒、暑、湿、燥、火六淫之气非时而侵袭人体。

pathogenic factors Refers to various Qi that does not move at the proper time， including wind Qi, cold Qi, summer Qi, dampness Qi, dryness Qi and fire Qi that attack the human body at the improper time.

客主【kè zhǔ】 上关的一个别称,为足少阳胆经中的一个穴位,位于颧弓上缘,距耳郭前缘约 1 寸处,为气功常用意守部位。

kezhu A synonym of Shangguan (GB 3), which is an acupoint in the gallbladder of foot Shaoyang, located on the upper of the zygoma and about 1 Cun to the upper of the auricle. This acupoint is a region usually used in practice of Qigong.

空【kōng】 佛家气功习用语,① 指中之意,即有与无之间,是与非之间;② 指一切现象,假而不实;③ 指静。

emptiness A common term of Qigong in Buddhism, referring to ① either the center, indicating the region between being and no being as well as the region between yes and no; ② or all phenomena, such as falseness without any fact; ③ or tranquility.

空不空,如来藏【kōng bù kōng rú lái cáng】 指既空又不空,在两者之中,能灭除烦恼,到达理想境界。

ideal emergence from vacuum A term of Qigong, referring to vacuum without absolute vacuum in order to eliminate annoyance and reach the ideal state.

空静无物【kōng jìng wú wù】 指习练气功时,精神内守,意在泥丸宫,自觉空虚而清静。

vacuum and tranquility without anything Refers to internal protection of the spirit, concentration of consciousness in the brain and feeling nothingness and tranquility in practicing Qigong.

空空【kōng kōng】 指虚静无为为空,至虚至静无为谓之空空。

vacuum Refers to tranquility, inactivity and nothingness after perfect practice of Qigong.

空空心【kōng kōng xīn】 指寂静的意识思维活动。

emptying the heart A term of Qigong, referring to the activities of consciousness and thought.

空窍【kōng qiào】 泛指机体开口于外的一切孔窍,如九窍、汗窍、津窍、精窍等。

opening orifice Refers to all the orifices lateral to the mouth, such as nine orifices, sweating orifice, fluid orifice and essence orifice etc.

空心静坐法【kōng xīn jìng zuò fǎ】 佛家气功功法。其作法为,静坐,导引入静,意识思维活动幽静,维持相对静止的状态。

exercise for stabilizing the heart and quiet sitting Refers to the exercise of Qigong in Buddhism, marked by sitting quietly, keeping the activity of thinking quiet and trying to reach the state of tranquility.

空中【kōng zhōng】 指习练气功,意识活动空寂明净,恰在身体之正中。

middle vacuum A term of Qigong, referring to tranquilized activity of consciousness that is just in the middle of the body in practicing Qigong.

孔德之容【kǒng dé zhī róng】 指从发的荣枯,可以观测人的健康情况。

manifestation of great morality Refers to observation of human health through hair vicissitude.

孔丘【kǒng qiū】 中华思想圣祖和气功圣祖孔子的另外一个称谓。

Kong Qiu Another name of Confucius

K

who was Shengren（sage）of traditional Chinese ideology and Qigong.

孔仲尼【kǒng zhòng ní】　中华思想圣祖和气功圣祖孔子的另外一个称谓。

Kong Zhongni　Another name of Confucius who was Shengren（sage）of traditional Chinese ideology and Qigong.

孔子【kǒng zǐ】　是文化圣人，重视修身论、动静论、中和论、正心论等，奠定了儒家气功养生理论，对后世气功学的发展产生了深远的影响。

Confucius　A great cultural sage, but also paid great attention to cultivation of health, tranquilization of mind, harmonization of the body and faithfulness of the heart, laying the theoretical foundation for Qigong in Confucianism, and greatly influencing Qigong in all the dynasties.

恐则气下【kǒng zé qì xià】　指恐惧伤肾，肾藏精，肾气伤则精气不升，心气不降、心肾不交则气下。

Fear reduces Qi.　This is a celebrated dictum, indicating that fear damages the kidney. The kidney stores essence. If kidney Qi is damaged, essential Qi cannot rise. If heart Qi does not descend and if the heart and the kidney are difficult to coordinate with each other, essential Qi certainly can only move downwards.

空闲【kòng xián】　指耳神。

leisure　Refers to the spirit in the ears.

口称三昧【kǒu chēng sān mèi】　为静功。其作法为，精神集中念佛，意识集中于佛，思维集中在佛。

stated Samadhi　A static exercise, marked by concentrating the spirit to read Buddhism, concentrating consciousness in Buddhism and concentra-

ting thinking inside Buddhism.

口齿治法【kǒu chǐ zhì fǎ】　为静功。其作法为，面向东坐，不息四通，叩齿三六次；常在与人生干支相值之日叩齿九次。

oral and dental exercise　A static exercise, marked by sitting to the east, stopping respiration in four ways, clicking the teeth for three and six times; or clicking the teeth for nine times in the day similar to life pole.

口臭【kǒu chòu】　为气功适应证，指由于五脏六腑失调，浊气上熏于胸。

foul breath　An indication of Qigong, referring to oral inflammation caused by disorder of the five Zang-organs（including the heart, the liver, the spleen, the lung and the kidney）and the six Fu-organs（including the gallbladder, the stomach, the small intestine, the large intestine, the bladder and the triple energizer）and accumulation of turbid Qi in the chest.

口功【kǒu gōng】　为动功。其作法为，张口呵气十数次，鸣天鼓九次，以舌口咽津，复呵复咽。可治疗口中焦干，喉痛。

oral exercise　A dynamic exercise, marked by opening the mouth to breathe out for dozens of times, pressing the back of the brain for nine times, stirring the mouth with the tongue for swallowing fluid, breating out again and swallowing again. Such a dynamic exercise can cure oral dryness and throat pain.

口舌疮【kǒu shé chuāng】　为气功适应证，指口舌发生糜烂，溃破、疼痛，多因心脾积热火体虚所致。

aphtha　An indication of Qigong, referring to erosion, ulceration and pain of the tongue caused by accumulation of heat or deficiency of the heart and spleen.

口舌疮候导引法【kǒu shé chuāng hòu dǎo yǐn fǎ】 为动功。其作法为，仰面，抬肩向七，头向左右转动各二十一次，暂停，待气血运行平静时再作。此法可祛风解表止痛，治外感寒热，脊腰颈项痛，风痹，口内生疮，牙齿痛，头眩晕。

exercise of Daoyin for oral ulcer A dynamic exercise, marked by raising up the face, raising the shoulders, turning the head to the right and the left and vice versa for twenty-one times respectively; stopping for a while, practicing again when the movement of Qi and the blood is quieted and balanced. Such a dynamic exercise can expel wind to relieve superficies, eliminate heat to stop pain and treat exogenous cold-heat, pain in the waist, neck and nape as well as wind impediment, oral sore, dental pain and dizziness.

口宜默【kǒu yí mò】 指习练气功期间，应少言语。

keeping silence A term of Qigong, referring to speaking less in practicing Qigong.

叩齿【kòu chǐ】 为动功，指上下牙互相叩击。

clicking teeth A dynamic exercise, referring to the upper teeth and the lower teeth clicking each other.

叩齿集神【kòu chǐ jí shén】 指每日早上起床后叩齿三十六遍，可防止牙龈萎缩，口腔溃疡。

clicking teeth for concentrating spirit Refers to clicking the teeth for thirty-six times every day when waking up in order to prevent gingival atrophy and

dental ulcer.

叩齿牙无疾法【kòu chǐ yá wú jí fǎ】 指凌晨醒来后叩齿三十六遍，可治齿疾。

exercise for preventing disease by clicking teeth Refers to clicking the teeth for thirty-six times every day when waking up in order to treat dental disease.

寇辅真【kòu fǔ zhēn】 北魏气功学家寇谦之的另外一个称谓，其研究气功导引，服气口诀，并得其法。

Kou Fuzhen Another name of Kou Qianzi, a master of Qigong in Northern Wei Dynasty (368 AD - 534 AD), who studied and analyzed Qigong, Daoyin, formulae for taking Qi and the exercises for practicing Qigong and Daoyin.

寇谦之【kòu qiān zhī】 北魏气功学家，研究气功导引，服气口诀，并得其法。

Kou Qianzi A master of Qigong in Northern Wei Dynasty (368 AD - 534 AD), who studied and analyzed Qigong, Daoyin, formulae for taking Qi and the exercises for practicing Qigong and Daoyin.

寇先生鼓琴【kòu xiān shēng gǔ qín】 为动功。其作法为，盘膝坐，以两手按膝，向左扭头项及背运气十二口，又向右转头项及背，亦运气十二口。治头疼与血脉不通。

Mr. Kou's exercise for music playing A dynamic exercise, marked by sitting with crossed legs, pressing the knees with both hands, turning the head, neck and back to the left side and moving Qi for twelve times; then turning the head, neck and back to the right side, and also moving Qi for twelve times. Such a dynamic exercise can cure headache and obstructed blood vessels.

枯木龙吟【kū mù lóng yín】 佛家气功习用语。木指灭绝一切妄念、妄想，维持思维活动的相对静止，身如枯木而不动。龙吟即阴之极而阳生。

loong sounding in fallen tree A common term of Qigong in Buddhism. In this term, tree refers to tranquility that eliminates wild fancy and delusion and controls the activity of thought. In practice Qigong, the body is just like a fallen tree without any movement. Loong sounding refers to the growth of Yang when Yin is extreme.

枯坐旁门【kū zuò páng mén】 指不识真种子，盲目习练气功，以邪术呆坐，毫无益处。

dull sitting at the side gate A term of Qigong, referring to failure to know the principles of Qigong, practicing Qigong blindly and dull sitting in a wrong way without any effect.

苦【kǔ】 佛家气功习用语，指神形失调，精神恼怒、躁忧、烦闷等，或自然因素，风、雨、寒热之灾。

suffering A common term of Qigong in Buddhism, referring to either imbalance of the spirit and the body with annoyance, dysphoria and irritancy; or natural factors, such as wind, rain, cold and heat.

快活无忧散【kuài huó wú yōu sǎn】 动静相兼功，即除烦恼，断妄想，使神气清爽，天君泰然。

happiness without any anxiety An exercise combined with a dynamic exercise and a static exercise, referring to eliminating annoyance and distracting thought in order to tranquilize the spirit and to stabilize the body.

矿去金存【kuàng qù jīn cún】 矿为杂质，金为冶炼后的纯金。指习练气功，排除杂念，神形和合。

elimination of mine and existence of gold A term of Qigong, in which mine refers to impurity while gold refers to pure gold, indicating that impurity must be eliminated and the spirit and the body must be combined with each other in practicing Qigong.

顗【kuí】 足太阳膀胱经之筋。

cheekbone The branch of the sinew in the bladder meridian of foot Taiyang.

愦愦【kuì kuì】 指昏乱。

confusion Refers to disordered mind.

愧【kuì】 ① 指精神活动，如愧心，对过错的反思；② 指感到羞耻，为佛家气功习用语。

ashamed Refers to ① either introspection of error; ② or shame, which is a common term of Qigong in Buddhism.

坤【kūn】 指坤卦，具体含义为① 指地；② 指腹；③ 指柔顺；④ 指母；⑤ 指静；⑥ 指西南方向。

kun Means Kun Trigram, referring to ① either the earth; ② or the abdomen; ③ or gentleness and agreeableness; ④ or mother; ⑤ or quietness; ⑥ or southwest.

坤鼎【kūn dǐng】 ① 指白虎，白虎指二十八宿中西方的七宿；② 内丹书中指"心中元神谓之龙，肾中元精谓之虎"。

kun cauldron Another appellation of white tiger, referring to ① either the seven constellations in the west among the twenty-eight constellations; ② or "the original spirit in the heart called Loong and the original essence in the kidney called tiger" mentioned in the books about internal Dan (pills of immortality).

坤位【kūn wèi】　指腹,即人身小腹或丹田。

kun position　A term of Qigong, referring to the abdomen, indicating the lower abdomen or Dantian which is divided into the upper Dantian (the region between the eyes), the middle Dantian (the region below the heart) and the lower Dantian (the region below the navel).

坤元【kūn yuán】　指地之德,顺天时以养长万物。亦指真阴,阴之本源。

kun origin　A term of Qigong, referring to either the function of the earth and following the celestial weather to nourish all things; or genuine Yin and the origin of Yin.

坤再索于乾而生离【kūn zài suǒ yú qián ér shēng lí】　即坤卦得乾卦之一阳爻,而生成离卦。

Kun Trigram obtaining a level from Qian Trigram to produce Li Trigram　Means that the Kun Trigram takes a level in the Qian Trigram to form the Li Trigram.

昆池【kūn chí】　昆池可以上接玉京,为气功习练时的一个重要概念。

chunchi pool　A term of Qigong, referring to a pool that can communicate with the moon, which is an important concept in practicing Qigong.

昆陵【kūn líng】　即昆仑的另外一个称谓。① 昆仑为泥丸之异名;② 指头;③ 为足太阳膀胱经中的一个穴位,在足外踝后。这一穴位为气功运行的一个常见部位。

kunling　A synonym of Kunlun which refers to ① either the mud bolus (the brain); ② or the head; ③ or Kunlun (BL 60), an acupoint in the bladder meridian of foot Taiyang located behind the external malleolus. This acupoint is a region usually used for keeping the essential Qi in practice of Qigong.

昆仑【kūn lún】　① 为泥丸之异名;② 指头;③ 为足太阳膀胱经中的一个穴位,在足外踝后。这一穴位为气功运行的一个常见部位。

kunlun　Refers to ① either a synonym of mud bolus (the brain); ② or the head; ③ or Kunlun (BL 60), an acupoint in the bladder meridian of foot Taiyang located behind the external malleolus. This acupoint is a region usually used for keeping the essential Qi in practice of Qigong.

昆仑五城【kūn lún wǔ chéng】　指头脑与五脏。

five cities in kunlun　Refer to the brain and the five Zang-organs (including the heart, the liver, the spleen, the lung and the kidney).

括囊【kuò náng】　喻人遇事闭目塞听,缄口不言,情绪稳定而不受干扰。

silence　Means to close the eyes, ears and mouth in order to prevent disturbance when encountering anything.

L

兰茂【lán mào】 明代医学家和气功学家,云南嵩明人。

Lan Mao A great doctor and master of Qigong in the Ming Dynasty (1368 AD - 1644 AD) who lived in Songming County, Yunnan Province.

兰台宫真人【lán tái gōng zhēn rén】指肝脏的神名。

Immortal in green chamber Refers to the spirit in the liver.

兰廷秀【lán tíng xiù】 明代医学家和气功学家兰茂的另外一个称谓。

Lan Tingxiu Another name of Lan Mao, a great doctor and master of Qigong in the Ming Dynasty (1368 AD - 1644 AD) who lived in Songming County, Yunnan Province.

蓝采和行歌城市【lán cǎi hé xíng gē chéng shì】 为动功。其作法为,自然站立,左边气血运行不畅,则举左手向前约与肩平,同时运气;右边气血不畅,则举右手,操作同前。主治气血运行不畅。

Lan Caihe's exercise for singing song in city A dynamic exercise, marked by standing naturally. If Qi and the blood in the left cannot move smoothly, the left hand should be raised to the shoulder for moving Qi; if Qi and the blood cannot move smoothly, the right hand should be raised to the shoulder for moving Qi. Such a dynamic exercise can cure stagnancy of Qi and the blood. Such a dynamic exercise can cure stagnancy of Qi and the blood.

蓝采和乌龙摆角法【lán cǎi hé wū lóng bǎi jiǎo fǎ】 为动功。其作法为,平地端坐,舒两脚,两手握拳,运身向前,运气二十四口,又以两脚踏定,低头,两手搬两脚尖,运气二十四口。主治遍身疼痛。

Lan Caihe's exercise of black Loong for moving horn A dynamic exercise, marked by sitting upright on the ground, holding the fists with both hands, moving the body forward, moving Qi for twenty-four times; then treading with the feet, lowering the head, pulling the tiptoes with both hands, moving Qi for twenty-four times. Such a dynamic exercise can cure body pain.

阆苑【láng yuàn】 指"三岛(顶、心、肾)之内,根源阆苑"。

immortal palace A term of Qigong, indicating that "the three islands (referring to the head, heart and kidney) are the sources of the essence, Qi and the spirit".

朗然子胎息诀【lǎng rán zǐ tāi xī jué】为静功。其作法为,静坐冥心,叩齿集神,意念与心神均放在丹田,可调节形神,预防治疗疾病。

Lang Ranzi's formula for fetal respiration A static exercise, marked by quietly sitting, tranquilizing the heart, clicking the teeth, concentration the spirit, entering consciousness and heart spirit into Dantian in order to regulate the body and spirit as well as to prevent and cure diseases. Dantian is divided into the upper Dantian (the region between the eyes), the middle Dantian (the region below the heart) and the lower Dantian (the region below the navel).

劳宫【láo gōng】　手厥阴心包经中的一个穴位,位于掌心横纹中,为气功中气感较强的部位之一。这一穴位为气功运行的一个常见部位。

Laogong（**PC 8**）　An acupoint in the pericardium meridian of hand Jueyin, located in the transverse line of the palm. This acupoint is a region usually used in practice of Qigong.

劳淋【láo lín】　为气功适应证,指小便淋沥不尽,遇劳即发。

stranguria due to overstrain　An indication of Qigong, referring to profuse dribbling urination that occurs when tired.

劳神【láo shén】　指烦劳精神。

spirit exhaustion　Refers to disorders that trouble the essence and the spirit.

劳神明【láo shén míng】　指调节精神意识。

stirring spiritual brightness　Refers to regulating the essence, the spirit and the consciousness.

劳神之位【láo shén zhī wèi】　指鼻。

location for stirring spirit　A term of Qigong, referring to the nose.

劳形【láo xíng】　指因事情繁杂,而损伤形体,致形疲。

somatic exhaustion　Refers to miscellaneous things that have injured the body.

劳瘵【láo zhài】　为气功适应证,由于劳伤正气,而感痨虫所致。

Consumptive disease　An indication of

Qigong, which is caused by pulmonary trematodiasis due to damage of the genuine Qi.

痨瘵治法【láo zhài zhì fǎ】　动静相兼功。其作法为,把两手交叉放在头上,长吸气即吐之,坐地慢慢伸展两脚,用两手从外边将膝抱起,急低头进入两膝间,这样两手交叉抱头上,行功十三遍。

exercise for curing tuberculosis　An exercise combined with dynamic exercise and static exercise, marked by crossing the hands to put over the head, inhaling for a long time to exhale, sitting on the ground to slowly stretch the feet, pulling the knees from the lateral sides with both hands, quickly lower the head between the knees, holding the head with both hands crossed and acting for thirteen times.

痨症治法【láo zhèng zhì fǎ】　动静相兼功。其作法为,侧卧,左手枕头,右手捏举向腹,往来擦抹,右脚在下微屈,左腿压上习睡,收气三十二口。

exercise for curing consumptive disease　An exercise combined with dynamic exercise and static exercise, marked by lying on one side, taking the left hand as pillow, pinching and raising the right hand to rub the abdomen to and fro, slightly bending the right foot, pressing the left foot for sleeping and inhaling Qi for thirty-two times.

老聃【láo dān】　是春秋末年伟大的思想家、哲学家,为道教的创始人老子的另外一个称谓。

Lao Dan　Another name of Lao Zi, a great thinker, a great philosopher and the founder of the most important Chinese thought known as Dao in the late Spring and Autumn Period（770 BC -

476 BC).

老复壮【lǎo fù zhuàng】 指返老还童之意。

rejuvenation Refers to renew one's youth after practicing Qigong.

老君【lǎo jūn】 即老子,又称为太上老君。

Lao Jun Refers Lao Zi, the great thinker, philosopher and the founder of the most important Chinese thought known as Dao, who was also called Taishang Laojun (the immortal in the universe).

老君导引法【lǎo jūn dǎo yǐn fǎ】 动静相兼功。指每凌晨时期,展两手于膝上,徐徐按捺两节。口吐浊气,鼻引清气,所谓吐故纳新。

great noble person's exercise of Daoyin An exercise combined with static exercise and dynamic exercise, marked by putting the hands on the knees and slowly pressing the two aspects in the early morning, vomiting turbid Qi from the mouth and inhaling clear Qi through the nose, known as to exhale the old and to inhale the new.

老君守一法【lǎo jūn shǒu yī fǎ】 为静功。夜半元气始生时,舌掠齿上下,舐唇,以鼻纳气,口咽之三九止,则生气通流于百脉。

great noble person's exercise for tranquilization A static exercise, marked by clicking the upper and the lower teeth with the tongue at midnight when the original Qi begins to appear, licking the lips, inhaling Qi through the nose and swallowing saliva through the mouth for three to nine times respectively in order to circulate Qi through all the meridians.

老君胎息法【lǎo jūn tāi xī fǎ】 为静功。其作法为,夜半时,日中前,自舒展脚手,拗脚咳嗽,长出气三两度即坐,握固摄心脐下。

great noble person's exercise for fetal respiration A static exercise, marked by stretching the feet and hands and coughing with fixed feet at the midnight and before the noon, usually sitting after exhaling for three or two degrees as well as concentrating and assimilating below the heart and the navel.

老君调气法【lǎo jūn tiáo qì fǎ】 为静功。其作法为,夜半候,日中前,取仰卧式,低枕,舒展双脚,双手握固,去身四五寸,两脚亦去四五寸。鼻微微引太阳气从鼻入,以意送此气通遍身体。

great noble person's exercise for regulating Qi A static exercise, marked by lying with a low pillow at the midnight or before the noon, relaxing the feet and holding the hands to extend the body and the feet for four or five Cun, inhaling the sunny Qi slightly through the nose and transmitting it to the whole body.

老郎【lǎo láng】 指气功锻炼群阴剥尽而成纯阳之体,故称为"老郎"。

great youth A term of Qigong, referring to the fact that Yin finally is transformed into pure Yang after sincere practice of Qigong. That is why it is called great youth.

老老恒言【lǎo lǎo héng yán】 《老老恒言》为气功养生学著作,由清代曹庭栋所著,谈老年人衣、食、住、行的养生方法。

Laolao Hengyan (*Permanent Analysis About Old People*) A monograph about Qigong entitled *Permanent Anal-*

ysis About Old People, written by Cao Tingdong in the Qing Dynasty (1636 AD - 1912 AD), discussing the way to cultivate life related to clothes, food, living and walking in old people.

老老恒言立式导引【lǎo lǎo héng yán lì shì dǎo yǐn】 为动功,方法多样。如正立,两手交叉置身后,提起左足前后摆功数遍,换右足,动作相同。

standing exercise of Daoyin based on permanent analysis A dynamic exercise with various methods, such as sitting with hands crossing over the back, lifting the left foot to move forwards and backwards for several times and then lifting the right foot in the same way.

老老恒言卧式导引【lǎo lǎo héng yán wò shì dǎo yǐn】 为动功,方法多样。如仰卧,竖屈两膝,膝盖相并,两足向外,用左手攀左足,右手攀右足,用力向外作数遍。

lying exercise of Daoyin based on permanent analysis A dynamic exercise with various methods, such as lying on the back, extending the knees connected with each other, stretching the feet externally, holding the left foot with the left hand and the right foot with the right hand externally for several times.

老老恒言坐式导引【lǎo lǎo héng yán zuò shì dǎo yǐn】 为动功,方法多样。如盘膝坐,腰伸直,两手握拳状,两手用力轮流,前作冲拳动作数遍。

sitting exercise of Daoyin based on permanent analysis A dynamic exercise with various methods, such as sitting with crossed legs, stretching the waist, clenching the fists, strongly taking turns with both hands and shaking the fists for several times.

老嫩【lǎo nèn】 指气功中药物生成时,嫩时需采,老时即枯。

old and tender Refers to the medicinal produced in Qigong, which should be collected when it is tender and withered when it is old.

老年导引法【lǎo nián dǎo yǐn fǎ】 为动功,方法多样。如调气、调神,即调匀呼吸,放松形神。

exercise of Daoyin for old people A dynamic exercise with various methods, such as regulating Qi and regulating the spirit which means to regulate respiration and to relax the body and the spirit

老彭【lǎo péng】 老子和彭祖的合称。老子是春秋末年伟大的思想家、哲学家,为道教的创始人。彭祖是上古时期气功养生学家。

Lao Peng Refers to Lao Zi and Peng Zu. Lao Zi was a great thinker, a great philosopher and the founder of the most important Chinese thought known as Dao in the late Spring and Autumn Period (770 BC - 476 BC). Peng Zu was a great master of Qigong and life cultivation.

老阳【lǎo yáng】 指九,九为阳数之极,故称为老阳。

Great Yang Refers to nine which is the highest number of Yang. That is why it is called great Yang.

老阴【lǎo yīn】 指六,六为阴数之极,故称为老阴。

Great Yin Refers to six which is the highest number of Yin. That is why it is called great Yin.

老庄【lǎo zhuāng】 指老子和庄子,为道家的代表。也指《老子》和《庄子》两书。

Lao Zhuang Refers to Lao Zi and

L

Zhuang Zi who were the founder of the most important Chinese thought known as Dao. It is also the titles of two important canons written by Lao Zi and Zhuang Zi.

老子【lǎo zǐ】 是春秋末年伟大的思想家、哲学家，为道教的创始人，也指《老子》一书，其中也有气功养生的精神。

Lao Zi A great thinker, a great philosopher and the founder of the most important Chinese thought known as Dao in the late Spring and Autumn Period (770 BC - 476 BC). Lao Zi is also the title of the great canon which is also entitled Dao De Jing (Canon of Dao and Morality).

老子想尔注【lǎo zǐ xiǎng ěr zhù】《老子》的注释本，据说为东汉末年张道陵所著。

Lao Zi's Thought and Annotation Explained to be a book written by Zhang Daoling in the late East Han Dynasty (25 AD - 220 AD), explaining Lao Zi, entitled the *Canon of Dao*.

乐天则寿【lè tiān zé shòu】 指不受外界刺激的干扰，精神内守，协调通达，内外和调，精神和调，体气至安。

happiness prolonging life A celebrated dictum, referring to no interference of external stimulus, internal concentration of the spirit, perforation through coordination, regulation of the internal and external, harmonization of the essence and spirit and stabilization of Qi in the body.

乐志【lè zhì】 指精神意识愉快、自在，神形合调，身体健康。

spiritual pleasure Refers to happiness and comfort in the spirit and the mind, integration of the spirit and the body,

and health cultivation.

雷车【léi chē】 指阴阳正合，水火共处，静中闻雷霆之声。

thunder cart Refers to hearing thunderbolt under tranquility with combination of Yin and Yang as well as water and fire.

雷电八振【léi diàn bā zhèn】 指胆气刚勇，有如雷电，威震八方。

Thunderbolt with eight vibrations A term of Qigong, referring to valor of gallbladder Qi like thunderbolt that shocks the eight directions.

雷鸣电激【léi míng diàn jī】 ① 指自然界的雷电；② 指叩齿。

thundering and electroporation A term of Qigong, referring to ① either thunderbolt in the natural world; ② or clicking the teeth.

雷霆府【léi tíng fǔ】 指鼻柱。

thunderbolt mansion A term of Qigong, referring to nasal septum.

类修要诀【lèi xiū yào jué】《类修要诀》为气功养生专著，由明代胡文焕所著，强调养生要旨在修炼精气神，收集了前人养生的歌诀、格言和警句。

Leixiu Yaojue（*Important Formulae of Cultivation in Various Categories*） A monograph of Qigong entitled *Important Formulae of Cultivation in Various Categories*, written by Hu Wenhuan in the Ming Dynasty (1368 AD - 1644 AD), emphasizing the importance of cultivating the essence, Qi and spirit; collecting the previous songs, and epigrams for cultivating life.

冷启敬【lěng qǐ jìng】 明代著名的气功养生家冷谦的另外一个称谓，著有气功专论，简明扼要地论述气功导引养生。

Leng Qijing Another name of Leng

Qian, an important master of Qiong and life cultivation in the Ming Dynasty (1368 AD – 1644 AD), who wrote a monograph about Qigong, concisely discussing the theory and practice of Qigong for cultivating health through Daoyin.

冷谦【lěng qiān】　明代著名的气功养生家,著有气功专论,简明扼要地论述气功导引养生。

Leng Qian　An important master of Qiong and life cultivation in the Ming Dynasty (1368 AD – 1644 AD), who wrote a monograph about Qigong, concisely discussing the theory and practice of Qigong for cultivating health through Daoyin.

冷热痢【lěng rè lì】　为气功适应证,包括痢疾中的寒痢和热痢。

cold and heat dysentery　An indication of Qigong, including cold dysentery and heat dysentery in the problems of dysentery.

冷热痢候导引法【lěng rè lì hòu dǎo yǐn fǎ】　为静功。其作法为,用鼻吸气,微微引气入腹,待气充满时,以吹字慢慢呼出。

exercise of Daoyin for cold and heat dysentery　A static exercise, marked by inhaling through the nose, mildly transmitting Qi into the abdomen, and slowly exhaling by reading the Chinese character Chui (blow) after Qi is full.

冷真集【lěng zhēn jí】　《冷真集》为气功专著,由宋代王吉昌所撰,主要论述习练气功的法诀及登堂境界。

Lengzhen Ji(*Collection of Coldness and Genuineness*)　A monograph of Qiong entitled *Collection of Coldness and Genuineness*, written by Wang Jichang

in the Song Dynasty (960 AD – 1279 AD), mainly describing the methods and states of Qigong practice.

冷注【lěng zhù】　为气功适应证,指风寒湿邪侵袭肢节、经络,其中又以寒证为主的病证。

cold attack　An indication of Qigong, referring to invasion of pathogenic wind, cold and dampness into the limbs, joints, meridians and collaterals, among which coldness is the most serious disease.

离【lí】　① 指卦名,为火;② 指日东升;③ 指智慧与柔和之性源于中正;④ 去类比象,离为目、为心、为大腹;⑤ 指方向。

li　Refers to ① either Li Trigram in the Eight Trigrams from Yijing (*Canon of Simplification, Change and No Change*), indicating fire; ② or sunrise in the east; ③ or the source of wisdom and gentleness in the center; ④ or analogy, in which Li refers to either the eyes or the heart or the upper abdomen; ⑤ or the directions.

离凡世【lí fán shì】　说明练功并非要身体"超离凡尘",长生不老,而是要让人的精神意识达到高级的境界。

ideal state　A term of Qigong, indicating that practice of Qigong should promote the spirit to the high state, not just reaching an otherworldly realm of life.

离宫【lí gōng】　指心脏。

fire palace　Refers to the heart.

离宫赤气【lí gōng chì qì】　指南方自然生发之气。亦指心的生发之气。

hot Qi in detached palace　Refers to natural Qi in the south. It also refers to Qi produced in the heart.

L

离宫腹内阴【lí gōng fù nèi yīn】 同坎内中心实,坎卦之中爻为阳爻,故称为"实"。练功中取肾阳(坎中之阳)与心阴(离中之阴)结合而产金丹。

internal Yin in detached palace The same as the central level of Kan Trigram, is a term of Qigong, in which the central level in the Kan Trigram is called Yang level. In practicing Qigong, combination of kidney Yang (Yang in the Kan Trigram) and heart Yin (Yin in the Li Trigram) can produce golden Dan (pills of immortality). Kan Trigram is in the Eight Trigrams from Yijing (*Canon of Simplification*, *Change and No Change*).

离中玄女【lí zhōng xuán nǚ】 指阳中有阴。

great woman in Li Trigram Means that there is Yin within Yang.

李伯阳【lǐ bó yáng】 指太上老君,是对老子的尊称。古人云:"太上老君,姓李名耳,字伯阳,一名重耳。"

Li Boyang The same of Supreme Great Immortal which is a celebration of Lao Zi who was the founder of the most important Chinese thought known as Dao. It was said in ancient China that Lao Zi was also named Li Boyang.

李博进火候法【lǐ bó jìn huǒ hòu fǎ】 为静功。其作法为,每日子后午前,若于五更初阳盛时更佳。就坐榻上,面东或南,握固盘足,合目,主腰正坐,澄心静虑,内视五脏,仰面合口,鼻中引出清气,可温补散寒。

Li Bo's exercise for entering duration of heating A static exercise, marked by practice before Zi (the period of the day from 11 p.m. to 1 a.m.) and after Wu (the period of the day from 11 a.m. to 1 p.m. in the noon) or at the early morning, sitting on the couch, turning the face to the east or south, holding the crossed feet, closing the eyes, stretching the waist in sitting, calming the heart and tranquilizing the mind, internally observing the five Zang-organs (including the heart, the liver, the spleen, the lung and the kidney), raising the face to close the mouth, inhaling pure air from the nose in order to warmly tonify the body and disperse cold.

李博内丹术【lǐ bó nèi dān shù】 源自气功学专论,深入系统地分析和说明了养心、养气、养神的方法和意义。

Li Bo's exercise for internal Dan Collected from a monograph of Qigong, mainly analyzing and introducing the methods and significance for nourishing the heart, Qi and the spirit through practice of Qigong.

李梴【lǐ chān】 明代医学家和气功家,应用气功养生防病,效果甚好。

Li Chan A great doctor and master of Qigong in the Ming Dynasty (1368 AD - 1644 AD), emphasizing the practice of Qigong for nourishing life and preventing disease with fine effect.

李淳风【lǐ chún fēng】 唐代学者,他撰写的学术著作对后世天文、历法、数学及气功学的发展,影响巨大。

Li Chunfeng A great scholar in the Tang Dynasty (618 AD - 907 AD). The monograph written by Li Chunfeng greatly influenced astronomy, calendar, mathematics and Qigong in the later generations.

李道纯【lǐ dào chún】 元代气功学家,著有多部气功学专著,对后世影响很大。

Li Daochun　A great master of Qigong in the Yuan Dynasty（1271 AD－1368 AD）, whose monographs of Qigong greatly influenced the later generations.

李东垣【lǐ dōng yuán】　金元四大医学家之一李杲的另外一个称谓。李杲重视气功学说, 以养神为主, 对后世医学气功的发展有一定的影响。

Li Dongyuan　Another name of Li Gao, one of the four great doctors in the Jin Dynasty（1115 AD－1234 AD）and Yuan Dynasty（1206 AD－1368 AD）. He paid great attention to nourishing the spirit in studying Qigong and influenced the development of medicine and Qigong in the later generations.

李耳【lǐ ěr】　春秋末年伟大的思想家、哲学家老子的另外一个称谓, 为道教的创始人；也指《老子》一书, 其中也有气功养生的精神。

Li Er　Another name of Lao Zi, a great thinker, a great philosopher and the founder of the most important Chinese thought known as Dao in the late Spring and Autumn Period（770 BC－476 BC）. Lao Zi is also the name of the great canon also entitled Dao De Jing（*Canon of Dao and Morality*）.

李奉时山人服气法【lǐ fèng shí shān rén fú qì fǎ】　为静功。其作法为, 功前先活动四肢, 然后以仰卧式调身, 无枕, 闭目, 安定神气。

Li Feng's exercise for respiration in mountains　A static exercise, marked by activating the four limbs before practicing Qigong, then lying supine without pillow, closing the eyes and stabilizing the spirit and Qi.

李杲【lǐ gǎo】　金元四大医学家之一, 其气功学说以养神为主, 对后世医学气功的发展有一定的影响。

Li Gao　One of the four great doctors in the Jin Dynasty（1115 AD－1234 AD）and Yuan Dynasty（1206 AD－1368 AD）. He paid great attention to nourishing the spirit in studying Qigong and influenced the development of medicine and Qigong in the later generations.

李含光【lǐ hán guāng】　唐代医学家, 为道家气功传人之一。

Li Hanguang　An important doctor in the Tang Dyansty（618 AD－907 AD）, also one of the important descendants of Qigong in Daoism.

李涵虚【lǐ hán xū】　宋代气功学家, 认真地研究和传播了气功学。

Li Hanxu　A great master of Qigong in the Song Dynasty（960 AD－1279 AD）who sincerely studied and propagated Qigong.

李简易【lǐ jiǎn yì】　宋代气功学家, 其气功专著对后世有一定的影响。

Li Jianyi　A master of Qigong in the Song Dynasty（960 AD－1279 AD）, whose monographs of Qigong influenced the later generations.

李明子【lǐ míng zǐ】　金元四大医学家之一李杲的另外一个称谓。李杲重视气功学, 以养神为主, 对后世医学气功的发展有一定的影响。

Li Mingzi　Another name of Li Gao, one of the four great doctors in the Jin Dynasty（1115 AD－1234 AD）and Yuan Dynasty（1206 AD－1368 AD）. He paid great attention to nourishing the spirit in studying Qigong and influenced the development of medicine and

L

Qigong in the later generations.

李千乘炼气法【lǐ qiān chéng liàn qì fǎ】 为静功。其作法为，常以生气时（夜半至日中为生气时），偃卧瞑目，握固闭气无息，意念集于身体之中。闭气良久时间约默数一百二十次，呼气从口中出之，以后逐日增加闭气时长。

Li Qiancheng's exercise for practicing Qigong A static exercise, marked by lying with closed eyes from the midnight to the noon, holding respiration, concentrating consciousness on the body, holding Qi for one hundred and twenty times, exhaling through the nose and eventually increasing the way to hold respiration.

李清庵【lǐ qīng ān】 元代气功学家李道纯的另外一个称谓，其著有多部气功学专著，对后世影响很大。

Li Qing'an Another name of Li Daochun, a great master of Qigong in the Yuan Dynasty (1271 AD - 1368 AD), whose monographs of Qigong greatly influenced the later generations.

李时珍【lǐ shí zhēn】 明代杰出的中医药学家，也是气功的重要研究人。

Li Shizhen A great medical scientist in the Ming Dynasty (1368 AD - 1644 AD), also making great contribution to the development of Qigong.

李元素【lǐ yuán sù】 元代气功学家李道纯的另外一个称谓，其著有多部气功学专著，对后世影响很大。

Li Yuansu Another name of Li Daochun, a great master of Qigong in the Yuan Dynasty (1271 AD - 1368 AD), whose monographs of Qigong greatly influenced the later generations.

李真人长生一十六字诀【lǐ zhēn rén cháng shēng yī shí liù zì jué】 与十六字诀法相同，为静功。其作法为，一吸便提，气气归脐；一提便咽，水火相见。

Li Zhenren's formula for prolonging life with sixteen characters A static exercise, the same as sixteen-characters method, referring to sixteen important ways for strengthening health and treating any disease, which are described with sixteen special Chinese characters. In practice, after inhalation, it must be enhanced. When any Qi is inhaled, it should be returned to the navel. When it is enhanced, it must be swallowed in order to coordinate with water and fire.

李真人海底捞月法【lǐ zhēn rén hǎi dǐ lāo yuè fǎ】 为动功。其作法为，将身曲如打恭形状，手足俱要交叉伏地，左右行功运气各一十二口，可和气养血。

Li Zhenren's exercise for dragging the moon from the bottom of the sea A dynamic exercise, marked by curving the body like salute, crossing the hands and feet over the ground and practicing Qigong from the left to the right and vice versa for twelve times in order to harmonize Qi and to nourish the blood.

李真人胎息诀【lǐ zhēn rén tāi xī jué】 为静功。其作法为，坐势，以心静立论，注意调节呼吸，不要有意憋气，以免偏差。

Li Zhenren's formula for fetal respiration A static exercise, marked by sitting quietly, tranquilizing the heart, regulating respiration and avoiding suffocation to prevent deviation.

理肺金诀【lǐ fèi jīn jué】 为动功。其作法为，先以左右单手向内转，伏于足前者三次；以左右单手向外转，伏于足前者三次；以左右双手向内转，次以左右双手向外转,伏于足前如之。

formula for regulating the lung metal　A dynamic exercise, marked by internally turning the left hand and the right hand singly; externally turning the left hand and right hand singly and keeping in front of the feet for three times; turning both hands internally and externally and keeping in front of the feet.

理肝木诀【lǐ gān mù jué**】**　为动功。其作法为,以左右两手次第下捺,思令气达掌心,行至指尖为度,不拘数;再以两手,如鸟舒翼状,左右各三;再以两手当胸,自上而下,复自下而上者三;再以两手,向左向右有各三,上下如当胸。

formula for regulating the liver　A dynamic exercise, marked by pressing the lower region with both hands, imagining to move Qi to the palms till the fingertips for several times; moving the hands like flying birds from the left to the right and vice versa for three times respectively; turning the hands to the chest and from the upper to the lower and vice versa for three times respectively; turning the hands from the left to the right and vice versa for three times respectively like touching the chest from the upper to the lower.

理脾土诀【lǐ pí tǔ jué**】**　为动功。其作法为,两足立定,以两手左右摇摆,手左目左,手右目右,意到足跟。脾土自然疏通。

formula for regulating spleen earth　A dynamic exercise, marked by standing up, swaying the hands from the left to the right and vice versa, turning the hands and eyes to the left and the right, and imagining to turn to the heels. Such a dynamic exercise can make the spleen earth naturally unobstructed.

理肾水诀【lǐ shèn shuǐ jué**】**　为动功。其作法为,握两拳,紧抵左右腰际,身向两边摇摆,使气达内肾,不拘数;再以两手垂睾丸之前,身向两边摇摆,使气达外肾,亦不拘数。

formula for regulating kidney water　A dynamic exercise, marked by holding the hands to reach the right side and left side of the waist, swaying the body from both sides to move Qi to the internal side of the kidney for several times; then drooping the front of testis with both hands, swaying the body from both sides to move Qi to the external side of the kidney for several times.

理五气于泥丸【lǐ wǔ qì yú ní wán**】**　指脑调节五脏之功能活动。

exercise for regulating five kinds of Qi in the mud bolus（**the brain**）　A celebrated dictum, referring to the functional activity of the five Zang-organs（including the heart, the liver, the spleen, the lung and the kidney）regulated by the brain.

理心火诀【lǐ xīn huǒ jué**】**　为动功。其作法为,先合两手,由胸前分排至脊后者三次;以左右两臂,各贴心窝者三次;以两手全伸,由胸前掷于背后者三次;以两手向地面,举过胸前,左持右掷,右持左掷,各三次。

formula for regulating heart fire　A dynamic exercise, marked by holding the hands to move from the chest to the spine for three times; pasting the precordium for three times with the left and right shoulders; raising the hands form the chest to the back for three times; stretching the hands towards the

L

ground and raising along the chest, keeping the left and throwing the right and vice versa for three times respectively.

理虚元鉴【lǐ xū yuán jiàn】 《理虚元鉴》为虚劳病专书,由明代绮石著,阐述虚劳病证、病机及预防措施。

Lixu yuanjian(*Originally Scrutinizing the Reason of Deficiency*) A monograph of consumptive disease entitled *Originally Scrutinizing the Reason of Deficiency*, written by Qi Shi in the Ming Dynasty(1368 AD - 1644 AD), describing the syndrome, pathogenesis and prevention of consumptive disease.

理圆【lǐ yuán】 指识玄妙中道不偏。

rational cycle Refers to impartiality in understanding the supreme middle way.

理瀹骈文【lǐ yuè pián wén】 《理瀹骈文》是外治专书,兼论气功,由清代吴师机著,详尽论述了临床各科的外治方法,对气功健身有独到见解。

liyue pianwen(*Rationale and Rhythmical Prose*) A monograph of external treatment with analysis of Qigong entitled *Rationale and Rhythmical Prose*, written by Wu Shiji in the Qing Dynasty(1636 AD - 1912 AD), thoroughly describing the external treatment of diseases in different clinical branches.

理瀹骈文导引法【lǐ yuè pián wén dǎo yǐn fǎ】 为动功,方法多样。如以两手掩耳,将第二指压中指弹脑后骨,去头脑疾。

exercise of Daoyin for rationale and rhythmical prose A dynamic exercise with various methods, such as covering the ears with both hands, pressing the middle finger with the second finger for filliping the occipital squama in or-

der to cure the disease in the brain.

醴泉【lǐ quán】 指甘美的泉水。在气功中即指唾液。

sweet spring Refers to sweet water in the spring, indicating saliva in Qigong practice.

立禅纳气法【lì chán nà qì fǎ】 动静相兼功,指静心息虑,不追思过去,不幻想未来,眼前事不留念。

exercise for standing meditation and normal inspiration An exercise combined with static exercise and dynastic exercise, marked by tranquilization of the heart without thinking about the past, imagining the future and remembering the present.

立春正月节后导引法【lì chūn zhēng yuè jié hòu dǎo yǐn fǎ】 为动功。立春正月节后,每日子丑二时,用于按摩两肾俞穴,左转身挺胸收腹,向上如扩胸,三十五次。

exercise of Daoyin for the days after festivals in January in beginning of spring A dynamic exercise, marked by pressing the acupoints located in the kidney meridians in Zi(the period of the day from 11 p.m. to 1 a.m.) and Chou(the period of a day from 1 a.m. to 3 a.m. in the morning), turning the body to the left in order to straighten the chest and adduct the abdomen for thirty-five times.

立春正月节坐功【lì chūn zhēng yuè jié zuò gōng】 为动功。每日子丑时叠手按髀,转身拗颈,左右耸引,各三五次,叩齿,吐纳,漱咽三次。

sitting exercise for the feast days in January in spring A dynamic exercise, marked by pressing the thigh with both hands in Zi(the period of the day from

11 p.m. to 1 a.m.) and Chou (the period of a day from 1 a.m. to 3 a.m. in
the morning), turning the body and
neck from the left to the right and vice
versa for three and five times, clicking
the teeth with inhalation and exhalation, and washing the mouth through
swallowing saliva.

立德【lì dé】 指神正、身正、左右正,不
受自然、社会的干扰而能处中得和。

moral composition A term of Qigong,
referring to straightening the spirit,
the body and all sides as well as balancing social disturbance.

立基【lì jī】 ① 指排除杂念,调节精神
与呼吸;② 指周天功练至百日,社会的
干扰能处中得和。

essential composition Refers to ① either elimination of distracting thought
and regulation of the spirit and respiration; ② or practicing celestial circuit
Qigong for one hundred days in order
to balance social disturbance.

立命直指地根章【lì mìng zhí zhǐ dì
gēn zhāng】 源自气功专论,主要阐述
"肾为北极之枢,精含万化,滋养百骸,赖
以永年"。

**taking the root in the earth as the shel-
ter** Collected from a monograph about
Qigong, mainly describing that "the
kidney is the root in the north pole, the
essence of which contains all the elements that nourish all the organs and
prolong life".

立秋七月节坐功【lì qiū qī yuè jié zuò
gōng】 为动功。每日丑寅时,正坐,两
手托地,缩体、闭息、耸身上踊,凡七八
次,叩齿、吐纳、咽液。

**sitting exercise for the feast days in July
in autumn** A dynamic exercise,

marked by sitting right in Chou (the
period of a day from 1 a.m. to 3 a.m.
in the morning) and Yin (the period of
a day from 3 a.m. to 5 a.m. in the
morning), pressing the ground with
both hands, shrinking the body, closing respiration, jumping up for seven
or eight times, clicking the teeth with
inhalation and exhalation, and swallowing saliva.

立夏四月节导引法【lì xià sì yuè jié
dǎo yǐn fǎ】 为动功。每日寅卯时,闭
息微闭双眼,左手向右上方导引,右手向
左上方导引各三十五次。

**exercise of Daoyin for the feast days in
the April in summer** A dynamic exercise, marked by suspending respiration
and slightly closing the eyes in Yin (the
period of a day from 3 a.m. to 5 a.m.
in the morning) and Mao (the period
of a day from 5 a.m. to 7 a.m. in the
morning), raising up the left hand to
the right and raising up the right hand
to the left for thirty-five times respectively.

立夏四月节坐功【lì xià sì yuè jié zuò
gōng】 为动功。每日寅卯时闭息瞑
目,反换两手,抑擎两膝,各五七次,叩
齿、吐纳、咽液。

**sitting exercise for the feast days in the
April in summer** A dynamic exercise,
marked by closing respiration and eyes
in Yin (the period of a day from
3 a.m. to 5 a.m. in the morning) and
Mao (the period of a day from 5 a.m.
to 7 a.m. in the morning), changing
the hands to press the knees for five to
seven times, clicking the teeth with inhalation and exhalation, and swallowing saliva.

L

立元神法【lì yuán shén fǎ】 为静功。其作法为，无为，安精养神，正性养神，稳定神形。

exercise for original spirit A static exercise, marked by keeping silent, pacifying the essence to nourish the spirit, rectifying the property to nourish the spirit and stabilizing the spirit and body.

历观五脏【lì guān wǔ zàng】 指以意念观五脏，与春夏秋冬自然之气相应。

mental observation of the five Zang-organs Refers to observation of the five Zang-organs with the thought and communication based on the natural Qi in the spring, summer, autumn an winter.

历兑【lì duì】 足阳明胃经的一个穴位，位于第二趾外侧。这一穴位为气功运行的一个常见部位。

Lidui（**ST 45**） An acupoint in the stomach meridian of foot Yangming, located in the external side of the second toe. This acupoint is a region usually used for keeping the essential Qi in practice of Qigong.

痢疾【lì jí】 为气功适应证，多因外受湿热疫毒之气，内伤饮食生冷，积滞于肠中所致。

Dysentery An indication of Qigong, usually caused by invasion of external dampness-heat and epidemic pathogenic factor, internal damage due to cold diet and dyspepsia in the intestines.

莲含华【lián hán huá】 指心外象如莲花之未开。

lotus containing magnificence A term of Qigong, indicating that the manifestation of the heart is just like the lotus not yet blooming.

莲华合掌【lián huá hé zhǎng】 佛家气功习用语，指竖左右十指，而指掌共合于胸前。

clasping fists with lotus A common term of Qigong in Buddhism, referring to erecting the ten fingers and stretching the fists to the chest.

莲华座【lián huá zuò】 佛家气功习用语，指盘腿坐。

lotus sitting A common term of Qigong in Buddhism, referring to sitting with crossed legs.

廉泉【lián quán】 任脉中的一个穴位，位于喉结上方。此穴位为气功习练之处。

lianquan（**CV 23**） An acupoint in the conception meridian, located above the Adam's apple. This acupoint is a region usually used in practice of Qigong.

炼【liàn】 ① 指苦行其当行之事；② 指熟行其当行之事；③ 指绝禁其不当为之事；④ 指精进励志而求气必成；⑤ 指割绝贪爱而不留余爱；⑥ 指禁止旧习而全不染习。

practice A term of Qigong, referring to ① either being penitential to do anything necessary; ② or being necessary to do anything familiar; ③ or being forbidden to do anything unnecessary; ④ or being encouraged to achieve the desires; ⑤ or being forbidden to be reluctant to part with anything desired; ⑥ or being forbidden to do anything backward.

炼丹【liàn dān】 指炼内丹和外丹。习练精气神为内丹，烧炼五金八石外丹。

refining Dan（**pills of immortality**） A term of Qigong, referring to refining the internal Dan（pills of immortality）and the external Dan（pills of immortality). The so-called internal Dan (pills of immortality) refers to refining the essence, Qi and the spirit; while the so-called external Dan (pills of immortality) refers to burning and refining the five metals and eight stones.

炼丹成神【liàn dān chéng shén】　即炼形养气,荣养神明,使之聪慧。

refining Dan (pills of immortality) to produce the spirit　A term of Qigong, referring to refining the body, nourishing the body, supporting the spirit and increasing wisdom in practicing Qigong.

炼丹出神【liàn dān chū shén】　指习练气功,可产生功能变化(出神)。

refining Dan (pills of immortality) to increase the spirit　Refers to formation of special function in practicing Qigong.

炼胆气法【liàn dǎn qì fǎ】　为静功。其作法为,常在四季之首月,端坐存神,意想北方黑气入胆九次,同时吞咽口中唾液。功效为气平体和,精全心逸。

exercise for refining gallbladder Qi　A static exercise, marked by sitting with concentrated spirit in the first month of every season, imagining to swallow black Qi from the north into the gallbladder for nine times, swallowing saliva in the mouth for stabilizing Qi, harmonizing the body, enriching essence and safeguarding the heart.

炼耳不听【liàn ěr bù tīng】　指练功时神守于内,耳不闻外声。

no hearing in refining ears　Refers to concentrating the spirit inside in practicing Qigong in order to avoiding listening to any voice in the external world.

炼肺气功【liàn fèi qì gōng】　为静功。

其作法为,立秋日寅时,面向西坐,鸣天鼓七次,口中唾液分三次咽下,两目微闭,心中存想西方白气入口中,吞入肺中,如此反复三次。功效使肺神安宁,延年益寿。

exercise for refining lung Qi　A static exercise, marked by sitting to the west in Yin (the period of the day from 3 a. m. to 5 a. m. in the early morning) at the beginning of autumn, clicking the teeth for seven times, swallowing saliva for three times, mildly closing the eyes, imagining to swallow white Qi through the mouth into the lung, repeatedly swallowing such a Qi for three times in order to stabilize the spirit in the lung and to prolong life.

炼肝气法【liàn gān qì fǎ】　为静功。其作法为,立春日寅时(清晨三至五时)面向东平坐,叩齿三次,闭气七息,存想东方青气吞入肝脏。功效为养肝明目,去眼疾。

exercise for refining liver Qi　A static exercise, marked by sitting to the east in Yin (the period of the day from 3 a. m. to 5 a. m. in the early morning) at the beginning of spring, clicking the teeth for three times, stopping respiration for seven times, imagining to swallow green Qi from the east into the liver in order to nourish the liver, to improve the eyes and to cure ocular disease.

炼功七无【liàn gōng qī wú】　指气功锻炼过程中,却除七种不利于稳定精神的因素,这样才能思想入静。

seven eliminations in practicing Qigong　Refer to expelling seven factors that affect the stability of the spirit. Only when these seven pathogenic factors are expelled can the mind be tranquilized.

练功效法四时阴阳升降【liàn gōng xiào fǎ sì shí yīn yáng shēng jiàng】源自气功专论,主要阐述人体气液相生与日月相应。

Ascent and descent of Yin and Yang in the four seasons reflect the effects of Qigong practice. This sentence is collected from a monograph of Qigong, mainly describing the mutual promotion and of Qi and humor in the human body, corresponding to the sun and the moon.

练功效验【liàn gōng xiào yàn】指练功后产生的各种生理效应。

effective experience in practicing Qigong A term of Qigong, referring to various physiological effects of Qigong practice.

练己【liàn jǐ】指气功锻炼中,调神排除杂念。

refining oneself A term of Qigong, referring to eliminate distracting thought in practicing Qigong.

练金丹大药法【liàn jīn dān dà yào fǎ】为静功。其作法为,端身静坐,凝神息虑,不越半个时辰,结成一粒,意念送入丹田。

exercise for refining golden Dan（pills of immortality）and large medicinal A static exercise, marked by sitting upright and quietly, concentrating the spirit, eliminating distracting thought, and forming a pill just in an hour and imagining to enter it into Dantian. Dantian is divided into the upper Dantian（the region between the eyes）, the middle Dantian（the region below the heart）and the lower Dantian（the region below the navel）.

练金精以固形【liàn jīn jīng yǐ gù xíng】指习练气功,炼养肺液,有强固形体,增进健康之功。

refining golden essence to strengthen the body A celebrated dictum, referring to refining and nourishing lung humor, strengthening the body and cultivating health in practicing Qigong.

练精【liàn jīng】① 指鼓漱搅海咽津;② 指咽津并叩齿。

refining essence A term of Qigong, referring to ① either rinsing the tongue, stirring the sea and swallowing the fluid; ② or swallowing the fluid and clicking the teeth.

练精补脑【liàn jīng bǔ nǎo】指练功中养精而不外泄,精气上承,可补脑安神。

refining the essence to tonify the brain A term of Qigong, referring to nourishing the essence without dispersion, raising essential Qi in practicing Qigong in order to tonify the brain and to stabilize the spirit.

练精法【liàn jīng fǎ】为静功。其作法为,正身端坐,宁神息虑,和调呼吸。

exercise for refining essence A static exercise, marked by sitting upright, stabilizing the spirit, tranquilizing the mind and regulating respiration.

练膜【liàn mó】即"务培其元气,守其中气,保其正气,护其肾气,养其肝气,调其肺气,理其脾气,升其清气,降其浊气,闭其邪恶不正之气"。

refining membrane A term of Qigong, referring to "enriching original Qi, stabilizing middle Qi, protecting healthy Qi, defending kidney Qi, nourishing liver Qi, regulating lung Qi, regulating spleen Qi, raising clear Qi, inducing turbid Qi and expelling pathogenic Qi".

炼脾气法【liàn pí qì fǎ】 为静功。其作法为,每日凌晨正坐,调气五息,鸣天鼓七次,存想中央黄气入口归脾,同时吞咽口中唾液。功效为百脉调畅,抗衰老。

exercise for refining spleen Qi A static exercise, marked by sitting upright every early morning, regulating respiration for five times, clicking teeth for seven times, imagining to swallow yellow Qi from the center through the mouth and into the spleen, and swallowing saliva in the mouth. The effect of such a static exercise is to smooth all the meridians and to prevent senility.

炼气【liàn qì】 指调节呼吸。

refining Qi A term of Qigong, referring to regulation of respiration.

炼气法【liàn qì fǎ】 为静功,即调身、调神、调气。其作法为,叩齿,咽津,搓面,仰卧,自然放松,冥心绝想,意识活动处于相对静止状态。

exercise for refining Qi A static exercise for regulating the body, spirit and Qi; marked by clicking the teeth, swallowing fluid, rubbing the face, lying on the back, naturally relaxing the body, tranquilizing the heart without any idea, keeping the activity of consciousness quiet.

炼气男女俱仙法【liàn qì nán nǔ jù xiān fǎ】 为静功。其作法为,委气三百六十息,正偃卧,握固、先调和、口中含唾莫咽,九息一展转,令足间相去五寸挽之,微还气时,身如委衣,骨节俱解,徐九十息止。男子左边,妇人右边,七十息一咽,此炼气男女俱宜之法也。

exercise for refining Qi enabling men and women to become immortals A static exercise, marked by breathing for three hundred and sixty times, lying supine, holding hands for regulating and harmonizing the body, keeping saliva in the mouth and turning it after nine times of respiration, keeping 5 Cun between the feet, mildly inhaling Qi, relaxing the body, loosening the condyles and mildly breathing for ninety times. Male practitioners stay in the left while female practitioners stay in the right, swallowing saliva once after seventy times of respiration. This is the best way for men and women to practice Qigong.

炼情【liàn qíng】 即调节意识思维活动。

refine disposition A term of Qigong, referring to regulating the activities of consciousness and thinking.

炼神【liàn shén】 指练神。

refining the spirit A term of Qigong, referring to regulation of the spirit.

炼肾气法【liàn shèn qì fǎ】 为静功。其作法为,立冬日寅时,面北而坐,叩齿五次,咽唾液三次,意想北方黑气吞入肾中。功效为神和体平。

exercise for refining kidney Qi A static exercise, marked by sitting to the north in Yin (the period of the day from 3 a.m. to 5 a.m. in the early morning) at the beginning of winter, clicking the teeth for five times, swallowing saliva for three times and imagining to swallow black Qi into the kidney in order to harmonize the spirit and to balance the body.

炼心气法【liàn xīn qì fǎ】 为静功。其作法为,立夏日寅时,而向南端坐,叩齿九次,用唾液在口中如漱口,然后分三次咽下。

exercise for refining heart Qi　A static exercise, marked by sitting to the south in Yin (the period of the day from 3 a.m. to 5 a.m. in the early morning) at the beginning of summer, clicking the teeth for nine times, keeping saliva in the mouth like rinsing the mouth and then swallowing for three times.

炼形【liàn xíng】　指气功锻炼中使形神协调的修炼方法。

refining the body　Refining the body is a term of Qigong, referring to the method for regulating the body and the spirit in practicing Qigong.

炼形六门【liàn xíng liù mén】　即玉液炼形,金液炼形,太阴炼形,太阳炼形,内观炼形,真空炼形。

refining the body with six gates　A term of Qigong, referring to refining the body with jade humor, golden humor, Taiyin, Taiyang, internal vision and genuine vacuum.

炼阳观【liàn yáng guàn】　在山东招远,世传为马丹阳炼丹之处。

temple for refining Yang　Located in Zhaoyuan County in Shandong Province. It was said in ancient China that Ma Danyang, a Daoist in the Song Dynasty (960 AD – 1279 AD), studied and developed alchemy in this temple.

炼药【liàn yào】　指气功炼元气、元精、元神,使之合三而一。

refining medicinal　A term of Qigong, referring to integrating the original Qi, the original essence and the original spirit into one in practicing Qigong.

炼液【liàn yè】　即舌搅齿内外,待有津液后,漱而吞咽之。

refining humor　A term of Qigong, referring to stirring the internal and external sides of the teeth, rinsing the tongue and swallowing saliva when there is fluid and humor.

良方除诸病法【liáng fāng chú zhū bìng fǎ】　为静功。其作法为,每腹空时,不拘昼夜,坐卧自便,使如木偶,可常自念言。

effective therapy for all diseases　A static exercise, marked by naturally sitting or lying at night or in daytime with normal reading of some important quotations.

梁丘子【liáng qiū zǐ】　唐代气功学家,在其注解的专著中论述了脑神、五脏神及其功能作用。

Liang Qiuzi　A master of Qigong in the Tang Dynasty (618 AD – 907 AD), describing the spirit and its functions in the brain and the five Zang-organs (including the heart, the liver, the spleen, the lung and the kidney) in his explanation and analysis of the monographs of Qigong.

两部【liǎng bù】　指两肾,肾主水,故称水王。

two parts　Refers to the two kidneys that control water and are known as the kings of water.

两扉【liǎng fēi】　指上、下眼睑。

two panels　Refer to upper and lower eyelids.

两颗梨【liǎng kē lí】　指睾丸。

two pears　Refer to testicles.

两仪【liǎng yí】　指事物含有的阴阳两个方面。

two sides　Refer to Yin and Yang contained in all the things.

疗肠鸣法【liáo cháng míng fǎ】　为动

功。其作法为，右胁著床，以右手支头，左手牵脚令屈，直身及直右脚，咽气令入右脚中，出肠中。

sound exercise for treating the intestines A dynamic exercise, marked by lying on the right side, holding the head with the right hand, bending the left foot with the left hand, stretching the body and the right foot and swallowing Qi deep into the right foot and out of the intestines.

疗精滑不禁术【liáo jīng huá bù jīn shù】 为静功。其作法为，行住坐卧兼可，缩胁腹，闭尾闾，先瞑目，头若带石，即引气自背直入泥丸，而后咽归丹田。可治滑精不禁、梦遗。

technique for curing spermatorrhea A static exercise, marked by walking or staying or sitting or lying, shrinking the hypochondrium and abdomen, closing the coccyx, closing the eyes first, transmitting Qi from the back directly into the mud bolus (the brain) if there is jade on the head, and finally swallowing saliva into Dantian in order to cure spermatorrhea and nocturnal emission. Dantian is divided into the upper Dantian (the region between the eyes), the middle Dantian (the region below the heart) and the lower Dantian (the region below the navel).

寥天【liáo tiān】 指人体的最上部位，即脑。

celestial space Refers to the brain which is the highest part of the body.

了【liǎo】 指三丹田精气合而为一，神、气、精相融为"了"。

integration Refers to integration of essence, Qi and the spirit in the upper Dantian (the region between the eyes),

the middle Dantian (the region below the heart) and the lower Dantian (the region below the navel).

了明篇【liǎo míng piān】 《了明篇》为气功学著作，由宋代毛日新编，介绍了气功的基本理论和方法。

Liaoming Pian（Gnosis Fascicl） A monograph entitled *Gnosis Fascicle* compiled by Mao Rixin in the Song Dynasty（960 AD - 1279 AD），introducing the basic theory and practice of Qigong.

了三得一经【liǎo sān dé yī jīng】 《了三得一经》为气功养生专著，阐述了气功的基本理论及实践应用技术，作者及成书年代不详。

Liaosan Deyi Jing（Canon For Analyzing Three Sections） Liaosan Deyi Jing is a monograph entitled *Canon For Analyzing Three Sections*, describing the basic theory and exercises of Qigong. The author and the time of compilation were unknown.

了悟【liǎo wù】 佛家气功习用语，指明心见性。

gnosis A common term of Qigong practice in Buddhism, referring to clearing the mind and human nature.

列仙赋【liè xiān fù】 《列仙赋》为气功专论，为晋代陆机所著。

Liexian Fu（Immortals Composition） A monograph about Qigong entitled *Immortals Composition*, written by Lu Ji, a great scholar in the Jin Dynasty（266 AD - 420 AD）.

列子【liè zǐ】 战国时的一个人名，也是先秦的一本书名。

Liezi Either a scholar's name in the Warring States; or the title of an important book written before the Qin

L

Dynasty (475 BC‐221 BC).

列子养生法【liè zǐ yǎng shēng fǎ】 为动功,指列子气功养生的方法,一是放松形体,二是和调精神。

Liezi's way for nourishing life A dynamic exercise, referring to Liezi's ways for nourishing life through practicing Qigong. The first way is to relax the body and the second way is to regulate the spirit.

捩身【liè shēn】 导引姿势,指扭转身体。

twisting body An exercise of Daoyin, referring to turning round the body.

林屋山人【lín wū shān rén】 宋末元初的气功理论家,著有多部气功学专著,精详阐述了气功的理论和方法,对后世颇有影响。

Linwu Shanren A theorist of Qigong in the late Song Dynasty (960 AD‐1279 AD) and early Yuan Dynasty (1271 AD‐1368 AD). He wrote several monographs about Qigong, particularly describing the theory and practice of Qigong, greatly influenced the later generations.

淋证导引法【lín zhèng dǎo yǐn fǎ】 动静相兼功,方法多样。如仰卧,曲腿,放两手于膝,脚跟尽量倾靠臀尾部,口吸气,鼻出气,使气达腹中,随呼吸起伏。

exercise of Daoyin for stranguria An exercise combined with dynamic exercise and static exercise with various methods, such as lying on the back, bending the legs, putting the hands on the knees, approaching the heels to the coccyx as far as possible, inhaling Qi through the mouth, exhaling Qi through the nose, reaching Qi to the abdomen and breathing with rise and fall.

灵【líng】 指神通万变。

soul A term of Qigong, referring to various changes of the spirit.

灵宝【líng bǎo】 灵指为神,宝指气,即神气。

soul treasure Soul refers to the spirit and treasure refers to Qi, indicating the spiritual Qi. So soul treasure actually refers to the spirit and Qi.

灵宝采药法【líng bǎo cǎi yào fǎ】 为静功。其作法为,戌时亥时,端身正坐,神识内守,鼻息绵绵,以肚腹微胁。

treasured exercise for collecting medicinals A static exercise, marked by sitting upright in Qu (the period of a day from 7 p.m. to 9 p.m. at night) and Hai (the period of a day from 9 p.m. to 11 p.m. at night), internally concentrating the spirit, slowly breathing through the nose and mildly turning the rib sides with the abdomen.

灵宝净明黄素书释义秘诀【líng bǎo jìng míng huáng sù shū shì yì mì jué】 《灵宝净明黄素书释义秘诀》为气功养生专著,作者不详。

Lingbao Jingming Hungsushu Shiyi Mijue (*Recipe Explanation of Yellow Plain Book with Soul Treasure and Clean Brightness*) A monograph of Qigong and life cultivation entitled *Recipe Explanation of Yellow Plain Book with Soul Treasure and Clean Brightness*. The author was unknown.

灵宝净明新修丸老神印伏魔秘法【líng bǎo jìng míng xīn xiū wán lǎo shén yìn fú mó mì fǎ】 《灵宝净明新修丸老神印伏魔秘法》为气功专著,由宋代何守证述。

Lingbao Jingming Xinxiuwan Laoshen

Yinfumo Mifa（*New Composition of Secret Exercise with Soul Treasure and Clean Brightness Support by Great Immortal for Controlling Demons*）　A monograph of Qigong entitled *New Composition of Secret Exercise with Soul Treasure and Clean Brightness Support by Great Immortal for Controlling Demons*, written by He Shouzheng in the Song Dynasty（960 AD - 1279 AD）.

灵宝静坐法【líng bǎo jìng zuò fǎ**】**动静相兼法。其作法为,晨起,披衣坐,绝念忘情。

treasured exercise for quiet sitting　An exercise combined with a dynamic exercise and a static exercise, marked by dressing the clothes, sitting in the morning and eliminating any desires and emotions.

灵宝聚火法【líng bǎo jù huǒ fǎ**】**为静功。其作法为,酉时入室静坐,咽气而揪外肾,收膀胱之气于内,纳心火于下,意念使上下相合。

treasured exercise for accumulating fire　A static exercise, marked by quietly sitting in the room in You（the period of a day from 5 p.m. to 9 p.m. at dusk）, swallowing Qi to twitch the external kidney, collecting Qi from the bladder inside the body, receiving heart fire in the lower and combining the upper and lower with consciousness.

灵宝三元用法【líng bǎo sān yuán yòng fǎ**】**为静功,方法多样。如静室中端身盘膝正坐,两手握固,蹲下腹肚,须臾升身,前出胸而微偃头于后,闭夹脊双关,肘后微扇一二伸腰。

exercise for absorbing three treasures　A static exercise with several methods,

such as sitting upright in a quiet room with crossed legs, holding the hands, squatting the abdomen, raising the body, turning the chest forwards and falling the head backwards, closing both sides of Jaji acupoint located on the lateral side of the spine, and mildly turning the elbows to straighten the waist.

灵宝咽法【líng bǎo yàn fǎ**】**为静功。其作法为,舌搅上腾两颊之间,先咽了恶浊之津,次退舌尖以满,玉池津生,不漱而咽。春三月,肝气旺而脾气弱,咽法日用离卦;夏三月,心气旺而肺气弱,咽法日用巽卦;秋三月,肺气旺而肝气弱,咽法日用艮卦;冬三月,肾气旺而心气弱,咽法日用震卦;四季之月,脾气旺而肾气弱,人以肾气为根源。

treasured exercise for swallow　A static exercise, marked by stirring the upper cheeks with the tongue, swallowing turbid fluid first, then returning the tip of the tongue in order to enrich the mouth and swallow when there is fluid in Yuchi（mouth）with rinsing. In the three months of spring, liver Qi is rich but spleen Qi is weak, the day for swallowing should follow Li Trigram; in the three months of summer, heart Qi is rich but lung Qi is weak, the day for swallowing should follow the Xun Trigram; in the three months of autumn, lung Qi is rich but liver Qi is weak, the day for swallowing should follow Gen Trigram; in the three months of winter, kidney Qi is rich but heart Qi is weak, the day for swallowing should follow Zhen Trigram; in the months in the four seasons, when spleen Qi is rich but kidney Qi is weak, men should depend on the kidney Qi.

灵根【líng gēn】 ① 指舌本；② 指脑神，为身体之本。

soul root Refers to ① either the origin of the tongue；② or the spirit in the brain which is the foundation of the body.

灵关【líng guān】 古人将心中藏元神的地方称为灵关。

soul joint Refers to the special region in the heart that contains the original spirit.

灵剑子【líng jiàn zǐ】《灵剑子》为气功养生专著，由晋代许逊所著，论述气功养生法的关键在于协调形神，协调形神的主要技术又是保持"正心"。

Lingjian Zi（*Soul Sword*） A monograph of Qigong entitled *Soul Sword*, written by Sun Xun in the Jin Dynasty (266 AD - 420 AD), mainly describing that the key of Qigong and life cultivation is regulation of the body and the spirit. The only technique for regulation of the body and the spirit is to keep the original and natural heart.

灵剑子导引子午记注【líng jiàn zǐ dǎo yǐn zǐ wǔ jì zhù】《灵剑子导引子午记注》为气功养生学专著，是对《灵剑子导引子午记》的注释性著作。作者不详。

Lingjianzi Daoyin Ziwu Jizhu（*Analysis and Explanation of Soul Sword Daoyin in Zi and Wu*） A monograph of Qigong entitled *Analysis and Explanation of Soul Sword Daoyin in Zi and Wu*. This monograph is a particular analysis and explanation of another monograph entitled Lingjianzi Daoyin Ziwu Ji, i. e. *Soul Sword Daoyin in Zi and Wu*. The author was unknown. In this title, Zi refers to the period of the day from 11 p. m. to 1 a. m. and Wu refers to the period of the day from 11 a. m. to 1 p. m.

灵剑子服气法【líng jiàn zǐ fú qì fǎ】为静功，即初习练时，开始凝神调息，静候气液。得气液后，气液同咽三十六次。

treasured exercise for moving Qi with sword A static exercise, marked by concentrating the spirit, regulating respiration and quieting Qi and humor at the beginning of practicing Qigong. When Qi and humor have appeared, they can be swallowed for thirty-six times.

灵门户【líng mén hù】 同九宫。古人认为人脑分为九部，也指天之八方加中央为九宫。

soul gate A term of Qigong, the same as nine palaces, which refer to the chamber of nine palaces and nine orifices in ancient China.

灵明一窍【líng míng yī qiào】 指脑和脑神。

a clear orifice A term of Qigong, refers the brain and the spirit in the brain.

灵山【líng shān】 指脑及脑神。

soul mountain A term of Qigong, referring to the brain and the brain spirit.

灵台【líng tái】 指脑及脑神。

soul platform A term of Qigong, referring to the brain and the brain spirit.

灵台盘固【líng tái pán gù】 指脑神稳定。

stable soul platform Refers to stability of the spirit in the brain.

灵台莹洁【líng tái yíng jié】 指脑神

莹洁,无一毫杂念纤尘。

pure soul platform　A term of Qigong, referring to purity of the spirit in the brain without any distracting thought.

灵台郁霭望黄野【líng tái yù ǎi wàng huáng yě】　指脑神用意内视黄庭。

When there is luxuriant brume in the soul platform, it is necessary to look at the yellow field.　This is a celebrated dictum, referring to internally observing Huangting (the region below the navel) with consciousness under the guidance of the spirit in the brain.

灵乌宿桂【líng wū xiǔ guì】　指阴阳和合。灵乌为心中真阴,桂喻肾中真阳。

spiritual bird lying in laurel　A term of Qigong, referring to combination of Yin and Yang. In this term, spiritual bird refers to the genuine Yin in the heart and laurel refers to the genuine Yang in the kidney.

灵仙观【líng xiān guàn】　在南昌,为晋代气功学家许旌阳隐居之处。

Immortal Temple　Located in Nanchang of Jiangxi Province, where Xu Jingyang, a great master of Qigong in the Jin Dynasty (266 AD - 420 AD), lived there in seclusion.

灵液【líng yè】　指唾液,专谓气功状态时增加的唾液。

soul humor　Refers to saliva increased during practice of Qigong.

灵宅【líng zhái】　眉、眼、鼻、口之所居,故名宅。

soul residence　Refers to the location of the eyebrows, the eyes, the nose and the mouth.

凌阴【líng yīn】　即冬天一昼夜间极冷的时刻。

cold Yin　Refers to the very cold period at night in winter.

陵阳子明垂钩【líng yáng zǐ míng chuí gōu】　为动功。其作法为,身体坐于席上,两脚自然向前伸,两手由前与足慢慢地前后来回运动,运气十九口。主治腰腿疼痛。

Ling Yangzi's fishing exercise　A dynamic exercise, marked by sitting on the bed, naturally stretching the feet, moving the hands from the front to the back slowly with the movement of the feet and moving Qi for nineteen times. Such a dynamic exercise can cure waist pain and leg pain.

刘操【liú cāo】　宋辽时期的气功学家,海蟾子的另外一个称谓。

Liu Cao　Another name of Hai Chanzi, a great master of Qigong in the Song Dynasty (960 AD - 1279 AD) and Liao Dynasty (907 AD - 1125 AD).

刘处玄【liú chù xuán】　金代气功学家,为全真随山派创始人。

Liu Chuxuan　A great master of Qigong in the Jin Dynasty (1120 - 1203) and the founder of the Shuishan Mountain School in Acme Genuine Dao.

刘道妙【liú dào miào】　金代气功学家刘处玄的另外一个称谓,为全真随山派创始人。

Liu Daomiao　Another name of Liu Chuxuan, a great master of Qigong in the Jin Dynasty (1120 AD - 1203 AD) and the founder of Suishan Mountain School in Acme Genuine Dao.

刘德仁【liú dé rén】　宋代大道教创始人、气功学家。

Liu Deren　The founder of Daoism and a greater master of Qigong.

刘海蟾【liú hǎi chán】　五代时著名的气功学家,著有多部气功专著。

L

Liu Haichan A great master of Qigong in the Five Dynasties (907 AD – 979 AD) who wrote several important monographs about Qigong.

刘海戏蟾【liú hǎi xì chán】 为动功。其作法为,自然立式,左脚向前半步,两手握拳,置于腰部,运气十二口,然后右脚向前,其余同。

Liu Hai playing toad Dynamic exercise, marked by natural standing up, moving the left foot forward for half a step, holding the fists with both hands over the waist, circulating Qi for twelve times, then moving the right foot forward. The following activities are the same.

刘京【liú jīng】 汉代气功学家,对气功养生的发展有一定的贡献。

Liu Jing A master of Qigong in the Han Dynasty (202 BC – 263 AD), contributing a great deal to the development of Qigong and life cultivation.

刘守真【liú shǒu zhēn】 金代医药学家和气功学家刘完素的另外一个称谓。

Liu Shouzhen Another name of Liu Wansu, a great doctor and master of Qigong in the Jin Dynasty (1120 AD – 1203 AD).

刘思敬【liú sī jìng】 明代气功学家,著有气功专著。

Liu Sijing A great master of Qigong in the Ming Dynasty (1368 AD – 1644 AD) who wrote an important monograph of Qigong.

刘思敬坐法【liú sī jìng zuò fǎ】 为静功。其作法为,子后午前,坐榻上,面东或南,握固盘足,合目伸腰,澄心静虑,内视五脏,仰面合口,鼻引清气,气极则生,要而咽之。

Liu Sijing's sitting exercise A static exercise, marked by sitting on the couch after Zi (the period of the day from 11 p.m. to 1 a.m.) and before the noon, turning the face toward the east or south, holding the knees and feet, closing the eyes, stretching the waist, stabilizing the heart, tranquilizing the mind, internally viewing the five Zang-organs (including the heart, the liver, the spleen, the lung and the kidney), looking up to close the mouth and inhaling clear Qi through the nose. Only when Qi is sufficient can life be cultivated. If necessary, Qi can be swallowed.

刘太玄【liú tài xuán】 汉代气功学家刘京的另外一个称谓。

Liu Taixuan Another name of Liu Jing, a great master of Qigong in the Han Dynasty (202 BC – 263 AD).

刘通妙【liú tōng miào】 金代气功学家刘处玄的另外一个称谓,其为全真随山派创始人。

Liu Tongmiao Another name of Liu Chuxuan, a great master of Qigong in the Jin Dynasty (1120 AD – 1203 AD) and the founder of Suishan Mountain School in Acme Genuine Dao.

刘完素【liú wán sù】 金代医药学家和气功学家。

Liu Wansu A great doctor and master of Qigong in the Jin Dynasty (1120 AD – 1203 AD).

刘无名【liú wú míng】 古代一位知名的气功学家,年代不详。

Liu Wuming A great master of Qigong in ancient China. But the related time and dynasty were unknown.

刘先玄【liú xiān xuán】 唐代气功学家刘知古的另外一个称谓,著有气功专论。

Liu Xianxuan　Another name of Liu Zhigu, a great master of Qigong in the Tang Dynasty（618 AD - 907 AD）who wrote an important monograph of Qigong.

刘一明【liú yī míng】　清代气功学家，撰写了多部专著，介绍了气功的基本理论和方法。

Liu Yiming　A great master of Qigong in the Qing Dynasty（1636 AD - 1912 AD）and wrote several monographs about Qigong to introduce the basic theory and practice of Qigong.

刘元靖【liú yuán jìng】　唐代气功学家，主要通过辟谷练气。

Liu Yuanjing　A great master of Qigong in the Tang Dynasty（618 AD - 907 AD）who refined Qi only with in-edibility.

刘真人胎息诀【liú zhēn rén tāi xī jué】　静功口诀，练气法的一种，认为保持身心安适、形体与精神安静，是习练的基础。

Liu Zhenren's fetal respiration formula　A static formula in practicing Qigong, indicating that stabilization of the body and mind as well as tranquilization of the body and spirit are the foundation for practicing Qigong.

刘政【liú zhèng】　汉代高才，博学，通气功，精通养生术。

Liu Zheng　A great scholar in the Han Dynasty（202 BC - 263 AD）, also familiar with Qigong and proficient in cultivating life.

刘知古【liú zhī gǔ】　唐代气功学家，著有气功专论。

Liu Zhigu　A great master of Qigong in the Tang Dynasty（618 AD - 907 AD）who wrote an important monograph of Qigong.

刘志渊【liú zhì yuān】　金代气功学家，有气功专著。

Liu Zhiyuan　A master of Qigong in the Jin Dynasty（1120 AD - 1203 AD）and wrote an important monograph of Qigong.

刘宗成【liú zōng chéng】　宋辽时期的气功学家海蟾子的另外一个称谓。

Liu Zongcheng　Another name of Hai Chanzi, a great master of Qigong in the Song Dynasty（960 AD - 1279 AD）and Liao Dynasty（907 AD - 1125 AD）.

留胎止精【liú tāi zhǐ jīng】　指习练胎息法，节制性欲。

avoiding conception and controlling semen　A term of Qigong, referring to controlling sexuality in practicing Qigong with fetal respiration exercise.

流水不腐，户枢不蠹【liú shuǐ bù fǔ hù shū bú dù】　说明经常运动锻炼身体的人，不会生病或少生病。

Running water will not be smelly and turning door will not be tattered.　This is a celebrated dictum, indicating that practitioners of Qigong will never be ill or seldom be ill.

流为华池【liú wéi huá chí】　指意念导引入丹田的津液。

flowing into Huachi pool　Refers to leading fluid and humor into Dantian with contemplation. Dantian is divided into the upper Dantian（the region between the eyes）, the middle Dantian（the region below the heart）and the lower Dantian（the region below the navel）.

流珠【liú zhū】　指心阴，或真阴。

flowing pearl　A term of Qigong, referring to heart Yin or genuine Yin.

瘤【liú**】** 为气功适应证，指长于体表的肿块和赘生物。

tumor An indication of Qigong, referring to lump and neoplasm in the body.

柳华阳【liǔ huá yáng**】** 清代气功学家，撰有气功专著，论述了内丹术和坐禅功法。

Liu Huayang A master of Qigong in the Qing Dynasty（1636 AD - 1912 AD）. He wrote several monographs of Qigong, analyzing the exercises of internal Dan（pills of immortality）and dhyana.

柳真人胎息诀【liǔ zhēn rén tāi xī jué**】** 静功口诀。习练本诀法，旨在养精爱气养神，法在安神养志，凝神固守。

Liu Zhenren's formula for fetal respiration A static exercise, the effect of which is to nourish the essence, protect Qi and nourish the spirit in order to stabilize the spirit, to nourish the mind, to concentrate the spirit and to straighten the body.

六【liù**】** 指老阴。

Six Refers to original Yin.

六不思【liù bù sī**】** 指习练气功期间，应稳定情绪，戒此六思，容易入静。

six ways without thought Refers to stabilizing the mood and eliminating six kinds of thought in order to tranquilize the mind in practicing Qigong.

六曹【liù cáo**】** 指的是六腑，即胆、胃、小肠、大肠、膀胱、三焦。

six organs A term of Qigong, refers to the six Fu-organs, including the gallbladder, the stomach, the small intestine, the large intestine, the bladder and the triple energizer.

六尘【liù chén**】** 佛家气功习用语。指色、声、香、味、触、法为六尘。

six dirties A common term of Qigong in Buddhism, referring to color, sound, fragrance, taste, contact and behavior.

六大【liù dà**】** 佛家气功习用语，指地、水、火、风、空、识。

six kinds of greatness A common term of Qigong in Buddhism, referring to the earth, water, fire, wind, vacuum and insight.

六丁【liù dīng**】** 指丁卯、丁丑、丁亥、丁酉、丁未、丁巳等六时，为六神主之。

six ding Refers to Ding Mao, Ding Chou, Ding Hai, Ding You, Ding Wei and Ding Ji, indicating six periods of time controlled by the six kinds of the spirit.

六法【liù fǎ**】** 佛家气功用语，指的是指地、水、火、风、空、识。

six conditions A common term of Qigong in Buddhism, referring to the earth, water, fire, wind, space and knowledge.

六腑精【liù fǔ jīng**】** 指胃、大肠、小肠、膀胱、三焦之精气。

essence in six Fu-organs Refers to the spirit and Qi in the stomach, the large intestine, the small intestine, the bladder and the triple energizer.

六根【liù gēn**】** 佛家气功习用语，指眼、耳、鼻、舌、身、意六宫。

six roots A common term of Qigong in Buddhism, referring to six kinds of palaces, such as the eyes, the ears, the tongue, the body and the mentality.

六根归道篇【liù gēn guī dào piān**】**《六根归道篇》为气功养生专著，作者不详。

Liugen Guidao Pian（*Canon About the*

Six Roots Returning to Dao） A monograph of Qigong and life cultivation entitled *Canon About the Six Roots Returning to Dao*. The author was unknown.

六根清净【liù gēn qīng jìng**】** 佛家气功习用语,指精神意识清净,六根相对稳定。

purified six roots A common term of Qigong in Buddhism, referring to purification of the spirit and consciousness and stabilization of the six root organs (including the eyes, the ears, the nose, the tongue, the body and the mind).

六根震动【liù gēn zhèn dòng**】** 佛家气功习用语,指练功中出现的六种生理效应。

vibration of six roots A common term of Qigong in Buddhism, referring to six physiological effects of Qigong practice.

六垢【liù gòu**】** 佛家气功习用语,指损伤情志的六种意识活动。

six disgraces A common term of Qigong in Buddhism, referring to six consciousness activities that have damaged the emotion.

六骸【liù hái**】** 指身、首、四肢。

six skeletons Refers to the body, the head and the four limbs.

六害【liù hài**】** 指欲、志、病、毒、邪、风六种损伤人体的因素。

six kinds of harm Refers to six pathogenic factors that have damaged the body, including desire, will, disease, toxin, evil and wind.

六行【liù háng**】** 指高尚精神作用下的行为,具体含义为六种善行与六种道德观,即仁、义、礼、智、信、乐兴。

six actions Refers to noble actions, especially six honest actions and six moral

actions, including benevolence, righteousness, propriety, wisdom, sincerity and happiness.

六合【liù hé**】** ① 指天地、四方;② 指十二经脉表里相对的六对组合;③ 指人体上下、左右、前后;④ 指二六相合,即六阴时与六阳时之合。

six combinations Refers to ① either the sky, the earth and the six directions; ② or the six combinations of the internal and the external from the twelve meridians; ③ or the upper side and the lower side, the left side and the right side, the front side and the back side; ④ or combination of six Yin periods and six Yang periods.

六和合【liù hé hé**】** 佛家气功习用语,指六根、六尘高度协调稳定,即"阴平阳秘"之意。

six harmonies A common term of Qigong in Buddhism, referring to six roots and six states that have highly coordinated and stabilized in accordance with equilibrium of Yin and Yang.

六慧【liù huì**】** 佛家气功习用语,指六种智慧,即闻慧、思慧、修慧、无相慧、照寂慧、寂照慧。

six wisdoms A common term of Qigong in Buddhism, referring to listening wisdom, thinking wisdom, regulating wisdom, invisible wisdom, quiet appraisal wisdom and appraising quiet wisdom.

六机【liù jī**】** 指六种情志意思活动,喜、怨、恶、悦、姻、媾。

six activities Refers to six emotional and mental activities, including happiness, resentment, wickedness, pleasure, love and copulation.

六极【liù jí**】** 指的是六种虚损病证及

六种不幸的事。

six extremities Refers to six kinds of deficiency diseases and six kinds of unfortunate things.

六甲【liù jiǎ】 指干支计时法。

six kinds of Jia Refers to chronometry of the Heavenly Stems and Earthly Branches.

六甲神【liù jiǎ shén】 指甲子、甲戌、甲申、甲午、甲辰、甲寅六时,有六神主之。

six Jia spirits Refers to six periods controlled by the six spirits, such as Jiazi, Jiaxu, Jiashen, Jiawu, Jiashen, Jiayin.

六界【liù jiè】 佛家气功用语,指地、水、火、风、空、识。

six states A common term of Qigong in Buddhism, referring to the earth, water, fire, wind, space and knowledge.

六界聚【liù jiè jù】 佛家气功习用语,即骨肉之地大,血之水大,暖热之火大,呼吸之风大,耳鼻空之空大,乐苦识之识大。

six states of communication A common term of Qigong in Buddhism, referring to the fact that the terrace of bones and muscles is large, water in the blood is large, fire in warm heat situation is large, wind in respiration is large, the space in the nose and the ears is large, and the recognition of happiness and bitterness is large.

六景【liù jǐng】 指习练气功时的六种景色显现,即丹田火炽、两肾汤煎、眼吐金光、耳后生风、身涌鼻搐、脑后莺鸣等。

six images Refers to six manifestations in practicing Qigong, such as flaming in Dantian, hot water in the kidneys, brightness in the eyes, wind produced behind the ears, fullness in the body and birdsong behind the brain. Dantian is divided into the upper Dantian (the region between the eyes), the middle Dantian (the region below the heart) and the lower Dantian (the region below the navel).

六境【liù jìng】 为气功习用语,指色、声、香、味、触、法六尘。

six states A term of Qigong, referring to color, sound, fragrance, taste, contact and behavior.

六龙【liù lóng】 指六腑之气。

six kinds of Loong Refer to Qi in the six Fu-organs (including the gallbladder, the stomach, the small intestine, the large intestine, the bladder and the triple energizer).

六律【liù lǜ】 古代乐器定音高低清浊的准则。

six principles Refers to the ancient principles for the high pitch, low pitch, clear pitch and sonant in accordatura.

六门【liù mén】 指眼、耳、鼻等器官,六窍为六门。

six gates Refers to the eyes, the ears and the nostrils which are the six orifices and called six gates.

六门紧闭【liù mén jǐn bì】 指结丹,须存神烹炼,存神应眼、耳、鼻、舌、口闭塞勿发通。

closure of six gates Refers to combination of internal Dan and external Dan, in order to maintain the spirit in practicing Qigong and keep the spirit in the eyes, ears, nose, tongue and mouth.

六念【liù niàn】 佛家六种气功功法,即念佛、念法、念戒、念施、念天。

six prayers　Refer to six methods in practicing Qigong in Buddhism, including reading Buddhism, reading Buddha dharma, reading Buddhist monastic discipline, reading performance and reading natural principles.

六气【liù qì】　① 指人体气、血、津、液、精、脉六种物质；② 指风、热（暑）、温、火、燥、寒六种气候。

six kinds of Qi　Refer to ① Qi, the blood, fluid, humor, essence and meridians; ② or wind, heat, dampness, fire, dryness and cold.

六气和合【liù qì hé hé】　指人体气、血、津、液、精、脉六种基本物质合而为一，协调稳定。

combination of six Qi　Refers to integration and stabilization of six basic substances, including Qi, blood, fluid, humor, essence and meridians.

六气精【liù qì jīng】　指天地、四时的精华。

six Qi and essence　Refers to the essence in the sky, in the earth and in the four seasons.

六情【liù qíng】　① 指六种情志活动，即喜、怒、哀、乐、爱、恶；② 指六种行为，即廉贞、宽大、公正三善，奸邪、阴贼、贪狼三恶；③ 指佛家气功习用语，眼、耳、鼻、舌、身、意为六情。

six emotions　Refer to ① six emotional activities, such as happiness, anger, sorrow, rejoicing, love and hatred; ② or six actions, such as chastity, leniency and justice as three moral actions, treacherousness, maliciousness and greediness as three immoral actions. ③ It also refers to the six concepts used in Buddhism in practice of Qigong, such as the eyes, the ears, the nose, the tongue, the body and the mentality.

六染心【liù rǎn xīn】　佛家气功习用语，指损伤情志的六种意识活动。

six ways to dye the heart　A common term of Qigong in Buddhism, referring to six consciousness activities that have damaged emotions.

六壬【liù rén】　指六十甲子中的六位。

six kinds of Ren　Refers to six years in a cycle of sixty years.

六入【liù rù】　① 指眼入色、耳入声、鼻入香、舌入味、身入触、意入法；② 指风、火、暑、湿、燥、寒六气互相作用以生化万物。

six kinds of entrance　Refer to ① color in the eyes, sound in the ears, fragrance in the nose, taste in the tongue, feeling in the body and emotion in the methods; ② or mutual functions of wind, fire, summer, dampness, dryness and cold that have promoted the growth and development of all things in the world.

六三【liù sān】　八卦之爻，从下数上，第三爻为阴爻，称为六三。

six-three　Refers to the Yao (levels) in the Eight Trigrams from the lower to the upper, among which the third one is Yin Yao (Yin level), also called six-three in the hexagram.

六神【liù shén】　指六甲神、六丁神、六腑神等。

six spirits　Refer to six kinds of Jia spirit, six kinds of Ding spirit and six kinds of the spirit in the six Fu-organs (including the gallbladder, the stomach, the small intestine, the large intestine, the bladder and the triple energizer).

L

六审【liù shěn】　指气功中调神所达到的境界。

six ideals　Refer to the ideal states for regulating the spirit in practicing Qigong.

六十甲子【liù shí jiǎ zǐ】　由天干配合地支所组成。

a cycle of sixty years　Refers to coordination between the ten Heavenly Stems and the twelve Earthly Stems that has formed sixty years.

六十六穴【liù shí liù xué】　指阳经之井荥输经合原三十六穴及阴经三十穴。

sixty-six acupoints　Refer to thirty-six acupoints related to Jing-well points, Ying-spring points, Shu-stream points, Jing-river points and He-sea points as well as thirty acupoins in the Yin meridians.

六十四卦【liù shí sì guà】　指《易》有八卦,两两相重,排列为六十四卦。

Sirty-four Trigrams　Refer to the doubled Ttrigrams in the Eight Trigrams. Originally there were just Eight Trigrams in Yijing. When the original Eight Trigrams were doubled by Ji Chang (姬昌, 1152 BC - 1056 BC), the first king in the Zhou Dynasty (1046 BC - 256 BC), the Eight Trigrams were increased to sixty-four Trigrams.

六十心【liù shí xīn】　佛家气功习用语,指六十种思维意识活动。

sixty hearts　A common term of Qigong in Buddhism, referring to sixty activities of thinking and consciousness.

六时【liù shí】　①指道家的六阳时和六阴时;②佛家的昼三时和夜三时。

six periods　Refer to ① either six Yang periods and six Yin periods in the Daoism; ② or three periods in the daytime

and three periods in the nighttime in Buddhism.

六识主帅【liù shí zhǔ shuài】　指眼、耳、鼻、舌、身、意六宫。

six commanders in chief　A term of Qigong, referring to six kinds of palaces, such as eyes, the ears, the tongue, the body and the mentality.

六事【liù shì】　指的是气功养生六事,即少看书、少思虑、反观内观、闭目养神、迟起床、早睡觉。

six matters　Refer to six matters in practicing Qigong for cultivating life, including reading less, contemplating less, internal observation, closing eyes to nourish the spirit, getting up late and sleeping early.

六衰【liù shuāi】　佛家气功习用语,指色、声、香、味、触、法六尘,损伤精神,破坏身体固有的稳定状态。

six declines　A common term of Qigong in Buddhism, referring to color, sound, fragrance, taste, contact and behavior that have damaged the spirit and destroyed the balance in the body.

六通【liù tōng】　指习练气功,一应通天文,二应通地理,三应通人事,四应通鬼神,五应通时机,六应通术数。

six communications　Refer to the ways for practicing Qigong, including communicating with the sky first, with the earth second, with the human affairs third, with the spirits fourth, with the times fifth and with the philosophy sixth.

六通四辟【liù tōng sì pì】　佛家气功习用语,其中的六通为风、雨、晦、明、阴、阳六气各行其时,四辟为四方开辟。另外,六也指六合,即上下四方的通达;四为春、夏、秋、冬四时顺畅。

L

six unobstructions and four establishments   A common term of Qigong in Buddhism，referring to wind，rain，nighttime，daytime，Yin and Yang，and so-called four establishments indicating to open up in the four directions. In this term，six also refers to six directions，i. e. the east，the west，the south，the north，the upper and the lower；four refers to the four seasons，i. e. spring，summer，autumn and winter.

六妄【liù wàng】 佛家气功用语，指意识思维混乱。

six avarices   A common term of Qigong in Buddhism，referring to disorder of consciousness and thinking.

六位【liù wèi】 指重卦的六爻。

six positions   Refer to the six levels in the important Trigrams in the Eight Trigrams.

六无为【liù wú wéi】 ① 指不妄为；② 指非姻缘和合形成；③ 指精神稳定。

six nothingness   Refers to ① either inactivity；② or absolute existence；③ or spiritual stability.

六相圆融【liù xiāng yuán róng】 佛家气功用语，指总相、别相、同相、异相、成相、坏相。

balance of six states   A common term of Qigong in Buddhism，referring to general state，special state，same state，different state，right state and wrong state.

六阳【liù yáng】 指六个阳卦、六个阳时、手足三阳经。

Six Yang   Refers to either six kinds of Yang Trigrams；or six periods of Yang；or three meridians of hand Yang and three meridians of foot Yang.

六阳会首【liù yáng huì shǒu】 指手三阳经脉从手走头，与足三阳经脉交会于头。

celebral accumulation of six Yang   Refers to accumulation of the three meridians of hand Yang and the three meridians of foot Yang over the head.

六阳时【liù yáng shí】 指子、丑、寅、卯、辰、巳六个时辰。

six Yang periods   A term of Qigong，referring to six periods of time in day，including Zi（the period of the day from 11 p. m. to 1 a. m.），Chou（the period of a day from 1 a. m. to 3 a. m. in the morning），Yin（the period of the day from 3 a. m. to 5 a. m.），Yin（the period of a day from 3 a. m. to 5 a. m. in the morning），Mao（the period of a day from 5 a. m. to 7 a. m. in the morning），Chen（the period of a day from 7 a. m. to 9 a. m. in the morning）and Si（the period of a day from 9 a. m. to 11 a. m. in the morning）.

六阳时法【liù yáng shí fǎ】 为静功。其作法为，夜半子时，服食生气九九八十一；平旦寅时，服八八六十四；食时辰时，服七七四十九；正中午时，服六六三十六；晡时申时，服五五二十五；黄昏戌时，服四四一十六。

six Yang methods   A static exercise，marked by taking Qi for eight-one times during Zi（the period of a day from 11 p. m. to 1 a. m.）in the midnight，sixty-four times during Yin（the period of a day from 3 a. m. to 5 a. m. in the morning），forty-nine times during Chen（the period of a day from 7 a. m. to 9 a. m. in the morning），thirty-six times during（the period of a day

L

from 11 a.m. in the morning to 1 p.m. in the afternoon), twenty-five times during Shen (the period of a day from 3 p.m. to 5 p.m. in the afternoon) and sixteen times during Xu (the period of a day from 7 p.m. to 9 p.m. in the evening).

六爻【liù yáo】 指八卦中每卦的六个爻。

six kinds of Yao Refer to the six levels of hexagram in all the Eight Trigrams.

六液【liù yè】 指精、泪、唾、涕、汗、溺,功在润泽周身。

six humors Refer to essence, tear, saliva, snivel, sweating and indulgence that have moistened the whole body.

六依【liù yī】 佛家气功习用语,指眼、耳、鼻、舌、身、意六宫。

six kinds of dependence A common term of Qigong in Buddhism, referring to the eyes, the ears, the nose, the tongue, the body and the mentality.

六意识【liù yì shí】 佛家气功习用语,指眼、耳、鼻、舌、身、意六识。

Six emotions A common term of Qigong in Buddhism, referring to the emotions related to the eyes, the ears, the nose, the tongue, the body, and the mind.

六阴【liù yīn】 ① 指六个阴卦;② 六个阴时;③ 手、足三阴经。

six Yin Refers to ① either six kinds of Yin Trigrams; ② or six periods of Yin; ③ or three meridians of hand Yin and three meridians of foot Yin.

六淫【liù yín】 指风、寒、暑、湿、燥、火六气变化太过,是引起外感病的致病因素。

six wastes Refer to wind, cold, summer-heat, dampness, dryness and fire

that have caused various changes and diseases.

六郁【liù yù】 气功适应证,指气、湿、热、痰、血、食等六种郁症的总称。

six stagnations An indication of Qigong, referring to Qi stagnation, dampness stagnation, heat stagnation, phlegm stagnation, blood stagnation and food stagnation.

六欲【liù yù】 ① 指生、死、耳、目、口、鼻;② 指引起情绪、意识不稳定的六种因素。

six desires ① Refers to life, death, ears, eyes, mouth and nose. ② It also refers to six factors that have caused instability of emotions and mentality.

六元【liù yuán】 六气,即风、热、湿、火、燥、寒,为三阴、三阳之本元,故称六元。

six originals Refer to six kinds of Qi, i.e. wind, heat, dampness, fire, dryness and cold which are the origin of the three Yin and three Yang. That is why it is called six originals.

六月节导引法【liù yuè jié dǎo yǐn fǎ】 为动功。其作法为,六月节每日丑寅时,取坐式调息半刻,消除积滞健身。

exercise of Daoyin in the feast days of June A dynamic exercise, marked by sitting for regulating respiration for fifteen minutes in Chou (the period of a day from 1 a.m. to 3 a.m. in the morning) and Yin (the period of a day from 3 a.m. to 5 a.m. in the morning) every feast day of June in order to eliminate stagnation and cultivate health.

六月中导引法【liù yuè zhōng dǎo yǐn fǎ】 为动功。其作法为,六月中每日丑寅时,双手握拳在臀、膝处按摩。

exercise of Daoyin in the middle of June　A dynamic exercise, marked by pressing and kneading the buttocks and knees with both hands in Chou (the period of a day from 1 a. m. to 3 a. m. in the morning) and Yin (the period of a day from 3 a. m. to 5 a. m. in the morning) every day in the middle of June.

六贼【liù zéi】　指眼、耳、鼻、舌、身、意。因器官接受外界的刺激,引起情志损伤,影响入静。

six thieves　Refers to the eyes, the ears, the nose, the tongue, the body and the mentality that are irritated by the external world and have damaged the mind, making it difficult to tranquilize the body.

六真观【liù zhēn guàn】　在河南修武北六真山。世传为丘处机、刘处玄、谭处端、王处一、郝大通、马珏等气功家讲道之处。

Liuzhen Temple　Located in the Liuzhen Mountain in Xiuwu County, Henan Province. It was said that the great masters of Qigong, such as Qiu Chuji, Liu Chuxuan, Tan Chuduan, Wang Chuyi, Hao Datong and Ma Jue, all preached sermon in this temple.

六种调伏法【liù zhǒng diào fú fǎ】　佛家气功习用语,指性调伏法、众生调伏法、行调伏法、方便调伏法、熟调伏法、熟调伏印法。

six adjustments　A common term of Qigong in Buddhism, refers to nature adjustment, all adjustment, active adjustment, convenient adjustment, ripe adjustment and stable adjustment.

六种散乱【liù zhǒng sǎn luàn】　佛家气功习用语,指自性散乱、外散乱、内散乱、相散乱、粗重散乱、作意散乱。

six disorders　A common term of Qigong in Buddhism, refers to self-existence disorder, external disorder, internal disorder, state disorder, rough disorder and mental disorder.

六字法【liù zì fǎ】　佛家气功功法,习练气功时,默念"南无阿弥陀佛"六字。

method with six characters　The method used to practice Qigong in Buddhism. In practicing Qigong, the six characters to read are Namomitabhaya buddhaya.

六字功【liù zì gōng】　是一种呼吸配合发音的治病方法。

formula with six characters　A therapeutic method marked by respiration combined with pronunciation for curing diseases.

六字气诀【liù zì qì jué】　是一种呼吸配合发音的治病方法。

qi formula with six characters　A therapeutic method marked by respiration combined with pronunciation for curing diseases.

六祖坛经【liù zǔ tán jīng】　《六祖坛经》为气功专著,禅宗六祖慧能在广州韶州大寺庙口述,弟子法海加以集录。

Liuzu Tanjing (*Liuzu's Altar Canon*)　A monograph of Qigong entitled *Liuzu's Altar Canon*, dictated by Dhyana Liuzu Huineng in a great temple located in Shaozhou City in Guanzhou Province, collected and compiled by his follower Fahai.

龙从火里出,虎向水中生【lóng cóng huǒ lǐ chū hǔ xiàng shuǐ zhōng shēng】　指习练气功,取阳中之阴入阴中,取阴中之阳归阳中。

loong coming out from fire and tiger appearing from water　A celebrated dictum, referring to promoting Yin from Yang to enter Yin and to promoting Yang from Yin to enter Yang in practicing Qigong.

龙虎【lóng hǔ】 ① 指精神活动；② 指以龙喻元神，以虎喻元精；③ 指水火。

loong and tiger A term in Qigong, referring to ① either spiritual activity; ② or Loong pertaining to the original spirit and tiger pertaining to the original essence; ③ or water and fire.

龙虎成象【lóng hǔ chéng xiàng】 指阴阳二气相感，结而成丹。

loong and tiger forming image A term of Qigong, referring to sympathy of Yin Qi and Yang Qi that has formed Dan (pills of immortality).

龙虎大丹【lóng hǔ dà dān】 指吞月华入腹所炼成的内丹。

Large Dan (pills of immortality) in Loong and tiger A term of Qigong, referring to the internal Dan (pills of immortality) produced by swallowing moonshine into the abdomen.

龙虎伏【lóng hǔ fú】 龙指的是肾，虎指的是肺，意为肾、肺之气保持稳定协调。

Harmony between Loong and tiger A term of Qigong, in which Loong refers to the kidney and tiger refers to the lung, indicating the balance and regulation of Qi in the kidney and the lung.

龙虎还丹诀【lóng hǔ huán dān jué】《龙虎还丹诀》为气功专著，为唐代吕洞宾所著，主要论述还丹之道。

Longhu Huandan Jue (*Formula of Loong and Tiger for Returning to Dan*) A monograph of Qigong entitled *Formula of Loong and Tiger for Returning to Dan*, written by Lǔ Dongbin in the Tang Dynasty (618 AD – 907 AD), mainly describing the way to return to Dan (pills of immortality).

龙虎会【lóng hǔ huì】 龙指肾，虎指肺。会为阴阳相交，意为肾、肺之气协调。

combination of Loong and tiger A term of Qigong, in which Loong refers to the kidney and tiger refers to the lung, indicating combination of Yin and Yang as well as regulation of Qi in the kidney and the lung.

龙虎交媾【lóng hǔ jiāo gòu】 指阴阳和合。

harmonization of Loong and tiger A term of Qigong, referring to harmonization of Yin and Yang.

龙虎亲【lóng hǔ qīn】 龙指神，虎指精气，神气凝合。

intimity of Loong and tiger A term of Qigong, in which Loong refers to the spirit and refers to the essential Qi, indicating combination of the spirit and Qi.

龙虎山【lóng hǔ shān】 位于江西省，为天师道创始人张道陵子孙世居之地。

loong and tiger mountain A mountain in the Jiangxi Province where the future generations of Zhang Daoling, the founder of Daoism, lived.

龙虎穴【lóng hǔ xué】 指左肾和右肾。

loong and tiger points Refers to the left kidney and right kidney.

龙虎之首【lóng hǔ zhī shǒu】 指神。

head of loong and tiger A term of Qigong, referring to spirit.

龙旌【lóng jīng】 指胆之象色青，言胆神真雄无极，阳盛之象。

loong banner Refers to the blue color

龙就虎【lóng jiù hǔ**】**　指龙与虎，即身体阴阳两个方面。

loong and tiger　Refers to the body and Yin and Yang.

龙烟【lóng yān**】**　指肝神。

loong smoke　A term in Qigong, referring to the liver spirit.

龙阳子【lóng yáng zǐ**】**　元代著名气功学家冷谦的另外一个称谓。

Long Yangzi　Another name of Leng Qian who was a great master of Qigong in the Yuan Dynasty(1271 AD‐1368 AD).

龙曜【lóng yào**】**　为胆神之名。

long brightness　A term of Qigong, referring to the spirit in the gallbladder.

隆晃【lóng huǎng**】**　指意念存想大雷电的巨大声响和亮光。

grand imagination　refers to imagined thundery sound and light.

癃闭【lóng bì**】**　为气功适应证，排尿困难，点滴而下，甚则闭塞不通。多因肺失肃降，脾失转输，肾气不足，导致三焦气化失常所致。

anuria and dysuria　An indication of Qigong, referring to difficulty in urination and block and congestion of meridians, usually caused by failure of the lung to depurate and descend, failure of the spleen to transport and insufficiency of kidney Qi, resulting in gasifying disorder of the triple energizer.

楼阁【lóu gé**】**　指喉。

pavilion　A term of Qigong, referring to the throat.

楼阁十二环【lóu gé shí èr huán**】**　指喉咙。

pavilion with twelve links　A term of Qigong, referring to the throat.

楼门【lóu mén**】**　即重楼，为中药名。

building gate　Refers to Rhizoma Paridis, which is a traditional Chinese medicinal.

漏【lòu**】**　佛家气功习用语，指烦恼。

leakage　A term of Qigong, referring to annoyance.

漏肩风治法【lòu jiān fēng zhì fǎ**】**　为动功。其作法为，立地闭气，双手微用力，如解木板状，左右各扯二十四，又转，汗出乃止，日行数次。

exercise for curing shoulder pain　A dynamic exercise, marked by standing up, stopping respiration, mildly forcing the hands like relieving board, pulling from the left to the right and vice versa for twenty-four times respectively, and stopping practice after sweating. Such a dynamic exercise can be performed for several times a day.

漏尽智证通【lòu jìn zhì zhèng tōng**】**　佛家气功习用语，指习练气功，可诸漏断尽，烦恼尽除，神形相适。

loss of leakage ensuring sophistication　A common term of Qigong in Buddhism, referring to obtaining special advantage for eliminating all leakage and annoyance in order to harmonize the body and the spirit.

卢间【lú jiān**】**　①指绛宫心；②指额卢之间，明堂中。

chamber　A term of Qigong, referring to ① either the middle Dantian (the region below the heart); ② or the region in the nose.

炉【lú**】**　①指神；②指肾；③指身；④指蓄火之具。

furnace　Refers to ① either the spirit;

② or the kidney；③ or the body；④ or the stove of fire.

炉鼎【lú dǐng】　外丹术中，炉为生火之器鼎，为炼药之具。内丹术中，炉鼎喻身体。

furnace cauldron　In the exercise of external Dan（pills of immortality），furnace refers to the cauldron for making fire，which is also a tool for making medicinal. In the exercise of internal Dan（pills of immortality），furnace cauldron is compared to the body.

胪【lú】　指腹壁，包括腹壁皮肤、筋膜、肌肉。

nape　Include the skin，sinews and fleshes in the napes.

陆地仙经【lù dì xiān jīng】　《陆地仙经》为气功专著，由清代马齐所著，以歌词形式阐述气功导引的养生方法。

Ludi Xianjing（*Immortal Canon in China*）　A monograph of Qigong entitled *Immortal Canon in China*，written by Ma Qi in the Qing Dynasty（1636 AD - 1912 AD），describing the ways of Qigong and Daoyin in cultivating life with poems.

陆地仙经歌【lù dì xiān jīng gē】　源自气功养生专论，主要阐述气功按摩导引、节饮食慎起居是防病祛邪健身之法。

songs of Immortal Canon in China　Collected from a monograph of Qigong，mainly describing that the practice of Qigong，Tuina and Daoyin as well as eating less，sitting and getting up carefully can prevent disease，expel pathogenic factors and cultivate life.

陆放翁【lù fàng wēng】　南宋时期伟大的诗人陆游的另外一个称谓，其对气功养生也有深入的研究，撰写了多部气功专著，记述了气功的理论、方法、经验和体会。

Lu Fangweng　Another name of Lu You，a great poet in the South Song Dynasty（1127 AD - 1276 AD）who also studied and practiced Qigong all his life. He wrote several monographs to introduce the theory，methods and experiences of Qigong.

陆潜阳【lù qián yáng】　宋代气功养生家，著有气功养生专著，精于道家气功。

Lu Qianyang　A master of Qigong and life cultivation in the Song Dynasty（960 AD - 1279 AD）. He wrote a monograph of Qigong and life cultivation，indicating that he was proficient in Qigong in Daoism.

陆务观【lù wù guān】　南宋时期伟大的诗人陆游的另外一个称谓，其对气功养生也有深入的研究，撰写了多部气功专著，记述了气功的理论、方法、经验和体会。

Lu Wuguan　Another name of Lu You，a great poet in the South Song Dynasty（1127 AD - 1276 AD）who also studied and practiced Qigong all his life. He wrote several monographs to introduce the theory，methods and experiences of Qigong.

陆修静【lù xiū jìng】　南朝气功学家，撰写了气功学专著，分析和研究了气功学的理论和方法。

Lu Xiujing　A great master of Qigong in South Dynasty（420 AD - 589 AD）who wrote a monograph of Qigong to analyze and to study the theory and practice of Qigong.

陆游【lù yóu】　南宋伟大的诗人，对气功养生也有深入的研究，撰写了多部气功专著，记述了气功的理论、方法、经验和体会。

Lu You A great poet in the South Song Dynasty（1127 AD - 1276 AD）who also studied and practiced Qigong all his life. He wrote several monographs to introduce the theory, methods and experiences of Qigong.

陆元德【lù yuán dé】 南朝气功学家陆修德的另外一个称谓,撰写了气功学专著,分析和研究了气功学的理论和方法。

Lu Yuande Another name of Lu Xiude, a great master of Qigong in South Dynasty（420 AD - 589 AD）who wrote a monograph of Qigong to analyze and study the theory and practice of Qigong.

鹿车【lù chē】 指从夹脊到玉枕关,气行宜速。

deer cart Refers to the region between Jiaji acupoints located on both sides of the spine and Yuzhen（BL 9）, along which Qi moves normally and rapidly.

闾丘方远【lǘ qiū fāng yuǎn】 唐代气功学家,对气功实践有一定的发挥。

Lǘqiu Fangyuan A master of Qigong in the Tang Dynasty（618 AD - 907 AD）, who well developed the practice of Qigong.

吕不韦【lǚ bù wéi】 战国末年的一位大商人,编撰了《吕氏春秋》,为气功的发展奠定了基础。

Lǚ Buwei A great merchant in the late Warring States who compiled *Lǚ's Spring and Autumn* which laid solid foundation for the development of Qigong.

吕纯阳【lǚ chún yáng】 唐代气功学家吕洞宾的另外一个称谓,撰有多部气功专著,对气功学的发展做出了特殊贡献。

Lǚ Chunyang Another name of Lǚ Dongbin, a great master of Qigong in the Tang Dynasty（618 AD - 907 AD）, who wrote several monographs of Qigong, contributing a great deal to the development of Qigong.

吕纯阳行气【lǚ chún yáng xíng qì】 为动功。其作法为,自然站立式,左手自然前伸,以右手自左手腕以上捏至左肩膀下,同时运气二十二口。

Lǚ Chunyang's regulation of Qi A static exercise, marked by naturally standing up, naturally stretching the left hand, pinching the region below the left shoulder with the right hand moving up from the left wrist, and directing Qi for twenty-two times.

吕纯阳真人沁园春丹词注解【lǚ chún yáng zhēn rén qìn yuán chūn dān cí zhù jiě】《吕纯阳真人沁园春丹词注解》为气功专著,由元代俞琰所著,解释丹词中的气功术语。

Lǚ Chunyang Zhenren Qinyuanchun Danci Zhujie（*Explanation of Immortal Lǚ Chunyang's Qinyuanchun Poetry*） A monograph about explanation of Qigong entitled *Explanation of Immortal Lǚ Chunyang's Qinyuanchun Poetry*, written by Yuyan in the Yuan Dynasty（1271 AD - 1368 AD）, explaining the terms of Qigong in the poems.

吕洞宾【lǚ dòng bīn】 唐代著名的气功学家,撰有多部气功专著,对气功学的发展做出了特殊贡献。

Lǚ Dongbin A great master of Qigong in the Tang Dynasty（618 AD - 907 AD）, who wrote several monographs of Qigong, contributing a great deal to the development of Qigong.

吕功成导引法【lǚ gōng chéng dǎo

L

yǐn fǎ】 动静相兼功,主要是调身、调气、调神,功效是补脑安神,调和脏腑功能。

Lǔ Gongcheng's exercise of Yaoyin An exercise combined with static exercise and dynastic exercise, mainly regulating the body, Qi and the spirit for tonifying the brain, stabilizing the spirit and regulating the functions of the viscera.

吕岩【lǔ yán】 唐代气功学家吕洞宾的另外一个称谓,撰有多部气功专著,对气功学的发展做出了特殊贡献。

Lǔ Yan Another name of Lǔ Dongbin, a great master of Qigong in the Tang Dynasty (618 AD - 907 AD), who wrote several monographs of Qigong, contributing a great deal to the development of Qigong.

吕真人小成导引法【lǔ zhēn rén xiǎo chéng dǎo yǐn fǎ】 为动功。其作法为,每夜半后,生气时,或五更睡觉,先呵出腹内浊气,或九次止,或三十次止,定心闭目,叩齿三十六通,以集心神。

Lǔ Zhenren's initial exercise of Daoyin A dynamic exercise, marked by generating Qi after midnight, or sleeping before dawn, exhaling turbid Qi in the abdomen first for nine times or thirty times, stabilizing the heart and closing the eyes, clicking the teeth for thirty-six times in order to concentrate the spirit in the heart.

吕祖【lǔ zǔ】 唐代气功学家吕洞宾的另外一个称谓,撰有多部气功专著,对气功学的发展做出了特殊贡献。

Lǔ Zu Another name of Lǔ Dongbin, a great master of Qigong in the Tang Dynasty (618 AD - 907 AD), who wrote several monographs of Qigong,

contributing a great deal to the development of Qigong.

膂【lǔ】 指脊柱两旁的肌肉。

sacrospinalis Refers to the muscles at lateral sides of the spine.

履霜【lǔ shuāng】 指事物的发展变化,由渐而来。

treading on frost Refers to the gradual development and changes of things.

虑其欲神将入舍【lǔ qí yù shén jiāng rù shè】 指排除欲念,才能内守意识、精神。

Only when desires are carefully considered can the spirit be concentrated in the body. This is a celebrated dictum, indicating that only when desires are eliminated can consciousness and the spirit be internally concentrated.

率谷【lǔ gǔ】 足少阳胆经中的一个穴位,位于耳尖上方,入发际1.5寸处,为气功中常用的意守部位。

shuaigu（GB 8） An acupoint in the gallbladder meridian of foot Shaoyang, located above the tip of auricle and 1.5 Cun into the hair line, which is the region for concentrating consciousness in practicing Qigong.

栾先生调气法【luán xiān shēng tiáo qì fǎ】 为动静功。其作法为,于净室内,施床枕与身平,布展手去身各三四寸,两足相去亦然,鸣天鼓三十二通,漱玉泉十五咽,以鼻吸入腹,数多为良,勿使耳闻气入声。

Mr. Luan's exercise for regulating Qi Dynamic and static exercise, marked by lying on the bed with pillow in a clear and quiet room, putting the hands over the body for three to four Cun with the same of the feet, sounding the celestial drum (rubbing the occipital) for thirty-two times, rinsing Yuquan (CV 3) for fifteen times, inhaling into the abdomen through the nose for several times, and avoiding the ears to listen the voice of Qi.

卵势【luǎn shì】　睾丸的另外一个别称。

scrotal style　A synonym of scrotum.

乱想【luàn xiǎng】　佛家气功习用语，指一切烦恼。

distracting thought　A common term of Qigong in Buddhism, referring to all annoyances.

乱心【luàn xīn】　佛家气功习用语，指精神意识活动躁动飞扬，不可抑止。

distracted heart　A term of Qigong, referring to active activity of consciousness that cannot be restrained.

论闭气不息长生【lùn bì qì bù xī cháng shēng】　气功专论,阐述长练行气法,闭气不息至气通,则可长生的道理。

discussion of always holding breath for prolonging life　Collected from a monograph of Qigong, mainly describing the rules for prolonging life by analyzing the methods for refining circulation of Qi and holding the breath to promote Qi circulation.

论朝元【lùn cháo yuán】　源自气功专论,主要阐述人身阳生之时,五脏之气朝于中元;阴生之时,五脏之液朝于下元;三阳上朝内院(顶)均称为朝元。

discussion of celebral origin　Collected from a monograph of Qigong, mainly describing that Qi from the five Zang-organs (including the heart, the liver, the spleen, the lung and the kidney) flows upwards to the middle origin when Yang grows in the body; that hu-

mor from the five Zang-organs flows downwards to the lower origin when Yin grows in the body; the three kinds of Yang are called celebral origin when they have reached the brain.

论抽添【lùn chōu tiān】　源自气功专论,主要阐述肾中真气为铅,炼而为汞,即抽铅添汞而生神。

discussion of extraction and addition　Collected from a monograph of Qigong, mainly describing the genuine Qi in the kidney as lead which becomes mercury after practice, indicating that extraction of lead and addition of mercury will produce the spirit.

论出神【lùn chū shén】　源自气功专论,阐述真气自凝,阳神自聚,以心运气,则气住神住,真积功满,调神出壳。

discussion of transmitting spirit　Collected from a monograph of Qigong, mainly describing natural coagulation of genuine Qi, natural accumulation of Yang spirit and circulation of Qi with the heart, which enables Qi and the spirit to stabilize genuine Qi to be sufficient, practice to be effective and the spirit to be regulated and transmitted externally.

论大道【lùn dà dào】　源自气功专论,主要阐述金丹大道就是阴阳的谐调、交媾。

discussion of the great way　Collected from a monograph of Qigong, mainly describing the golden pellet way for regulating Yin and Yang and improving coitus.

论丹药【lùn dān yào】　源自气功专论,主要阐述"内丹之药材,出于心肾""本于龙虎交媾而变黄芽"。

discussion of cinnabar medicinal　Collected from a monograph of Qigong, mainly describing that " the internal cinnabar medicinal comes from the heart and the kidney" and that "it originates from the intercourse of Loong and tiger that has transformed into essence".

论道家功【lùn dào jiā gōng**】**　源自气功专论,阐述道家功的基本理论、作法及其特点。

discussion of Daoism exercise　Collected from a monograph of Qigong, mainly describing the basic theory, methods and characteristics of Qigong practice in Daoism.

论调气【lùn diào qì**】**　源自气功专论,主要阐述了"气"与"形"的关系。

discussion of regulating Qi　Collected from a monograph of Qigong, mainly describing the relationship between Qi and the body.

论鼎器【lùn dǐng qì**】**　源自气功老子,主要阐述了"鼎器"的涵义以及"内鼎""外鼎""玄牝"等的具体内容。所谓"内鼎",指的是下丹田;所谓"外鼎",指的是"玄牝之门";所谓"玄牝"指的是有天与地、鼻与口、上与下、父精与母血和肾、元神、中丹田、心之左右二窍等诸说。

discussion of cauldron　Collected from a monograph of Qigong, mainly describing the meaning and content of cauldron as well as the internal cauldron, the external cauldron, the nose and the mouth. The so-called internal cauldron refers the lower Danian (the region below the navel); the so-called external cauldron refers to the gate of Xuanpin; the so-called Xuanpin refers to the sky and the earth, or the nose and the mouth, or the upper and the lower, or

the paternal semen and the maternal blood, or the kidney, the original spirit, the middle Dantian (the region below the heart) and the left and the right orifices of the heart.

论功夫【lùn gōng fū**】**　源自气功专论,解释了功夫的含义。

discussion of skills　Collected from a monograph of Qigong, explaining the actual meaning of skills.

论还丹【lùn huán dān**】**　源自气功专论,主要阐述气在上、中、下三丹田既往而有归就是还丹。

discussion of returning Dan　Collected from a monograph of Qigong, mainly describing returning Qi to the upper Dantian (the region between the eyes), the middle Dantian (the region below the heart) and the lower Dantian (the region below the navel).

论河车【lùn hé chē**】**　源自气功专论,主要阐述河车有搬运阴阳之妙用。

discussion of river cart　Collected from a monograph of Qigong, mainly describing the wonderful effect of the river cart for transmitting Yin and Yang.

论黑铅黑汞【lùn hēi qiān hēi gǒng**】**源自气功专论,解释了"黑铅""黑汞"的含义,即"要知是气之名,须究内外之道。气之在外者曰黑铅,气之在内者曰黑汞"。

discussion of black lead and black mercury　Collected from a monograph of Qigong, mainly describing the meaning of black lead and black mercury. To know the name of Qi, one must first well understand the internal way and external way. Thus Qi in the external is called black lead and Qi in the internal is called black mercury.

论活子时【lùn huó zǐ shí】 源自气功专论,主要阐述练功中一阳来复之时便是活子时。

discussion of life time Collected from a monograph of Qigong, mainly describing the time when Yang returns in practicing Qigong.

论金液还丹【lùn jīn yè huán dān】 源自气功专论,认为"金液还丹"的实质,仍为炼精、气、神。

discussion of golden humor returning to Dan（pills of immortality） Collected from a monograph of Qigong, mainly describing the fact that the substance of golden humor returning to Dan（pills of immortality）means to refine the essence, Qi and the spirit.

论炼九还【lùn liàn jiǔ huán】 源自气功专论,主要阐述服日月精华,能易气、血、脉、肉、髓、骨、发、筋、形。

discussion of nine points Collected from a monograph of Qigong, mainly describing taking the essence of the sun and the moon in order to improve Qi, the blood, the meridians, the fleshes, the marrows, the bones, the hairs, the sinews and the body.

论炼形【lùn liàn xíng】 源自气功专论,精炼地论述了形与神的关系及炼形与养神的关系。

discussion of refining the body Collected from a monograph of Qigong, mainly describing the relationship between the body and the spirit as well as refining the body and nourishing the spirit.

论龙虎【lùn lóng hǔ】 源自气功专论,主要阐述龙虎及龙虎交媾。龙本肝之象,虎乃肺之神。

discussion of Loong and tiger Collected from a monograph of Qigong, mainly describing Loong and tiger as well as the intercourse of Loong and tiger. In this term, the so-called Loong refers to the shape of the liver and the so-called tiger refers to the spirit in the lung.

论内观【lùn nèi guān】 源自气功专论,主要阐述内观可以使神识自住,同时介绍了阳升、阴降、匹配阴阳等内观法。

discussion of internal meditation Collected from a monograph of Qigong, mainly describing the fact that internal mediation can enable the spirit to concentrate itself. It has also introduced the internal meditation of Yang ascending, Yin descending and connection of Yin and Yang.

论铅汞【lùn qiān gǒng】 源自气功专论,主要阐述内丹中之铅即父母之真气,隐于肾。汞即心液中正阳之气。

discussion of lead and mercury Collected from a monograph of Qigong, mainly describing that the so-called lead in the internal Dan（pills of immortality）refers to genuine Qi in parents hidden in the kidney. The so-called mercury refers to genuine Yang Qi in the heart humor.

论日月【lùn rì yuè】 源自气功专论,主要阐述气功锻炼要效法天地阴阳升降之道,日月交合之理,说明人与自然的关系。

discussion of the sun and moon Collected from a monograph of Qigong, mainly describing the fact that practice of Qigong should follow the communicating principle of the sun and moon as well as the ascending and descending ways of the sky and the earth, Yin and Yang, indicating the relationship between man and nature.

L

论儒家功【lùn rú jiā gōng】 源自气功专论,阐述儒家功的基本理论、作法及其特点。

discussion of Confucianism exercise Collected from a monograph of Qigong, mainly describing the basic theory, methods and characteristics of Qigong practice in Confucianism.

论神室铅汞【lùn shén shì qiān gǒng】源自气功专论,阐述了"下丹田""大海(亦名大中极)""丹田(亦名金胎神室)"的部位及介绍了"铅汞"的多种代名词。

discussion of lead and mercury in the spirit chamber Collected from a monograph of Qigong, mainly describing the positions of the lower Dantian (the region below the navel), great sea (also called great middle extremity) and Dantian (also called golden embryo and spirit chamber) as well as the different names of Qian (lead) and Gong (mercury). Dantian is divided into the upper Dantian (the region between the eyes), the middle Dantian (the region below the heart) and the lower Dantian (the region below the navel).

论肾间动气【lùn shèn jiān dòng qì】源自气功专论,主要阐述肾间动气上蒸脾土而化饮食,荣养一身。故气功锻炼强调意守下腹部。

discussion of active Qi in the kidney Collected from a monograph of Qigong, mainly describing the active Qi in the kidney that flows up to the spleen to transform into diet to nourish the body. That is why Qigong practice emphasizes the importance of concentrating mentality on the lower abdomen.

论释家功【lùn shì jiā gōng】 源自气功专论,阐述释家气功的基本理论、作法及特点。

discussion of Buddhism exercise Collected from a monograph of Qigong, mainly describing the basic theory, methods and characteristics of Qigong practice in Buddhism.

论水火【lùn shuǐ huǒ】 源自气功专论,主要阐述水火在气功中的运用,论述甚为精辟。

discussion of water and fire Collected from a monograph of Qigong, mainly describing the application of water and fire in practicing Qigong.

论天地【lùn tiān dì】 源自气功专论,主要阐述天地阴阳交合而生万物,人身阴阳升降交合效法天地。

discussion of the sky and the earth Collected from a monograph of Qigong, mainly describing the fact that combination of the sky and the earth as well as Yin and Yang has produced everything in the universe; and that the ascent and descent of Yin and Yang in the human body should follow the rules of the sky and the earth.

论吐纳【lùn tǔ nà】 源自气功专论,主要阐述六气的应用。

discussion of exhalation and inhalation Collected from a monograph of Qigong, mainly describing the application of six kinds of Qi.

论往来【lùn wǎng lái】 源自气功专论,指阴阳一消一长、一往一来的自然变化。

discussion of going and coming Collected from a monograph of Qi, referring to the natural changes of Yin and Yang, including growth and decline as well as coming and going.

论我命在我【lùn wǒ mìng zài wǒ】源自气功专论,强调了人的精神、情绪和意志对人体健康的影响。

discussion of my life with myself　Collected from a monograph of Qigong, mainly emphasizing the influence of the spirit, emotion and thought on life health.

论修炼合丹【lùn xiū liàn hé dān】　源自气功专论,强调"修炼合丹"即指炼精、气、神。

discussion of practicing and combining Dan　Collected from a monograph of Qigong, mainly describing the fact that practicing and combining Dan means to refine the essence, Qi and the spirit.

论行气当和气调息【lùn xíng qì dāng hé qì tiáo xī】　源自气功专论,强调了初练行气法时的注意事项。

discussion of circulating Qi, harmonizing Qi and regulating respiration　Collected from a monograph of Qigong, mainly emphasizing matters needing attention in preliminarily practicing Qigong.

论玄牝【lùn xuán pìn】　源自气功专论,主要阐述下丹田为玄牝,练功者伏其气于下丹田。

discussion of Xuanpin aspect　Collected from a monograph of Qigong, mainly describing that the so-called Xuanpin refers to the lower Dantian (the region below the navel) where Qi is concentrated in practicing Qigong.

论养神【lùn yǎng shén】　源自气功专论,主要阐述养神的前提。

discussion of nourishing sprit　Collected from a monograph of Qigong, mainly describing the precondition for nourishing the spirit.

论真铅【lùn zhēn qiān】　源自气功专论,所阐述者为天地真一之气。

discussion of genuine lead　Collected from a monograph of Qigong, mainly describing the genuine Qi in the sky and the earth.

论证验【lùn zhèng yàn】　源自气功专论,主要阐述练功后的各种效验,对练功者有很好的参考价值。

discussion of experience　Collected from a monograph of Qigong, mainly describing various efficacies of Qigong practice which will provide the references for practitioners.

论子午卯寅【lùn zǐ wǔ mǎo yín】　源自气功专论,主要阐述子为六阳之首,阴极阳生之时;午为六阴之首,阳极阴生之时;卯寅二时,为心肾二气交分之时。阐明四时,在练功中的地位。

discussion of Zi, Wu, Mao and Yin　Collected from a monograph of Qigong, mainly describing that Zi (the period of the day from 11 p. m. to 1 a. m.) is the first position of the six kinds of Yang and the time when Yin has developed to the extremity and Yang has grown; that Wu (the period of the day from 11 a. m. to 1 p. m.) is the first position of the six kinds of Yin and the time when Yang has developed to the extremity and Yin has grown; that Yin (the period of the day from 3 a. m. to 5 a. m. in the early morning), Mao (the period of the day from 5 a. m. to 7 a. m. in the early morning) are the first time when Qi from the heart and the kidney begins to coordinate with each other. These four periods are the states for practicing Qigong.

罗达夫【luó dá fū】　明代的一位学者

L

罗洪先的另外一个称谓,对气功也非常精通。

Luo Dafu Another name of Luo Hongxian, a great scholar in the Ming Dynasty（1368 AD – 1644 AD）, quite familiar with Qigong.

罗浮翠虚吟【luó fú cuì xū yín】 源自气功专论,阐述炼丹的基本知识,介绍炼丹的方法、过程及注意事项。

singing thorough flowing and green illusion Collected from a monograph of Qigong, mainly describing the basic knowledge, methods, procedure and attentions in practicing alchemy.

罗浮山【luó fú shān】 位于广东省,为东晋时期葛洪炼丹之处。

Luofu Mountain Located in the Guangdong Province, where Ge Hong, a great scholar in the East Jin Dynasty （317 AD – 420 AD）studied and practiced alchemy.

罗福至【luó fú zhì】 清代气功学家,撰写多部专著,推崇气功,讲究动静结合。

Luo Fuzhi A master of Qigong in the Qing Dynasy（1636 AD – 1912 AD）who wrote several monographs, emphasizing Qigong and combination of dynamic exercise and static exercise.

罗洪先【luó hóng xiān】 明代的一位学者,对气功也非常精通。

Luo Hongxian A great scholar in the Ming Dynasty（1368 AD – 1644 AD）, quite familiar with Qigong.

罗念庵【luó niàn ān】 明代学者罗洪先的另外一个称谓,对气功也非常精通。

Luo Nian'an Another name of Luo Hongxian, a great scholar in the Ming Dynasty（1368 AD – 1644 AD）, quite familiar with Qigong.

罗钦顺【luó qīn shùn】 明代学者,认为气为宇宙万物之根本。

Luo Qinshun A great scholar in the Ming Dynasty（1368 AD – 1644 AD）, believing that Qi is the root of all things in the universe.

罗允升【luó yǔn shēng】 明代学者罗钦顺的另外一个称谓,认为气为宇宙万物之根本。

Luo Yunsheng Another name of Luo Qinshun, a great scholar in the Ming Dynasty（1368 AD – 1644 AD）, believing that Qi is the root of all things in the universe.

罗整庵【luó zhěng ān】 明代学者罗钦顺的另外一个称谓,认为气为宇宙万物之根本。

Luo Zheng'an Another name of Luo Qinshun, a great scholar in the Ming Dynasty（1368 AD – 1644 AD）, believing that Qi is the root of all things in the universe.

螺蚌生珠【luó bàng shēng zhū】 喻人在气功状态下,吸日月精华之气而作丹,与自然相应,顺其理法。

mussel producing pearl A term of Qigong, indicating to inhale essential Qi from the sun and the moon to form Dan（pills of immortality）for corresponding to the natural world and complying with the principles in practicing Qigong.

瘰疬【luǒ lì】 为气功适应证,多因肺肾阴亏,阴虚火旺,情志不畅,肝气郁结,气滞伤脾,脾失健运,痰热内生,结于颈项,腋下或胯间所致。

scrofula An indication of Qigong, usually caused by consumption of Yin in the lung and the kidney, deficiency of Yin and exuberance of fire, gloomy mood, stagnation of liver Qi, spleen damage due to Qi stagnation，failure of the spleen to transport normally，and internal existence of phlegm-heat in the neck，armpit or crotch.

瘰疬瘘候导引法【luǒ lì lòu hòu dǎo yǐn fǎ**】** 为动功。其作法为，张腿屈膝而坐，用两手从腿弯处伸入按地上，把脚放在手上，抬起臀部，同时行气。消肿散结，治瘰疬，乳痈。

exercise of Daoyin for scrofula A dynamic exercise，marked by sitting with stretched legs and bent knees，pressing the ground with both hands along the leg elbow，putting the foot on the hand，lifting the buttocks and moving Qi. Such a dynamic exercise can subside swelling to dissipate indurated mass and cure scrofula and breast abscess.

L

M

麻姑仙磨疾诀【má gū xiān mó jí jué】
为动功。其作法为,站立定,左边气脉不
通,右手行功,意引在左;右边气脉不通,
左手行功,意引在右,各运气五口。主治
气脉不通。

**female Immortal Ma's formula for elimi-
nating disease** A dynamic exercise,
marked by sitting quietly, appearing
obstructed Qi meridian in the left side,
moving the right hand, imagining to
lead it to the left side and moving Qi
for five times; appearing obstructed Qi
meridian in the right side, moving the
left hand, imagining to lead it to the
right side, and moving Qi for five
times. This dynamic exercise can cure
obstructed Qi meridian.

麻衣真人和调真气【má yī zhēn rén
hé tiáo zhēn qì】 为静功。其作法为,
侧卧,炼神入静,令神息相依。治疗失
眠、多梦、梦游等。

**Immortal Ma Yi pacifying and regulating
genuine Qi** A static exercise, marked
by lying on one side, refining and tranquilizing the spirit, and coordinating
the spirit and respiration. This static
exercise can cure insomnia, dreaminess
and sleepwalking.

马从义【mǎ cóng yì】 金代针灸家和
气功专家马丹阳的另一称谓,著有多部
专著。

Ma Congyi Another name of Ma Danyang, a great master of acupuncture,
moxibustion and Qigong in the Jin Dy-

nasty (1123 - 1183), who wrote several
monographs.

马丹阳周天火候法【mǎ dān yáng
zhōu tiān huǒ hòu fǎ】 为动功。其作
法为,平地坐定,用两手擦热揉目,然后
拄定两胁下行气,令其气上升,主治元气
衰败。

**Ma Danyang's dynamic dhyana
exercise** A dynamic exercise, marked
by sitting on the ground, rubbing the
hands hot to knead the eyes, and enabling Qi in the hypochondrium to flow
up. Such a dynamic exercise can cure
decline of original Qi.

马丹阳【mǎ dān yáng】 金代针灸家
和气功家,著有多部专著。

Ma Danyang A great master of acupuncture, moxibustion and Qigong in
the Jin Dynasty (1123 - 1183), who
wrote several monographs.

马王堆汉墓导引图【mǎ wáng duī
hàn mù dǎo yǐn tú】《马王堆汉墓导引
图》为气功导引专著,1973 年于湖南长
沙马王堆三号汉墓出土。

**Mawangdui Hanmu Daoyin Tu (*Daoyin
Pictures in the Mawangdui Tomb of the
Han Dynasty*)** A monograph of
Qigong entitled *Daoyin Pictures in the
Mawangdui Tomb of the Han Dynasty*,
discovered in 1973 from the third tomb
of the Han Dynasty (202 BC - 263 AD)
in Bawangdui area in Changsha City,
Hunan Province.

马玄宝【mǎ xuán bǎo】 金代针灸家

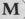

和气功家，著有多部专著。

Ma Xuanbao Another name of Ma Danyang, a great master of acupuncture, moxibustion and Qigong in the Jin Dynasty (1123－1183), who wrote several monographs.

马宜甫【mǎ yí fǔ】　金代针灸家和气功家，著有多部专著。

Ma Yifu Another name of Ma Danyang, a great master of acupuncture, moxibustion and Qigong in the Jin Dynasty (1123－1183), who wrote several monographs.

马钰【mǎ yù】　金代针灸家和气功专家马丹阳的另一称谓，著有多部专著。

Ma Yu Another name of Ma Danyang, a great master of acupuncture, moxibustion and Qigong in the Jin Dynasty (1123－1183), who wrote several monographs.

马自然醉卧雪溪【mǎ zì rán zuì wò zhà xī】　为动功。其作法为胸、腹贴床而卧，两手向后上举，两脚也往上举，运行十二口。主治肠炎和腹痛。

dynamic horse-lying exercise A dynamic exercise, marked by lying with the chest and abdomen on the bed, raising up the hands and the feet for twelve times. Such a dynamic exercise can treat enteritis and abdominal pain.

脉【mài】　① 指气血运行的通道；② 指脉象。

meridian Refers to ① either the channels through which Qi and blood move; ② or pulse.

脉气【mài qì】　指脉中精气。

Meridian Qi Refers to the essential Qi in the meridians.

脉舍神【mài shě shén】　指心中脉，脉为血之府，神舍于其中。

meridian containing spirit Refers to the meridian in the heart which is the palace of the blood and the spirit.

脉望论火候【mài wàng lùn huǒ hòu】源自气功专论，主要阐述火候，即意念，重点谈得药时之火候。

observation and discussion of heat according to the meridian Collected from a monograph of Qigong, mainly describing the thought as the heat level and the heat level as the advantage for obtaining medicinal.

芒种五月节坐功【máng zhòng wǔ yuè jié zuò gōng】　为动功。其作法为，每日寅卯时正立仰身，两手上托，左右力举，各五七次，定息、叩齿、吐纳、咽液。

sitting exercise of Daoyin in the feast days in May A dynamic exercise, marked by standing up in Yin (the period of a day from 3 a. m. to 5 a. m. in the morning) and Mao (the period of a day from 5 a. m. to 7 a. m. in the morning) every day, raising up the hands from the left to the right for five or seven times in order to stabilize respiration, click the teeth, inhale and exhale as well as swallow saliva.

毛际【máo jì】　指阴阜上长阴毛处与皮肤的边缘部。

pubic margin Refers to the area between the pubes and the margin of skin.

毛玄汉降伏龙虎【máo xuán hàn xiáng fú lóng hǔ】　为静功。侧卧，凝神令性定、情忘，而龙虎自降伏。

loong and tiger conquering exercise A static exercise, referring to lying on the side, tranquilizing the emotion and harmonizing the whole body.

M

茅季伟【máo jì wěi】 汉代精研气功的学者茅三君的另外一个称谓,其学术著作后世一直传承。

Mao Jiwei Another name of Mao Shushen, a scholar of Qigong in the Han Dynasty (202 BC - 263 AD), whose monograph was inherited by the later generations.

茅三君【máo sān jūn】 汉代精研气功的学者,其学术著作后世一直传承。

Mao Sanjun A scholar of Qigong in the Han Dynasty (202 BC - 263 AD), whose monograph was inherited by the later generations.

茅山派【máo shān pài】 西汉时形成的一个重要的气功流派。

Maoshan school An important school of Qigong, developed in the West Han Dynasty (202 BC - 8 AC).

茅山贤者服气法【máo shān xián zhě fú qì fǎ】 为静功,方法多样。如先侧卧,右胁著地,微缩两足,著头向南面东,两手握固,傍其颐。

exercise of Maoshan Mountain immortal respiration A static exercise with several ways to practice, such as lying on one side with the region from the armpit to the rib over the ground, slowly shrinking the feet, turning the head to the southeast, holding the fists with both hands and closing to the cheek.

茅叔申【máo shū shēn】 汉代精研气功的学者茅三君的另外一个称谓,其学术著作后世一直传承。

Mao Shushen Another name of Mao Sanjun, a scholar of Qigong in the Han Dynasty (202 BC - 263 AD), whose monograph was inherited by the later generations.

茅思和【máo sī hé】 汉代精研气功的学者茅三君的另外一个称谓,其学术著作后世一直传承。

Mao Sihe Another name of Mao Sanjun, a scholar of Qigong in the Han Dynasty (202 BC - 263 AD), whose monograph was inherited by the later generations.

茅衷【máo zhōng】 汉代精研气功的学者茅三君的另外一个称谓,其学术著作后世一直传承。

Mao Zhong Another name of Mao Sanjun, a scholar of Qigong in the Han Dynasty (202 BC - 263 AD), whose monograph was inherited by the later generations.

卯酉【mǎo yǒu】 ① 指卯时和酉时; ② 指左右。

Mao and You Refers to ① either Mao (the period of a day from 5 a.m. to 7 a.m. in the morning) and You (the period of a day from 5 p.m. to 7 p.m. in the afternoon); ② or the left and right.

卯酉周天功【mǎo yǒu zhōu tiān gōng】 为静功,指调身、调气、调神,其功效为补脑安神,调节脏腑功能。主要用治头痛头眩,心悸怔忡,健忘失眠,胸肋胀痛,脘痞腹胀。

Mao and You cycle exercise A static exercise, referring to regulating the body, Qi and spirit in order to effectively tonify the brain, to stabilize the spirit and to regulate the functions of viscera. It is mainly used to treat headache, dizziness, palpitation, amnesia, insomnia, distending pain of the chest and hypochondrium, epigastrium stuffiness and abdominal distension. Mao refers to the time from 5 a.m. to 7 a.m. in the morning and You refers to the time from 5 p. m. to 7 p. m. in the afternoon.

冒风鼻塞导引法【mào fēng bí sāi dǎo yǐn fǎ**】** 为动功。其作法为，先清肺经，用两手指擦鼻两旁，使其内外俱热，如虚火升两眼，双目看两脚底，治感冒鼻塞。

exercise of Daoyin for mild cough and nasal congestion A dynamic exercise, marked by clearing the lung meridian, rubbing the nasal sides with both hands for warming the internal and the external of the nose like raising mild fire to the eyes, and observing the soles with both eyes in order to cure common cold and nasal congestion.

眉本【méi běn**】** 足太阳膀胱经中的一个穴位，原名攒竹，位于眉毛内侧端。这一穴位为气功运行的一个常见部位。

Meiben A synonym of an acupoint in the bladder meridian of foot Taiyang, originally called Cuanzhu（BL 2）, located in the depression of the medial and of the eyebrow. This acupoint is a region usually used for keeping the essential Qi in practice of Qigong.

眉头【méi tóu**】** 足太阳膀胱经中的一个穴位，原名攒竹，位于眉毛内侧端。这一穴位为气功运行的一个常见部位。

Meitou A synonym of an acupoint in the bladder meridian of foot Taiyang, originally called Cuanzhu（BL 2）, located in the medial and of the eyebrow. This acupoint is a region usually used for keeping the essential Qi in practice of Qigong.

梅核气【méi hé qì**】** 为气功适应证，多因情志郁结，肝气夹痰所致。

obstruction sensation in the throat（globus hystericus） An indication of Qigong, usually caused by emotional depression and phlegm accumulation in the liver Qi.

门牖【mén yǒu**】** 指耳目犹如门窗，可以从里洞观外界一切。

gate window Refers to the eyes and the ears similar to the gates and windows that can observe all the things in the world.

蒙以养正【méng yǐ yǎng zhèng**】** 指头脑思维如童蒙，纯一无杂，即能育养正气。

purely nourishing healthy Qi Refers to pure consciousness without any distracting thought, which can rear and nourish healthy Qi.

孟轲【mèng kē**】** 战国时期的思想家、政治家和教育家孟子的另外一个称谓，也发展了儒家的气功。

Meng Ke Another name of Mencius, a great thinker, politician and educator in the Warring States Period（475 BC - 221 BC）, who well developed Qigong in Confucianism.

孟子【mèng zǐ**】** 战国时期的思想家、政治家和教育家，发展了儒家的气功。

Mencius A great thinker, politician and educator in the Warring States Period（475 BC - 221 BC）, who well developed Qigong in Confucianism.

孟子舆【mèng zǐ yú**】** 战国时期的思想家、政治家和教育家孟子的另外一个称谓，也发展了儒家的气功。

Meng Ziyu Another name of Mencius, a great thinker, politician and educator in the Warring States Period（475 BC - 221 BC）, who well developed Qigong in Confucianism.

弥罗天【mí luó tiān**】** 指脑。
The whole sky Refers to the brain.

M

迷坑【mí kēng】 指迷妄的意识思维活动引起精神失调。

delusion A term of Qiong, referring to imbalance of the spirit due to delusive activities of consciousness and thinking.

迷真性说【mí zhēn xìng shuō】《迷真性说》为气功专论，主要阐述迷真性则神形失调，形神疾病随之而生的道理。

idea about confusing genuine nature Collected from a monograph of Qigong, mainly describing imbalance of the spirit and body due to confusion of genuine nature, eventually causing diseases in the body and spirit.

密户【mì hù】 指肾元，亦指命门。

secret household Refers to nephric origin or life gate.

绵绵若存用之不勤【mián mián ruò cún yòng zhī bù qín】 指调节呼吸时，入息绵绵，出息微微，缓和自然，适中。

vague existence with slight use A celebrated dictum, referring to vague inhalation and slight exhalation with natural relaxation for regulating respiration.

面壁【miàn bì】 佛家气功习用语，指习练气功，亦指传授佛家气功。

facing the wall A common term of Qigong in Buddhism, referring to either practice of Qigong; or teaching about how to practice Qigong in Buddhism.

面功【miàn gōng】 为动功。其作法为，用两手相摩使热，随向面上高低处揩之，定要周到，再以口中津唾于掌中，擦热揩面多次。

facial exercise A dynamic exercise, marked by rubbing the hands hot, wiping the upper and lower of the face, vomiting fluid from the mouth over the palms and repeatedly rubbing the palms hot.

面王【miàn wáng】 指鼻头部位。

facial king Refers to the tip of the nose.

妙观法【miào guān fǎ】 为静功，即用意识一次又一次观阴心，协调和稳定全身各部。

exquisite exercise of vision A static exercise, referring to coordinating and stabilizing all parts of the body according to continuous vision of the Yin heart with consciousness.

妙静之道【miào jìng zhī dào】 指神形和合的处世境界。

ideal quite state Refers to the irreproachable state of integration of the spirit and the body.

妙觉【miào jué】 佛家气功习用语，指通过习练气功，神形放松，静寂生慧，意识活动保持较长时间的稳定。

magic sense A common term of Qigong in Buddhism, referring to relaxation of the spirit and the body, tranquilization for increasing wisdom and stabilization of consciousness activity in practicing Qigong.

灭【miè】 佛家气功习用语，① 指灭除烦恼，为调节精神活动的方法；② 指灭为解脱、涅槃。

eradication A common term of Qigong in Buddhism, referring to either eliminating annoyance which is the method to regulate spirit activities; or disengagement and nirvana.

灭病【miè bìng】 佛家气功习用语，指防治神形性疾病。

eradication of disease A common term of Qigong in Buddhism, referring to preventing and treating diseases related to the spirit and the body.

灭谛【miè dì】　佛家气功习用语,指断灭世俗诸苦产生的原因,是佛家气功要达到的目的。

careful eradication　A term of Qigong in Buddhism, referring to the reason why all the secular problems should be expelled. This is the aim of Buddhism about Qigong practice.

灭定【miè dìng】　意为平静精神活动,使神形安定。

fixed eradication　Refers to tranquilizing the spirit activity and stabilizing the spirit and the body.

民火【mín huǒ】　指膀胱。

human fire　Refers to the gallbladder.

民散则国亡气竭则身死【mín sàn zé guó wáng qì jié zé shēn sǐ】　气在人身至为重要,犹如一国之民,无民则无国,无气则无身。故修炼气功十分重视元气的充养。

Confusion of people defeats the country and exhaustion of Qi causes death.　This is a celebrated dictum. Qi in the human body is very important, just like the people in a country. If there are no people, no country can exist; if there is no Qi, no body can exist. So to enrich and to cultivate the original Qi is very important in practicing Qigong.

闵苕叓【mǐn tiáo fū】　清代气功学家闵一得的另外一个称谓,著有多部气功专著。

Min Tiaofu　Another name of Min Yide, a great master of Qigong in the Qing Dynasty (1636 AD – 1912 AD), who wrote several monographs of Qigong.

闵小艮【mǐn xiǎo gèn】　清代气功学家闵一得的另外一个称谓,著有多部气功专著。

Min Xiaogen　Another name of Min Yide, a great master of Qigong in the Qing Dynasty (1636 AD – 1912 AD), who wrote several monographs of Qigong.

闵一得【mǐn yī dé】　清代气功学家,著有多部气功专著。

Min Yide　A great master of Qigong in the Qing Dynasty (1636 AD – 1912 AD), who wrote several monographs of Qigong.

泯其念【mǐn qí niàn】　即思维活动专一,未有杂念。

eliminating whims　Indicates that the activity of thinking is concentrated without any distracting thought.

名【míng】　佛家气功习用语,① 指精神活动;② 指称谓义。

fame　A common term of Qigong in Buddhism, referring to ① either spiritual activity; ② or righteousness.

明【míng】　佛家气功习用语,① 指智慧;② 指真言;③ 指光明;④ 指明心、悟性。

brightness　A common term of Qigong in Buddhism, referring to ① either wisdom; ② or genuine words; ③ brightness in the natural world and social world; ④ clear-heartedness and consciousness.

明道篇【míng dào piān】　《明道篇》为气功专著,由元代王惟一撰,阐述了习练气功的重要问题。

Mingdao Pian (*Accurate Cognition of Dao*)　A monograph of Qigong entitled *Accurate Cognition of Dao*, written by Wang Weiyi in the Yuan Dynasty(1271 AD – 1368 AD), describing the major problems in practicing Qigong.

明耳目诀【míng ěr mù jué】 为动功。其作法为，常以手按两眉后小穴中二十一次，又以手心及手指摩两目，以手旋耳，三十次。然后以手拭额，从眉中开始，止入发际中，二十七次，口咽津液，不拘数遍。

exercise for promoting the eyes and ears A dynamic exercise, marked by pressing two small acuppoints behind the eyes with both hands, rubbing the eyes with the palms and fingers, revolving the ears with hands for thirty times; then wiping the forehead with hands from the center of the eyes till the hair line for twenty-seven times, and swallowing fluid and humor with many times.

明目法【míng mù fǎ】 为静功。其作法为，即正坐调节呼吸，平顺三焦之气，然后意想南方之火照耀全身，自觉通身温暖。久行之可明目曲翳。

exercise for brightening the eyes A static exercise, marked by sitting upright with regulation of respiration, pacifying the movement of Qi from the triple energizer, imagining the fire from the south shining the body and feeling warm in the whole body. Such a way of practicing Qigong will improve vision and cure nebula after a long time of practice.

明上【míng shàng】 与英玄同，指眼神，即目光精彩。

supreme brightness The same as outstanding supremeness, refers to the spirit in the eye, indicating brilliant vision.

明石【míng shí】 明石为白，肺金所主，位在西方，故明石指西方自然太和之气。

light stone In this term, light stone refers to white color controlled by lung metal and located in the west. So light stone refers to natural and harmonious Qi in the west.

明堂【míng táng】 ① 指脑中九宫之一；② 指心；③ 指鼻。

light chamber Refers to ① either one of the nine chambers in the brain; ② or the heart; ③ or the nose.

明堂四达法海源【míng táng sì dá fǎ hǎi yuán】 指心肾相交，坎离同宫，神形合一。

bright chamber combined with the sea origin in four ways Refers to communication of the heart and kidney, combination of the Kan (Trigram) and Li (Trigram) and integration of the spirit and the body.

明淫心疾【míng yín xīn jí】 指思虑烦多，情志失调，劳而生疾。

obsceneness causing heart problems Refers to disease caused by excessive anxiety and maladjustment of emotion.

明映之术【míng yìng zhī shù】 为动功，指用手按耳郭以聪耳。

exercise for brightening and shining A dynamic exercise, referring to pressing the ears in order to sharpen the ears.

明珠【míng zhū】 指眼目。

light pearl Refers to the eyes.

鸣法鼓【míng fǎ gǔ】 指叩正中上下牙齿。

beating right drum Refers to clicking the upper and the lower central teeth.

鸣谦【míng qiān】 指有名望而谦虚。

expressing modesty Means that a famous person should be very modest.

鸣天鼓【míng tiān gǔ】 为动功，指叩门牙。

beating celestial drum　A dynamic exercise, referring to clicking the front teeth.

冥上玄【míng shàng xuán】　指心肾相交，心与肾连。

concentrating the upper　Refers to communication and connection of the heart and the kidney

冥守【míng shǒu】　指闭目内守。

concentrated defense　Refers to closing the eyes and concentrating the internal.

冥心【míng xīn】　指专心于一境，达到不想任何事物的境地。

concentrated the heart　Means to concentrate the heart（mind）in just one state in order to reach the tranquil circumstance without anything.

冥心法【míng xīn fǎ】　为静功。其作法为，深居静室，端拱默然，一尘不染，万虑俱忘，无思无为，任运自如，无视无听，抱神以静，无内无外，无将无迎，离相离空，离迷离妄，体含虚寂，常觉常明。

exercise for concentrating the heart　A static exercise, marked by staying silently in a quiet room; maintaining the original pure character without any desires, thought, vision, and listening; keeping the spirit quiet without any external change, internal change, deviation, confusion and attempt. Only when all parts in the body are pure and tranquil can the heart be clear and the eyes be bright.

冥心绝想【míng xīn jué xiǎng】　指习练气功时，意守虚无，保持精神意识活动相对静止的状态。

vacuum trance　Refers to vacuuming consciousness, tranquilizing the activities of the spirit and consciousness in practicing Qigong.

瞑目【míng mù】　即闭目，为习练气功的一个重要功法。

closing the eyes　One of the important ways to practice Qigong.

瞑目观容【míng mù guān róng】　指闭目内视自己的容貌，为汉时练功的方法。

closing the eyes with inspection　Refers to inward vision of oneself features after closing the eyes, which is an exercise for practicing Qigong.

瞑目则至【míng mù zé zhì】　指习练气功，闭目静候则气自至，神光自然而来。

acme of closing the eyes　Indicates that Qi has reached the acme of perfection and spiritual brightness has naturally arrived when the eyes are closed and the mind is tranquilized in practicing Qigong.

命功【mìng gōng】　调节呼吸为主的功法。

life exercise　Refers to the exercise mainly for regulating respiration.

命窟【mìng kū】　指脑。

life cave　Refers to the brain.

命门【mìng mén】　① 指下丹田；② 指脐；③ 指肾；④ 指眼睛；⑤ 指右肾；⑥ 为经穴名；⑦ 为石门穴的别名。

life gate　Refers to ① either the lower Dantian（the region below the nave）; ② or the navel; ③ or the kidney; ④ or the eyes; ⑤ or the right kidney; ⑥ or the name of an acupoint known as Mingmen（GV 4）, which is an acupoint in the governor meridian; ⑦ or a synonym of Shimen（CV 5）, which is an acupoint in the conception meridian.

命门火【mìng mén huǒ】　即肾阳，为

M

生命本元之火，寓于肾阴之中，有温养五脏六腑之功能。

life gate fire Refers to kidney Yang which is the fire in the origin of life, also containing in kidney Yin, effectively warming and nourishing the five Zang-organs (including the heart, the liver, the spleen, the lung and the kidney) and the six Fu-organs (including the gallbladder, the stomach, the small intestine, the large intestine, the bladder and the triple energizer).

命之蒂【mìng zhī dì】 指脐。

pedicel of life Refers to the navel.

命宗【mìng zōng】 指习练气功时呼吸为主的气功流派。

life school Refers to a school of Qigong characterized by paying great attention to regulation of respiration, taking it as the priority in studying and practicing Qigong.

摩腹【mó fù】 为动功，指经常按摩腹部，能健脾胃，帮助消化，防治水谷积滞不化。为内伤调中之法。

rubbing the abdomen A dynamic exercise, marked by rubbing the abdomen for fortifying the spleen and stomach, digesting food, preventing and curing indigestion of food. Such a dynamic exercise is for curing internal damage and regulating the middle.

摩火养神【mó huǒ yǎng shén】 指温养肾阳，能以生神养神。

rubbing fire for nourishing the spirit Refers to warming and nourishing kidney Yang as well as promoting the spirit and nourishing the spirit.

摩目【mó mù】 为动功，即用手指或手掌擦热候揉摩两眼，明目去翳。

rubbing eyes A dynamic exercise, referring to rubbing the fingers or fists hot for kneading the eyes in order to improve the eyesight and eliminate nebula.

摩手熨目法【mó shǒu yùn mù fǎ】 为动功，即两手侧立摩掌如火，开目熨睛数遍，能明目，祛风，不生障翳，亦能补肾气。

exercise for rubbing the hands and warming the eyes A dynamic exercise, marked by raising the hands at lateral sides to rub the fists like fire, opening and warming the eyes for several times to improve the eyesight, expelling wind and nebula. Such a dynamic exercise can tonify kidney Qi.

摩眼【mó yǎn】 熨目的另外一个称谓，为动功，指经常按摩腹部，能健脾胃，帮助消化，防治水谷积滞不化。为内伤调中之法。

ocular rubbing A synonym of rubbing the abdomen, is a dynamic exercise, marked by rubbing the abdomen for fortifying the spleen and stomach, digesting food, preventing and curing indigestion. Such a dynamic exercise is for curing internal damage and regulating the middle.

魔【mó】 即入魔。指损伤情志的行为，影响气功入静的杂念及虚妄的景象。

demon The same as entering demon, referring to either the activity that damages emotion; or distracting thought that affects tranquility in practice of Qigong; or image of fabrication.

莫若啬【mò ruò sè】 指修身治国，当爱惜精神，积蓄力量。

difference from stinginess Refers to treasuring the spirit and accumulating the energy in cultivating the body and ruling the country.

莫向天边寻子午，身中自有一阳生

【mò xiàng tiān biān xún zǐ wǔ shēn zhōng zì yǒu yī yáng shēng】 强调说明行功时意念的专一，胜过于行功时辰的选择。

Don't look for Zi and Wu in the horizon because there is Yang produced in the Body. Emphasizes the importance of single-minded consciousness in practicing Qigong, which is better than the periods of time selected for practicing Qigong.

漠虚静【mò xū jìng】 指形神稳定状态。

calmness and quietness Refers to stability of the body and the spirit.

墨子行气法【mò zǐ xíng qì fǎ】 为静功，其作法为，调身、调气、调神。调身时，取自然坐式或仰卧式，作好功前准备，如宽衣解带，先行大小便等；调气时，坐定或卧好后即可行功，先嗽津咽液三至五次；调神时，行气之先，即当安其身，不与意争，常守勿倦。

Mo Zi's exercise for moving Qi A static exercise for regulating the body, Qi and spirit, marked by naturally sitting or lying on the back for regulating the body and well preparing the practice of Qigong, such as taking off coat, untying belt and finishing defecation and urination; sitting quietly or lying quietly for regulating Qi, rinsing fluid and swallowing humor first for three or five times; stabilizing the body before moving Qi for regulating the spirit, avoiding struggle against consciousness and often keeping the spirit without any fatigue.

默存【mò cún】 指默想存念，内守精神。

contemplation Refers to silent thinking as a keepsake for concentrating the spirit.

默默【mò mò】 指恍惚，即弹之极也。

silence Refers to integrated state of the spirit and body.

母玄父元【mǔ xuán fù yuán】 指父精母血之意。

maternal abstruseness and paternal origin Refers to the paternal sperm and the maternal blood.

木并金【mù bìng jīn】 指身体内阴阳两个方面，即气功产药、作丹的基本物质。

wood with metal Refers to Yin and Yang in the human body, the primary substance of Qigong in producing medicinal and Dan (pills of immortality).

木朝元【mù cháo yuán】 指五脏之气上朝天元。

wood leading to origin Refers to Qi from the five Zang-organs (including the heart, the liver, the spleen, the lung and the kidney) that flows up to the celestial origin.

木火位侣【mù huǒ wèi lǚ】 木为肝，火为心，五行为木生火，子母相生，指肝心相互作用，混融为一。

interaction of wood and fire Wood refers to the liver and fire refers to the heart. Among the five elements (including wood, fire, earth, metal and water), wood produces fire like interaction between child and mother, indicating the interaction and integration of the liver and heart.

木火刑金【mù huǒ xíng jīn】 指五行学说用以阐释五脏病变相互影响的一种。

wood and fire impairing metal Refers to one way to explain the pathological changes of the five Zang-organs (including the heart, the liver, the spleen, the lung and the kidney) according to the five elements (including wood, fire, earth, metal and water).

木金【mù jīn】 五行之木、金二行,文中木金即指肝、肺二脏。

wood and metal Refer to the movement of wood and metal among the five elements(including wood, fire, earth, metal and water), referring to the liver and lung in traditional Chinese medicine.

木金间隔【mù jīn jiàn gé】 木为肝,金为肺,指肝、肺为阴阳两个不同的方面。

differentiation of wood and metal Wood refers to the liver and metal refers to the lung, indicating that the liver and the lung refer to the two different sides of Yin and Yang.

木位【mù wèi】 运气术语,风木所主之位。

wood direction A term of Qigong practice, referring to the location of wind wood.

木性金情配合【mù xìng jīn qíng pèi hé】 性在肝属木,情在肺属金,木性爱金,金情恋木,金木和合,肺肝协调。

combination of wood and metal The liver pertains to wood and the lung pertains to metal. Wood loves metal and metal loves wood. Integration of wood and metal indicates regulation of the lung and the liver.

木运【mù yùn】 运气术语,为五运之一。

wood motion A term of Qigong prac-

tice, referring to one of the five movements (including wood, fire, earth, metal and water).

木运临卯【mù yùn lín mǎo】 运气术语。丁为木运,卯为木的正位,即丁卯年为岁会。

action of wood to Mao (**the period of a day from 5 a. m. to 7 a. m. in the morning**) A term of Qigong. Wood movement is related to Ding and the position of wood is related to Mao, indicating that Ding Mao year is the summarization of a whole year among the sixty years.

目暗不明候导引法【mù àn bù míng hòu dǎo yǐn fǎ】 为动功,方法多样。如蹲下如坐,用两手搬起两脚的五趾,尽力低头,使五脏之气皆上至头。明目聪耳,治耳聋,视物不明。

exercise of Daoyin for blurred vision A dynamic exercise with various methods, such as squatting like sitting with both hands holding all the toes, lowering the head and promoting Qi from the five Zang-organs to flow up to the head. Such a way of practice will improve the sight and hearing and relieve deafness and blurred vision.

目胞【mù bāo】 指眼睑,遮盖在眼球的前方。

eyelid Located in front of the eyeball.

目风泪出候导引法【mù fēng lèi chū hòu dǎo yǐn fǎ】 为动功,方法很多。如两足底和臀部着地,两膝上耸而坐,伸右脚,两手抱左膝盖,伸直腰,用鼻吸气至极限,然后慢慢呼于出,作七息,利关节,通经络,治下肢难以屈伸,起坐困难,小腿麻木疼痛,迎风流泪,耳聋。

exercise of Daoyin for treating wind and tear in the eyes A dynamic exercise with various methods, such as touching the ground with the soles and buttocks, sitting with the knees turning up, stretching the right foot, holding the knees with both hands, strengthening the waist, inhaling with the nose to the extremity, slowly exhaling for seven times in order to disinhibit the joints, unobstructing the meridians and collaterals. Such a dynamic exercise can relieve stiffness of the legs, difficulty in sitting, numbness and pain of the shanks as well as tearing and deafness when facing wind.

目风内出【mù fēng nèi chū】　气功适应证，由肝肾两虚，经穴耗散所致。

epiphora due to wind　An indication of Qigong practice, usually caused by deficiency of the liver and the kidney and dissipation of acupoints in the meridians.

目功【mù gōng】　为动功。其作法为，每睡醒且勿开目，用大两指背相合擦热，揩目十四次，转眼珠左右七次，紧闭少时，忽大睁开。

eye exercise　A dynamic exercise, marked by closing the eyes after waking up, wiping the dorsum warm with both thumbs, wiping the eyes for fourteen times, returning the eyeballs for seen times, tightly closing the eyes for a short period of time and then suddenly opening the eyes.

目髎【mù liáo】　手少阳三焦经中丝竹空穴位的别称，位于眉毛外侧段凹陷处。这一穴位为气功运行的一个常见部位。

Muliao　A synonym of Sizhukong (TE 23) which is an acupoint in the triple energizer meridian of hand Shaoyang, also called Juliao or Muliao, located in the lateral depression of the eyebrow. This acupoint is a region usually used for keeping the essential Qi in practice of Qigong.

目内眦【mù nèi zì】　即内眼角，位上下眼睑于鼻侧连接部，是足太阳膀胱经的起点。

inner canthus　Located between the upper and lower eyelids connected with the nasal side, which is the origin of the bladder meridian of foot Taiyang.

目青盲【mù qīng máng】　气功适应证，本病多因五脏六腑的精气不能上荣目系所致。

blue blindness　An indication of Qigong practice, usually caused by failure of essence and Qi from the five Zang-organs (including the heart, the liver, the spleen, the lung and the kidney) and six Fu-organs (including the gallbladder, the stomach, the small intestine, the large intestine, the bladder and the triple energizer) to flow to the ocular systems.

目听【mù tīng】　即目能听见声音。指练气功后出现的特异功能。

ocular listening　Means that the eyes can hear certain sound, which is an extrasensory perception and psychokinetic power in practicing Qigong.

目外眦【mù wài zì】　即小眦。

outer canthus　Located in the region connected with the lower eyelid and temple.

目为神候【mù wéi shén hòu】　指目能反映人体内在的精神意识活动。

eye as spiritual emotion　Refers to the fact that the eyes can reflect the activities of the spirit and consciousness.

沐浴【mù yù】　①指清静安神；②指

行动中调节意识思维活动；③ 指行动中吞津咽液，溉润脏腑；④ 指习练气功，平秘阴阳。

bathing Means several manifestations in practicing Qigong, referring to ① either tranquilization of the spirit; ② or regulation of the activities related to consciousness and thought; ③ or taking fluid and swallowing saliva in practicing Qigong in order to moisten the five Zang-organs（including the heart，the liver，the spleen，the lung and the kidney）and the six Fu-organs（including the gallbladder，the stomach，the small intestine，the large intestine，the bladder and the triple energizer）；④ or harmonization of Yin and Yang in practicing Qigong.

沐浴法【mù yù fǎ】 动静相兼功，方法多样。其作法为，① 静心调气：静心于室内，端身正坐，先调其气；② 按摩导引：以左右手搓令热摩面，然后起立，左右手叉之，翻掌向上过顶上托于天，足尽力踏地，耸身；③ 调五脏气：先补其肝，想肝之中有青龙盘旋并青龙之目有光，从我之目出，乃出嘘之气，咽嘘之气皆九过；④ 收功，开合双目，鸣天鼓左三右四，按摩肾区，左三右四。

exercise for bath An exercise combined with dynamic exercise and static exercise with various methods，marked by ① sitting upright in the room and regulating Qi first in order to tranquilize the heart and regulate Qi; ② rubbing the hands hot for kneading the face，then standing up，crossing both hands，turning the palms upwards to the top，treading the ground with the feet and jumping up the body in order to practice Daoyin by rubbing; ③ tonifying the liver first，imagining a blue Loong in the liver spiraling up with ocular brightness through the eyes，breathing out Qi and swallowing Qi for nine times respectively in order to regulate Qi from the five Zang-organs（including the heart，the liver，the spleen，the lung and the kidney）；④ opening the eyes，sounding the celestial drum（rubbing the occipital）for three times at the left side and for four times at the right side，kneading the kidney region for three times at the left side and for four times at the right side at the end of practice.

沐浴之功【mù yù zhī gōng】 即子午卯寅，源自气功专论，主要阐述子为六阳之首，阴极阳生之时；午为六阴之首，阳极阴生之时；卯寅二时，为心肾二气交分之时。阐明四时，在练功中的地位。

function of bath The same as discussion of Zi，Wu，Mao and Yin，is collected from a monograph of Qigong，mainly describing that Zi（the period of the day from 11 p.m. to 1 a.m.）is the first position of the six kinds of Yang and the time when Yin has developed to the extremity and Yang has grown; that Wu（the period of the day from 11 a.m. to 1 p.m. in the noon）is the first position of the six kinds of Yin and the time when Yang has developed to the extremity and Yin has grown; that Yin（the period of the day from 3 a.m. to 5 a.m. in the early morning），Mao（the period of the day from 5 a.m. to 7 a.m. in the morning）are the first time when Qi from the heart and the kidney begins to coordinate with each other. These four periods are the states for practicing Qigong.

牧宫【mù gōng】 指五脏中的肾。

herd chamber Refers to the kidney in the five Zang-organs (including the heart, the liver, the spleen, the lung and the kidney).

M

N

纳甲说【nà jiǎ shuō】 源自气功专论，主要阐述乾坤往复、阴阳变化作用。

idea of receiving Jia Collected from a monograph of Qigong, mainly describing going out and coming in of Qian (Trigram) and Kun (Trigram), indicating to change the effect of Yin and Yang.

纳律法【nà lǜ fǎ】 为静功。其作法为，正坐，以舌柱上腭，觉口内外液自生，漱满咽会神口，存念心下有一孩，开口方致之。

exercise of receiving law A static exercise, marked by sitting upright, holding the upper jaw with the tongue, feeling production of internal and external humor in the mouth, rinsing the mouth and pharynx with spirit, imagining embryo in the heart and opening the mouth to devote it.

捺耳窍【nà ěr qiào】 为动功，指按捺并摇动耳窍，可去邪保聪，治耳鸣、耳聋。

exercise for pressing the ears A dynamic exercise, referring to pressing and shaking the ears to expel evils, to keep wisdom and to cure tinnitus and deafness.

南北宗【nán běi zōng】 指道家气功影响深远的两大宗派。

south and north schools Refer to two important schools of Qigong in Daoism.

南方不以意思意【nán fāng bù yǐ yì si yì】 指意识思维活动和畅于起念之前，慧发于忘知之后。

It is not to contemplate consciousness with consciousness in the south. Indicates that the activities of consciousness and thought start before thinking and wisdom increases after being tranquilized.

南宫岩守炉鼎【nán gōng yán shǒu lú dǐng】 为静功。其作法为，正身端坐，凝神入静。精神身体端正后，炉鼎（阴阳）自坚牢。治失眠、多梦、梦游等。

keeping furnace and cauldron with stone in south palace A static exercise, marked by sitting upright, concentrating the spirit and tranquilizing the mind. When the spirit and body are normalized, the furnace and cauldron (Yin and Yang) will be straightened. This way of practice can cure insomnia, dreaminess and sleepwalking.

南华真经【nán huá zhēn jīng】 战国时期的哲学家和气功学家庄子的另外一个称谓。

Nanhua Zhenjing Another name of Zhuang Zi, a great philosopher and a great master of Qigong in the Warring States Period (475 BC - 221 BC).

南华真人【nán huá zhēn rén】 战国时期的哲学家和气功学家庄子的另外一个称谓。

Nanhua Zhenren Another name of Zhuang Zi, a great philosopher and a great master of Qigong in the Warring States Period (475 BC - 221 BC).

南柯子【nán kē zǐ】　源自气功专论，描述习练静功的基本方法。

Nan Kezi　Collected from a monograph of Qigong, describing the basic methods for practicing static exercise.

南离【nán lí】　指心脏。习练气功，取坎中之阳，补离中之阴。气功学中，坎指肾，离指心。

South Li（Trigram）　Refers to the heart. In practicing Qigong, Yang from Kan（Trigram）tonifies Yin in Li（Trigram）. In Qigong, Kan（Trigram）refers to the kidney and Li（Trigram）refers to the heart.

南山【nán shān】　终南山之别称，为秦岭主峰之一，相传为全真派北五祖中的吕洞宾、刘海蟾修炼之处。

South Mountain　A synonym of Zhongnan Mountain in Shaanxi Province where Lǚ Dongbin and Zhang Haichan, two important immortals in ancient China and founder of entire genuine school, practiced Qigong.

南五祖【nán wǔ zǔ】　指全真派张伯端、石泰、薛道光、陈楠、白玉蟾五位祖师。

five ancestors in the south　Refers to the five ancestors of entire genuine school, including Zhang Boduan, Shi Tai, Xue Daoguang, Chen Nan and Bai Yuchan.

南宗内丹【nán zōng nèi dān】　指南宗气功养生法。

internal Dan（pills of immortality）in south school　Refers to the exercise for cultivating life in the south school of Qigong.

难禅【nán chán】　佛家气功功法，即久习胜妙之禅定，于诸三昧，心得自在，哀愍众生，欲使成熟，故舍第一禅之东而生于欲界。依禅而出生无量无数不可思议之诸深三昧。依禅而得无上菩提。

difficult dhyana　An exercise of Qigong in Buddhism, marked by long time well practice according to the dhyana meditation with samadhi for commiserating all the people, and reaching the realms of desire after abandoning the first dhyana in the east in order to mature oneself; then producing innumerable and inconceivable Samadhi based on dhyana; finally obtaining supreme Bodhi based on dhyana.

脑【nǎo】　① 指脑的生成；② 指脑在人体之上部；③ 指脑内有九宫；④ 指脑为髓之海；⑤ 指人有七窍权归脑；⑥ 指脑主神明；⑦ 指脑主感觉和知觉；⑧ 指脑与全身各部相连；⑨ 指脑藏五脏神及全身各部神；⑩ 指脑调节五脏六腑的而功能；⑪ 指脑与心神通；⑫ 指脑实则神全。

brain　Refers to ① either the production of the brain; ② or the brain locates in the upper side of the body; ③ or the nine palaces in the brain; ④ or the sea of marrow; ⑤ or the source of seven orifices; ⑥ or the brain controlling overall spirituality; ⑦ or the brain responsible for sensation and consciousness; ⑧ or the brain connected with all parts of the body; ⑨ or the brain storing the spirit from five Zang-organs（including the heart, the liver, the spleen, the lung and the kidney）and the six Fu-organs（the gallbladder, stomach, small intestine, large intestine, bladder and triple energizer）as well as all parts of the body; ⑩ or the brain regulating the functions of the five Zang-organs and the six Fu-organs；⑪ or the brain and combined with the heart spirit；⑫ or the perfection of the spirit due to reality of the brain.

脑发相扶【nǎo fā xiāng fú】 指胆神与脑、发相通。

hair manifesting the brain Means that the spirit in the gallbladder communicates with the brain and hair.

脑风【nǎo fēng】 属头风，症见项背寒，脑户极冷，剧痛。

brain wind Refers to wind head syndrome / pattern characterized by coldness and sharp pain of the neck, back and brain.

脑宫【nǎo gōng】 指脑神所居之宫。

brain palace Refers to the region where the brain spirit is stored.

脑户【nǎo hù】 督脉中的一个穴位，位于枕骨粗隆上缘之凹陷处，为气功中常用的意守部位。

Naohu（GV 17） An acupoint in the governor meridian, located in the depression on the upper border of the external occipital protuberance, which is the region for concentrating consciousness in practicing Qigong.

脑减则发素【nǎo jiǎn zé fà sù】 指脑气不足，精血亏损，则头发变白。

brain deficiency causing white hair Means that insufficiency of Qi in the brain and depletion and detriment of the essence and blood make the hair white.

脑渐空【nǎo jiàn kōng】 指脑随着年龄的增加，脑功能逐渐衰退。

gradual decaying of the brain Indicates that the brain gradually declines with the increasing of age.

脑潜于阴【nǎo qián yú yīn】 指阳中有阴，脑中生真阴。

the brain concealing in Yin Means that there is Yin within Yang and so there is genuine Yin in the brain.

脑清脑浊【nǎo qīng nǎo zhuó】 指脑清静则智慧生，脑浊乱则愚钝出。

clear brain and turbid brain Indicates that wisdom and intelligence exist when the brain is clear and tranquil, while stupidity and obtuseness appear when the brain is turbid and chaotic.

脑散动觉之气【nǎo sàn dòng jué zhī qì】 源自气功专论，阐述脑的组织结构、生理功能，脑与全身各部的联系。

movement of the brain promoting the flow of Qi Collected from a monograph of Qigong, describing the structure and physiological functions of the brain, indicating the communication of the brain with all parts of the body.

脑神【nǎo shén】 指头中之神，居头之中央。

brain spirit Refers to the spirit in the center of the brain.

脑神精根字泥丸【nǎo shén jīng gēn zì ní wán】 指脑神为精根，字泥丸，精根即阴阳之根。

The brain spirit is the essential root and the manifestation of the mud bolus（the brain）. Indicates that the brain spirit is the essential root and the essential root is the root of Yin and Yang.

脑生细微动觉之气【nǎo shēng xì wēi dòng jué zhī qì】 指脑是运动、感觉、知觉之本根。

The brain produces the subtle and active Qi. Indicates that the brain is the original root of movement, sensation and consciousness.

脑实神全【nǎo shí shén quán】 指脑

及脑髓充盈,精神饱满,意识思维活动健全。

perfection of the spirit with reality of the brain Refers to exuberance of the brain and brain marrow, fullness of the essence and spirit, and perfect activities of consciousness and thought.

脑髓生【nǎo suǐ shēng】 指脑髓为精所生,是精的生长发展。

generation of brain marrow Means that the marrow in the brain is produced by the essence, indicating the development of the essence.

脑为贵【nǎo wéi guì】 指脑为身之元首,为万神汇集之都,主意识思维活动,是全身各部之主,生命之根本。

importance of the brain Indicates that the brain is the original source of the human body, the region with the collection of all the spirits and the root of life that controls the activities of consciousness and thought as well as all parts of the body.

脑为髓海真气之所聚【nǎo wéi suǐ hǎi zhēn qì zhī suǒ jù】 指脑主髓而为之海,是一身真气汇集的处所。

The brain is the combination of marrow sea and genuine Qi. Indicates that brain controls the sea of marrow and is the region to store the genuine Qi in the whole body.

脑为髓之海【nǎo wéi suǐ zhī hǎi】 源自气功专论,阐述脑与髓的联系,说明脑与全身各部有细络相通。

The brain is the sea of marrow. This sentence is collected from a monograph of Qigong, describing the relation between the brain and marrow, indicating that the brain thoroughly communicates with all parts of the body.

脑为一身之灵【nǎo wéi yì shēn zhī líng】 指脑为神之舍,一身之灵根。

The brain is the soul in the whole body. Indicates that the brain is the source of the spirit and the root of the whole body.

脑为元神之府【nǎo wéi yuán shén zhī fǔ】 指脑主意识思维活动,是记忆产生的地方。

brain as the palace of the original spirit Means that the brain controls the activities of consciousness and thought and is the foundation of memory.

脑血之琼房【nǎo xuè zhī qióng fáng】 指脑内元神所居之宫。

fine chamber of brain blood Refers to the chamber in the brain that stores the original spirit.

脑与周身连系【nǎo yǔ zhōu shēn lián xì】 指脑与全身各部相连系。

brain connected with the whole body Means that the brain communicates with all parts of the body.

脑中九房【nǎo zhōng jiǔ fáng】 指脑的内部结构,谓脑中有九室,为脑神归藏之所。

nine chambers in the brain Refers to structure of the brain, in which there are nine regions to store the spirit in the brain.

脑转目眩【nǎo zhuǎn mù xuàn】 气功适应证,指脑神为自然和社会心理因素的干扰、躁动不宁则头目昏眩。

vertigo and blurred vision An indication of Qigong, referring to the brain spirit disturbed by the natural, social and psychological factors that cause vertigo, and blurred vision due to dysphoria.

臑骨【nào gǔ】 指肱骨,是上肢最粗壮的骨。

forelimb bone Refers to humerus, which is the strongest bone in the upper limbs.

内安其神,内去其欲【nèi ān qí shén nèi qù qí yù】　其意有二,一是要安定精神,保持情志活动的正常;二是生活上要节制欲念。

internally tranquilizing the spirit and externally eliminating craving A celebrated dictum, referring to the fact that only when the spirit is stabilized can the emotional activity be normal and that only when the mind is tranquilized can desires be controlled.

内丹【nèi dān】　"气能存生,内丹也。药能固形,外丹也。"即内丹与外丹相对。

internal Dan (pills of immortality) Internal Dan (pills of immortality) refers to Qi that can protect life and external Dan (pills of immortality) refers to medicinals that can strengthen the body.

内丹大道【nèi dān dà dào】　为静功。常使精、气、神内三宝不逐物而游,耳、目、口外三宝不透中而扰。

great way for internal Dan (pills of immortality) A static exercise, referring to constantly promoting the essence, Qi and the spirit as well as protecting the ears, the eyes and the mouth.

内丹说【nèi dān shuō】　源自气功专论,阐述"内丹之说,不过心肾交会,精气搬运,存神闭息,吐故纳新"。

discussion about internal Dan (pills of immortality) Collected from a monograph of Qigong, mainly describing the idea of internal Dan (pills of immortality) related to combination of the heart and the kidney as well as transportation of the essence and Qi.

内丹之基【nèi dān zhī jī】　"生于肾中,以育元精,补续元气,续续不耗,日益月强。"指内丹修炼中,神与气合为内丹之基础。

foundation of internal Dan (pills of immortality) Refers to coordination of the spirit and Qi in practicing Qigong based on the kidney for nourishing the original essence, replenishing original Qi and strengthening the body. This term indicates that the combination of the spirit and Qi is the foundation for refining the internal Dan (pills of immortality).

内丹之术【nèi dān zhī shù】　指练气功时要静心、养气、提神、健身。

skills for internal Dan (pills of immortality) Refers to the skills of Qigong practice for tranquilizing the heart, nourishing Qi, increasing the spirit and cultivating health.

内德【nèi dé】　指脏腑、筋骨、血肉之象。

internal stability Refers to the manifestations of the five Zang-organs (including the heart, the liver, the spleen, the lung and the kidney) and the six Fu-organs (including the gallbladder, the stomach, the small intestine, the large intestine, the bladder and the triple energizer), the sinews, the bones, the blood and the muscles.

内鼎外鼎【nèi dǐng wài dǐng】　指内鼎为丹田中之气;外鼎为丹田之形。

internal cauldron and external cauldron Refers to the fact that the so-called internal cauldron refers to Qi in Dantian while the so-called external cauldron refers to the form of Dantian.

Dantian is divided into the upper Dantian (the region between the eyes), the middle Dantian (the region below the heart) and the lower Dantian (the region below the navel).

内府【nèi fǔ】　指人体内胆、胃、大肠、小肠、膀胱、三焦六府。

internal fu-organs　Refers to the gallbladder, stomach, large intestine, small intestine, bladder and triple energizer.

内功【nèi gōng】　指习练气功，练精气神，结丹于内，强壮身体，不露形貌。

internal strength　Refers to strengthening the body and showing no styles in practicing Qigong and refining the essence, Qi and the spirit.

内功图说【nèi gōng tú shuō】　《内功图说》为气功专著，清代王祖源著。

Neigong Tushuo (*Explanation About Internal Qigong with Pictures*)　A monograph of Qigong entitled *Explanation About Internal Qigong with Pictures*, written by Wang Zuyuan in the Qing Dynasty (1636 AD‐1912 AD).

内关【nèi guān】　是手厥阴心包经的一个穴位，位于腕横纹 2 寸，为气功学重要体表标志之一。

Neiguan (**PC 6**)　An acupoint in the pericardium meridian of hand Jueyin, located 2 Cun to the rasceta, which is one of the important symbols in Qigong.

内观【nèi guān】　① 指精神内守而逐步稳定；② 指精神内守而两目内视。

internal view　Refers to either keeping the spirit inside for stabilizing the body; or keeping the spirit inside to observe the internal with both eyes.

内观存想【nèi guān cún xiǎng】　练功时，心中存想一形象，而使心不狂而意不乱，而神识自住，属于调神的方法。

vipassana with imagination　Refers to keeping a concentrated imagination in the heart in order to tranquilize the heart and the mind, which is a good method to regulate the spirit.

内观坐忘【nèi guān zuò wàng】　指绝念无想，真空一境，然后入恍惚之境。

vipassana with vacuum　Refers to no special thought and idea in the mind in order to completely tranquilize the mind and the heart.

内呼吸【nèi hū xī】　指身体内阴阳和平，自呼自吸，一开一阖，息息、归根。

internal respiration　Refers to harmonization of Yin and Yang as well as normal inhalation and exhalation of Yin and Yang in the body.

内踝【nèi huái】　即胫骨下端向内之夹起处。

malleolus medialis　Located in the lower part and the inner side of the tibia.

内楗【nèi jiàn】　指关门，内不出，外不入。

internal closure　Refers to keeping the healthy Qi inside in order to avoid invasion of pathogenic factors.

内交真气【nèi jiāo zhēn qì】　指胎息妙疑，内气不出，外气不入的宁谧呼吸状态。

internal maintenance of genuine Qi　Refers to practice of fetal respiration in order to prevent internal Qi flowing externally and external Qi flowing internally.

内界【nèi jiè】　佛家气功习用语，① 指精神活动为内界；② 指六识界为内界。

internal state　A common term of Qigong in Buddhism, referring to ① either the spirit activity in the internal; ② or the sixth state of consciousness in the internal.

内境【nèi jìng】 ① 指内脏及腑生理功能、病理变化；② 指思维活动内向，以意存观脏腑组织。

intrinsic manifestation Refers to ① either physiological functions and pathological changes of the five Zang-organs (including the heart, the liver, the spleen, the lung and the kidney) and the six Fu-organs (including the gallbladder, the stomach, the small intestine, the large intestine, the bladder and the triple energizer); ② or spiritual observation of the five Zang-organs and the six Fu-organs through the activity of consciousness.

内炼法【nèi liàn fǎ】 为静功。其作法为，以目视鼻，以鼻对脐，降心火入于气海。

internal exercise method A static exercise, marked by seeing the nose with the eyes, aligning the navel with the nose and descending heart fire into Qihai (the sea of Qi) which is an acupoint located below the navel.

内练功【nèi liàn gōng】 为静功。其作法为，入室端坐，澄心静虑，息调气定，寂然良久。

internal exercise A static exercise, marked by sitting in the house quietly to tranquilize the mind, to regulate respiration and to keep silent for a long time.

内魔障【nèi mó zhàng】 指习练气功时，杂念从内而生（非外感而来），影响入静。

internal obstruction Refers to appearance of distracting thoughts in practi-

cing Qigong, making it difficult to tranquilize the mind.

内气洗身【nèi qì xǐ shēn】 指用意念引吸入之气洗去身上之污浊邪气。

internal Qi bathing body Refers to washing foul pathogenic factors in the body by absorbing Qi through the mind.

内遣三害【nèi qiǎn sān hài】 指邪念、烦恼、填恚。此三害，均有碍于调神。

internal elimination of three obstacles Refers to evil thought, annoyance and anger which all affect the regulation of the spirit.

内热【nèi rè】 ① 指内热所致之病；② 指烦躁体内闷热。

internal heat Refers to ① either a disease caused by internal heat; ② or stuffiness due to irritability.

内三宝【nèi sān bǎo】 指精、气、神。

three internal essences Refers to the essence, Qi and the spirit.

内三要【nèi sān yào】 主要指头、心、肾。

three internal essentials Mainly refers to the head, the heart and the kidney.

内三要论【nèi sān yào lùn】 源自气功专论，主要阐述头、心、命门在气功修炼中的重要作用。

discussion about three internal essentials Collected from a monograph of Qigong, mainly describing the importance of the head, the heart and the life gate in practicing Qigong.

内视【nèi shì】 习练气功时，意识活动使目光注视身体某个部分，如心、肝、肾等。只是意视，并非眼的视线达到内在脏腑。

internal vision Refers to enabling the eyes to look at certain organs inside the body (such as the heart, the liver and the kidney) mentally, not visually, in practicing Qigong in order to tranquilize the mind. Such a exercise of Qigong practice is just mentally observation, not really reaching the eyesight into the five Zang-organs (including the heart, the liver, the spleen, the lung and the kidney) and the six Fu-organs (including the gallbladder, the stomach, the small intestine, the large intestine, the bladder and the triple energizer).

内视返听【nèi shì fǎn tīng】 指习练气功时,意识(不是眼睛)向内而视脏腑、听声音。目的守神于内,不使外越。

intrinsic inspection and listening Refers to consciousness (not the eyes) that observes the five Zang-organs (including the heart, the liver, the spleen, the lung and the kidney) and the six Fu-organs (including the gallbladder, the stomach, the small intestine, the large intestine, the bladder and the triple energizer), and listens to sound inside the body. Such a practice of Qigong can keep the spirit inside and prevent it flowing outwards.

内守【nèi shǒu】 指守精于内而不泄,守神于舍而不散。

internal concentration Refers to constantly keeping the spirit inside and avoiding the spirit to leak.

内胎【nèi tāi】 佛家气功习用语,指头脑。

internal fetus A common term of Qigong in Buddhism, referring to the brain.

内调气法【nèi tiáo qì fǎ】 指行吐故纳新调气法,渐习至千息。

method for intrinsic regulation of Qi Refers to gradually getting rid of the stale and taking in the fresh.

内外八卦【nèi wài bā guà】 指头为乾,足为坤,膀胱为艮,胆为巽,肾为坎,心为离,肝为震,肺为兑。

eight internal and external Trigrams Refers to the fact that the head pertains to Qian Trigram, the foot pertains to Kun Trigram, the bladder pertains to Gen Trigram, the gallbladder pertains to Xun Trigram, the kidney pertains to Kan Trigram, the heart pertains to Li Trigram, the liver pertains to Trigram, the lung pertains to Dui Trigram.

内外大药【nèi wài dà yào】 源自气功专论,主要阐述虽有内、外、大、药之名,都是由神、气、精锻炼而得。

internal and external big medicinals Collected from a monograph of Qigong, describing the fact that the so-called internal and external big medicinal are all obtained by the essence, Qi and the spirit in practicing Qigong.

内外丹【nèi wài dān】 ① 指炼精气神为内丹,炼五金八石为外丹;② 指习练精气神,均可称为内外丹。

internal and external Dan (pills of immortality) Refers to either tempering the essence, Qi and the spirit as the internal Dan (pills of immortality), and tempering the five kinds of metals and eight kinds of stones as the external Dan (pills of immortality); or tempering the essence, Qi and the spirit all known as the internal Dan (pills of immortality) and the external Dan (pills of immortality).

内外丹论【nèi wài dān lùn】 源自气功专论,主要阐述内外丹的修炼。

discussion about internal and external Dan (pills of immortality) Collected from a monograph of Qiong, mainly describing the principles, rules and methods about how to practice Qigong through flourishing the essence in the internal and the external.

内外金浆【nèi wài jīn jiāng】 指漱咽之津液为内金浆,坚持"养神明,补元气""固形体,坚脏腑"。

internal and external golden plasma Refers to fluid and humor in the saliva that nourish the spirit, tonify the original Qi, strengthen the body and protect the the five Zang-organs (including the heart, the liver, the spleen, the lung and the kidney) and the six Fu-organs (including the gallbladder, the stomach, the small intestine, the large intestine, the bladder and the triple energizer).

内外六入【nèi wài liù rù】 佛家气功习用语,① 指眼、耳、鼻、舌、身、意六根,为内之六入,从内引起相应的意识思维活动;② 指色、声、香、味、触六境,为外之六入,因外而入内,引起相应的意识思维活动。

six internal and external entrances A common term of Qigong in Buddhism, refer to ① either the six roots like the eyes, the ears, the nose, the tongue, the body and the mind that start the activities of consciousness and thinking; ② or the six states like color, sound, fragrance, taste, external and internal states that start the activities of consciousness and thinking.

内象【nèi xiàng】 指脏腑、筋骨、血肉之象。

intrinsic demonstration A term of Qigong, refers to the manifestations of the viscera, sinews, bones, blood and muscles.

内心【nèi xīn】 ① 指思维意识活动;② 指用意于内。

internal heart Refers to ① mental activity; ② also refers to consciousness inside.

内省端操【nèi xǐng duān cāo】 指内自思量审察,以调节意识思维活动,端正行为。

upright practice with introspection Refers to internal thinking and investigating in order to regulate the activities of consciousness and thinking and to normalize the physical activities.

内修形神【nèi xiū xíng shén】 指内调神形,使之合而为一。

somatic and spiritual integration Refers to internal regulation of the spirit and the body in order to integrate with each other.

内阳三神【nèi yáng sān shén】 指内阳为乾首,三神指三丹田之神。喻脑神。

internal Yang and three spirits Refers to the spirit in the three kinds of Dantian, which is compared to the celebral spirit. Dantian is divided into the upper Dantian (the region between the eyes), the middle Dantian (the region below the heart) and the lower Dantian (the region below the navel).

内养三阴【nèi yǎng sān yīn】 指习练气功,内养少阴、厥阴、太阴。

intrinsic cultivation of three Yin Refers to nourishing Shaoyin, Jueyin and Taiyin in practicing Qigong.

内养形神除嗜欲【nèi yǎng xíng shén chú shì yù】 指除嗜欲能稳定情绪,稳定情绪即能内守精神,外养形体。

internally cultivating the body and spirit in order to eliminate craving　Refers to the fact that elimination of appetitive action can stabilize the mind and that stabilization of the mind can keep the spirit and nourish the body.

内药【nèi yào】　指元精、元气、元神。

internal medicinal　Refers to the original essence, the original Qi and the original spirit taken as medicinals in practicing Qigong in order to cultivate health and prolong life.

内药运动【nèi yào yùn dòng】　源自气功专论，主要阐述真阴真阳交合而生丹。

movement of internal medicinals　Collected from a monograph of Qigong, mainly describing accumulation of genuine Yin and genuine Yang in order to produce essence.

内因【nèi yīn】　指喜、怒、忧、思、悲、恐、惊七情过度，致气机紊乱，损伤脏腑而成为致病因素。

internal cause　Refers to disorder of Qi and damage of the five Zang-organs (including the heart, the liver, the spleen, the lung and the kidney) and the six Fu-organs (including the gallbladder, the stomach, the small intestine, the large intestine, the bladder and the triple energizer) due to excess of happiness, anger, anxiety, contemplation, sorrow, fear and horror.

内院【nèi yuàn】　泥丸宫之别称。

internal mansion　A synonym of the chamber in the mud bolus (the brain).

内阅【nèi yuè】　通过观七窍（眼、鼻、口、耳）以内察五脏。

intrinsic inspection　Refers to analyzing the five Zang-organs (including the heart, the liver, the spleen, the lung and the kidney) through observing the eyes, the ears, the nose and the mouth.

内脏【nèi zàng】　指五脏六腑。

internal viscera　Refers to the five Zang-organs (including the heart, the liver, the spleen, the lung and the kidney) and the six Fu-organs (including the gallbladder, the stomach, the small intestine, the large intestine, the bladder and the triple energizer).

内照图【nèi zhào tú】　指练功中入静内观自身之内脏。

internal inspection picture　Refers to internal observation of the internal viscera through tranquilization of the mind in practicing Qigong.

内芝【nèi zhī】　指五脏之液。

internal ganoderma　Refers to humor in the five Zang-organs (including the heart, the liver, the spleen, the lung and the kidney).

内治【nèi zhì】　指内因引起的内环境失调所致之病，应以气功调节内气治疗。

internal therapy　Refers to disease caused by disorder of the internal environment which can be cured by regulation of internal Qi by practice of Qigong to normalize the internal environment.

内珠【nèi zhū】　指内丹，"调冲和之气，补肝，下气海，添内珠尔"。

internal pearl　Refers to internal Dan (pills of immortality) used to harmonize Qi, improve the liver and regulate Qihai (the sea of Qi).

内拙【nèi zhuō】　指外重于物，为之诱惑，内则意识活动紊乱，精神失调，昏拙沉闷。

N

intrinsic faint　Refers to disorder of mental activity and spirit due to temptation of things in the society.

内自省【nèi zì xǐng】　指内省，自我观察以调节精神思维活动及行为。

internal introspection　Refers to regulation of the spirit and the activities of the spirit and thinking through self-observation.

内眦【nèi zì】　即内眼角，位上下眼睑于鼻侧连接部，是足太阳膀胱经的起点。

inner canthus　Located between the upper eyelid and the lower eyelid connected with the nasal side, which is the origin of the bladder meridian of foot Taiyang.

能守一而弃万疴【néng shǒu yī ér qì wàn kē】　指精神意识专一，并能守之而不分散，可以调节神形，预防治疗各种神形失调引起的疾病。

ability to keep one and eliminate all diseases　Indicates that concentration of the spirit and consciousness can keep the spirit and consciousness without any dispersion, regulate the spirit and body, and prevent all diseases caused by imbalance of the spirit and the body.

能恬能静【néng tián néng jìng】　指古代仙家习练气功，重在调节精神，使意识活动保持恬静。

to be tranquil and quiet　Indicates that the immortals in ancient China paid great attention to regulation of the spirit in order to tranquilize the activity of consciousness.

能一【néng yī】　指调节呼服，使神形合而为一。

concentrating one　Means to regulate respiration and to combine the spirit and the body.

能隐能彰【néng yǐn néng zhāng】　指习练气功到一定的精度，能隐身隐物，或能使身体或物显现并昭著。

ability to conceal and emerge　Means that practice of Qigong to a certain degree can conceal the body and all things, or obviously emerge the body and all things.

能知药而取火【néng zhī yào ér qǔ huǒ】　即练功中明白什么时候生药，什么时候应用什么火候来烹炼，是练功中至关重要的问题。

ability to understand medicinal and take fire　Indicates that understanding how to produce medicinal and knowing how to smelt with certain fire duration are the important issues in practicing Qigong.

泥丸【ní wán】　指脑，脑藏神，一般称泥丸亦指脑神。

mud bolus（the brain）　Refers to the spirit in the brain.

泥丸百节皆有神【ní wán bǎi jié jiē yǒu shén】　即脑各部都有神。

There are all the spirits in the hundred joints in mud bolus（the brain）.　Indicate that there is the spirit in every part of the brain.

泥丸夫人【ní wán fū rén】　指脑中阴神。

mud bolus（the brain）lady　Refers to Yin spirit in the brain.

泥丸宫【ní wán gōng】　指脑中的一部分。脑中有九宫，泥丸宫为九宫之一，为人体之神所汇聚的地方。

mud bolus（the brain）chamber　A part of the brain. In the brain there are nine chambers. Mud bolus chamber, one of the nine chambers, is the region in which the spirit in the human body concentrates in it.

泥丸九真皆有房【ní wán jiǔ zhēn jiē yǒu fáng】　指脑内九宫皆有房舍，每一宫中的神称谓真神。

There are all the chambers in the nine palaces of the mud bolus（the brain）.　In the brain, there are chambers all the nine palaces and the spirit in each palace is called genuine spirit.

泥丸君【ní wán jūn】　指脑，脑藏神，一般称泥丸亦指脑神。

Mud bolus（the brain）immortal　Refers to the spirit in the brain.

泥丸君，总众神也【ní wán jūn zǒng zhòng shén yě】　指脑为神明之舍，是精神意识活动的枢纽。

Immortals in the mud bolus（the brain）are all spirits.　Indicates that the brain is the storage of the spirit and the pivot of the activities of the spirit and consciousness.

泥丸通百节【ní wán tōng bǎi jié】　百节指全身即脑与全身各部相通。

Mud bolus（the brain）opens up hundred joints.　Hundred joints refer to the whole body, indicating that the brain is connected with all parts of the body.

泥丸为神之府，气精之原【ní wán wéi shén zhī fǔ qì jīng zhī yuán】　指脑为众神之府，气精之渊源。

The mud bolus（the brain）is the chamber of the spirit and the origin of Qi and essence.　Indicates that the brain is the palace of all the spirits and the original source that has produced Qi and the essence.

泥垣【ní yuán】　指头中，两目直入的部位。

mud wall　Refers to a region in the head through which the eyes directly enter the brain.

逆来顺受【nì lái shùn shòu】　指进行气功养生法，排除杂念，调节神形，将逆转顺，任其自然。

resigning oneself to adversity　Refers to eliminating distracting thought, regulating the spirit and body, changing contrary condition naturally into clockwise condition.

逆气【nì qì】　气功适应证，即体内之气上逆，多因大怒所致。

reversed Qi　An indication of Qigong, referring to upward counterflow of Qi from the body caused by rage.

逆气候导引法【nì qì hòu dǎo yǐn fǎ】　为静功。其作法为，用左脚跟勾住右脚踇趾，用鼻吸气，至极限时慢慢呼出，作七息。

exercise of Daoyin for reversed Qi　A static exercise, marked by catching the big toe of the right foot with the left heel, inhaling Qi through the nose and finally exhaling it slowly for seven times.

年病【nián bìng】　由于身心保养失宜，恣情纵意，散失元阳，耗散其气所致。

yearly disease　Caused by failure to nourish the body and heart due to distracting thought, dispersion of original Yang and dissipation of Qi.

念【niàn】　① 指念头、意念；② 指记忆，为佛家气功习用语；③ 指诵念；④ 指默念。

idea　Refers to ① either intention and thought; ② or memory, which is a common term of Qigong in Buddhism; ③ or recitation; ④ or contemplation.

念鼻【niàn bí】　指精神意识活动集中于鼻。

idea in nose　Indicates that the activity of the essence, the spirit and the consciousness concentrates in the nose.

念必祛【niàn bì qū】 指习练气功,应用意念排除杂念。

elimination of idea Refers to elimination of distracting thought with consciousness in practicing Qigong.

念肺五叶【niàn fèi wǔ yè】 指意念活动集中于肺中五叶。

concentration of five parts in the lung Indicates that the activity of thought should concentrate on the five parts of the lung.

念可蔽性之光【niàn kě bì xìng zhī guāng】 指杂念火邪念可遮蔽神明的慧光。

Idea can cover the manifestations of human nature. Indicates that distracting thought and wicked idea can expel the wisdom and brightness of the mind.

念口鸿赤【niàn kǒu hóng chì】 指精神意识活动集中于目。

opening idea with grand redness Refers to concentration of the activities of the essence, the spirit and the consciousness in the eyes.

念力【niàn lì】 佛家气功习用语,指意念的力量。

Strength of idea A common term of Qigong in Buddhism, referring to the power of thought.

念心不动【niàn xīn bú dòng】 指意识思维活动的稳定。

idea in tranquilized heart Refers to stability of the activities of consciousness and thought.

鸟迹【niǎo jì】 佛家气功习用语,指习练气功,有感觉而无实体,譬如鸟飞空中,有迹而不可见。

bird flying A common term of Qigong in Buddhism, referring to Qigong prac-

tice characterized by sensation without substance like bird flying that really exists but is difficult to observe.

鸟申【niǎo shēn】 动功之一势,仿鸟颈之申。

bird stretching A way of dynamic exercise, imitating the bird to stretch its neck in practicing Qigong.

鸟戏【niǎo xì】 五禽戏之一。双立手,翘一足,伸两臂,扬眉鼓力,右十四次。

bird frolic One of the frolics of five animals, marked by holding up both hands, raising one foot, stretching both arms, raising the brows to the right for fourteen times.

尿血【niào xiě】 气功适应证,多因肾阴不足,心肝火旺,下移小肠,或脾肾两亏,血失统摄所致。

hematuria An indication of Qigong, usually caused by insufficiency of kidney Yin, effulgent heart and liver fire that moves downwards into the small intestine, or deficiency of the spleen and kidney, and failure of the blood to control any aspects.

捏目四眦法【niē mù sì zì fǎ】 为动功。其作法为,以手按目内眦,闭气为之,气通即止,终而复始,数遍,常行之,眼能洞见。

exercise for pressing inner canthus A dynamic exercise, marked by pressing the inner canthus with the hands for stopping respiration. When Qi movement is unobstructed, such a way of practice can be stopped. To practice for several times can enable the eyes to observe deeply and thoroughly.

捏中指中节法【niē zhōng zhǐ zhōng jié fǎ】 为动功。其作法为,手握拳,拇指捏住中指中节,两掌面相合,置于两大腿之间,两腿用力紧挟,治伤寒无汗。

exercise for pinching the middle of the middle finger A dynamic exercise, marked by holding the fists with hands, pinching the middle of the middle finger, holding the palms in the middle of two thighs held by two legs in order to cure cold damage and adiaphoresis.

聂商恒【niè shāng héng】　明代气功养生家,著有气功养生专著。

Nie Shangheng A master of Qigong and life cultivation in the Ming Dynasty (1368 AD – 1644 AD), who wrote a monograph of Qigong and life cultivation.

涅槃【niè pán】　① 即圆寂,为佛家气功习用语,指消除烦恼;② 指精神活动相对静止;③ 指达到健康安乐境界;④ 指坐忘。

nirvana A common term of Qigong in Buddhism, referring to ① either eliminating annoyance; ② or tranquilizing spirit activity; ③ or reaching the state of health, peace and happiness; ④ or sitting without memorizing anything.

涅槃乐【niè pán lè】　佛家气功习用语,指学习佛理,应用佛家功法,消除外界对人引起的各种精神损伤的因素,使人神形合调。

nirvana state A common term of Qigong in Buddhism, referring to studying the theory of Buddhism and using the exercises of Buddhism to eliminate factors from the external world that damage human spirit in order to balance the spirit and the body.

颞颥【niè rú】　指眉弓后外侧,耳前上方的部位。

tempus Refers to the lateral backside of the eyebrow at the upper part of the ear.

宁先生导引法【níng xiān shēng dǎo yǐn fǎ】　为动功,子后午前,解发,东向握固,不息,举手左右导引,手掩两耳,令发黑不白。卧引为三。以手指捎项边脉,三通,令人目明。

Mr. Ning's exercise of Daoyin A dynamic exercise, marked by releasing hair after Zi (the period of the day from 11 p.m. to 1 a.m.) and before Wu (the period of the day from 11 a.m. to 1 p.m.), holding strictly toward the east, suspending respiration, keeping one unobstruction, raising up the hands to practice Daoyin from the left to the right, covering the ears with hands, keeping the hair black not white; or lying to practice for three times with the hands pinching the meridians along the neck, keeping three unobstructions in order to brighten the eyes.

宁先生导引图之导引法【níng xiān shēng dǎo yǐn tú zhī dǎo yǐn fǎ】　动静相兼功,方法多样。如稍低头,微息,但抱手左右,不息,十二通,消食,令人轻身,益精神,邪气不得入。

Mr. Ning's exercise of Daoyin with techniques An exercise combined with static exercise and dynamic exercise with various methods, such as slightly lowering the head, mildly respiring, holding the hands in the left and right, suspending respiration, keeping twelve unobstructions, relaxing the body and improving the spirit in order to prevent invasion of pathogenic factors.

宁先生论导引行气【níng xiān shēng lùn dǎo yǐn xíng qì】　源自气功专论,主要阐述导引行气的作用,导引治于四肢,行气可补于里，导引行气能除百病，令人长寿。

Mr. Ning's discussion about Daoyin for directing Qi Collected from a monograph about Qigong, mainly describing the effect of Daoyin for directing Qi. Daoyin can relieve disorders in the four limbs and directing Qi can tonify the organs inside the body. Thus Daoyin for directing Qi can treat various diseases and prolong life.

凝抱固丹田【níng bào gù dān tián】为静功。其作法为静坐，存想元神，入于丹田，随意呼吸，旬日丹田完固，百日灵明渐通，不可或作或辍。

Concentrated and stabilized Dantian A static exercise, marked by sitting quietly, imagining to lead the original spirit to Dantian, breathing with free rein, solidly finishing Dantian in ten days, normalizing the spirit in one hundred days and avoiding now practicing and then stopping. Dantian is divided into the upper Dantian (the region between the eyes), the middle Dantian (the region below the heart) and the lower Dantian (the region below the navel).

凝固【níng gù】 指气功中意识思维活动集中而不分散。

concretion Refers to concentration of the activities of consciousness and thinking without any dispersion.

凝结之所【níng jié zhī suǒ】 即祖窍，指位于心与脐之正中。

concentrated region The same as ancestral orifice, referring to the central region between the heart and the navel.

凝神【níng shén】 指排除杂念，精神安宁，意念专一的练功状态。

concentrated spirit Refers to elimina-

ting distracting thought, stabilizing the spirit and concentrating consciousness in practicing Qigong.

凝神合气【níng shén hé qì】 指神气合而为一，为习练气功进入理想境界后神形和合的状态。

concentrated spirit and integrated Qi Refers to integration of the spirit and Qi, which is the ideal state of the spirit and body in practicing Qigong.

凝神内照【níng shén nèi zhào】 源自其中专论，阐述调身、调气、调神的方法及气功中自身的感受。

Internal view of concentrated spirit Collected from a monograph of Qigong, describing the methods and experiences of regulating the body, Qi and spirit in practicing Qigong.

凝神气穴，息息归根【níng shén qì xué xī xī guī gēn】 源自气功专论，要阐述神驭气，神定息定的道理。

concentrating the spirit into Qi point and constantly entering the root Collected from a monograph of Qigong, mainly describing the spirit for controlling Qi and the principle for stabilizing the spirit and respiration.

凝神乾顶【níng shén qián dǐng】 指凝神入脑，调节阴阳而成丹。

concentrated spirit on the celestial top Refers to concentrating the spirit in the brain and regulating Yin and Yang to form Dan (pills of immortality).

凝神入气穴【níng shén rù qì xué】 即将调神所得之元神下藏于下丹田之内。气穴即指丹田。

concentrated spirit in the Qi point Refers to storing the original spirit obtained from regulation of the spirit into the lower Dantian (the region below the navel). The so-called Qi point refers to Dantian which is divided into the upper Dantian (the region between the eyes), the middle Dantian (the region below the heart) and the lower Dantian (the region below the navel).

凝神须知窍【níng shén xū zhī qiào】指凝神须知意守之窍,窍即玄关。神存乎窍内,即是凝神入气穴。

concentrating the spirit in aperture Refers to understanding the aperture of consciousness for concentrating the spirit. Storing the spirit in the aperture means to concentrate the spirit in Qi point. The so-called aperture refers to Xuguan acupoint located between the eyes. Storage of the spirit in the aperture refers to concentration of the spirit in the Qi point.

牛车【niú chē】 指由玉枕关到泥丸,力大方能过关。

oxcart Refers to entrance from the back of the head into the mud bolus (the brain) with great power.

牛车大乘【niú chē dà chéng】 为静功,意为闭鼻息而不呼,回天风以合神灵。

oxcart Mahayana A static exercise, referring to the way to close the nose and to stop respiration in order to return the celestial Qi and to combine it with the spirit.

牛眠地【niú mián dì】 古人将牛眠地以为风水宝地。

cattle sleeping spot Refers to a very important area which was traditionally called treasure place of wind and water.

牛女相逢【niú nǚ xiāng féng】 喻气功真阴、真阳相逢,阴平阳秘,合为一处。

meeting of cowherd and maid Refers to

integration of genuine Yin and genuine Yang in practice of Qigong and harmony between Yin and Yang.

牛皮癣【niú pí xuǎn】 气功适应证,多发于颈项部。

psoriasis An indication of Qigong, usually appears in the neck and nape.

拗颈【niù jǐng】 指反折颈部。

obstinate neck Refers to reflexing the neck.

努腰就肚【nǔ yāo jiù dù】 指向前挺腰,使之靠近此肚皮的导引动作。

bending posture Refers to the Daoyin act for straightening the waist forward near the belly.

女偊闻道法【nǚ yǔ wén dào fǎ】 为静功。其作法为,坐式,意守道后入静,守之又守,逐渐深化,导引入静,提高认识,增加智慧。

static female dhyana A static exercise, marked by sitting with tranquility and quietness, tranquilizing the mind constantly in order to keep physical and mental quietness, increasing knowledge and improving wisdom.

女子贵炼形【nǚ zǐ guì liàn xíng】 指女性习练气功以养形益血为贵。

female physique exercise Refers to importance of nourishing the body and invigorating the blood for women to practice Qigong.

疟疾治法【nüè jí zhì fǎ】 为静功。其作法为,身体朝向东北方,正身端坐,两手掌心相互擦热极,抱住阴囊运气,八口乃止。

treatment of malaria A static exercise, marked by sitting upright toward the northeast, rubbing the palms hot with each other, and holding the scrotum to move Qi for eight times.

O

欧公愈足疮【ōu gōng yù zú chuāng**】**
为静功。其作法为，重足坐，闭目握固，
缩谷道，摇飑为之两足如气球状，气极即
休，气平复为之。
Ou Gong's exercise for treating toot furuncle　A static exercise, marked by sitting with pounding the feet, closing the eyes and holding the hands, shrinking the grain trail (anus), shaking the feet like a balloon. In such a practice, if Qi is extreme, rest is necessary; if Qi is stable, the practice can be continued.

呕吐【ǒu tù**】**　气功适应证，多因饮食积滞，肝气犯胃，胃失和降，或寒邪犯胃，脾胃虚弱，痰饮内伏等因素所致。
vomiting　An indication of Qigong, usually caused by stagnation of food, liver Qi attacking the stomach, failure of stomach Qi to descend, or pathogenic cold attacking the stomach, weakness of the spleen and stomach, and internal retention of phlegmatic rheuma.

呕吐候导引法【ǒu tù hòu dǎo yǐn fǎ**】**
为动功，可通过正坐，两手向背后，或仰卧，伸展四肢，健胃和中，治食不下，吐逆。
exercise of Daoyin for vomiting　A dynamic exercise, marked by sitting upright with both hands turning to the back, or lying on the back with the four limbs stretched in order to strengthen the stomach, to harmonize the center, to relieve difficulty in taking food and to cure vomiting.

P

潘师正【pān shī zhèng】 隋唐时期气功学家,认真研究和传播气功学理论与方法。

Pan Shizheng A master of Qigong in the late Sui Dynasty (581 AD - 618 AD) and the early Tang Dynasty (618 AD - 907 AD), who studied and disseminated the theory and practice of Qigong.

潘体玄【pān tǐ xuán】 隋唐时期气功学家潘师正的另外一个称谓,其认真研究和传播气功学理论与方法。

Pan Tixuan Another name of Pan Shizheng, a master of in the late Qigong and the early Sui Dynasty (581 AD - 618 AD) and Tang Dynasty (618 AD - 907 AD), who studied and disseminated the theory and practice of Qigong.

潘子真【pān zǐ zhēn】 隋唐时期气功学家潘师正的另外一个称谓,认真研究和传播气功学理论与方法。

Pan Zizhen Another name of Pan Shizheng, a master of in the late Sui Dynasty (581 AD - 618 AD) and the early Tang Dynasty (618 AD - 907 AD), who studied and disseminated the theory and practice of Qigong.

盘膝坐【pán xī zuò】 同结跏趺坐,即吉祥座,为佛家气功坐式,方式有二,一为吉祥,二为降魔。

sitting with crossed legs Refers to auspicious sitting which is an exercise of sitting for practicing Qigong in Bud-

dhism with two ways, one is to be auspicious, the other is to expel evil.

膀胱【páng guāng】 六腑之一,位小腹,居脏腑之最下部,是水液汇聚之处。

bladder One of the six Fu-organs (including the gallbladder, the stomach, the small intestine, the large intestine, the bladder and the triple energizer), is located in the lower abdomen and the lowermost region of the viscera, where fluid in the body accumulates.

膀胱病【páng guāng bìng】 气功适应证,主要表现为排尿的功能失常。

bladder disease An indication of Qigong, mainly manifested as abnormal urination

膀胱病候导引法【páng guāng bìng hòu dǎo yǐn fǎ】 为动功。其作法为,斜身蹲坐,尽力把两手前伸,仰掌,左右转倒腰部二十一次,通阳散寒,治膀胱内冷血风,骨节拘强;两膝跪地,入静,以意引心气向下达涌泉,存想气流布全身,然后,两手舒展放在两胁旁,意想掌心吸气呼气不止,待面部有紧缩感时,站立,向下弯腰十四次。温阳通络,治膝头冷,膀胱旧疾,脊腰强硬,脐下冷闷。

exercise of Daoyin for bladder disease A static exercise, marked by slanting and squatting, extending the hands forcefully forwards, raising the fists and turning from the left and right to the waist for twenty-one times, dredging Yang and expelling cold, curing internal cold and blood wind in the bladder as well as spasm of bones and joints; kneeling with both knees on the ground, tranquilizing the mind, imagining to lead Qi to the lower Yongquan (KI 1) and to flow in the whole body, then stretching both hands to put over the rib-sides, imagining to constantly breathe in and out in the palms, standing up when the face is felt tightened, and bending the waist for fourteen times. Such a dynamic exercise can warm Yang to open collaterals, cure knee coldness, chronic bladder disease, stiffness of the spine and waist as well as coldness and stuffiness below the navel.

培养正气法【péi yǎng zhèng qì fǎ】为静功。其作法为，端身正坐，先想脑如日；次想黄气自脾而出，存于中央，化作土。

exercise for cultivating healthy Qi A static exercise, marked by sitting upright, imagining that the brain is just like the sun and that yellow Qi emerges from the spleen, existing in the center and transforming into the earth.

裴玄静驾云升天【péi xuán jìng jià yún shēng tiān】动静相兼功。其作法为，身体盘膝端坐，以手擦下丹田，同时凝神运气四十九口。主治小肠虚冷，腹腔疼痛。

Pei Xuanjing's exercise for flying up to the clouds and the sky An exercise combined with dynamic exercise and static exercise, marked by sitting upright with crossed knees, rubbing the lower Dantian (the region below the navel) with hands, concentrating the spirit and moving Qi for forty-nine times. Such an exercise combined with dynamic exercise and static exercise can cure deficiency and coldness of the small intestine and abdominal pain.

彭嬾翁收放丹枢【péng lǎn wēng shōu fàng dān shū】为静功，本法为右侧卧式睡法。治失眠、多梦、梦游等。

Peng Lanweng's exercise for collecting and releasing court A static exercise, marked by lying on the right side for curing insomnia, dreaminess and sleepwalking.

彭晓【péng xiǎo】五代时期的气功学家，精内丹说。

Peng Xiao A master of Qigong in Five Dynasties (907 AD – 979 AD), quite proficient in Dan (pills of immortality).

彭祖【péng zǔ】上古时代气功养生学家。

Peng Zu A great master of Qigong and life cultivation in ancient China.

彭祖导引法【péng zǔ dǎo yǐn fǎ】为动功，方法多样。如凡解衣披卧，伸腰，瞑少时，五息止，引肾气，去消渴，利阴阳。

Peng Zu's exercise of Daoyin A dynamic exercise with various methods, such as taking off clothes, lying on the bed with clothes thrown on, closing the eyes for a while, stopping respiration for five times, leading kidney Qi, relieving consumptive thirst and profiting Yin and Yang.

彭祖导引图【péng zǔ dǎo yǐn tú】为动功。其作法为，解发，东向坐，握固不息，一通，举手左右导引，以手掩两耳，以指捏两眉梢，五通，令人目明，发黑不白，治头风。

Peng Zu's illustration of Daoyin A dynamic exercise, marked by freeing hair, sitting to the east, holding the body, stopping respiration for once, raising the hands to lead Qi from the left to the right and vice versa, covering the ears with both hands, pinching the tips of the brows for five times. Such a dynamic exercise can improve the eyesight, blacken hair and cure headache.

彭祖明目法【péng zǔ míng mù fǎ**】**为动功。其作法为,平地坐定,以两手反背,伸左胫,右膝压左腿上,行五息,引肺去风。

Peng Zu's exercise for improving eyesight　A dynamic exercise, marked by sitting on the ground, turning the hands to the back, stretching the left shank, pressing the left leg with the right knee, breathing for five times and leading the lung to relieve wind.

彭祖摄生养性论【péng zǔ shè shēng yǎng xìng lùn**】**《彭祖摄生养性论》为气功养生学专著,主张养生要淡泊平和以保神。作者不详。

Pengzu Shesheng Yangsheng Lun (*Discussion about Peng Zu's Regimen and Life Cultivation***）**　A monograph of Qigong and life cultivation entitled *Discussion about Peng Zu's Regimen and Life Cultivation*, mainly suggesting simplicity, placidity and balance for protecting the spirit. The author was unknown.

彭祖养生治身法【péng zǔ yǎng shēng zhì shēn fǎ**】**动静相兼功。其作法为,常闭气纳息,从旦至中,正坐拭目,摩搦身体,舐唇咽唾,服气数千。功效为调和身之血脉,强壮形体,延年益寿。

Peng Zu's exercise for nourishing life and curing the body　An exercise combined with dynamic exercise and static exercise, marked by often closing Qi, inhaling Qi, sitting upright from the morning to the noon, rubbing the eyes, kneading the body, licking the lips, swallowing saliva and taking Qi for thousands of times. Such an exercise combined with dynamic exercise and static exercise can regulate blood vessels and meridians, strengthen the body, prolong life and cultivate health.

蓬岛【péng dǎo**】**　指头,亦指脑。

legendary island　Refers to the head or the brain.

披衣正形法【pī yī zhèng xíng fǎ**】**为静功。其作法为,正身端坐,专一视觉形体静定象枯槁的枝术;内守精神,集中意念,精神意识活动象息灭的灰烬。

exercise for dressing clothes and straightening the body　A static exercise, marked by sitting upright, concentrating vision, tranquilizing the mind, stabilizing the spirit, centralizing consciousness and keeping the activities of the spirit and consciousness like quenching ashes.

被褐怀玉【pī hè huái yù**】**　指有德行的人,外练形体,内养精神。

poor man with genuine jade　Means that that a man with virtue externally exercises the body and internally nourishes the spirit.

脾【pí**】**　五脏之一。气功中常为意守部位,其功能运化水谷精微,输布全身,供人体生长发育和生命活动的需要。

spleen　One of the five Zang-organs (including the heart, the liver, the spleen, the lung and the kidney). In Qigong, the spleen is the region for keeping consciousness, the function of

P

which is to move and transform nutrients of food and water to the whole body for the development of the body and the activities of life.

脾病导引【pí bìng dǎo yǐn】 动静相兼功，方法多样。如坐于床上，右腿伸直，左腿上屈，双手放于身后，稍用力左右拉，然后左腿伸直，右腿上屈，手仍做上述动作三五次。

exercise of Daoyin for spleen disease An exercise combined with dynamic exercise and static exercise with various methods, such as siting on the bed, stretching the right foot, bending upward the left foot, putting both hands on the body for mildly pulling from the left to the right and vice versa, then stretching the left foot, bending upward the right foot, moving the hands in the previous way for 3 to 5 times.

脾病候导引法【pí bìng hòu dǎo yǐn fǎ】 为静功。其中法为，无声用嘻字出气，运脾除湿，治肌表游风微微作痛，身痒，烦闷疼痛。

exercise of Daoyin for spleen disease A static exercise, marked by exhaling Qi without any sound through the Chinese character giggle, moving the spleen to expel dampness and curing hypodynia, pruritus, annoyance and pain.

罢极之本【pí jí zhī běn】 指肝。

root with great tolerance Refers to the liver.

脾经导引法【pí jīng dǎo yǐn fǎ】 为静功。其作法为，安静脏腑，调顺血脉，食必以时，快必以节。宽胃养气。

exercise of Daoyin for spleen meridan A static exercise, marked by quieting the five Zang-organs (including the heart, the liver, the spleen, the lung and the kidney) and the six Fu-organs (including the gallbladder, the stomach, the small intestine, the large intestine, the bladder and the triple energizer), regulating blood in the six Fu-organs, eating quickly in a certain time. Such a static exercise can relax the stomach and nourish Qi.

脾神【pí shén】 指脾脏之神，为脾物质的精微结构和功能作用。

spleen spirit Refers to the refined structure and function of the spleen.

脾神去【pí shén qù】 指脾神损伤，意出身外，食不甘味。

loss of spleen spirit Refers to damage of the spleen spirit. Under such a condition, consciousness is dispersed and food is tasteless.

脾俞【pí shū】 足太阳膀胱经中的一个穴位，位第十一胸椎棘突下旁开 1.5 寸处，为气功中常用的意守部位。

Pishu（BL 20） An acupoint in the bladder meridian of foot Taiyang, located 1.5 Cun lateral to the region below the spinous process of the eleventh thoracic vertebra, which is the region for concentrating consciousness in practicing Qigong.

脾胃肚腹症导引法【pí wèi dù fù zhèng dǎo yǐn fǎ】 为动静相兼功。其作法为，端坐，两手抱脐下，待丹田暖热，运气四十九口止。

exercise of Daoyin for spleen, stomach and abdominal diseases An exercise combined with dynamic exercise and static exercise, marked by sitting upright, embracing the region below the navel and moving Qi for forty-nine times when Dantian is warm and hot. Dantian is divided into the upper Dantian (the region between the eyes), the middle Dantian (the region below the heart) and the lower Dantian (the region below the navel).

脾胃气不和不能饮食候导引法【pí wèi qì bù hé bù néng yǐn shí hòu dǎo yǐn fǎ】

为动功。其作法为,身侧屈,两手向屈侧舒展,互相牵拉,用力,左右各二十一次。然后,两手从颈项前后向左右慢慢伸开,似向外扒,全身放松,动摇二十一次,左右交替。健胃和中,通络止痛。

exercise of Daoyin for disharmony of Qi in the spleen and stomach with inability to take food A dynamic exercise, marked by bending the body to one side, stretching and pulling the bending side from the left to the right and vice versa for twenty-one times respectively, then slowly stretching the hands from the front and back of the neck to the left and right as pulling to the lateral side, relaxing the whole body and shaking the body for twenty-one times with alternation of the left and right. Such a dynamic exercise can fortify the stomach, harmonize the center, dredge the collaterals and relieve pain.

脾胃治法【pí wèi zhì fǎ】
为动功。其作法为,斜身,两手偏向一侧,急挺身,舒松头和手,两手相抓互相牵拉,尽量保持姿势不变。

exercise for curing the spleen and the stomach A dynamic exercise, marked by slanting the body, stretching both hands to one side, quickly straightening the body, relaxing the head and hands, mutually grasping and pulling the hands to keep the posture without any change.

脾脏导引法【pí zàng dǎo yǐn fǎ】
为动功。其作法为,大坐,伸一脚,屈一脚,以两手向后反掣,各三五度。去脾脏积聚、风邪、喜食。

exercise of Daoyin for the spleen A dynamic exercise, marked by sitting down, stretching one foot, bending the other foot, drawing the hands backward for three to five degrees respectively. Such a dynamic exercise can eliminate spleen mass, pathogenic wind and preference of diet.

脾脏修养法【pí zàng xiū yǎng fǎ】
为静功。其作法为,常以季夏之月朔旦并及四季之月十八日旭旦,坐中宫,禁气五息,鸣天鼓十二通,吸坤宫之黄气入口十二咽,以补之。

exercise for cultivating and nourishing the spleen A static exercise, marked by sitting in the central palace on the first day in every month in summer and at sunrise on the eighteenth day in every month in the four seasons, stopping respiration for five times, sounding the celestial drum (rubbing the occipital) for twelve times, inhaling yellow Qi from Kun palace through the mouth and swallowing it for twelve times for tonification.

痞块导引法【pǐ kuài dǎo yǐn fǎ】
为动功。其作法为,左手向前上伸,右手向后下伸,闭气一口,抽身转项,左右旋转各七十回。

exercise of Daoyin for abdominal lump A dynamic exercise, marked by stretching the left hand forward, stretching the right hand backward, stopping respiration for a while, extricating oneself and turning the neck, and rotating from the left to the right and vice versa for seventy times respectively.

癖【pǐ】　气功适应证,指两胁下的结块。

mass　An indication of Qiong, referring to scleroma at the rib-sides.

癖候导引法【pǐ hòu dǎo yǐn fǎ】　为动功。其作法为,两于按地蹲坐,两膝高举、夹在两颊旁,久坐,消痞破积。

exercise of Daoyin for abdominal mass　A dynamic exercise, marked by squatting with hands pressing the ground, raising the knees against the cheeks and sitting for a long time. Such a dynamic exercise can relieve abdominal mass and expel indigestion.

辟却虚羸【pì què xū léi】　指脾消谷磨食,运化水谷精微于全身,防治身体虚羸之病。

stopping diet to prevent weakness　Refers to the spleen digesting and grinding food; and transforming nutrients of food and water in the whole body for preventing and treating disease due to weakness.

偏风【piān fēng】　气功适应证,指风邪偏客于人体一边,乘虚而伤害人体。

hemiplegia　An indication of Qigong, caused by invasion of pathogenic wind into one side of the body to damage the body.

偏风候导引法【piān fēng hòu dǎo yǐn fǎ】　为动功。其作法为,一手长伸,手掌向上,另一手握住下颌尽力向外拉,左右各十四次。然后,手不动,头尽量向两侧转动,左右各快速牵引十四次。

exercise of Daoyin for paralysis　A dynamic exercise, marked by stretching one hand, raising the palm, holding the lower jaw with the other hand to pull it hard laterally from the left to the right and vice versa for fourteen times respectively, then stopping moving the hands, quickly turning the head to the left side and right side and vice versa for fourteen times respectively.

偏跏【piān jiā】　即盘膝而坐时,一足压于对侧大腿上的练功姿势。

sitting on one foot　Refers to sitting with crossed legs and pressing the thigh with one foot in practicing Qigong.

牝静胜牡【pìn jìng shèng mǔ】　指以弱制强,以柔克刚。气功文献中,牝为静,牡为动。

quiet female superior to male　Refers to weakness controlling strength and softness and restraining hardness. In the literature of Qigong, Pin (female) means quiet while Mu (male) means active.

牝牡四卦【pìn mǔ sì guà】　指乾坤坎离四卦,可统摄阴阳。牝为阴物的总称,牡为阳物的总称。

four female and male Trigrams　Refer to Qian Trigram, Kun Trigram, Kan Trigram and Li Trigram that control Yin and Yang. In this term, Pin (female) refers to all the things pertaining to Yin and Mu (male) refers to all the things pertaining to Yang.

牝牡相从【pìn mǔ xiāng cóng】　指思虑之神与呼吸之气所结的丹。

combination of female and male　Refers to Dan (pills of immortality) formed by the spirit in consideration and Qi in respiration. In this term, Pin (female) refers to all the things pertaining to Yin and Mu (male) refers to all the things pertaining to Yang.

平陂之质在于神【píng bēi zhī zhì zài

yú shén】　指神具有调节阴阳两方面，使之协调平衡的作用。

peace and harmony depending on the spirit　Refers to the fact that the spirit can regulate Yin and Yang in order to coordinate and balance these two aspects.

平旦【píng dàn】　指寅时，即凌晨三至五时。

early morning　Refers to Yin (the period of a day from 3 a.m. to 5 a.m. in the early morning) in the early morning.

平气【píng qì】　① 指调节阴阳；② 指运气平和。

normal respiration　Refers to ① either regulation of Yin and Yang; ② or harmony in moving Qi.

平人【píng rén】　指阴阳气血和平的无病之人。

normal people　Refers to those whose Yin and Yang, Qi and blood are harmonized in the body without any disease.

平易【píng yì】　指精神思维活动安稳。

stability　Refers to stability of the spirit and consciousness activities.

平易穴【píng yì xué】　指尾间穴，位于尾骨端与肛门之间，经属督脉、督脉之络穴。

Pingyi acupoint　An acupoint located between the coccyx and the anus, belonging to the governor meridian and its collateral.

平正擅匈【píng zhèng shàn xiōng】指人秉天地之气以生，精神意识平正中和，乃可长寿。

pure peace　Refers to the fact that human beings depend on Qi from the sky and the earth. Only when the spirit and

consciousness are harmonized can life be prolonged.

屏尽万缘【píng jìn wàn yuán】　指练功过程中自始至终要排除外界的一切干扰和杂念。

stopping various karma　Refers to eliminating all kinds of disturbance and distracting thought in practicing Qigong.

婆罗门导引十二法【pó luó mén dǎo yǐn shí èr fǎ】　为动功，方法多样，如两手用力上举兼作拉弓姿势，左右相同，两手相握高举过头。

Brahman's twelve exercises of Daoyin　A dynamic exercise with various methods, such as raising the hands forcefully above the head like drawing a bow with the same activity in the left side and right side.

婆娑【pó suō】　指安闲自得。

breeze　Refers to being carefree and contented.

破车【pò chē】　指八邪五疫搬入真气，元阳难以抵挡，使人既老且病而死。

broken cart　Refers to senescence, disease and death caused by invasion of eight pathogenic factors and five kinds of pestilence into the genuine Qi, which is difficult to be prevented by original Yang.

破迷正道歌【pò mí zhèng dào gē】《破迷正道歌》为气功学养生专著，由唐代钟离权所著，论述气功的原理与功效。

Pomi Zhengdao Ge (*Right Way of Songs for Clarifying Riddles*)　A monograph of Qigong entitled *Right Way of Songs for Clarifying Riddles*, written by Zhong Liquan in the Tang Dynasty (618 AD – 907 AD), describing the theory and effects of Qigong.

魄门【pò mén】　指肛门。

corporeal soul gate   Refers to the anus.

菩提【pú tí】 佛家气功习用语，指觉悟。

Bodhi   A common term of Qigong in Buddhism, referring to consciousness.

菩提心【pú tí xīn】 佛家气功习用语，指求正觉之心，为稳定神形的精神活动。

Bodhi heart   A common term of Qigong in Buddhism, referring to seeking the purified heart in order to stabilize the activity of the spirit.

蒲虔贯【pú qián guàn】 宋代养生学家，通气功，著有气功养生专著。

Pu Qianguan   A master of life cultivation in the Song Dynasty (960 AD - 1279 AD), familiar with Qigong. He wrote a monograph of Qigong and life cultivation.

普照【pǔ zhào】 指练功中经过精、气、神的修炼而成乾阳丽天之象，无不光照。

illumination   Refers to beautiful celestial scene with enlightenment after refining the essence, Qi and the spirit in practicing Qigong.

P

Q

七不【qī bù】　指不杀、不欲、不盗、不偷、不邪、不妄、不颠不狂。

seven kinds of no　Refers to no killing，no desire，no stealing，no robbing，no evil，no absurd and no bumping.

七常住果【qī cháng zhù guǒ】　佛家气功习用语，指佛家气功所要达到的理想境界。

seven ideal boundaries　A common term of Qigong in Buddhism，referring to the ideal state of the spirit in Buddhism.

七冲门【qī chōng mén】　指消化系统中的七个冲要之门，即飞门（唇）、户门（齿）、吸门（会厌）、贲门（胃上口）、幽门（胃下口）、阑门（大小肠交界处）、魄门（肛门）。

seven rushing gates　Refers to seven important gates in the digestive system，including the lip，tooth，epiglottis，cardia，pylori，ileocecal conjunction and anus.

七返【qī fǎn】　指耳、目、口、鼻七窍内观为七返。

seven vipassana　Refers to the introspection in the seven orifices including ears，eyes，nostrils and mouth.

七返还丹【qī fǎn huán dān】　即心之阳，复还于心，而在中丹。

returning of seven kinds to Dan（**pills of immortality**）　Refers to Yang from the heart that returns to the heart and enters the middle Dan（the middle of the chest）.

七宝【qī fǎn】　指人体津、水、唾、血、神、气、精七种物质。

seven treasures　Refers to fluid，water，saliva，blood，spirit，Qi and essence.

七门【qī mén】　指身有七门，即泥丸为天门，尾闾为地门，夹脊为中门，明堂为前门，玉枕为后门，重楼为楼门，绛宫为房门。

seven gates　Refers to the mud bolus（the brain）known as celestial gate，the coccyx known as earthly gate，the back and the waist known as middle gate，the nose known as front gate，the posterior hairline known as back gate，the trachea known as building gate and the precordium known as house gate.

七元【qī yuán】　指七窍之元，及七元甲子。

seven origins　Refers to either seven stars；or seven orifices；or seven Jiazi（sixty years）.

七魄【qī pò】　指肺神及损伤情志的因素。

seven corporeal souls　Refers to either lung spirit；or the factors that have damaged emotion.

七窍【qī qiào】　指人身眼、耳、口、鼻七孔。

seven orifices　Refers to the eyes，the ears，the nostrils and the mouth.

七情【qī qíng】　指七种情感，即喜、怒、哀、乐、爱、恶、欲。

seven emotions　Refers to seven mental activities，including happiness，anger， anxiety, contemplation, sorrow, fear and surprise.

七日之五【qī rì zhī wǔ】　指五脏之气，七日来复。

five in seven days　Refers to reflex of Qi from the five Zang-organs (including the heart, the liver, the spleen, the lung and the kidney) in seven days.

七蕤玉龠【qī ruí yù yuè】　指七窍开合。

seven flowers and jade instrument　Refers to opening and closing the seven orifices.

七伤【qī shāng】　指七种劳伤，男子肾气亏损的七种表现，道教对修道者的七种禁忌。

seven impairments　Refers to either seven kinds of internal lesion caused by overexertion; or seven manifestations of kidney Qi loss in men; or seven taboos in Daoism.

七神去【qī shén qù】　指损伤五脏六腑的情况。肝神损伤于魂散失目不明，心神损伤于神散失唇见青白，肺神损伤于魄不在身鼻不通，肾神损伤于意出身外食不甘味，头神损伤于神出泥丸头目眩晕，腹神损伤于胃肠神散，四肢神损伤于骨关节重滞不动。

loss of seven spirits　Refers to different ways to damage the spirit from the five Zang-organs (including the heart, the liver, the spleen, the lung and the kidney) and the six Fu-organs (the gallbladder, stomach, small intestine, large intestine, bladder and triple energizer). The spirit in the liver is damaged by dispersion of the ethereal soul; the spirit in the heart is damaged by loss of the spirit and change of the lips; the spirit in the lung is damaged by dispersion of the corporeal soul and obstructed nose; the spirit in the kidney is damaged by no pure emotion and no good food; the spirit in the brain is damaged by dispersion of the spirit from the mud bolus (the brain) and dizziness; the spirit in the abdomen is damaged by dispersion of the spirit in the stomach and intestines; the spirit in the four limbs is damaged by stagnation of the joints.

七十二候【qī shí èr hòu】　古代以五日为一候，一月六候。三候为一节气。一年分为二十四节气，共七十二候。

seventy-two Hou (five days)　A traditional Chinese concept. In ancient China the period of five days was called Hou and altogether there were six Hou in a month. Traditionally there is one festival in three Hou. In a whole year there are twenty-four festivals and seventy-two Hou.

七漱玉泉【qī shù yù quán】　指一日七次漱唾液咽之，有益于神形。

gargling saliva for seven times　The term of gargling saliva for seven times refers to chewing and swallowing saliva for seven times daily, effectively benefiting the spirit and body.

七星【qī xīng】　指北斗星。

seven stars　The term of seven stars refers to the Big Dipper.

七玄【qī xuán】　指七窍流通之象。

seven mysteries　Refers to circulation of the seven orifices.

七曜【qī yào】　即日、月、金、木、水、火、土七大星球。常用配七窍，说明七窍的生理功能与自然的关系。

seven kinds of sunlight　Refers to the sun, the moon, the Venus, the Jupiter, Mercury, Mars and Saturn, usually connected with the seven orifices to explain the physiological function and the relation with the natural world.

七液【qī yè】 指七窍之液；也指心液、肝液、脾液、肺液、肾液、气液、血液。

seven humors Refers to either fluid in the seven orifices; or heart humor, liver humor, spleen humor, lung humor, kidney humor, Qi humor and blood humor.

七阴【qī yīn】 指的是涕、唾、精、津、气、血、液。

seven kinds of Yin Refers to tear, saliva, essence, fluid, Qi, blood and humor.

七月节导引法【qī yuè jié dǎo yǐn fǎ】 为动功。其作法为，七月节每日丑寅时正坐，两手握住阴囊，闭气引气向上，口中唾液咽下三五口。可治劳伤、除积聚。

exercise of Daoyin in the feast days of July A dynamic exercise, marked by sitting upright in Chou (the period of a day from 1 a.m. to 3 a.m. in the morning) and Yin (the period of a day from 3 a.m. to 5 a.m. in the morning) every day in July for practicing Qigong, holding the scrotum with both hands, leading Qi to flow upwards and swallowing saliva for three or five times. Such a dynamic exercise can cure internal lesion caused by overexertion.

七月中导引法【qī yuè zhōng dǎo yǐn fǎ】 为动功。其作法为，七月中每日丑寅时，正坐片时，转头左右摇二十四遍。可祛病邪，健身。

exercise of Daoyin in the middle of July A dynamic exercise, marked by sitting upright in Chou (the period of a day from 1 a.m. to 3 a.m. in the morning) and Yin (the period of a day from 3 a.m. to 5 a.m. in the morning) every day in July for practicing Qigong, shaking the head to the left and right and vice versa for twenty-four times respectively. Such a dynamic exercise can relieve pathogenic factors and cultivate health.

七正之一【qī zhèng zhī yī】 专指目。在气功锻炼中，目在七窍中特别重要。

one of the seven orifices Refers to the eye, which is the most important orifice in practicing Qigong.

七知【qī zhī】 即① 知法，知十二部经能诠之法；② 知义，知经中一切文字语言所诠之义理；③ 知时，知可修寂静、精进、舍定、般若等；④ 知足，对饮食、衣、药、行、住、坐、卧等知止知足；⑤ 知自，知悉自己之戒；⑥ 知众；⑦ 知信者不信之别。

seven cognitions Refers to ① either cognizing laws, related to twelve meridians; ② or cognizing information, related to the characters in describing the twelve meridians; ③ or cognizing time, related to cultivation of the mind and the spirit and understanding officials and wisdom; ④ or cognizing satisfaction, related to understanding about how to take food, dress clothes, take medicine and start the activities of walking, staying, sitting and lying; ⑤ or self-cognition, related to benevolence; ⑥ or cognizing others; ⑦ or cognizing belief, related to different from unbelief.

七种舍【qī zhǒng shě】 指七种舍去烦恼，稳定精神，维持神形相对平衡的行为。

seven kinds of truncation Refers to the

seven ways to relieve annoyance and to keep the stability of the spirit and the body.

期门【qī mén**】** 足厥阴肝经中的一个穴位,位于乳头直下,为气功中常用的意守部位。

Qimen（LR 14） An acpuoint in the liver meridian of foot Jueyin, located directly below the breast, which is the region for concentrating consciousness in practicing Qigong.

栖心凝神【qī xīn níng shén**】** 指练功中平心安神,以使之意念入静的一个法则。

tranquilizing the heart and concentrating the spirit Refers to the principle for tranquilizing the mind by pacifying the heart and stabilizing the spirit.

栖真【qī zhēn**】** 指应用气功养生法,导引入静。

genuine perch Refers to tranquilization in practicing Qigong and life cultivation.

其大元外,其小无内【qí dà yuán wài qí xiǎo wú nèi**】** 源自《管子》,指灵气之大,广漠无垠;言灵气其小"一分为二",万世不竭。

as big as no external side and as small as no internal side Collected from Guanzi, a great canon compiled in the Spring and Autumn Period（770 BC - 476 BC）. It means that the spiritual Qi is so large without any boundary and so small with just two stages, absolutely inexhaustible.

其生五,其气三【qí shēng wǔ qí qì sān**】** 源自《黄帝内经》,指天气衍生金、木、水、火、土五行,阴阳之气又依盛衰消长而各分为三阴(太阴、少阴、厥阴)三阳(太阳、阳明、少阳)。

Production of five categories with three kinds of Qi. Collected from the most important Chinese canon Hangdi Neijing（entitled *Yellow Emperor's Internal Canon of Medicine*）, indicating that the celestial Qi evolves into the five elements（including metal, wood, water, fire and earth）, while the wax and wane of Yin and Yang can be divided into three Yin（including Taiyin, Shaoyin and Jueyin）and three Yang（including Taiyang, Yangming and Shaoyang）.

奇经八脉【qí jīng bā mài**】** 指督脉、任脉、冲脉、带脉、阴维脉、阳维脉、阴跷脉、阳跷脉八条经脉。此经脉为气功习练之处。

extraordinary eight meridians Refers to the governor meridian, conception meridian, thoroughfare meridian, belt meridian, Yin link meridian, Yang link meridian, Yin heel meridian and Yang heel meridian. These meridians are the regions usually used in practice of Qigong.

奇经八脉考【qí jīng bā mài kǎo**】** 中医专著,兼论气功,由明代李时珍所撰。

Qijing Bamai Kao（*Study of Extraordinary Eight Meridians***）** A comprehensive monograph of traditional Chinese medicine with the discussion about Qigong entitled *Study of Extraordinary Eight Meridians*, written by Li Shizhen, a great scientist of traditional Chinese medicine in the Ming Dynasty（1368 AD - 1644 AD）.

歧骨【qí gǔ**】** ① 泛指两骨连接成角之处;② 指胸骨下角。

bone juncture Refers to ① either the connected joint of two bones; ② or the

Q

lower part of the sternum.

脐呼吸【qí hū xī**】**　指应用腹肌鼓凹作为气体变换的动力,呼吸的枢机在脐,口鼻仅是呼吸之气出入的通道。

Navel respiration　Indicates that plucking up the abdomen is the power for changing Qi, the key of respiration is in the navel and the mouth and nose are the ways for inhalation and exhalation.

踑踞【qí jù**】**　指屈膝张腿而坐的导引姿势。

stretching feet　Refers to feature of Daoyin marked by sitting, bending the knees and stretching the feet.

启真集【qǐ zhēn jí**】**　《启真集》为气功专著,由金代刘志渊所撰,叙述了习练气功的基本理论与方法。

Qizhen Ji(*Collection of Activation of Truth*)　A monograph of Qigong entitled *Collection of Activation of Truth*, written by Liu Zhiyuan in the Jin Dynasty (1115 AD – 1234 AD), discussing the theory and methods of Qigong practice.

起髀法【qǐ bì fǎ**】**　为动功。其作法为,静坐存中气,挺身,以两手相叉,用力向左右伸出各七次,手向左侧头向右,向右侧则头向左,如此三五次,静坐片刻,善和脾胃,增进食欲,治腰背拘挛,与开关法配合行之更好。

exercise for raising the high　A dynamic exercise, marked by sitting quietly, keeping Qi in the middle, straightening the back, crossing the hands, stretching to the left and right for seven times respectively, turning the hand to the left and the head to the right and vice versa for three or five times respectively. Such a way of quiet sitting for a while can harmonize the spleen

and stomach, increase appetite, cure spasm in the waist and back and cooperate with the exercise for opening joints.

起火得长安法【qǐ huǒ dé cháng ān fǎ**】**　为静功。其作法为,子午二时,存想真火自涌泉穴起,先从左足行,上玉枕,过泥丸,降入丹田,三遍。次从右足,亦行三遍。复从尾闾起,又三遍。

exercise of increasing fire for longevity　A static exercise, marked by starting from Zi (the period of the day from 11 p.m. to 1 a.m.) and Wu (the period of the day from 11 a.m. to 1 p.m. in the noon), imagining to start genuine fire from Yongquan (KI 1), rising first from the left foot to Yuzhen (BL 9) through mud bolus (the brain) and entering Dantian for three times, then rising from the right foot in the same way for three times, finally rising from the coccyx for three times. Dantian is divided into the upper Dantian (the region between the eyes), the middle Dantian (the region below the heart) and the lower Dantian (the region below the navel).

起火法【qǐ huǒ fǎ**】**　为静功。其作法为,入静室,散发披衣,闭目瞑心,正坐握固,叩齿集神,升身起火,微以意留息,少入迟出,默想脐下,火轮大如斗,须臾焰起,照定自身。

exercise for breaking out fire　A static exercise, marked by entering a quiet room, loosening clothes, closing the eyes, tranquilizing the heart, sitting upright, holding the hands, clicking the teeth, concentrating the spirit, raising the body to increase fire, mildly keeping respiration, seldom inhaling

Q

and slowly exhaling, imagining to increase great fire below the navel to illuminate the whole body.

气【qì】 ① 指呼吸出入之气；② 指脏腑功能；③ 指气候、气色；④ 指气味；⑤ 指古代哲学概念。

Qi Refers to ① either all kinds of air in the natural world; ② or respiration; ③ or functions of the viscera; ④ or climate; ⑤ or taste; or concept of philosophy.

气痹【qì bì】 气功适应证，指由情志不遂等因素启发的痹证。

Qi impediment An indication of Qigong, refers to emotional frustration that has caused various impediments.

气出于脑【qì chū yú nǎo】 指人体正气从脑出。

Qi originating from sea Refers to the healthy Qi in the body that comes out of the brain.

气传子母【qì chuán zǐ mǔ】 五行相生，生者为母，所生者为子。

Qi passing on to child and mother Refers to the relations among the five elements (including wood, fire, earth, metal and water) during which to promote means mother and to be promoted means child.

气法【qì fǎ】 为静功。即从子时到午时为阳，可吸气；从午时到子时为阴，可闭气。

Qi exercise A static exercise, referring to either the time from Zi (the period of the day from 11 p.m. to 1 a.m.) to Wu (the period of the day from 11 a.m. to 1 p.m.) which belongs to Yang, during which Qi can be absorbed; or the time from Wu (the period of the day from 11 a.m. to 1 p.m.)

to Zi (the period of the day from 11 p.m. to 1 a.m.) which belongs to Yin, during which Qi cannot be absorbed.

气法景象【qì fǎ jǐng xiàng】 源自气功专论。指日夜存心，节候自成。一日著身，二日如梦，三日小腹觉知，四日腹鸣，五日两眼热，六日两足热，七日神见，八日气如云行，九日上下通，十日神光行形中。

manifestation of Qi exercise Collected from a monograph of Qigong, referring to the method usually used to practice Qigong, indicating that the body is cultivated in the first day; dream is felt in the second day; the lower abdomen appears clear in the third day; the abdomen sounds in the fourth day; the eyes feel warm in the fifth day; the feet feel hot in the sixth day; the spirit appears in the seventh day; Qi moves like cloud in the eighth day; the upper and lower are unimpeded in the ninth day; and spiritual brightness emerges in the tenth day, etc.

气法要妙至诀【qì fǎ yào miào zhì jué】《气法要妙至诀》为气功养生专著，作者不详。主要论述气功养生法中的深奥道理。

Qifa Yaomiao Zhijue (*Perfect Formula for Exercise of Qigong*) A monograph of Qigong and life cultivation entitled *Perfect Formula for Exercise of Qigong*, mainly discussing the profound truth of Qigong practice in cultivating health.

气功【qì gōng】 ① 指调身、调气、调神；② 指调节呼吸的功夫。

Qigong Refers to ① either regulation of the body, Qi and the spirit; ② or regulation of the functions of respiration.

气功保固神气【qì gōng bǎo gù shén qì**】**源自气功专论,指习练气功,不费针药,又不辛劳,取之自身实际,如坚持不懈,有保固神气之功。

qigong protecting the spirit and Qi Collected from a monograph of Qigong, referring to the fact that practice of Qigong should not take medicinal, should avoid hardness and should preserve in order to stabilize the function of spiritual Qi.

气功工夫说【qì gōng gōng fu shuō**】**源自气功专论,阐述习练气功出现的练功者的感受。

idea about Qigong practice Collected from a monograph of Qigong, mainly describing the experience of Qigong practice.

气功声法【qì gōng shēng fǎ**】**为静功。其作法为,在练气功过程中,口中发出特定的音响或在行功的同时,口念咒语等,称气功声法。

exercise of Qigong with sound A static exercise, marked by pronouncing a special sound in practicing Qigong or reading incantation in staging any activity.

气共力调【qì gòng lì tiáo**】**指导引时,气和力的使用要协调,不能力大于气,或气大于力。

balance between Qi and strength Refers to coordination of Qi and power in practicing Daoyin, ensuring the fact that Qi should not be greater than power and power should not be greater than Qi.

气归丹田法【qì guī dān tián fǎ**】**为动功。其作法为,半夜子时以后,床上瞑目盘坐面东,呵出腹内旧气两三口,然后停息,便于鼻内微纳清气数口。

exercise for Qi entering Dantian A dynamic exercise, marked by referring to sitting quietly to the east on the bed with closed eyes after Zi (the period of the day from 11 p. m. to 1 a. m.), breathing out obsolete Qi from the abdomen for two or three times, then suspending respiration for clear Qi in the nose to clean the mouth. Dantian is divided into the upper Dantian (the region between the eyes), the middle Dantian (the region below the heart) and the lower Dantian (the region below the navel).

气归髓满【qì guī suǐ mǎn**】**指气归丹田,自然髓海满盈。

entrance of Qi fulfilling marrow Refers to entrance of Qi into Dantian and exuberance of the brain. Dantian is divided into the upper Dantian (the region between the eyes), the middle Dantian (the region below the heart) and the lower Dantian (the region below the navel).

气归元海【qì guī yuán hǎi**】**指气功现象,为行功者晴感受。即气归丹田,精气盈满则溢之状。

Qi entering original sea Refers to entrance of Qi into Dantian and exuberance of essential Qi. Dantian is divided into the upper Dantian (the region between the eyes), the middle Dantian (the region below the heart) and the lower Dantian (the region below the navel).

气海【qì hǎi**】**即"元阳在肾,肾为气之海"。

Qi sea Refers to the fact that the original Qi is in the kidney and the kidney is the sea of Qi.

气海门【qì hǎi mén】 精气聚散常在此处,水火发端也在此处,阴阳变化也在此处,有无出入也在此处。

gate of Qi sea Refers to the region where the essential Qi concentrates and disperses there, water and fire appear there, Yin and Yang change there, exit and entrance exist there.

气化【qì huà】 ① 指阴阳之气的变化;② 指身体脏腑器官、经络精气功能活动;③ 指自然界六气的变化。

Qi transformation Refers to ① either the changes of Qi from Yin and Yang; ② or functional activities of the essence and Qi in the viscera and meridians; ③ or changes of six kinds of air in the natural world.

气化神【qì huà shén】 指习练气功,导引入静后,神气合而为一。

Qi blending spirit Refers to tranquilization and quietness in practicing Qigong, leading to integration of Qi and spirit.

气街【qì jiē】 ① 指经气通行的路径;② 指腹股沟动脉搏动处,又称气冲。

Qi passage Refers to ① either the way for Qi in the meridians to flow; ② or an acupoint named Qichong (ST 30).

气口【qì kǒu】 指手太阴肺经及其所过之寸口部位。

Qi port Refers to the lung meridian of hand Taiyin with its pulse on the wrist.

气淋【qì lín】 气功适应证,指少腹胀满较明显,小便艰涩疼痛,尿有余沥。多因肝气郁结,膀胱气化不利所致。

Qi stranguria An indication of Qigong, refers to the fact that the lower abdomen is swollen and urination is difficult due to depression of the liver and difficulty of the bladder to transform Qi.

气淋候导引法【qì lín hòu dǎo yǐn fǎ】 为动功。其作法为,用两足跟交替放在膝上,能通阳利水,治隆闭;指仰卧,两手放膝头,脚跟放臀下,用口吸气,鼓腹,待气充满腹部时,用鼻呼出,作七息。

exercise of Daoyin for Qi stranguria A dynamic exercise, marked by crossing the heels and alternately putting on the knees in order to unobstruct Yang and to promote water for curing frequent micturition; then lying on the back with both hands pressing on the knees and both feet stretching under the buttocks, breathing in through the mouth, increasing the abdomen and exhaling with the nose for seven times if Qi is sufficient in the abdomen.

气瘤【qì liú】 气功适应证,多因肺气失宣,复感外邪,痰气凝结,营卫不和所致。

Qi tumor An indication of Qigong, is usually caused by disorder of lung Qi, invasion of external pathogenic factors and disharmony of nutrient Qi and defense Qi.

气轮【qì lún】 指眼科五轮之一,白睛(包括球结膜及前部巩膜)。

Qi wheel Refers to one of the five kinds of wheels, indicating the white part of the eye (including bulbar conjunctiva and sclera).

气满任督自开【qì mǎn rèn dū zì kāi】 指习练周天气功,意守丹田,精气盈满,任督二脉自然开通。

fullness of Qi dredging the conception meridian and governor meridian Refers to the fact that only when consciousness is concentrated on the Dantian and the essential Qi is exuberant can the conception meridian and the governor meridian naturally be opened. Dantian is divided into the upper Dantian（the region between the eyes）, the middle Dantian（the region below the heart）and the lower Dantian（the region below the navel）.

气门【qì mén】　指腧穴，"知补虚泻实，上下气门"。

Qi gate　Refers to the acupoint called Shuxue which is the special location for Qi and blood in the viscera and meridians to flow in and out.

气逆治法【qì nì zhì fǎ】　为动功。其作法为，两手向后，尽力向上把托腰；指两足趾相对，行气五息，引气入心肺。

Qi reversing exercise　A dynamic exercise, marked by turning the hands to the back, forcefully holding up the waist, keeping the toes from both feet related to each other, moving Qi for five times and leading Qi into the heart and the lung.

气入丹田火自生【qì rù dān tián huǒ zì shēng】　源自气功专论，主要阐述气功炼就阳神景象。

natural appearance of fire after entrance of Qi into Dantian　Collected from a monograph about Qigong, mainly describing the image of Yang spirit in practicing Qigong. Dantian is divided into the upper Dantian（the region between the eyes）, the middle Dantian（the region below the heart）and the lower Dantian（the region below the navel）.

气神调匀【qì shén tiáo yún】　指神气合而为一，即气与思维活动协调统一。

harmony between Qi and spirit　Refers to coordination and unity of Qi and

consciousness activity for the purpose of succeeding the practice of Qigong.

气神相应【qì shén xiāng yìng】　指神气相依，互为照应。

correspondence between Qi and spirit　Refers to the fact that Qi and spirit depend on each other and coordinate with each other for the purpose of cultivating health and protecting the body.

气数【qì shù】　指一年二十四节气的常数，用以标志万物的生化。

Qi numbers　Refers to the twenty-four festivals in a year, indicating the growth and transformation of all things in the universe.

气香兰【qì xiāng lán】　即习练气功时，气功状态下，口中津液甘香，而身体有异香发出。

fragrant saliva　Refers to the fact that fluid and humor in the mouth feels sweet and there is sweet taste in the body in practicing Qigong.

气邪【qì xié】　指损气、滞气、逆气的八种因素，即风、寒、暑、湿、饥、饱、劳、逸。

Qi evils　Refers to eight pathogenic factors that damage Qi, stagnate Qi and retrograde Qi, including wind, cold, summerheat, dampness, hunger, fullness, labor and leisure.

气形相应【qì xíng xiāng yìng】　指气与形体协调相依。

correspondence between Qi and body　Refers to correspondence and dependence between Qi and the body.

气穴【qì xué】　① 指下丹田；② 指经穴名，别名胞门、子户。

Qixue　Refers to ① either lower Dantian（the region below the navel）, ② or an acupoint named Qixue（KI 13）or Baomen（KI 13）or Zihu（KI 13）.

Q

气血源头【qì xuè yuán tóu】 指神定息定，调息也在其中。

origin of Qi and blood Refers to tranquilizing the spirit and respiration.

气液相济【qì yè xiāng jì】 源自气功专论，说明心肾相交，水火既济的作用过程。

communication between Qi and humor Collected from a monograph of Qigong, referring to the procedure of coordination between the heart and the kidney as well as balance between water and fire.

气瘿【qì yǐng】 气功适应证，指颈前结喉处肿块，多因情志内伤或水土因素所致。

Qi wart An indication of Qigong, is usually caused by lump of throat and internal damage due to emotional activities or water and earth factors.

气郁【qì yù】 气功适应证，指由于情志内伤，肝气郁结所致。症见精神抑郁，情绪不宁，胸胁胀痛。

Qi depression An indication of Qigong, refers to depression caused by mental activity damaging the internal organs and stagnation of liver Qi, characterized by deprementia, thoracic pain and abdominal anorexia.

气钟于子【qì zhōng yú zǐ】 指子时一阳之气生。

Qi appearance in noon Refers to appearance of Yang Qi in Zi (the period of the day from 11 p.m. to 1 a.m.).

气足神全丹始成【qì zú shén quán dān shǐ chéng】 源自气功专论，主要阐述气功学中的药是先天气，火是神。

sufficiency of Qi and exuberance of the spirit ensuring formation of Dan (pills of immortality) Collected from a monograph about Qigong, mainly describing that in Qigong the medicinal is the prenatal Qi and fire is the spirit.

弃损淫欲专守精【qì sǔn yín yù zhuān shǒu jīng】 即抛弃不利于机体的淫欲念头和行为，专志一意守精神。

Only when lust is abandoned can the essence be concentrated. Suggests to eliminate the idea and behavior of lust for concentrating the consciousness in the essence and the spirit.

炁【qì】 同气，指气含阴阳两个方面。

qi Refers to Yin and Yang in Qi and the righteousness in Daoism.

千法明门【qiān fǎ míng mén】 佛家气功习用语，指引练各种佛家功法。

all schools of Qigong A term of Qigong in Buddhism, referring to practice of Qigong with various methods in Buddhism.

千金方【qiān jīn fāng】 《千金方》为中医经典著作，由唐代药王孙思邈所作。

Qian Jin Fang (Thousand Golden Formula) A canon of traditional Chinese medicine entitled *Thousand Golden Formula*e, written by Sun Simiao, the king of traditional Chinese medicine in the Tang Dynasty (618 AD – 907 AD).

千金翼方【qiān jīn yì fāng】 《千金翼方》为中医经典著作，由唐代药王孙思邈所作。

qian Jin Yi Fang (A Supplement to Thousand Golden Formula) A canon of traditional Chinese medicine entitled *A Supplement to Thousand Golden Formulae*, written by Sun Simiao, the king of traditional Chinese medicine in the Tang Dynasty (618 AD – 907 AD).

铅鼎【qiān dǐng】 ① 即下丹田，指气海；② 指脐下。

lead cauldron　① The same as lower Dantian（the region below the navel）, refers to either Qihai（CV 6）located below the navel；② or the region below the navel.

铅汞【qiān gǒng**】**　同水中银，① 喻心，属火，为正阳之精；② 指神气。

lead and mercury　The same as silver in water，referring to ① either the heart that belongs to fire；② or spiritual Qi.

铅汞相投【qiān gǒng xiāng tóu**】**　铅指精，汞指神，以神炼精，称铅汞相投。

combination of lead and mercury　Refers to combination of the essence and the spirit. In this term，lead refers to the essence and mercury refers to the spirit.

铅汞异炉【qiān gǒng yì lú**】**　同龙虎交媾，指阴阳和合。

unusual furnace with lead and mercury　The same as harmonization of Loong and tiger，referring to harmonization of Yin and Yang. In this term，lead and mercury refer to Yin and Yang.

前关【qián guān**】**　足少阳胆经中的一个穴位瞳子髎的另外一个称谓，位于目外眦外侧 0.5 寸。

Qianguan　A synonym of Tongziliao（GB 1）which is an acupoint in the gallbladder meridian of foot Shaoyang，located 0.5 Cun lateral to the outer canthus.

前后相随【qián hòu xiāng suí**】**　指在自然、社会之中，前后之事对立而出现，前后之事相互依赖，彼此转化。

interrelation of the front and the back　Refers to the fact that all the things around in the natural world and social world are opposite to each other and dependent on each other，and naturally transforming each other.

前三三【qián sān sān**】**　指练功中的腹部三关。

front three and three　Refers to three joints in the abdomen in practicing Qigong.

前识【qián shí**】**　指意识于先事之行而行，先理之动而功。

precognition　Refers to consciousness starting before the activities of anything and moving before the movement of any factors.

前弦【qián xián**】**　即上弦之时，为阴中阳半。

principal rafter　Refers to half of Yin being Yang.

前弦半轮月【qián xián bàn lún yuè**】**　指的是白虎。白虎指二十八宿中西方的七宿；内丹书中指"心中元神谓之龙，肾中元精谓之虎"。

front chord with half moon　Refers to the white tiger. Traditionally white tiger refers to either the seven constellations in the west among the twenty-eight constellations；or "the original spirit in the heart called Loong and the original essence in the kidney called tiger" mentioned in the books about internal Dan (pills of immortality).

乾【qián**】**　① 卦名，指天；② 指首；③ 指日；④ 指有道德精神意识稳定的人；⑤ 指阳气；⑥ 指刚、动。

qian（Trigram）　The Qian Trigram in the Eight Trigrams from Yijing（*Canon of Simplification*，*Change and No Change*），referring to ① either the sky；② or the head；③ or the sun；④ or the man with stable virtue, spirit and consciousness；⑤ or Yang Qi；⑥ or firmness and activity.

Q

乾顶【qián dǐng】　指头顶。乾指的是头。

top of Qian（Trigram）　Refers to the top of the head. In this term, Qian（Trigram）refers to the head.

乾宫【qián gōng】　即乾顶，指头顶。乾指的是头。

Qian（Trigram）palace　The same as top of Qian（Trigram）, referring to the top of the head. In this term, Qian（Trigram）refers to the head.

乾坤【qián kūn】　① 指宇宙之内的阴阳两方面及其变化；② 指人身的阴阳两方面及其变化；③ 指气功药物；④ 指天地；⑤ 指乾坤相互为根。

Qian（Trigram）and Kun（Trigram）　Refers to ① either Yin and Yang and their changes in the universe；② or Yin and Yang and their changes in the human body；③ or medicinal in Qigong；④ or the sky and earth；⑤ or mutual root of Qian（Trigram）and Kun（Trigram）.

乾坤交媾【qián kūn jiāo gòu】　指气功状态下，身体阴阳相交，和合协调。

intercourse of Qian（Trigram）and Kun（Trigram）　Refers to integration and coordination of Yin and Yang in the body under the condition of Qigong practice.

乾坤交泰【qián kūn jiāo tài】　指阴阳相交，相互作用而化生万物。

interaction between Qian（Trigram）and Kun（Trigram）　Refers to integration of Yin and Yang that has produced all things in this world.

乾坤坎离【qián kūn kǎn lí】　① 气功学名词，喻身体上下左右；② 乾坤为经，坎离为纬，运动变化，交相作用，以成金丹大药；③ 卦名，即乾、坤、坎、离四卦。

Qian（Trigram）, Kun（Trigram）, Kan（Trigram）and Li（Trigram）　① A term of Qigong, referring to either the upper, the lower, the left and the right sides of the body；② or movement, changes and integration of meridians and collaterals that have produced golden Dan（pills of immortality）, in which Qian（Trigram）and Kun（Trigram）refer to the meridians while Kan（Trigram）and Li（Trigram）refer to the collaterals；③ or the names of four Trigrams, i. e. Qian Trigram, Kun Trigram, Kan Trigram and Li Trigram.

乾坤体成【qián kūn tǐ chéng】　指气功中，金丹之成，由阴阳两类药物组成。

formation of Qian（Trigram）and Kun（Trigram）　Indicates that formation of golden Dan（pills of immortality）is made by Yin medicinal and Yang medicinal in Qigong.

乾马【qián mǎ】　指心，喻心阳。

celestial horse　Refers to the heart, comparing to heart Yang.

潜龙【qián lóng】　① 指君子隐居不出，处静不动；② 指精神意识活动保持稳定，不受外来因素的影响。

hidden Loong　Refers to ① either living in seclusion and keeping tranquility；② or stabilized activities of the spirit and consciousness without being affected by anything in the external world.

潜心下照【qián xīn xià zhào】　指习练气功时，意识活动集中于肾之意。

Carefully illuminating the lower　Refers to concentration of consciousness activity in the kidney.

遣之踵前说【qiǎn zhī zhǒng qián shuō】　源自气功专论，重点讨论踵息的特点和方法。

idea about sending the heel Collected from a monograph of Qigong, mainly discussing the characteristics and methods of heel respiration.

敲爻歌【qiāo yáo gē】 《敲爻歌》为气功著作,由唐代吕洞宾著,书中认为进行气功锻炼,平时宜放松形体,逍遥自在,顺应自然,注意精神稳定平和。

Qiaoyao Ge (*Qiaoyao Song*) A monograph of Qigong entitled *Qiaoyao Song*, written by Lü Dongbin in the Tang Dynasty (618 AD - 907 AD), suggesting relaxing the body, being carefree, following natural environment and stabilizing and harmonizing the essence and the spirit in practicing Qigong.

敲竹唤龟吞玉芝【qiāo zhú huàn guī tūn yù zhī】 指气功清静脑神,调节呼吸,吞津咽液。

knocking bamboo, calling tortoise and taking jade Ganoderma Refers to quieting the brain spirit, regulating respiration and swallowing fluid and humor.

侵气【qīn qì】 ① 指引气;② 指损害。

invading Qi Refers to ① either leading Qi; ② or damage.

秦越人【qín yuè rén】 即扁鹊,战国时杰出医学家,通气功。

Qin Yueren Another name of Bian Que, a great doctor in the Warring States Period (475 BC - 221 BC), who was very proficient in Qigong.

琴心三叠【qín xīn sān dié】 指意识思维活动如琴音和谐,则三丹田之气和合而为一。

three sides of music centers Indicates that the activities of consciousness and thinking are just like harmonious music, enabling Qi from the three kinds of

Dantian to be harmonized and integrated. The three kinds of Dantian refer to the upper Dantian (the region between the eyes), the middle Dantian (the region below the heart) and the lower Dantian (the region below the navel).

勤【qín】 佛家气功习用语,指努力修行(习练)气功,不懈怠。

diligence A common term of Qigong in Buddhism, referring to practicing Qigong without any slacking.

勤求【qín qiú】 即刻苦磨炼,坚持不懈。

diligence with efforts Means to temper forcefully and make unremitting efforts.

勤行【qín xíng】 ① 佛家气功习用语,指刻苦操行;② 指不择行、住、坐、卧、一切时间而修行。

diligent movement A common term of Qigong in Buddhism, referring to ① either conducting hard; ② or practicing not only by moving, staying, sitting or lying at any time.

擒元赋【qín yuán fù】 《擒元赋》为气功学专著,论述简易明白,有实用价值。作者不详。

Qinyuan Fu (*Collection of Original Composition*) A monograph of Qigong entitled *Collection of Original Composition*, describing the theory and practice of Qigong very clear and valuable. The author was unknown.

青城山【qīng chéng shān】 位于四川省,相传为东汉张道陵修道之处。

Qingcheng Mountain Located in Sichuan Province. According to traditional legendary story, Zhang Daoling, the founder of Daoism, studied and created Daoism in this mountain.

Q

青娥【qīng é】 喻真意。

green moth Compares to genuine idea.

青锦【qīng jǐn】 指肝之外象。

green brocade Refers to the external image of the liver.

青锦披裳佩玉铃【qīng jǐn pī shang pèi yù líng】 指肝的外部结构、征象。肝之色为青锦,白脉垂肝之象而曰玉铃。

dressing green brocade with decoration of jade bell Refers to the structure and symbol of the liver. In this celebrated dictum, Green brocade refers to the color of the liver, jade bell refers to the white meridian connected with the liver.

青龙【qīng lóng】 指二十八宿中东方七宿,即角、亢、氐、房、心、尾、箕组成龙像,位于东方,五行配五色属青色,故称青龙。

green Loon Refers to seven lunar mansions in the east among the twenty-eight lunar mansions, i.e. Jiao, Kang, Di, Fang, Xin, Wei and Qi that form the image of Loong. When the five elements (including wood, fire, earth, metal and water) match with the five colors, the east is green. That is why Loong is called green Loong.

青龙探爪【qīng lóng tàn zhǎo】 为动功,即两手握拳置于两腰,上体偏转,一手沿胸壁伸向对侧,五指伸开,掌心向上,再旋臂翻掌,握拳收回到腰际。

green Loong exploring paws A dynamic exercise, marked by holding the fists with both hands to put them over the two sides of the waist and to turn laterally upwards, stretching to the opposite region of the chest with one hand, spreading the five fingers, raising up the palms, turning the palms by revolving the arms, and finally clenching the fists to return to the waist.

青龙与白虎相拘【qīng lóng yǔ bái hǔ xiāng jū】 青龙为阳,白虎为阴,喻身阴阳两方面。此指身体内阴阳两方面相互制约。

mutual control of green Loong and white tiger A celebrated dictum, in which the green Loong means Yang and the white tiger means Yin, referring to Yin and Yang in the human body. This sentence means that Yin and Yang in the human body control each other.

青天歌注释【qīng tiān gē zhù shì】 《青天歌注释》为气功专著,由元代混然子所注,阐述性命双修奥旨,使后人易学。

Qingtian Ge Zhushi (*Annotation of Green Celestial Song*) A monograph of Qigong entitled *Annotation of Green Celestial Song*, explained by Hun Ranzi in the Yuan Dynasty(1271 AD – 1368 AD), describing the important ways to cultivate life, making it easy for later generations to study.

青童【qīng tóng】 指肝神。

green boy Refers to the liver spirit.

青霞子【qīng xiá zǐ】 晋隋时期著名气功学家苏元朗的另外一个称谓,其著有三部气功专著,据说活了三百多年。

Qing Xiazi Another name of Su Yuanlang, a great master of Qigong in the Jin Dynasty (266 AD – 420 AD) and Sui Dynasty (581 AD – 618 AD), who wrote three monographs of Qigong. It was said that he lived for three hundred years.

青心【qīng xīn】 佛家气功习用语,指静虑。

green heart A common term of Qigong

in Buddhism, referring to dhyana (tranquility and meditation).

青牙【qīng yá】 指肝之真气，亦指肝神。

green tooth Refers to genuine Qi in the liver or the spirit in the liver.

轻撮谷道【qīng cuō gǔ dào】 指提肛收腹。

lightly gathering the grain trail（anus） Refers to lifting the anus and fixing the abdomen.

清光太初生辉内景【qīng guāng tài chū shēng huī nèi jǐng】 为静功。其作法为，于夏历每月初二日夜间，清净的室内坐定，入静，意想自己身坐昆仑山顶，遥望远方，海边月亮初出，其形如钩，叩齿咽津各二十七。

internal state of clarity, light and primary brightness A static exercise, marked by sitting quietly in a clear room at night on the second day in every month in summer, tranquilizing the mind, imagining to reach the top of Kunlun Mountain, looking to the distant place with moonrise like hook, clicking the teeth and swallowing fluid for twenty-seven times respectively.

清净【qīng jìng】 佛家气功习用语，① 指涤除杂念，清静神形，无烦无扰；② 指消除意识活动中的污秽，避免精神刺激。

lustration A common term of Qigong in Buddhism, referring to ① either eliminating distracting thought, clearing and tranquilizing the spirit and the body, avoiding any annoyance and disturbance; ② or eliminating filth from the activity of consciousness and avoiding stimulation of the spirit.

清净净禅【qīng jìng jìng chán】 佛家气功功夫，指修禅定的十种方法，即① 清净净不昧不染污禅；② 出世间清净净禅；③ 方便清净净禅；④ 得根本清净净禅；⑤ 根本上胜进清净净禅；⑥ 住起力清净净禅；⑦ 拾复入力清净净禅；⑧ 神通所作力清净净禅；⑨ 离一切见清净净禅；⑩ 烦恼智库断清净净禅。此法调节精神意识活动，保持神形安静、协和。

pure and tranquil dhyana An exercise of Qigong in Buddhism, referring to ten kinds of exercises, including ① avoidance of contamination with pure and tranquil dhyana, ② staying in the external world with pure and tranquil dhyana, ③ facilitating with pure and tranquil dhyana, ④ obtaining the root with pure and tranquil dhyana, ⑤ going up from the root with pure and tranquil dhyana, ⑥ increasing energy with pure and tranquil dhyana, ⑦ rounding up and inputing energy with pure and tranquil dhyana, ⑧ dredging the spirit with pure and tranquil dhyana, ⑨ leaving everything with pure and tranquil dhyana, and ⑩ eliminating annoyance and improving wisdom with pure and tranquil dhyana. This exercise can regulate the activities of the spirit and consciousness and protect the stability, tranquility and coordination of the spirit and body.

清净明了【qīng jìng míng liǎo】 指内感觉身心空，外感觉万物空，弃除一切妄想杂念，无所牵挂的意思。

clear and tranquil state Refers to feeling of vacuum inside the body and outside the external world, and eliminating any distracting thought and worry.

Q

清净心【qīng jìng xīn】　佛家气功习用语,指脱尽烦恼、忧思、淫欲、贪婪、污秽的意识思维活动。

clear and tranquil heart　A common term of Qigong in Buddhism, referring to eliminating annoyance, anxiety, desire, avarice and filth from the activities of consciousness and thinking.

清净业处【qīng jìng yè chù】　佛家气功习用语,指纯洁、明净的意识活动所生之处。

clear and tranquil residence　A common term of Qigong in Buddhism, referring to the pure, bright and clear place where the activity of consciousness is performed.

清静补气法【qīng jìng bǔ qì fǎ】　为静功。其作法为,定心端坐,调息归根,候一阳之初生,采先天之正气聚于丹田,久则丹田俱满,充于五脏,五脏气足,散于百骸,百骸气全,自然撞透三关,由前降入黄庭,以身中之坎,填身中之离。

exercise for tonifying Qi with clarity and tranquility　A static exercise, marked by tranquilizing the heart, sitting upright, regulating respiration, ensuring primary production of one kind of Yang, obtaining innate healthy Qi and concentrating it in Dantian, contenting it in Dantian, enriching it in the five Zang-organs (including the heart, the liver, the spleen, the lung and the kidney) and all the skeletons, penetrating the three joints, descending to the yellow chamber (the region below the navel) from the front, filling Li Trigram (the heart) from Kan Trigram (the kidney) in the human body. Dantian is divided into the upper Dantian (the region between the eyes), the

middle Dantian (the region below the heart) and the lower Dantian (the region below the navel).

清静可以为天下正【qīng jìng kě yǐ wéi tiān xià zhèng】　喻气功中脑神情虚宁静,全身各部自然安适端正。

Clarity and tranquility can surpass everything in the world.　This is a celebrated dictum, indicating that tranquilized and clarified the brain spirit in practicing Qigong will naturally stabilize and balance all parts of the body.

清静妙经【qīng jìng miào jīng】　《清静妙经》为气功专著,作者不详。主要从清心除欲谈气功养神,认为人心本自清净,常为物欲干扰而不得清静。

Qingjing Miaojing (*Marvelous Canon of Clarity and Tranquility*)　A monograph about Qigong entitled *Marvelous Canon of Clarity and Tranquility*, mainly describing the fact that only when the heart is tranquilized and desires are eliminated can the spirit be nourished through practicing Qigong, and that only when the heart is tranquilized can disturbance be avoided. The author was unknown.

清冷宫【qīng lěng gōng】　肝的译名。

clear and cold palace　The synonym of the liver.

清明三月节坐功【qīng míng sān yuè jié zuò gōng】　为动功。其作法为,每日丑寅时(一至五时),正坐定,换手左右如引硬弓,各七八次,叩齿、纳清吐浊、咽液各三次。主治腰肾肠胃等多种疾病。

exercise of sitting in March with Pure Brightness festival　A dynamic exercise, marked by sitting upright in Chou (the period of a day from 1 a.m. to 3 a.m. in the early morning) and Yin （the period of a day from 3 a. m. to 5 a. m. in the early morning）every day，exchanging the hands from the left to the right and vice versa for seven to eight times respectively；clicking the teeth，inhaling clear Qi，exhaling turbid Qi，and swallowing humor for three times respectively. Such a dynamic exercise can cure the waist，kidney，intestines and stomach diseases.

清微丹诀【qīng wēi dān jué**】**《清微丹诀》为气功学专著，此书为宋代道家清微派修炼内功功法的经典。作者不详。

Qingwei Danjue（*Clear and Subtle Dan Formula***）** A monograph of Qigong entitled *Clear and Subtle Dan（Pills of Immortality）Formula*. This monograph was a canon of internal practice of Qigong with the clear and subtle school of Daoism Qigong in the Song Dynasty（960 AD‑1279 AD）. The author was unknown.

清心【qīng xīn**】** 指清净神明。

purifying the heart Refers to clear and tranquil divinities.

清心静坐法【qīng xīn jìng zuò fǎ**】** 为静功。其作法为，"清心静坐，凝神定息，收视返听，内不知乎我身，外不忘乎宇宙"。

exercise for clearing the heart and sitting quietly A static exercise，marked by "clearing the heart，sitting quietly，concentrating the spirit，stabilizing respiration，avoiding vision and hearing and idea，internally dismembering oneself body and externally remembering the universe".

清虚府【qīng xū fǔ**】** 上丹田的异名。

clear and deficient mansion The synonym of the upper Dantian（the region between the eyes）.

清虚元妙真君【qīng xū yuán miào zhēn jūn**】** 喻张三丰，为明代气功学家，深入系统地研究和发展了气功的理论和方法。

Qingxu Yuanmiao Zhenju（Clear，Pure，Original，Fine and Genuine Immortal） A celebration of Zhang Sanfeng，a great master of Qigong in the Ming Dynasty（1368 AD‑1644 AD），who thoroughly and systematically studied and developed the theory and practice of Qigong.

清源【qīng yuán**】** 指脑及脑神。

clear source Refers to the brain and brain spirit.

清浊【qīng zhuó**】** 指清阳升，浊阴降。

purity and turbidity Refers to ascent of clear Yang and descent of turbid Yin.

情变【qíng biàn**】** 喻气功功法习练，可以改变人的性格。

disposition change Means that exercise for practicing Qigong can change the character of the practitioners.

情识两忘【qíng shí liǎng wàng**】** 指意识生境、生情。内无外念，不生外境，外境不生，内境不出，内外两忘而安静。

oblivion of double disposition Means that consciousness produces state and disposition. According to Qigong，if there is no external idea in the internal，external state will not be formed；if there is no external state，internal state will not be formed；if both the external and the internal are disremembered，stability and tranquility will be kept.

情欲【qíng yù**】** 指人体情感、思想上的念头。

Q

emotional desire Refers to the idea of disposition and thought.

邛疏寝右【qióng shū qǐn yòu】 为动功。其作法为,右侧身卧式,右手曲肘置于枕边,用右手指掩住右鼻孔。

alienation with right hand A dynamic exercise, marked by lying on the right side with the right hand bending the elbow and stretching to the pillow side and with the right hand finger to press the right nostril.

穷理尽性【qióng lǐ jìn xìng】 指根据人体向外的精神意识活动,能穷尽物理,认识本性。

clarification of truth and perfection of nature Refers to fully understanding the principles and cognizing the original nature of all things.

穷取生身处【qióng qǔ shēng shēn chù】 源自气功专论,主要阐述生身处,即产药之地,返此之本,还此之源则龙虎降。

universal cognition of life background Collected from a monograph of Qigong, mainly describing the region of life conception as the place of medicinal production. When returning to this region and place, Long and tiger will descend. Loong refers to the kidney and tiger refers to the lung.

穷戊己【qióng wù jǐ】 戊己即中央土。穷戊己,是说练功者必须弄清土的功用。即水火分为上下,木金列于西东。

clarification of Wu and Ji In this term, Wu and Ji refer to the central ground, and clarification of Wu and Ji means to clear the function of the ground. In order to clear the function of the ground, water and fire can be divided into the upper and the lower, wood and metal can be listed into the west and east.

穹苍【qióng cāng】 即天,气功学借以喻人头。

welkin Refers to the sky. In Qigong, it refers to the head.

琼浆玉液【qióng jiāng yù yè】 指神水,即唾液。

fine syrup and pure humor Refers to saliva known as the spiritual water.

琼山道人【qióng shān dào rén】 即白玉蟾(1194—1229),为宋代的一位气功学家。

Qiongshan Daoren（Daoist in the Fine Mountain） Refers to Bai Yuchan, a great master of Qigong in the Song Dynasty(960 AD - 1279 AD).

琼室【qióng shì】 指脑。

fine chamber Refers to the brain.

琼液【qióng yè】 即仙人之粮,指吞咽口中唾液。

fine humor The same as immortal grain, referring to swallowing saliva.

丘长春既济法【qiū cháng chūn jì jì fǎ】 为静功,方法多样。如金精入顶,紧闭两耳,使肾气不出,并入天宫,造化金精下降,如淋雨相似。

Qiu Changchun's harmonizing exercise A static exercise with various methods, such as ascending to the golden essence into the head, closing the ears, preventing kidney Qi to flow out and promoting it to enter the brain in order to descend the golden essence like raining.

丘长春搅辘轳势【qiū cháng chūn jiǎo lù lú shì】 为动功。其作法为,高坐,放松形体,将左右脚斜舒,两手掌按膝,行功运气一十二口。治背膊疼痛。

Qiu Changchun's knee-rubbing exercise A dynamic exercise, marked by sitting high, relaxing the body, slanting the feet, holding the knees with both hands and moving Qi for twelve times. Such a dynamic exercise can relieve back pain and arm pain.

丘处机【qiū chù jī**】** 宋元时期气功学家长春真人的另外一个称谓。

Qiu Chuji Another name of Qiu Chuji, also known as Changchun Zhenren, who was a great scholar and master of Qigong in the late Song Dynasty (960 AD - 1279 AD) and Yuan Dynasty (1271 AD - 1368 AD).

丘通密【qiū tōng mì**】** 宋元时期气功学家长春真人，即丘处机的另外一个称谓。

Qiu Tongmi Another name of Qiu Chuji also known as Changchun Zhenren, who was a great scholar and master of Qigong in the Song Dynasty (960 AD - 1279 AD) and Yuan Dynasty (1271 AD - 1368 AD).

秋分八月中坐功【qiū fēn bā yuè zhōng zuò gōng**】** 为动功。其作法为，每日丑寅时，盘足而坐，两手掩耳，左右反侧，各三五次，叩齿、吐纳、咽液。

exercise of sitting in the middle of August in autumn A dynamic exercise, marked by sitting with crossed feet in Chou (the period of a day from 1 a.m. to 3 a.m. in the morning) and Yin (the period of a day from 3 a.m. to 5 a.m. in the morning), covering the ears with both hands to turn from the left to the right and vice versa for three to five times, clicking the teeth, breathing in and out, and swallowing humor.

秋令导引法【qiū lìng dǎo yǐn fǎ**】** 为动功。其作法为，用呬字导引，可正坐，以两手据地，缩身曲脊向上三举，又当反手搥背上，左右各三度。

exercise of Daoyin in autumn A dynamic exercise, marked by Daoyin with the Chinese character Xi (breath), sitting upright, pressing the ground with both hands, shrinking the body and bending the spine for three times, returning the hands to thump the back from the left to the right and vice versa for three degrees respectively.

秋石【qiū shí**】** 指先天一气萌生，亦指肺气萌发。

autumn stone Refers to the production of innate qi or germination of lung Qi.

求生之道当知二山【qiú shēng zhī dào dāng zhī èr shān**】** 源自气功专论，主要论述太元之山脑及其调节精神所达到的境界。

The way for survival is to understand two mountains. This sentence is collected from a monograph of Qigong, which mainly describes the original brain in the mountain and the state of spirit regulation.

求玄珠法【qiú xuán zhū fǎ**】** 为静功。其作法为，静坐，宁神息虑，意念继而全无，日久神气相合即得。

exercise for obtaining mystic pearls A static exercise, marked by sitting quietly and calming the spirit to consider respiration. After a period of time to practice such a static exercise, consciousness eventually will disappear, the spirit and Qi will integrate with each other.

求玄珠赋【qiú xuán zhū fù**】** 《求玄珠赋》为气功专论，由唐代白居易所作，全文旨在分析研究"以心忘心，以智去智"的基本方法。

Qiu Xuanzhu Fu (*Composition of Obtai-***

ning Mystic Pearls) A monograph of Qigong entitled *Composition of Obtaining Mystic Pearls*, written by a great poet and scholar in the Tang Dynasty (618 AD - 907 AD), mainly analyzing "neglecting the heart from the heart and eliminating wisdom from wisdom" which is the basic method of Qigong.

驱二物【qū èr wù】 指意念导引精气之意。

expelling two things Means to lead the essence and Qi with consciousness.

屈舌【qū shé】 导引津液的一种方法。

bending tongue A method for leading fluid and humor.

屈原【qū yuán】 战国时期诗人和政治家,为气功的发展做出了积极贡献。

Qu Yuan A great poet and politician in the Warring States Period (475 BC - 221 BC), contributing a great deal to the development of Qigong.

胠【qū】 人体部位,指腋下腰上的部位,也指胁肋。

Qu Refers to either the part between the axilla and the waist; or lateral thorax.

瞿上辅炼魂魄【qú shàng fǔ liàn hún pò】 为静功。其作法为,天以日为魂,地以月为魄,日中寻兔髓,月内取乌血。本法为右侧卧式睡法。治疗失眠、多梦、梦游等。

Mr Qu's exercise for refining the ethereal soul and the corporeal soul in the upper bunk A static exercise, marked by lying on the right side, selecting rabbit marrow in the daytime and obtaining crow blood at nighttime. The sky takes the sun as the ethereal soul while the earth takes the moon as the corporeal soul. Such a static exercise can cure in-

somnia, dreaminess and sleepwalk.

瞿佑【qú yòu】 明代医学家、诗人,兼通气功。其专著中阐述养生应注意的事项,重视气功养生。

Qu You A doctor of traditional Chinese medicine and poet in the Ming Dynasty who was also proficient in Qigong. In his monographs, he described the principles and practice of Qigong for cultivating life.

瞿佑养生法【qú yòu yǎng shēng fǎ】 源自气功专论,主要阐述养生的关键是养神,神和则能归真返朴。

Qu You's exercise for cultivating life Collected from a monograph of Qigong, mainly describing the importance of nourishing the spirit for cultivating life and harmonizing the spirit for returning to the original nature.

瞿宗吉【qú zōng jí】 明代医学家、诗人,兼通气功,瞿佑的另外一个称谓。其专著中阐述养生应注意的事项,重视气功养生。

Qu Zongji Another name of Qu You, a doctor of traditional Chinese medicine and poet in the Ming Dynasty who was also proficient in Qigong. In his monographs, he described the principles and practice of Qigong for cultivating life.

曲鬓【qǔ bìn】 足少阳胆经中的一个穴位,位于耳前上方。这一穴位为气功运行的一个常见部位。

Qubin(GB 7) An acupoint in the gallbladder meridian of foot Shaoyang, located in the region above the preauricule. This acupoint is a region usually used for keeping the essential Qi in practice of Qigong.

曲池【qǔ chí】 手阳明大肠经的一个

穴位,位肘横纹桡侧端。这一穴位为气功运行的一个常见部位。

Quchi（LI 11） An acupoint in the large intestine meridian of hand Yangming, located on the radialis in the transverse line of the elbow. This acupoint is a region usually used for keeping the essential Qi in practice of Qigong.

曲骨【qū gǔ】 任脉中的一个穴位,位于前正中线,脐下5寸。这一穴位为气功运行的一个常见部位。

Qugu（CV 2） An acupoint in the conception meridian, located in the middle line at the front and 5 Cun below the navel. This acupoint is a region usually used for keeping the essential Qi in practice of Qigong.

曲甲【qū jiǎ】 指人体的一个部位,即肩甲冈,为肩胛骨背面上三分之一处。

mesoscapula A part of the body, located one third upwards to the back of the scapula.

曲江【qū jiāng】 ① 指肾中之水; ② 指肠。

crooked river Refers to ① either water in the kidney; ② or the intestines.

曲泽【qū zé】 手厥阴心包经中的一个穴位,位于肘横纹上。这一穴位为气功运行的一个常见部位。

Quze（PC 3） An acupoint in the pericardium meridian of hand Jueyin, located in the transverse line of the elbow. This acupoint is a region usually used for keeping the essential Qi in practice of Qigong.

取【qǔ】 佛家气功习用语,① 指爱的别称;② 烦恼的总称。

taking A common term of Qigong in Buddhism, referring to ① either a synonym of love; ② or the general term of annoyance.

取法天地【qū fǎ tiān dì】 指人与天地相适应,气功之理取法自然。

following the sky and the earth Refers to the fact that human adapt to the sky and the earth and that the principle of Qigong follows the law of the natural world.

取坎填离【qǔ kǎn tián lí】 指练功中取肾阳(即坎中之阳)与心阴(即离中之阴)结合而产金丹。

taking Kan Trigram and stuffing Li Trigram Refers to combination of kidney Yang (referring to Yang in the Kan Trigram) and hear Yin (referring to Yin in the Li Trigram) that has produced golden Dan (pills of immortality).

取阳时法【qǔ yáng shí fǎ】 为静功。其作法为,常取六阳时食气,半夜子时服八十一次;平旦寅时服六十四次;食时辰时服四十九次;正中午时服三十六次;哺时申时服二十五次;黄昏戌时服一十六次。

exercise for taking Yang A static exercise, marked by taking Qi in the period of six Yang (from November to April) and during which Qi is taken eighty-one times at midnight every day; taking Qi in Yin period (the period of a day from 3 a.m. to 5 a.m. in the morning) the early morning for sixty-four times; taking Qi in Shi period or Chen period (the period of a day from 7 a.m. to 9 a.m. in the morning) for forty-nine times; taking Qi in the noon for thirty-six times; taking Qi in Bu period, also called Shen period, (the period of a day from 3 p.m. to 5 p.m. in the afternoon）；taking Qi in Wu period（the period of a day from 7 p. m. to 9 p. m. at night）.

去嗔之法【qù chēn zhī fǎ**】** 为动功。嗔恚即发怒，怒之发，必有诱因。

exercise for rage eradication A dynamic exercise, referring to getting angry due to certain reason.

全道说【quán dào shuō**】** 源自气功专论，主要阐述形、神、气合一而激发全能的道理。

idea about entire Daoism Collected from a monograph, mainly describing the integration of the body, spirit and Qi that activates the all-round ability.

全形【quán xíng**】** 指人体健康，形体完整无损。

healthy body Means that the body is quite healthy without any prejudice.

全阳子【quán yáng zǐ**】** 金代气功学家王处一的另外一个称谓，为全真道嵛山派的创始人。

Quan Yangzi Another name of Wang Chuyi, a great master of Qigong in the Jin Dynasty（1142－1217），who was the founder of Yushan school in Acme Genuine Dao.

全真【quán zhēn**】** 保守本性，为道家之一派。

entire genuineness Refers to either keeping the original property; or a school in the Daoism.

全真派【quán zhēn pài**】** 气功流派之一，大定七年（1167）由王重阳所创立。

school of entire genuineness One of the schools in Qigong, established by Wang Chongyang in 1167 in the Jin Dynasty （1115 AD－1234 AD）.

颧【quán**】** 指颧骨，位于眼眶外下方。

cheekbone Located below the lateral

side of the orbital cavity.

颧髎【quán liáo**】** 手太阳小肠经中的一个穴位，位于目外眦直下。

Quanliao（ST 12） An acupoint in the small intestine meridian of hand Taiyang, located directly below the outer canthus.

缺盆【quē pén**】** ① 指锁骨上窝；② 指足阳明胃经中的一个穴位，位锁骨中点上方之凹陷处，为气功中常用的意守部位。

Quepen Refers to ① either subclavicular fossa；② or Quepen（ST 12），an acpuoint in the stomach meridian of foot Yangming, located in the depression above the middle of subclavicular fossa, which is the region for concentrating consciousness in practicing Qigong.

却病延年法【què bìng yán nián fǎ**】** 为动功，指通过调身、调气和调神以却病延年，调节形神，疏通经络，畅利气机。

exercise for eradicating disease and prolonging life A dynamic exercise, referring to regulating the body, Qi and the spirit for eradicating disease, prolonging life, regulating the body and the spirit, dredging the meridians and the collaterals and freeing the activities of Qi.

却谷【què gǔ**】** 指少食或不食。古代养生家在进行气功锻炼的同时，减少食五谷，甚至在一定时间内不食五谷。

diet reduction Refers to eating less or non-eating. In ancient China, scholars for health cultivation reduced diet in practicing Qigong, or even stopped taking food in a certain period of time.

却谷食气法【què gǔ shí qì fǎ**】** 为静功。其作法为，每日早晚起床后，入睡前，用鼻吸气，口呼气，以调和五脏，排除体内浊气和宿食。

diet reduction exercise for taking Qi　A static exercise，marked by inhaling through the nose and exhaling through the mouth when getting up early or late and before sleeping in order to regulate the five Zang-organs（including the heart，the liver，the spleen，the lung and the kidney）and eliminate turbid Qi and dyspepsia.

却谷食气篇【què gǔ shí qì piān】《却谷食气篇》为古代气功著作，作者不详，提出了一年四季进行气功锻炼的方法和要求。

Quegu Shiqi Pian（*A Book about Reducing Diet and Taking Qi*）　A monograph of Qigong in ancient China entitled *A Book about Reducing Diet and Taking Qi*，proposing the methods and requirements for practicing Qigong in the four seasons. The author was unknown.

却粒【què lì】　即辟谷，不饮食。练功到一定程度出现不感饥饿，不进饮食而精神不减，身体轻快而无不适。

inedia（stopping diet）　Refers to the marvel in practicing Qigong，characterized by no hunger in practicing Qigong to a certain level. Although food is not taken in practicing Qigong,

the spirit is still energetic and the body is still brisk.

却走马以补脑【què zǒu mǎ yǐ bǔ nǎo】　指习练气功，固涩止精，能于补脑安神。走马即男女媾合泻精。

stopping horse running to tonify the brain　Refers to astringing seminal emission in order to tonify the brain and to stabilize the spirit. In this term，the so-called horse running refers to copulation of man and woman that reduce semen.

鹊桥【què qiáo】　指舌顶上腭，交通任督二脉。

magpie bridge　Refers to the upper jaw and transportation of the conception meridian and the governor meridian.

阙【què】　即两眉之间。

glabella　Refers to the region between the eyebrows.

阙庭【què tíng】　指发际于眉间的部位。

middle of forehead　Refers to the region between the hair line and glabella.

群阴剥尽【qún yīn bō jìn】　喻丹熟后成为纯阳之体。

elimination of all Yin　Refers to a body with pure Yang after perfect formation of Dan（pills of immortality）.

R

染污【rǎn wū】 佛家气功习用语,指烦恼引起意识思维活动失调。

contamination A term of Qigong, referring to disorder of the activities of consciousness and thinking caused by annoyance.

热痹【rè bì】 气功适应证,①指热毒流注关节或内有蕴热,复感风寒湿邪,与热相搏的痹证;②指脉痹。

heat impediment An indication of Qigong, referring to ① either migration of heat toxin into the joints or with intrinsic heat, eventually attacked by wind-heat and pathogenic dampness combating with heat; ② or meridian impediment.

热痢【rè lì】 气功适应证,指痢疾之属热者。

heat dysentery An indication of Qigong, referring to dysentery related to heat.

热淋【rè lín】 气功适应证,多因温热蕴结下焦,膀胱气化失司所致。

heat strangury An indication of Qigong, usually caused by warmth and heat accumulating and binding in the lower energizer as well as disorder of Qi transformation in the bladder.

人定【rén dìng】 即人安定之时,为亥时,即夜九至十时。

human stability Refers to quietness of human life, usually indicating the time from 9 p.m. to 11 p.m. at night.

人间世【rén jiān shì】 ①《庄子》篇之一;② 也指人世间关系纷繁复杂。

human world era Refers to ① either the title of an article in Zhuang Zi; ② or complexity in the world.

人门【rén mén】 指的是虚危穴,精气聚散常在此处,水火发端也在此处,阴阳变化也在此处,有无出入也在此处。此穴位为气功习练之处。

human gate Refers to an acupoint known as Xuwei, referring to the region where the essential Qi concentrates and disperses there, water and fire appear there, Yin and Yang change there, exit and entrance exist there. This acupoint is a region usually used in practice of Qigong.

人气【rén qì】 指人体生发之气,即平旦人气生,日中而人气隆,日西而阳气已虚。

human Qi Refers to Qi in the human body that is prosperous in the noon and declines after sunset.

人人本有长生药【rén rén běn yǒu cháng shēng yào】 源自气功专论,主要阐述长生之药,人人固有。

elixir in everyone's life Collected from a monograph of Qigong, mainly describing the discussion about the medicinals effective for prolonging life.

人神【rén shén】 ①指人体身内之神;②指人体的精神周期,显示人体精神差。

human spirit Refers to ① either the spirit inside the body; ② or the cycle of the spirit in the human body, indicating difference of the spirit at different time.

人生消天地【rén shēng xiāo tiān dì】指人与自然相应，与天地阴阳变化的规律相同。

correspondence of man to the sky and earth Refers correspondence between man and the universe.

人体元气消长说【rén tǐ yuán qì xiāo zhǎng shuō】 源自气功专论，主要阐述人体生命活动中元气消长的过程，提示人们习练气功宜早，即蓄养元气，调节阴阳，返老为壮。

growth and decline of original Qi in human body Collected from a monograph of Qigong, mainly describing the procedure of the original Qi that now declines and then grows, suggesting that the practice of Qigong should be done early. Early practice of Qigong means to concentrate and to nourish the original Qi, to regulate Yin and Yang, and to strengthen the body after being aged.

人性【rén xìng】 指人的本性，即人固有的天性，本性有静有躁，性静宜练动功，性动者应练静功。

human nature Refers to the original nature of human beings, indicating that the original human nature is sometimes quiet and sometimes rash. Those who are quiet can practice dynamic exercise while those who are active should practice static exercise.

人性方圆【rén xìng fāng yuán】 指人的性情可以通过后天的教育而改变。喻人的情性可以通过气功功法而调节。

circumference of humanity Refers to the fact that human nature can be changed by postnatal education, indicating that human nature can be regulated by practice of Qigong.

人有七窍权归脑【rén yǒu qī qiào quán guī nǎo】 指头面部七窍为脑所主。

The brain controls seven orifices in the human body. Indicates that the seven orifices on the complexion are controlled by the brain.

人与天地相参【rén yǔ tiān dì xiāng cān】 指人与自然界有很密切的关系，四时气候及环境变化影响人体阴阳平衡。

coherence between man and the sky and earth Refers to the close relationship between man and the natural world, which is very important for cultivating health and prolonging life. The environmental changes in the four seasons affect the balance between Yin and Yang in the human body.

人之大宝，只此一息真阳【rén zhī dà bǎo zhǐ cǐ yī xī zhēn yáng】 真阳即命门之火，指人身最宝贵的是命门火。此言强调阳气的重要性。

The great treasure for human beings is the genuine Yang in respiration. The genuine Yang refers to fire in the life gate which is the most important treasure in the human body. This celebrated dictum actually emphasizes the importance of Yang Qi.

人中【rén zhōng】 ① 指人中穴在鼻下唇上，鼻唇沟之正中；② 也指身体九窍中，单窍与双窍的分界点。此穴位为气功习练之处。

renzhong Refers to ① either an acupoint located in the area between the upper lip and nose；② or the cut-off

R

point between the single orifice and double orifice among the nine orifices. This acupoint is a region usually used in practice of Qigong.

壬癸【rén guǐ】 指元气所生之时。

ren gui Refers to the ninth of the ten Heavenly Stems and the last of the ten Heavenly Stems.

壬水之腑【rén shuǐ zhī fǔ】 指膀胱。

water viscus Refers to the bladder.

壬子【rén zǐ】 指的是十天干中的第九和十二地支中的第一。

ren Zi Refers to the ninth of the ten Heavenly Stems and the first of the twelve Earthly Branches.

仁者寿【rén zhě shòu】 指精神内守，清静中正平和，取天地之美以养生，所以能和调神形，延年益寿。

purified mind ensuring longevity Refers to spirit concentration, tranquilization, justice and peace for obtaining beauty from the sky and the earth to nourish life, to regulate the spirit and the body, to cultivate health and to prolong life.

忍【rěn】 佛家气功习用语，① 指忍受违逆之境而不起嗔心；② 指认识道理之后，能定志守神而不分散。

toleration A common term of Qigong in Buddhism, referring to ① either tolerance of disobeyed state without any annoyance; ② or stabilizing the will and maintaining the spirit without any dispersion after cognition of the truth.

忍怒以全阴气【rěn nù yǐ quán yīn qì】 指调节精神使志勿怒，可保全阴气。

tolerance of annoyance to fulfill Yin Qi Refers to well regulating the essence and the spirit in order to avoid any annoyance and secure Yin Qi.

忍喜以全阳气【rěn xǐ yǐ quán yáng qì】 指通过调节精神，不过分喜悦，可保全阳气。

tolerance of rejoicing to fulfill Yang Qi Refers to regulating the essence and the spirit in order to avoid exultancy and to secure Yang Qi.

任督二脉导引秘旨【rèn dū èr mài dǎo yǐn mì zhǐ】 源自气功专论，说明任督二脉在习练周天功时的作用。

purpose of Daoyin for conception and governor meridians Collected from a monograph about Qigong, explaining the effect of the conception and governor meridians in refining the celestial cycle (a term of Qigong).

任督交接之处【rèn dū jiāo jiē zhī chù】 即九灵铁鼓，精气聚散常在此处，水火发端也在此处，阴阳变化也在此处，有无出入也在此处。

connection of the conception and governor meridians The same as nine genius-fire drums, referring to the region where the essential Qi concentrates and disperses there, water and fire appear there, Yin and Yang change there, exit and entrance exist there.

任脉【rèn mài】 奇经八脉之一，是气功中常用的经脉之一。

conception meridian One of the eight extraordinary meridians and one of the commonly used meridians in practicing Qigong.

日晡所【rì bū suǒ】 指申时，约下午三至五时，"日晡所发潮热，不恶寒"。

late afternoon Late afternoon refers to 3 – 5 hours in the afternoon during which it is warm, not cold.

日乘四季【rì chéng sì jì】 指一日一夜之际。古人讲一日一夜划分为四季。

four seasons in a day Refers to the fact that in ancient China one day was divided into four seasons.

日出【rì chū】 即卯时,约早晨五至七时。

sunrise Refers to 5 - 7 hours in the early morning.

日华【rì huá】 即日之光华。瞑目握固,存想日中五色流霞来绕,于是日光流霞,俱入口中。

sunshine Refers to closing the eyes, holding the fists, tranquilizing the mind and imagining five kinds of brightness from the sun flowing into the mouth.

日华胎【rì huá tāi】 即指竹笋,"服日月之精华者,欲得常食竹笋"。

bamboo shoot Refers to the fact that absorption of sun brightness enables people to normally take bamboo shoot.

日魂月魄【rì hún yuè pò】 指日魂为阳,喻肝;月魄为阴,喻肺。

sun ethereal soul and moon corporeal soul Refers to Yin and Yang in the body, indicating the liver and the lung.

日魂月魄真要【rì hún yuè pò zhēn yào】 源自气功专论,主要阐述魂魄即是阴阳,也指人的神、气,以及在练气功时,守魂魄、调阴阳的重要性。

importance of sun ethereal soul and moon corporeal soul Collected from a monograph of Qigong, referring to the importance of keeping the ethereal soul and the corporeal soul as well as regulating Yin and Yang in practicing Qigong.

日精【rì jīng】 即日之精光,"服食日精,金华充盈"。

brightness of the sun Refers to the fact that absorbing the brightness of the sun will exuberate anything.

日精月华【rì jīng yuè huá】 指心中真液,肾中真气。指日、月之精光华采。

essence and brightness of the sun and the moon Refers to either genuine humor in the heart and genuine Qi in the kidney; or sunshine and moonshine.

日想观【rì xiǎng guān】 佛家气功功法。习练气功时,盘膝正坐,面向西。

solar contemplation An exercise of Qigong in Buddhism, referring to sitting regularly with face turning to the west for practicing Qigong.

日新【rì xīn】 指洗除精神意识中的积垢,才能奋发自新。

renew Refers to constant elimination of distracting thoughts in the spirit and consciousness in order to rouse and renew life.

日昳【rì yì】 即午后一至三时,"脾病者,日昳慧,平旦甚"。

afternoon Refers to 1 - 3 hours in the afternoon during which spleen disease can be relieved.

日用五行的要【rì yòng wǔ xíng dí yào】 主要阐述何为日用,何为五行,及其气、神、形皆在五行相聚时才能成丹的道理。

importance of applying the five elements every day Refers to the principle that only when Qi, the spirit and the body are accumulated in the five elements can health be cultivated and life be prolonged.

日用之神【rì yòng zhī shén】 指平素的意识思维活动。

general use of the spirit Refers to normal mental activities.

日月【rì yuè】 指阳中含阴,也指乳头下方足少阳胆经的一个穴位。这一穴位为气功运行的一个常见部位。

R

sun and moon Refers to either Yin within Yang; or an acupoint in the gallbladder meridian of foot Shaoyang located below the breast. This acupoint is a region usually used for keeping essential Qi in practice of Qigong.

日月精【rì yuè jīng】 指日月之精华。

sunshine and moonshine Refers to the essence and brightness of the sun and the moon.

日月之光求老残【rì yuè zhī guāng qiú lǎo cán】 指气功中,采日月之精光,有调节阴阳,抗衰老的作用。

avoiding senility with the brightness of the sun and moon Refers to absorbing the brightness of the sun and the moon for regulating Yin and Yang and relieving senility.

日月之祖【rì yuè zhī zǔ】 指神。

ancestor of sun and moon Refers to the original Qi in the sky and the earth.

荣观燕处【róng guān yān chù】 圣人身处荣耀繁华的环境,而超然独处,不沉溺于其中。

splendid observation of swallow place Refers to a splendid and prosperous place where the great sage lived and surpassed it.

容成公静守谷神【róng chéng gōng jìng shǒu gǔ shén】 为动功。其作法为,端坐身体,咬牙闭气,两手掌心按于耳上,手指轻弹头枕部三十六下,叩齿三十六下。

rong Chenggong's quiet protection of ravine spirit A dynamic exercise, marked by sitting upright, gritting the teeth, stopping respiration, pressing the ears with the palms, mildly pulling the pillow for thirty-six times and clicking the teeth for thirty-six times.

容主【róng zhǔ】 上关的一个别称,为足少阳胆经中的一个穴位,位于颧弓上缘,距耳郭前缘约1寸处,为气功常用意守部位。

Rongzhu A synonym of Shangguan (GB 3), which is an acupoint in the gallbladder of foot Shaoyang, located on the upper of the zygoma and about 1 Cun to the upper of the auricle. This acupoint is a region usually used in practice of Qigong.

柔心弱骨【róu xīn ruò gǔ】 指神情和缓,筋骨柔韧。

softening the heart and weakening the bones Means that the spirit and the emotion should be gentle and the sinews and the bones should be pliable.

肉分【ròu fēn】 肌肉之间的间隙。

muscular space Refers to the space between muscles.

肉瘤【ròu liú】 气功适应证,指瘤体肿块软如绵,肿如馒,如肉隆起。

sarcoma An indication of Qigong, referring to soft and steamed swelling as if the fleshes were bulged.

肉轮【ròu lún】 眼部五轮之一,指眼睑(胞睑)。在脏属脾,其疾患多从脾胃论治。

flesh wheel One of the five wheels in the eyes, referring to the eyelid. Among the viscera, it pertains to the spleen. The related diseases are usually treated from the spleen and stomach.

肉瘿【ròu yǐng】 气功适应证,指瘤体肿块软如绵,肿如馒,如肉隆起。

sarcoma An indication of Qigong, marked by soft and steamed swelling as if the fleshes were bulged.

肉之一【ròu zhī yī】 指肠胃。

one of fleshes Refers to the intestines

and the stomach.

如来空藏【rú lái kōng cáng**】**　即七常住果，为佛家气功习用语。指佛家气功所要达到的理想境界。

tathagata inspecting vacuum　The same as seven ideal boundaries, the common term of Qigong in Buddhism, referring to the ideal state of the spirit in Buddhism.

如影随形【rú yǐng suí xíng**】**　即形影相随不离。

as the shadow following the person　Refers to close association of the body and shadow.

儒道释论性命【rú dào shì lùn xìng mìng**】**　源自气功专论，主要阐述儒、道、释三家气功学的特点。

discussion of life by Confucianism, Daoism and Buddhism　Collected from a monograph of Qigong, mainly describing the characteristics of Qigong in Confucianism, Daoism and Buddhism.

儒家功【rú jiā gōng**】**　源于儒家的功法。

Confucian exercise　Refers to the exercise originating from the Confucianism.

臑【rú**】**　即臂内侧肌肉。

forelimb　Refers to muscles in the interior sides of the shoulders.

臑会【rú huì**】**　手少阳三焦经中的一个穴位，位于尺骨鹰嘴与肩髎(位于肩峰外后下方)的连线上。此穴位为气功习练之处。

Naohui（TE 13）　An acupoint in the triple energizer meridian of hand Shaoyang, located in the line between olecroanon and Jianliao (TE 14). This acupoint is a region usually used in practice of Qigong.

臑交【rú jiāo**】**　手少阳三焦经中的一个穴位臑会的另外一个称谓，位于尺骨鹰嘴与肩髎(位于肩峰外后下方)的连线上。此穴位为气功习练之处。

Naojiao　A synonym of Naohui（TE 13）, which is an acupoint in the triple energizer meridian of hand Shaoyang, located in the line between olecroanon and Jianliao (TE 14). This acupoint is a region usually used in practice of Qigong.

臑髎【rú liáo**】**　手少阳三焦经中的一个穴位臑会的另外一个称谓，位于尺骨鹰嘴与肩髎(位于肩峰外后下方)的连线上。此穴位为气功习练之处。

Naoliao　A synonym of Naohui（TE 13）, which is an acupoint in the triple energizer meridian of hand Shaoyang, located in the line between olecroanon and Jianliao (TE 14). This acupoint is a region usually used in practice of Qigong.

臑俞【rú shù**】**　手太阳小肠经中的一个穴位，位于上臂内后方。此穴位为气功习练之处。

Naoshu（SI 10）　An acupoint in the small intestine meridian of hand Taiyang, located at the interior side and backside of the shoulders. This acupoint is a region usually used in practice of Qigong.

蠕动处则默合神气于命根【rú dòng chù zé mò hé shén qì yú mìng gēn**】**　指意念导引神气归于丹田。

peristalsis silently coordinates essential Qi with life root　Indicates that consciousness leads the spirit and Qi to Dantian that is divided into the upper Dantian (the region between the eyes), the middle Dantian (the region below the heart) and the lower Dantian (the region below the navel).

乳蛾治法【rǔ é zhì fǎ】 动静相兼功。其作法为,用左手托右膊,更换,服气十一口,呵气三十一口,左右二十遍。

treatment of tonsillitis An exercise combined with dynamic exercise and static exercise, marked by raising the right elbow with the left hand and raising the right elbow with the left hand, taking Qi for eleven times, exhaling Qi for thirty-one times, and from the left to the right and vice versa for twenty times respectively.

乳结核后导引法【rǔ jié hé hòu dǎo yǐn fǎ】 为动功。其作法为,臀部与足掌同时着地而坐,用两手从脚弯处伸入按地上,把脚弯曲放在手上,抬起臀部,也可行气。

exercise of Daoyin for breast tuberculosis A dynamic exercise, marked by sitting on the ground with the buttocks and the soles, pressing the ground with the hands from the foot joint, putting the bending part of the foot on the hand, lifting the buttocks and moving Qi.

乳癖【rǔ pǐ】 气功适应证,指乳房部出现形状大小不一的硬结肿块。

breast mass An indication of Qigong, indicating various forms of hard lump in the breast.

乳养【rǔ yǎng】 指像乳养小孩一样温养精气神。

nursing Indicates that nourishing the essence, Qi and the spirit in the human body is just like nourishing the baby.

入道【rù dào】 ① 泛指信奉道家之学并实践之,称为入道;② 泛指学习气功知识,应用气功方法;③ 也指入佛家修行,亦谓学习佛家气功并实践之为入道。

entering Dao Refers to ① ether believing the study and practice of Qigong in Daoism, indicating to study the knowledge and to practice the exercises and techniques for practicing Qigong in Daoism; ② or following the ways of practicing Qigong in Buddhism; ③ studying the theory and practice of Qigong in Buddhism.

入定【rù dìng】 佛家气功习用语,指入于禅定,使精神意识思维活动专注一境,止息身、口和意之三业(行为)。

sitting quietly to meditate A common term of Qigong in Buddhism, referring to concentrating the emotion and thought in a special state in order to control the body, mouth and consciousness.

入定说【rù dìng shuō】 源自气功专论。主要说明习练气功出现遥视、遥感力后,应用入定之法,继续使慧定加强。

idea of meditation Collected from a monograph of Qigong, referring to remote vision and remote sense in practicing Qigong which can be changed by tranquilization.

入观【rù guān】 佛家气功习用语。气功中,现想虚静,排出粗放散乱的意识活动。

contemplation of truth A common term of Qigong in Buddhism, referring to quietness and tranquility in practicing Qigong in order to eliminate distracting thought in consciousness activity.

入火垂两臂,不息不伤火法【rù huǒ chuí liǎng bì bù xī bù shāng huǒ fǎ】 为动功,方法多样。如向南方蹲踞,以两手从屈膝中入掌足五指,令内曲,利腰尻完,治淋遗,溺愈等。此动功指多法运动手臂四肢以静心安神、养生长寿。

technique for drooping arms with fire and without damage The dynamic exercise with various methods, such as squatting to the southern direction, holding the toes with the hands stretching forward along the knees, bending the interior sides and improving the waist and buttocks in order to cure strangury and weakness. Such a dynamic exercise can tranquilize the heart and spirit, nourish the body and prolong life through various ways to move the hands, arms and fingers.

入静【rù jìng】 指行功中,意识活动的宁静,也指作气功。

tranquility Refers to either tranquilization of mental activity; or practice of Qigong.

入魔【rù mó】 指损伤情志的行为,影响气功入静的杂念及虚妄的景象。

entering demon Refers to either the activity that damages emotion; or distracting thought that affects tranquility in practice of Qigong; or image of fabrication.

入神【rù shén】 指气功调神时,意识活动达到理想境界。

entering spirituality Refers to the fact that mental activity should reach the ideal state in practicing Qigong, indicating that the activity of consciousness should reach the ideal state after regulation of the spirit in practicing Qigong.

入室炼形【rù shì liàn xíng】 指精通气功,炼养形体。

cultivating life with mastered skills Refers to proficiency in practicing Qigong and constant exercise for nourishing the body.

入水举两手臂,不息不没(水)法【rù shuǐ jǔ liǎng shǒu bì bù xī bù mò(shuǐ)fǎ】 为动功。其作法为,面向北,箕踞,以手挽足五指,以两手从曲脚入据地,曲脚加其手举尻,其可用行气;举脚交叉项,以两手握据地,举尻持任息极,交脚项上,愈腹中愁满,去三虫,利五脏,快神气;蹲踞,以两手举足,蹲极横,治气冲痛、寒疾入上下致肾气;蹲踞,以两手举足五指,低头,自极,则五脏气总至,治耳不闻,目不明;正偃卧,卷两手即握,不息,顺脚据床,治阴结筋脉痿累;以两手据膝上,仰头像鳖取气,致大黄元气至丹田,令腰脊不知痛。通过静站静坐、屈腿伸腿、举手拿握以养心安神、驱邪除病。

technique for raising two arms without water A dynamic exercise, marked by naturally squatting toward the north, drawing the five toes in a foot with one hand, putting the hands to the ground along the heels, raising the hands to the buttocks with the heels for moving Qi; raising the hands and crossing them to the neck, holding the place for practicing Qigong with both hands, raising the buttocks for improving respiration, crossing the feet with the neck in order to relieve anxiety in the abdomen, to expel three insects, to promote the five Zang-organs (including the heart, the liver, the spleen, the lung and the kidney), and to increase the spirit and Qi; squatting again, lifting the feet with both hands, squatting in the transverse way in order to cure pain due to attack of Qi and disease located in the upper and the lower due to disorder of kidney Qi; squatting again, lifting the five toes in the foot with both hands, lowering the head forcefully and fortifying the

R

Qi in the five Zang-organs in order to cure deafness and blindness; lying on the back, holding the hands, stopping respiration and keeping the feet on the bed in order to cure flaccidity of sinews and muscles; pressing the knees with both hands, raising the head like a turtle to obtain Qi in order to enter the yellow original Qi in Dantian for curing waist pain and spine pain. Through quiet standing and sitting, bending and stretching leg, raising hands and pressing with hands, the heart will be nourished, the spirit will be stabilized, pathogenic factors will be expelled and disease will be cured. Dantian is divided into the upper Dantian (the region between the eyes), the middle Dantian (the region below the heart) and the lower Dantian (the region below the navel).

入胎定观【rù tāi dìng guān】 胎即胎息,定观即心定内观。

respiration and tranquilization Refers to mental observation of pure sides when fetal respiration starts.

入药镜【rù yào jìng】《入药镜》为气功专著,为唐代崔希范所著,主要阐述身体阴阳二气相互作用而成丹的道理及金丹形成后身体内的感受。

ruyao Jing（*Entering Drug Mirror*） A monograph of Qigong entitled *Entering Drug Mirror*, written by Cui Xifan in the Tang Dynasty (618 AD - 907 AD), mainly describing the principles for interaction of Yin and Yang for developing into Dan (pills of immortality) and the experience of forming golden Dan (pills of immortality).

阮籍【ruǎn jí】 三国时期的七贤之一,主张保自然的性,而养自然的神。

Ruan Ji One of the seven sages in the Three Kingdoms Period (220 AD - 280 AD), suggesting to keep natural property and to nourish natural spirit.

阮嗣宗【ruǎn sì zōng】 三国时期七贤之一阮籍的另外一个称谓,主张保自然的性,而养自然的神。

Ruan Sizong Another name of Ruan Ji, one of the seven sages in the Three Kingdoms Period (220 AD - 280 AD), suggesting to keep natural property and to nourish natural spirit.

蕊珠【ruǐ zhū】 指天上仙宫,喻脑中至精之处。

pistil and pearl Refers to immortal palace in the sky, comparing to the essential chamber in the brain.

锐眦【ruì zì】 即目外眦,亦即小眦。

outer canthus Located in the region connected with the lower eyelid and temple.

若能常守弯弯窍,神自灵明气自充【ruò néng cháng shǒu wān wān qiào shén zì líng míng qì zì chōng】 阐述守神与养气的关系。

If the flexed orifices are often protected, the spirit will certainly be flexible and Qi will naturally be enriched. Describes the important relationship between protection of the spirit and cultivation of Qi.

若要长生,肠中常清【ruò yào cháng shēng cháng zhōng cháng qīng】 指大便通畅对健康、长寿的重要性。

Only when the intestines are clear can life be prolonged. Emphasizes the importance of smooth defecation for health and longevity.

若一志【ruò yī zhì】 指练功时,意念

R

要专一。

just one will　Refers to sincerity in practicing Qigong.

若有如无【ruò yǒu rú wú**】**　指习练气功意守景物或人体的某一部分时，意念活动处于若有若无，若即若离，恍恍惚惚的状态。

trance　Refers to trance or maintaining a lukewarm relationship or vague situation of consciousness activity made by concentration of consciousness on a certain state or a certain part of the body in practicing Qigong.

若欲长生，神气相注【ruò yù cháng shēng shén qì xiāng zhù**】**　源自《遵生八笺》，指神与气不相离散。

Only when the spirit and Qi are protected can life be prolonged.　Collected from a monograph entitled Zunsheng Bajian or *Eight Annotations of Life Cultivation*, indicating that the spirit and Qi cannot be dispersed.

若欲存身，先安神气【ruò yù cún shēn xiān ān shén qì**】**　源自气功专论《孙思邈存神炼气铭》，主要阐述神气存则身健，神气相依。

Only when the spirit and Qi are protected can life be cultivated.　This is a celebrated dictum collected from a monograph entitled Sunsimiao Cunshen Mingqi Ming or *Sun Simiao's Inscription about Protecting the Spirit and Refining Qi*, mainly describing that only when the spirit is protected can health be cultivated and the spirit and Qi be connected.

弱其恶志【ruò qí è zhì**】**　指排查杂念，或邪念。

softening the evil will　Means to eliminate distracting thought or evil idea.

R

S

洒心【sǎ xīn】 指安静精神意识活动，弃除外物的刺激。

Tranquilized heart Refers to tranquilization of the activities of the spirit and consciousness in order to expel stimulation of things in the external world.

塞兑垂帘默默窥【sāi duì chuí lián mò mò kuī】 即静候子时，不劳心，内自相交。

tranquilizing the heart，closing the eyes and glimpsing silently Refers to tranquilize the heart and mind in Zi（the period of the day from 11 p. m. to 1 a.m.）for relaxing the body and communicating the internal.

塞其兑【sāi qí duì】 指闭口，呼吸之气从鼻出入。

tranquilizing the heart Refers to closing the mouth and breathing in and out Qi in respiration all through the nose.

三宝【sān bǎo】 ① 指慈、俭、逊；② 指三丹田；③ 指精、气、神。

three treasures Refer to ① either kindness，frugality and abdication；② or three kinds of Dantian, i. e the region between the eyes，the region below the heart and the region below the navel；③ or essence，Qi and spirit. Dantian is divided into the upper Dantian（the region between the eyes），the middle Dantian（the region below the heart）and the lower Dantian（the region below the navel）.

三宝归身说【sān bǎo guī shēn shuō】 源自气功专论，主要阐述耳、目、口（外三宝），与精、神、气（内三宝）的关系及精、神、气内聚不散对人的重要性。

discussion about three treasures in human body Collected from a monograph of Qigong，mainly describing the relationship of the external Triratna（including the ears，the eyes and the mouth）and the internal Triratna（including the essence，the spirit and Qi）as well as the important accumulation of the essence，the spirit and Qi.

三晡【sān bū】 晡为午后申时，指傍晚时分。

dusk Refers to the period of the day from Shen（3 p. m. to 5 p. m. in the afternoon）.

三不善根【sān bù shàn gēn】 即三毒，佛教认为贪、嗔、痛三种烦恼最能损害人体健康，是产生其他烦恼的根本。

triple inability to protect the root Refers to greed，anger and stupidity that annoy the brain and damage health.

三不使【sān bù shǐ】 指健康无病，必须先调节精神，正意识思维活动，一不使呼吸急促，二不使狂妄乱思，三不使贪欲迷惑本性。

three avoidances Refer to health without disease，regulation of the spirit first and purifying the activities of consciousness and thinking. The first requirement is no tachypnea，the second is no bad dream and the third is no greed.

三才【sān cái】 指天、地、人,或天地、人、万物,或体、神、气。

three talents Refer to either sky, earth and man; or sky-earth, man and all things; or the body, the spirit and Qi.

三岔骨【sān chà gǔ】 指尾闾。尾闾穴是人体穴位之一,位于尾骨端与肛门之间,为督脉、督脉之络穴,别走任脉。这一穴位为气功运行的一个常见部位。

caudal bone Refers to occyx. It also refers to an acupoint located between the occyx and the anus related to the governor meridian and its collaterals. This acupoint is a region usually used in practice of Qigong.

三岔口【sān chà kǒu】 指尾闾穴。此穴位为气功习练之处。

triple divergence Refers to an acupoint between the caudal bone and the anus. This acupoint is a region usually used in practice of Qigong.

三车【sān chē】 指羊车、鹿车、牛车,或指小河车、大河车、紫河车,或使者车、雷车、破车。

three carts Refer to either sheep cart, deer cart and cow cart; or small river cart, large river cart and purple cart; or attack cart, thunder cart and broken cart.

三池【sān chí】 指口为玉池,泥丸为天池,胃为中池;或胆为中池,舌下为华池,小腹胞为玉池。

three ponds Refer to either the mouth, mud bolus (the brain) and stomach; or the gallbladder, tongue and lower abdomen.

三虫【sān chóng】 ① 指引起精神失调的因素;② 指三尸;③ 指肠内寄生虫。《洞神玄诀》说,"上虫居上丹田脑心

也""使人好嗜欲痴滞";"中虫居中丹田,使人贪财好喜怒,浊乱真气";"下虫居下丹田""使人爱衣服,耽酒好色"。

three insects Refers to ① the pathogenic factors that cause psychataxia; ② or three insects harming the body or three pathogenic factors in the brain, abdomen and foot; ③ or parasite in the intestines. In Dongshen Xuanjue (*Supreme Formulae for Appreciating the Spirit*), it says that "the upper insect is in the upper Dantian and the brain, making people appetitive and sluggish"; "the middle insect is in the middle Dantian, making people greedy and turbid"; "the lower insect is in the lower Dantian, making people like clothes, alcohol and lechery." The upper Dantian refers to the region between the eyes, the middle Dantian refers to the region below the heart and the lower Dantian refers to the region below the navel.

三虫病【sān chóng bìng】 气功适应证。指长虫病、赤虫病、蛲虫病的合称。

three insect diseases Refers to an indication of Qigong, including long insect disease, red insect disease and oxyurid disease.

三虫候导引法【sān chóng hòu dǎo yǐn fǎ】 为动功。其作法为,两手交叉放在头上,深长吸气后吐出,坐地上,慢慢伸展下肢,用两手外抱住膝部,迅速低头进入两膝间,两手再交叉放上十三次;印齿十四次,咽气十四次。此法可祛虫,治三虫症。

exercise of Daoyin for eliminating three insects A dynamic exercise, marked by crossing the hands and putting them on the top of the head, breathing out

S

after deeply breathing in sitting on the ground, slowly stretching the legs, holding the knees with both hands, quickly lowering the head into the region between the knees, again crossing the hands and then pressing them on the top of the head for thirteen times, knocking the teeth for fourteen times and inhaling for fourteen times. Such a dynamic exercise can eliminate insects and cure three insect diseases.

三春【sān chūn】 指春季三个月, 或指三年。

three springs   Refer to three months in the spring or three years.

三寸【sān cùn】   指三丹田中、上、下三处。

three Cun   Refers to the chamber in the upper Dantian (the region between the eyes), the middle Dantian (the region below the heart) and the lower Dantian (the region below the navel).

三丹三田论【sān dān sān tián lùn】 源自气功专论。主要阐述三丹田位置及其为精、气、神所藏之处。

discussion about three kinds of Dan (pills of immortality)   Collected from a monograph of Qigong, mainly describing the location of three kinds of Dantian as well as the storage of essence, Qi and spirit. Three kinds of Dantian include the upper Dantian (the region between the eyes), the middle Dantian (the region below the heart) and the lower Dantian (the region below the navel).

三岛【sān dǎo】   指神仙所居之山, 指头顶、心、肾。《钟吕传道记·论水火》中说, "顶曰上岛, 心曰中岛, 肾曰下岛"。

three islands   Refers to either the mountain where immortals stay; or the top of the head, the heart and the kidney. In Zhonglü Chuandao Ji (entitled *Zhonglü's Records for Transmission of Dao*), an ancient Chinese monograph related to Qigong, it says that "The head is the upper island, the heart is the middle island and the kidney is the lower island".

三盗【sān dào】   指的是万物盗天地, 人盗物, 物盗人。万物从自然得到滋生、补养, 人与万物相互补益。

three absorptions   Refers to the fact that all things absorbing from the sky and the earth, human beings absorbing from all things and all things absorbing from human beings.

三道【sān dào】   佛家气功习用语, 指烦恼道、业道、苦道, 三道相互作用, 紊乱精神意识思维活动。

three kinds of Dao   A common term of Qigong in Buddhism, referring the way of annoyance, the way of control and the way of anger, the combination of which disturbs the spirit and the activities of consciousness and thinking.

三德【sān dé】   佛家气功习用语, 为调节精神意识活动的三种方法。

three moralities   A common term of Qigong in Buddhism, referring to three ways to regulate mental and spiritual activities.

三叠【sān dié】   指三丹田之气, 使之和积如一。

accumulation of pubic region   Refers to accumulation in the three kinds of Dantian, including the upper Dantian (the region between the eyes), the middle Dantian (the region below the heart) and the lower Dantian (the region below the navel).

三冬【sān dōng】 指的是三年,或曰三个冬天。也指冬季三月。

three winters Refer to either three years; or three months in winter.

三洞枢机杂说【sān dòng shū jī zá shuō】《三洞枢机杂说》为气功专著,作者不详。主要强调,练气功旨在"想身于无身之中,存心于无为之境"。

sandong Quji Zashuo（*Different Versions About Three Caves*） A monograph of Qigong entitled *Different Versions About Three Caves*. The author was unknown. This monograph mainly describes that "the body should be cultivated in the place without any body and the heart should be maintained in the state without any realm."

三毒【sān dú】 佛教认为贪、嗔、痛三种烦恼最能损害人体健康,是产生其他烦恼的根本。

three poisons Refer to greed, anger and stupidity that annoy the brain and damage health according to Buddhism.

三而一【sān ér yī】 三为儒、释、道三家,指道、儒、释三家气功,源流不同,理法一致。

three and one Refers to integrated theory and methods of Qigong in the Daoism, Confucianism, and Buddhism, which are different in sources, but are the same in theory and exercises.

三房【sān fáng】 即黄庭、元海、丹田。

three houses Refer to Huangting（the region below the navel）, Yuanhai（the region below the heart）and Dantian which is divided into the upper Dantian（the region between the eyes）, the middle Dantian（the region below the heart）and the lower Dantian（the re-

gion below the navel）.

三丰祠【sān fēng cí】 在丰都山,明永乐年间,气功家张三丰曾住于此。

Sanfeng Temple Located in the Fengdou Mountian where Zhang Sanfeng, a great master of Qigong in the Ming Dynasty（1368 AD – 1644 AD）, stayed.

三丰筑基歌【sān fēng zhù jī gē】 源自气功专论,主要论述习练气功时心静神静,则阴精永固,气神健全,人体康泰。

essential cantus about triple abundance Collected from a monograph of Qigong, mainly describing that only when the heart and the spirit are tranquilized in practicing Qigong can Yin essence be stabilized, Qi and the spirit be strengthened and the body be cultivated.

三伏【sān fú】 即初伏、中伏、末伏,为一年中最热的时候。初伏指夏至后第三庚日起,中伏指第四庚日起,末伏指立秋后第一庚日起。

three periods of summer Refers to three hottest periods in a year, i.e. the first dog-days, the middle dog-days and the last dog-days. According to traditional Chinese calendar, the first dog-days refers to the period beginning from the third ten days in summer, the middle dog-days refers to the period beginning from the fourth ten days in summer, and the last dog-days refers to the period beginning from the first ten days in summer.

三缚【sān fù】 指贪、嗔、痴捆缚,引起精神失调。

three indulgences Refers to avarice, anger and stupidity which imbalance the spirit.

三更【sān gēng】 指一夜分为五更,其

S

中子时为三更，丑时为四更，寅时为五更。

the third period of midnight Means that one night is divided into five periods, Zi (the period of a day from 11 p.m. to 1 a.m.) is the third period, Chou (the period of a day from 1 a.m. to 3 a.m. in the morning) is the fourth period and Yin (the period of a day from 3 a.m. to 5 a.m. in the morning) is the fifth period.

三宫【sān gōng】　指的是丹田，分为上丹田、中丹田、下丹田。

three palaces Refers to Dantian, which is divided into upper Dantian (the region between the eyes), the middle Dantian (the region below the heart) and the lower Dantian (the region below the navel).

三垢【sān gòu】　佛家气功习用语。佛教认为贪、嗔、痛三种烦恼最能损害人体健康，是产生其他烦恼的根本。

three dirts A common term of Qigong in Buddhism, referring to greed, anger and stupidity that annoy the brain and damage health according to the Buddhism.

三关【sān guān】　① 指口、足、手；② 指玉枕、夹脊、尾闾；③ 指耳、目、口；④ 指脐下关元，亦谓之三关；⑤ 指精关、气关、神关；⑥ 指明堂、洞房、丹田；⑦ 指泥丸为天关，丹田为地关，绛宫为人关；⑧ 指初关、中关、下关；⑨ 指头、足、手。

three passes Refer to ① either the mouth, the foot and the hand; ② or Yuzhen (BL 9) (an acupoint in the bladder meridian), Jiaji (EX - B2) (an acupoint located in the spine) and coccyx; ③ or the ears, the eyes and the mouth; ④ or Guanyuan (CV 4) (an acupoint in the conception meridian) also known as three passes; ⑤ or the essence pass, Qi pass and the spirit pass; ⑥ or bright chamber (nose), nuptial chamber (chamber in the brain) and Dantian; ⑦ or the mud bolus (brain) as the celestial pass, the Dantian as the earthly pass and the precordium as human pass; ⑧ or the original pass, the middle pass and the lower pass; ⑨ or the head, the foot and the hand.

三关修炼【sān guān xiū liàn】　指气功锻炼中，炼精化气、炼气化神、炼神还虚三个阶段为三关修炼。

three stages of cultivation A term of Qigong, referring to three stages of Qigong practice, including refining the essence to transform Qi, refining Qi to transform the spirit and refining the spirit to relieve deficiency.

三观【sān guān】　为静功，指的是空观、假观、中观。

three reflections A static exercise, referring to either hallow observation; or false observation; or middle observation.

三光【sān guāng】　指的是目。《黄庭外景经》说，"三光者，眼是也"。

three lights Refers to the eyes. In Huangting Waijing Jing (entitled *Canon of External Images in the Yellow Mansion*), an ancient Chinese monograph related to Qigong, it says that "the three kinds of light refer to the eyes".

三贵【sān guì】　指的是阳热、血、气。《内镜·敬身格言》说："身内有三贵，热以为生，血以为养，气以为动觉。"

three values Refer to Yang heat, blood and Qi. In Neijing (entitled *Internal Images*), an ancient Chinese monograph related to Qigong, it says that "There are three great elements in the human body, among which heat indicates growth, blood indicates cultivation and Qi indicates activity and consciousness."

三害【sān hài】　指的是邪念、烦恼、嗔恚。

three harms　Refer to wicked idea, annoyance and anger.

三和【sān hé】　指阳和、阴和、泰和。《五厨经气法注》说："在天为阳和,在地为阴和,交合为泰和也。"

three harmonies　Refer to Yang harmony, Yin harmony and Tai harmony. In Wuchu Jingqifa Zhu (entitled *Annotation of Meridian Qi in the Five Kitchenes*), an ancient Chinese monograph related to Qigong, it says that "Yang harmony is in the sky, Yin harmony is in the earth and peaceful harmony is in the integration of all things."

三候【sān hòu】　指的是指春、夏、秋三候。气功文献中认为,了解时令、季节、气候变化对疾病的影响,有利于应用气功调摄。

three seasonal climates　Refer to the spring, the summer and the autumn, which are the three seasons in a year. The literature of Qigong suggests that understanding the influence of seasons and climates upon disease is beneficial to the application of Qigong for cultivating life.

三壶【sān hú】　指海中三山,是习练气功的理想地方。《搜神记》说："三壶者,海中三山也。一曰方壶,二曰蓬壶,三曰

瀛壶。"

three pots (ideal places)　Refer to three mountains in the sea that are the ideal places for practicing Qigong. In Soushen Ji (entitled *Records of Collecting the Spirits*), an ancient Chinese monograph related to Qigong, it says that "The so-called three pots refer to the three mountains in the sea. The first mountain in the sea is called Square Mountain, the second is called the Fleabane Mountain and the third is called Ocean Mountain."

三花聚顶【sān huā jù dǐng】　指肾气、真气、心液,合而为一,上聚于脑;指神、气、精合而为一,上聚于脑。

accumulation of three flowers in the top　Refers to either integration of kidney Qi, genuine Qi and heart humor in the brain; or integration of the spirit, Qi and the essence in the brain.

三黄【sān huáng】　指雄黄、雌黄、硫黄。

three kinds of yellow　A noun of external Dan (pills of immortality), referring to realgar, gamboge and sulfur.

三慧【sān huì】　指的是开慧、思慧、修慧。

three wisdoms　Refer to starting wisdom, considering wisdom and cultivating wisdom.

三魂【sān hún】　指爽灵、胎光、幽精三魂,为精神意识活动之一,属阳神。

three ethereal souls　Refer to Yang spirit, including great spirit, fetal brightness and serene essence, which is one of the spiritual and mental activities, belonging to Yang spirit.

三火【sān huǒ】　① 指君火、臣火、民火,即以心为君火,以气为臣火,以精为

民火；② 指三阳，即太阳、少阳、阳明。

three fires Refer to ① either monarch fire, minister fire and human fire, in which the heart is monarch fire, Qi is minister fire and the essence is human fire； ② or the three kinds of Yang, i. e. Taiyang, Shaoyang and Yangming.

三惑【sān huò】 指酒、色、财三种损伤情志的因素。

three seductions Refer to alcohol, sex and property that damage the mental factors.

三极至命筌蹄【sān jí zhì mìng quán tí】《三极至命筌蹄》为气功专著，为宋代王庆升述，深入分析介绍了气功学的基本理论、方法和功效。

Sanji Zhiming Quanti (*Tripolar Achievement of Life*) A monograph of Qigong entitled *Tripolar Achievement of Life*, compiled by Wang Qingsheng in the Song Dynasty (960 AD – 1279 AD), thoroughly analyzing and introducing the basic theory, methods and effects of Qigong.

三家相见【sān jiā xiāng jiàn】 指神形相互作用下，全身各部处于相对稳定状态。

convergence of three aspects Refers to integration of the spirit and the body, stabilizing all parts of the whole body.

三焦【sān jiāo】 六腑之一。指上、中、下三焦，上焦在胃上口，中焦在胃脘，下焦在脐下。

triple energizer Refers to one of the six Fu-organs (the gallbladder, stomach, small intestine, large intestine, bladder and triple energizer) among which the upper energizer is located in the epigastric coelom, the middle energizer is located in the gastric cavity and

the lower energizer is located below the navel.

三教【sān jiào】 指的是儒教、道教、释教。三教均研究气功。《北史》说："帝生高座，辨释三教先后，以儒为先，道教次之，释教为后。"

three religions Refers to Confucianism, Daoism and Buddhism. These three religions all studied Qigong. In Beishi (entitled *History of the North*), an ancient Chinese monograph related to Qigong, it says that "The Emperor has analyzed the order of the three religions, suggesting that the Confucianism is the first, Daoism is the second and the Buddhism is the third".

三教合一【sān jiào hé yī】 指儒、释、道三教，合一指气功理论及实践方法基本相同。

combination of three religions Refers to the combination of the theory and practice of Qigong in Daoism, Confucianism and Buddhism.

三教无异说【sān jiào wú yì shuō】指道、儒、释三家气功，殊途同归。

no heterodoxy in three religions Refers to Qigong similar to each other in Daoism, Confucianism and Buddhism, concluding as all rivers running into sea.

三结【sān jié】 ① 指经气结聚的头、胸、腹三部；② 指胸结、肢结、便结。

three kinds of stasis Refer to ① either stasis in the chest, the limbs and defecation； ② or the chest, the limbs and defecation.

三戒【sān jiè】 指戒色、戒斗、戒得。色、斗、得三者，损伤形体，破坏神形的稳定。

three commandments Refer to abstaining sex, fight and avarice which damage the body and destroy the spirit and body.

三界【sān jiè】　佛家气功习用语，指的是欲界、色界、无色界。

three stages A common term of Qigong in Buddhism，referring to the stages of avarice，natural world and tranquility.

三界唯心【sān jiè wéi xīn】　指欲界、色界、无色界的一切所由，都是心造，即意识思维。

three stages from the heart Refers to avarice，lust and colorlessness caused by the heart，indicating the changes of consciousness and thought.

三精【sān jīng】　在天指日、月、星；在人指精、气、神。

three essences Refer to either the sun，the moon and the stars in the sky；or the essence，Qi and the spirit in the human body.

三精气【sān jīng qì】　佛家气功习用语，指自然的精气、人的精气、气功功法的精气。

three essential Qi A common term of Qigong in Buddhism，referring to the spiritual Qi in the natural world，in the human body and in the Qigong exercise.

三觉【sān jué】　佛家气功习用语，指自觉、觉他、觉行穷满；或指本觉、始觉、知觉。

three senses A common term of Qigong in Buddhism，referring to either personal sense，other sense and full sense；or original consciousness，initial consciousness and advanced consciousness.

三老【sān lǎo】　指的是上寿、中寿、下寿。亦指古代天子养老。

three longevities Refer to upper longevity，middle longevity，and lower longevity. It also refers to the ways of the emperors in ancient China to cultivate and to prolong their life.

三老同坐各有朋【sān lǎo tóng zuò gè yǒu péng】　指身体各部相互为用，上、中、下三部协调平衡。

mutual balance among three stages Refers to coordination of all parts in the body and regulation and balance between the upper region，the middle region and the lower region.

三乐【sān lè】　佛家气功习用语，指天乐、禅乐、涅槃乐。

three enjoyments A common term of Qigong in Buddhism，referring to enjoyment of the sky，dhyana and nirvana.

三炼【sān liàn】　指的是炼精、炼气、炼神。

three exercises Refer to essence exercise，Qi exercise and spirit exercise.

三轮【sān lún】　佛家气功习用语。三轮指的是神通轮、记心轮和教诫轮。即以佛之身业，现种种之神变，使人相信佛理及佛法；以佛之意业，分辨人的精神与形体、行为的不同；以佛之口业教诫人而使之相信义理，实践气功功法。

three cycles A common term of Qigong in Buddhism，referring to understanding the spirit，the heart and the commandments. These three cycles actually refer to three ways. The first cycle is to depend on the body state in Buddhism in order to enable others to believe the theory and practice of Qigong in Buddhism；the second cycle is to depend on the consciousness state in Buddhism in order to differentiate the spirit，the

S

body and the activity of different people; the third cycle is to depend on the oral state in Buddhism in order to enable others to believe the moral texture and practical exercise of Qigong.

三论元旨【sān lùn yuán zhǐ】《三论元旨》为气功学专著,其作者不详。

Sanlun Yuanzhi (*Three Discussions About Primordial Sense*) A monograph of Qigong entitled *Three Discussions About Primordial Sense*. The author was unknown.

三脉【sān mài】 指的是足阳明胃经、足厥阴肝经、足少阴肾经三条经脉。

three meridians Refer to the stomach meridian of foot Yangming, the liver meridian of foot Jueyin and the kidney meridian of foot Shaoyin.

三毛【sān máo】 又称为丛毛、聚毛,生于足大趾爪甲后皮肤上。

three hairs Also called feathering or accumulated hair, growing on the skin over the hallux.

三茅真君【sān máo zhēn jūn】 指茅盈、茅固、茅衷三兄弟。传说三茅兄弟修道,有仙术,通气功。

three sincere gentlemen Refer to three brothers of Mao Sheng, Mao Gu and Maozhong who were great masters of Qigong in Daoism.

三茅真君诀【sān máo zhēn jūn jué】源自气功专论,主要阐述神与气的关系及其重要性。

discussion about sincere gentlemen in three aspects Collected from a monograph of Qigong, mainly describing the relationship and importance of spirit and Qi.

三昧【sān mèi】 指的是义为正定、正心行处。《大智度论》说:"善心一处住不

动,是各三昧。"

samadhi Refers to rectifying the will and heart for ensuring all magic power and activity. In Dazhi Dulun (entitled *Discussion about Great Wisdom and Degrees*), an ancient Chinese monograph related to Qigong, it says that "No change of the purified heart is called Samahi."

三昧法【sān mèi fǎ】 为功法。其作法为,跏趺坐,正身,头身平正,调节呼吸,使之平稳。

samadhi exercise A dynamic exercise, marked by sitting in lotus position, stretching the body, balancing the head and body, regulating respiration in order to stabilize the whole body.

三昧印【sān mèi yìn】 指的是小周天。

samadhi image Refers to small circulatory cycle.

三昧真火【sān mèi zhēn huǒ】 气功学术语,指心、肾、膀胱之元气。

three primordial fires Refers to the original Qi from the heart, kidney and bladder.

三眠【sān mián】 指习练卧功的三种姿势,即病龙眠,拳其膝;家猿眠,抱其膝;龟息眠,手足曲而心思定。

three sleeps Refer to three styles in practicing Qigong, i. e boxing the knee, embracing the knee and twisting the hands and feet in order to tranquilize the heart and the mind.

三眠魂自安【sān mián hún zì ān】 指龙、猿、龟三眠。龙眠弯曲膝关节,猿眠抱住膝关节,龟眠手足弯曲、心神呼吸宁静。

three sleeping postures Refer to Loong sleeping (bending the knee joints), ape sleeping（clasping the knee points）and turtle sleeping（bending the feet）for quieting respiration.

三明【sān míng】 ① 指天三明，为日、月、星；② 指地三明，即文、章、华；③ 指人三明，即耳、目、口。

three kinds of brightness Refers to ① either the sun，the moon and the stars in the sky；② or the scenery，jade and magnificence in the earth；③ or the ears，the eyes and the mouth in the human body.

三摩地【sān mó dì】 即三昧法，为功法。其作法为，跏趺坐，正身，头身平正，调节呼吸，使之平稳。

samadhi technique The same as Samadhi exercise，is a dynamic exercise，marked by sitting in lotus position，stretching the body，balancing the head and body，regulating respiration in order to stabilize the whole body.

三男三女【sān nán sān nǚ】 三男指的是震、坎、艮，三女指的是巽、离、兑。

three men and three women In this term，the so-called three men refers to Zhen Trigram，Kan Trigram and Gen Trigram known as three men；and the so-called three women refers to Xun Trigram，Li Trigram and Dui Trigram known as three women.

三品【sān pǐn】 指的是精、气、神。

three kinds of genuineness Refer to essence，Qi and spirit，which are three most important factors in the human body.

三奇【sān qí】 ① 主要指的是精、气、神；② 三宫之神；③ 乾卦；④ 乙、丙、丁。

three kinds of unusualness Refers to ① either essence，Qi and spirit；② or the spirit in the three chambers；③ or

Qian Trigram in Yijing；④ or Yi（the second of the ten Heavenly Stems），Bing（the third of the ten Heavenly Stems）and Ding（the fourth of the ten Heavenly stems）.

三气【sān qì】 ① 指的是太初、太始、太素之气，太初为气之始，太始为形之始，太素为质之始；② 指玄气、元气、始气；③ 指三丹田之气；④ 指元气，即太阴、太阳、中和三气共为理。

three kinds of Qi Refer to ① either Qi from the origin which is the start of Qi，beginning which is the start of formation and simplicity which is the start of quality；② or the supreme Qi，the original Qi and the initial Qi；③ or Qi in the three kinds of Dantian；④ or only the original Qi，which is formed from the Qi from Taiyin，Taiyang and neutralization.

三千威仪【sān qiān wēi yí】 佛家气功习用语，指佛家气功身法之多，数在三千。

three thousands of fine comportments A common term of Qigong in Buddhism，referring to the fact that there are over three thousand methods of Qigong practice in Buddhism.

三窍【sān qiào】 指眼为神窍，耳为精窍，口为气窍。

three orifices Refer to the eyes known as spiritual orifices，ears known as essential orifices and mouth known as Qi orifice.

三清【sān qīng】 玉清、上清、太清。指天上仙人所居之清静境界。喻脑神所居之处应清静。

three purities Refer to jade purity，upper purity and great purity which are the pure states where the immortals

S

stay, also comparing to the tranquilized chamber where the spirit in the brain exists.

三秋【sān qiū】 指的是秋季三个月，也指三年。

three autumns Refer to three months in the autumn or three years.

三去【sān qù】 指的是去甚、去奢、去泰，即去掉叹端的、过分的、奢侈的情志和行为，以保持意识思维活动的稳定。

three eliminations Refer to eliminating extreme, excessive and extravagant emotions and activities in order to stabilize the activities of consciousness and thinking.

三全【sān quán】 指的是精全、气全、神全。《脉望》说："修行不用太急，久而不得心变。戒思虑，神全；戒言语，气全；戒色欲，精全。神圆不思睡，气圆不思食，精圆不思欲。"

three fulfillments Refers to fulfillment of the essence, Qi and the spirit. In Maiwang (*Observation of Meridians*), it says that "Practice of Qigong should not be anxious and the heart will not be changed if stability is kept for a long time. Giving up contemplation will perfect the spirit; giving up speech will perfect Qi; and giving up concupiscence will perfect the essence. When the spirit is perfect, sleep is not emphasized; when Qi is perfect, diet is not emphasized; when the essence is perfect, desire is not emphasized."

三全三圆【sān quán sān yuán】 指戒思虑神全，戒言语气全，戒色欲精全。

triple fullness and triple perfection Refer to abstaining contemplation to perfect the spirit, abstaining speech to perfect Qi and abstaining lust to perfect

the essence.

三热【sān rè】 佛家气功习用语。三热指①热风，热沙著身，烧及皮肉、骨髓引起的苦恼；② 或指恶风、厉风骤起，吹伤形体、衣饰引起的苦恼；③ 或指兽入室，欲夺饮食，引起惊惧苦恼。

three kinds of hotness A common term of Qigong in Buddhism, referring to ① either hot wind that burns the muscles and damages the marrows; ② or evil wind that damages the body and breaks the clothes; ③ or monsters that enter the room, plundering food and terrifying people.

三神【sān shén】 指的是元神、识神、真神。

three spirits Refer to the original spirit, the knowledgeable spirit and the genuine spirit.

三乘【sān shèng】 所谓三乘，佛学以车乘喻佛法，学者接受能力不一，称三乘；道家称第一洞上乘，第二洞为中乘，第三洞为下乘。

three classes Refers to either comparing Buddhism to a cart, different studying abilities, which are called three carts; or three cavities in Daoism, which are divided into the first class, the second class and the third class.

三尸【sān shī】 ① 即三虫，为引起精神失调的因素；② 指三彭，即居脑中、腹中、足中，损害人体健康的邪气。

three pathogenic factors Refer to ① either three insects that harm the spirit and the body; ② or three pathogenic factors in the brain, abdomen and foot that have damaged physical health.

三十六【sān shí liù】 指一月的天数。古代太阳历将一年分为十月，每月三十六天。

thirty-six days Refer to the days in a month because in ancient China one year was composed of ten months and one month was composed of thirty-six days.

三十六咽说【sān shí liù yān shuō】 源自气功专论。详细阐述了"三十六咽"的具体做法及其要求。

discussion about thirty-six swallows Collected from a monograph of Qigong, thoroughly describing the methods and requirements of thirty-six swallows in practicing Qigong.

三时【sān shí】 佛家气功习练时间，指白天早晨、中午、黄昏三时，夜间初夜、中夜、后夜三时。

three periods Refer to the time to practice Qigong in Buddhism, indicating the early night, middle night and late night. It also refers to the early period, middle period and late period in the night.

三识【sān shí】 佛家气功习用语，主要是认识人与自然、人与社会的联系，从而平调神志意识。具体指的是，真识，即自性洁净心，通真不通妄，妄者染，真者净；现识，即变现之义，含藏一切善恶种子，而变现为现时世界；分别识，即于六尘种种诸境而起分别，由传送第六意识而起分别。

three realizations A common term of Qigong in Buddhism, referring to realization of human-nature relationship and human-society relationship, making it possible to pacify and to regulate emotion and consciousness. These three realizations actually refer to three ways. The first is genuine recognition, indicating to naturally purify and tranquilize the heart without any delusion and distracting thought; the second is ordinary recognition, indicating to emphasize reality and to maintain both moral and wicked ideas, especially caring about the present world; the third is differential recognition, indicating to separate and to transmit the six kinds of states.

三寿【sān shòu】 ① 指上、中、下三寿；② 指将高年期分为三个等级。

three longevities ① Refers to upper longevity, middle longevity, and lower longevity. ② It also divides longevity into three levels.

三素云【sān sù yún】 ① 指目中有三色；② 指肺、肝、脾三脏之气。

three plain features Refer to ① either three colors in the eyes; ② or Qi in the lung, the liver and the spleen.

三台【sān tái】 指的是三焦。《道枢》说："五藏五岳也，三焦三台也，四水四渎也。"

three platforms Refers to triple energizer. In Dao Shu (entitled *Pivot of Dao*), an ancient Chinese monograph related to Qigong, it says, "the five mountains are the comparisons of the five Zang-organs (including the heart, the liver, the spleen, the lung and the kidney), the three platforms are the comparisons of the triple energizer and the four rivers or the four ditches are the comparisons of four kinds of water."

三天门【sān tiān mén】 指两眉正中处出现的精光。

three celestial gates Refers to brightness in the center of the eyes.

三天易髓【sān tiān yì suǐ】 《三天易髓》为气功专著，深入地阐述了气功的理论和方法。李道纯撰，成书于元代。

Santian Yisui（*Three Days to Change Marrow*）　A monograph of Qigong entitled *Three Days to Change Marrow*, written by Li Daochun in the Yuan Dynasty(1271 AD－1368 AD), thoroughly describing the theory and practice of Qigong.

三田【sān tián】　即三丹田，指的是脑、心和气海。即脑为上丹田，心为中丹田，气海为下丹田。

three fields　Refers to the three kinds of Dantian, related to the brain, heart and Qihai (the lower part of the abdomen). In this term, the brain refers to the upper Dantian, the heart refers to the middle Dantian and Qihai refers to the lower Dantian. In fact the upper Dantian refers to the region between the eyes, the middle Dantian refers to the region below the heart and the lower Dantian refers to the region below the navel.

三田升降一条【sān tián shēng jiàng yī tiáo】　源自气功专论。主要阐述练功即是修炼神气于三丹田升降交合。

promotion and demotion of the triple energizer　Collected from a monograph of Qigong, mainly discussing ascent, descent and combination of the spirit and Qi in the three kinds of Dantian in practicing Qigong. The three kinds of Dantian include the upper Dantian (the region between the eyes), the middle Dantian (the region below the heart) and the lower Dantian (the region below the navel).

三无为【sān wú wéi】　指的是不妄为、非姻缘和合形成、精神稳定。

three inactions　Refers to inactivity, absolute existence and spiritual stability.

三五【sān wǔ】　① 指人体的五色、五音、五味，称为三五；② 指外界刺激引起意识活动紊乱，精神失调。

three-five　A term of Qigong, referring to ① either the five colors, the five sounds and the five tastes; ② or stimulation in the external world that has disordered the activity of consciousness and dislocated the spirit.

三五合气【sān wǔ hé qì】　① 指三丹田与五脏之气和合为一；② 指心、肾、肺合而为一，相互作用。

integration of three and five　Refers to ① integration of three levels of Dantian and Qi in the five Zang-organs (including the heart, the liver, the spleen, the lung and the kidney); ② or integration of the heart, the kidney and the lung. Dantian is divided into the upper Dantian (the region between the eyes), the middle Dantian (the region below the heart) and the lower Dantian (the region below the navel).

三五气合九九节【sān wǔ qì hé jiǔ jiǔ jié】　在这一概念中，三为三丹田，五为五脏之气，九为脑中九宫与自然九宫之气节。也指天地人合而为一。

combination of three and five kinds of Qi with nine integrities　Refer to either the three kinds of Dantian, the five Zang-organs (including the heart, the liver, the spleen, the lung and the kidney) and the nine chambers in the brain; or integration of the sky, the earth and human beings. Dantian is divided into the upper Dantian (the region between the eyes), the middle Dantian (the region below the heart) and the lower Dantian (the region below the navel).

三五玄【sān wǔ xuán】 指三丹田和五脏。

three-five mysteries Refers to three Dantian (including upper Dantian, the region between the eyes; middle Dantian, the region below the heart; lower Dantian, the region below the navel) and the five Zang-organs (including the heart, the liver, the spleen, the lung and the kidney).

三五一【sān wǔ yī】 ① 指三阳，五行，一气为三五一；② 或指五脏之气，内聚中土。

three-five-one aspects Refers to ① either three Yang, five elements (including wood, fire, earth, metal and water) and one Qi; ② or accumulation of Qi from the five Zang-organs (including the heart, the liver, the spleen, the lung and the kidney) in the middle.

三五一枢要【sān wǔ yī shū yào】 源自气功专论。主要阐述三五一的含义，及其在习练气功中的重要性。

discussion about the essentials of three-five-one Collected from a monograph of Qigong, mainly describing the meaning of three, five and one as well as the importance of Qigong practice.

三息【sān xī】 指的是息缘、息气、息心。《中和集》认为："息缘达本禅之机，息心明理儒之极，息气凝神道之玄，三息相须无不克。"

three senses Refer to destiny sense, mentality sense and Qi sense. In Zhonghe Ji (entitled *Collection of Neutralization and Harmonization*), an ancient Chinese monograph related to Qigong, it says that "Sense of destiny

means to reach the state of dhyana, sense of mentality means to understand the truth of Confucianism, and sense of Qi means to supremely concentrate the spirit. These three senses are interrelated, not different."

三息论【sān xī lùn】 源自气功专论，主要阐述释、儒、道三家气功学之特点。

discussion of three respirations Collected from a monograph of Qigong, mainly describing the characteristics and functions of Qigong in Buddhism, Confucianism and Daoism.

三夏【sān xià】 指夏天三个月或三年。

three summers Refer to either three months in the summer, or three years.

三想【sān xiǎng】 佛家气功习用语，指的是欲想、嗔想、害想、怨想、亲想、亲爱父母、兄弟之想。

three thoughts A common term of Qigong in Buddhism, referring to either avarice, including greed, anger, victimization and hatred; or love, including lovely parents, elder brothers and sisters as well as younger brothers and sisters; or disharmony of the spirit and mind.

三象【sān xiàng】 指气动而清，神静而宁，智因而明等三种气功现象。《至游子》说："气功而清者，天之象也；心静而宁者，地之象也；智圆而明者，月之象也。三者和会则自然见吾神灵之妙用矣。"

three phenomena Refers to the fact that the movement of Qi is clear, tranquility of the spirit is serene, and pure wisdom is bright. In Zhi Youzi (entitled *Sincere Travelers*), an ancient Chinese monograph related to Qigong, it says that "Active and clear Qi represents the

S

phenomenon of the sky, tranquil and stable heart represents the phenomenon of the earth, and perfect and pure wisdom represents the phenomenon of the moon. Harmonization of these three phenomena naturally reflects the intelligence of the spirit and the soul."

三星【sān xīng】　阴茎、两睾丸合称三星。

three stars　Refer to penis and scrota which are called the three stars in the human body.

三性【sān xìng】　指元气、元精、元神。

three properties　Refer to the original Qi, the original essence and the original spirit.

三虚【sān xū】　指的是念虚、月虚、时虚。

three insufficiencies　Refer to year insufficiency, month insufficiency and hour insufficiency.

三玄【sān xuán】　指的是《老子》《庄子》《周易》三书为玄学之经典。古代气功文献多有引用三书以为说理。

three canons　Refer to three important classics entitled *Lao Zi*, *Zhuang Zi* and *Zhou Yi*. In ancient Chinese literature of Qigong, these three important canons were often used to study and to analyze the basic theory and practice of Qigong.

三学【sān xué】　佛家气功习用语,指戒学、定学、慧学,即三类气功功法。

three studies　A common term of Qigong in Buddhism, referring to three kinds of Qigong practice, including commandment study, stability study and wisdom study.

三阳【sān yáng】　指心液之气为阳中之阴,肾中之气为阴中之阳,丹田中真气

为阳中之阳,故谓之三阳。

three Yang　Refers to Qi in the heart known as Yin within Yang, Qi in the kidney known as Yang within Yin and genuine Qi in Dantian known as Yang within Yang. Dantian is divided into the upper Dantian (the region between the eyes), the middle Dantian (the region below the heart) and the lower Dantian (the region below the navel).

三阳聚顶【sān yáng jù dǐng】　① 指丹田、泥丸、绛宫之阳聚于头脑;② 指太阳、少阳、阳明之气聚于大脑。

accumulation of three Yang in the top　① Refers to concentration of Yang from Dantian, the mud bolus (the brain) and the heart in the brain; and concentration of Taiyang, Shaoyang and Yangming, three Yang in the brain. ② Dantian is divided into the upper Dantian (the region between the eyes), the middle Dantian (the region below the heart) and the lower Dantian (the region below the navel).

三阳开泰【sān yáng kāi tài】　指冬至一阳生,农历十二月二阳生,农历正月三阳生,三阳开泰,春天开始。

beginning of spring　Refers to the fact that in the traditional Chinese calendar, the first Yang appears in the winter solstice, the second Yang appears in December and the third Yang appears in the January, activating the spring.

三阳五会【sān yáng wǔ huì】　① 指百会,百会指督脉中的一个穴位;② 指气功常见意守部位;③ 指百神之会。这一穴位为气功运行的一个常见部位。

Sanyang Wuhui　① A synonym of Baihui (GV 20) which refers to either an acupoint in the governor meridian;

② or the region where consciousness maintains in practicing Qigong; ③ or convergence of hundred spirits. This acupoint is a region usually used in practice of Qigong.

三要【sān yào】 指内三要、外三要。也指一要炼精,第二要调息,第三要养心。

three essentials Refer to either the internal essentials and the external essentials; or practicing essence, regulating breath and nourishing the heart.

三要达到篇【sān yào dá dào piān】《三要达到篇》为气功专著。本文意在说明习练气功要获得成功,首先应具备三要,即省言语、去邪视、除淫声。作者不详。

Sanyao Dadao Pian (*Discussion About Three Essentials*) A monograph of Qigong entitled *Discussion About Three Essentials*, mainly describing three important requirements, i. e. speaking less, eliminating evil vision and lewd voice. The author was unknown.

三一【sān yī】 ① 指三丹田合一;② 指精气神合而为一;③ 指泥丸、绛宫、丹田。

three-one Refers to ① either combination of three kinds of Dantian, referring to the upper Dantian (the region between the eyes), the middle Dantian (the region below the heart) and the lower Dantian (the region below the navel); ② or integration of the essence, Qi and the spirit; ③ or the mud bolus (the brain), crimson palace (the heart) and Dantian.

三一长存【sān yī cháng cún】 指三为身之元神,一为身之真精,炼之神真精,健康益寿延年。

combination of three and one Refers to integration of three original spirits and one genuine essence in the human body, practice of which is beneficial to cultivating health and prolonging life.

三一法【sān yī fǎ】 练气功的静法。其作法为,常以生气之时,静卧瞑目,握固闭口,不息,心数至二百,乃口中微吐气出之,日增其数。

three-one technique A static exercise of Qigong practice, marked by lying quietly during the production of Qi, closing the eyes and mouth, stopping respiration till the heart beating for two hundred times, slowly breathing out through the mouth and increasing it every time.

三一服气法【sān yī fú qì fǎ】 为静功。其作法为,"夫欲长生,三一当明。上一在泥丸中,中一在绛宫中,下一在丹田中。人生正在此也"。

three-one ways of inhalation Means that for prolonging life one must be clear about three-one ways of inhalation. The first inhalation is in the mud bolus (the brain), the second is in the heart and the third is in the Dantian. Dantian is divided into the upper Dantian (the region between the eyes), the middle Dantian (the region below the heart) and the lower Dantian (the region below the navel).

三一机要【sān yī jī yào】 源自气功专论,主要阐述气功锻炼精及气神之机要。

confidentiality based on integration of three essentials Collected from a monograph of Qigong, mainly describing the right ways to practice Qigong and to enrich essence, Qi and spirit.

S

三医【sān yī】 佛家气功习用语,指上、中、下三种医师。上医诊断听音,中医诊断相色,下医诊断切脉。

three grades of doctors A common term of Qigong in Buddhism, referring to great doctors, ordinary doctors and backward doctors. According to the traditional Chinese medicine theory and treatment, the first-class doctors diagnose patients by listening to the sound, the middle-class doctors diagnose patients by observing the complexion and the lower-class doctors diagnose patients by taking the pulse.

三易【sān yì】 指《连山》《归藏》《周易》。《连山》为夏之《易》,《归藏》为商之《易》,二书已失传。

three Yi Refers to three important books about Yijing including *Lianshan* compiled in the Xia Dynasty (2070 BC‐1600 BC), *Guizang* compiled in the Shang Dynasty (1600 BC‐1046 BC) and *Zhouyi* compiled in the Zhou Dynasty (1046 BC‐256 BC), both of which disappeared in ancient China.

三阴交【sān yīn jiāo】 属足太阴脾经,位内踝尖上 3 寸,胫骨后缘。此穴位为气功习练之处。

Sanyinjiao(SP 6) An acupoint in the spleen meridian of foot Taiyin, located about 3 Cun above the medial malleolus and behind the tibia. This acupoint is a region usually used in practice of Qigong.

三元【sān yuán】 指的是农历正月、七月、十月的十五日,或指日月星,或指三丹田,或指元精、元气、元神。

three initiatives Refer to either fifteen important days in January, July and October; or three kinds of Dantian; or

the original essence, the original Qi and the original spirit in the body. Three kinds of Dantian refers to the upper Dantian (the region between the eyes), the middle Dantian (the region below the heart) and the lower Dantian (the region below the navel).

三元混一【sān yuán hùn yī】 即摄三归一。三指精、气、神;摄精、气、神而为一,可炼成丹。

integration of three and one Refers to integration of the essence, Qi and the spirit into one for refining Dan (pills of immortality) in practice of Qigong.

三元全陆地仙【sān yuán quán lù dì xiān】 指练气功保全精、气、神,则可延年益寿。

three primordial immortals in the world Refers to protecting the essence, Qi and the spirit in practicing Qigong for prolonging life.

三元用事【sān yuán yòng shì】 指精气流向三丹田,三丹田之气相互作用。

management of three origins Refers to the essential Qi flowing into the three kinds of Dantian and interaction of Qi in the three kinds of Dantian. The three kinds of Dantian include the upper Dantian (the region between the eyes), the middle Dantian (the region below the heart) and the lower Dantian (the region below the navel).

三月清明节后导引法【sān yuè qīng míng jié hòu dǎo yǐn fǎ】 为动功。其作法为,三月清明节后,每日丑寅时,正身端坐,两手交叉如托天状,引下腹部气向上七八次,口中唾液咽下,身中浊气呼出。其功效可强腰肾。

exercise of Daoyin after Qingming Festival A dynamic exercise, marked by sitting upright in Hou (the period of a day from 1 p. m. to 3 p. m. in the afternoon) and Yin (the period of a day from 3 a. m. to 5 a. m. in the morning) after the Spring Festival, crossing hands to rise up like reaching the sky, promoting Qi from the lower abdomen to flow upwards for seven to eight times, swallowing saliva in the mouth, and breathing out turbid Qi in the body. Such a dynamic exercise can strengthen the waist and the kidney.

三月中导引法【sān yuè zhōng dǎo yǐn fǎ**】** 为动功。其作法为, 每日丑寅时, 腰伸直而坐, 左手在右腰身俞处向上按摩十五次, 右手在左腰身俞处按摩十五次, 引口中唾液下咽中丹田二三次。功效为去脾胃之淤血。

exercise of Daoyin in the middle of March A dynamic exercise, marked by sitting up from Chou (the period of a day from 1 a. m. to 3 a. m. in the morning) and Yin (the period of a day from 3 a. m. to 5 a. m. in the morning) every day, stretching the waist, pressing and kneading the kidney acupoint on the right side of the waist with the left hand for fifteen times, pressing and kneading the kidney acupoint on the left side of the waist with the right hand, swallowing saliva in the mouth to the middle Dantian (the region below the heart) for two or three times. Such a dynamic exercise can relieve blood stasis in the spleen and the stomach.

三障【sān zhàng**】** 佛家气功习用语, 指的是烦恼障, 为贪欲、嗔毒、愚痴等损伤情志的精神活动现象; 业障, 为五逆十恶引起的精神活动现象。

three obstructions A common term of Qigong in Buddhism, referring to either avarice, anger and stupidity that damage the mind and spirit; or abnormal spirit activity caused by five diversities and ten nauseas.

三止法【sān zhǐ fǎ**】** 为静功。其作法为, 一是体直止, 意想性空, 止息一切攀缘妄想; 二是随缘止, 意想空中, 安住假谛之理而不动, 静定守神; 三是制心止, 意想知真非真而入寂静, 住心于内, 不分散注意力。

three tranquil techniques A static exercise. The first is to be righteousness without any desires and delusion; the second is to naturally accept without any optional activities in order to tranquilize the mind and to stabilize the spirit; the third is stabilization without any dispersion of the spirit and the mind.

三住铭【sān zhù míng**】** 指脑神御气, 气住神宁。形、气、神三住合而为一。

triple sovereign cores Refers to the spirit in the brain that controls Qi. Only when Qi is controlled can the spirit be stabilized. Only under such a condition can the body, Qi and the spirit be integrated.

三足金蟾【sān zú jīn chán**】** 指的是虚危穴, 为精气聚散常在此处, 水火发端也在此处, 阴阳变化也在此处, 有无出入也在此处。

three sufficient golden toads Refers to an acupoint known as Xuwei, referring to the region where the essential Qi concentrates and disperses water and fire appear, Yin and Yang change, exit and entrance exist.

三足乌【sān zú wū**】** 在气功文献中以"三足乌""金乌"称太阳。

S

three deities　Refers to the sun in the literature of Qigong.

散化五形变万神【sàn huà wǔ xíng biàn wàn shén】　泛指气功的中和平衡作用。

disseminating and transforming five shapes can change all kinds of the spirit. Indicates the effects of balance and peace in Qigong practice.

散为精沴【sàn wéi jīng zhuó】　指三焦布散周身的津液,有安神养脑,润泽皮肤毛发之功。

disseminating essence　Refers to disseminating fluid and humor in the whole body, the effect of which is to stabilize the spirit, to nourish the brain, and to moisten skin and hair.

丧神【sàng shén】　指损伤精神,即损伤脑神。

depletion of the spirit　Refers damage of the essence and the spirit, indicating injury of the spirit in the brain.

扫除不洁,神乃留处【sǎo chú bù jié shén nǎi liú chù】　指扫除情欲,精神内守而不外散。

Only when impurity is eliminated can the spirit be kept.　Refers to the fact that only when libido is eliminated can the spirit be concentrated inside without dispersion.

扫除六贼净心基【sǎo chú liù zéi jìng xīn jī】　源自气功专论,主要阐述净心炼气是练功中至关重要的地方。

eliminating six thieves to tranquilize the heart　Collected from a monograph of Qigong, mainly describing the important place for practicing Qigong in order to tranquilize the heart.

色【sè】　佛家气功习用语,① 指有形物质,如身体、树木、土地等;② 指精神活动;③ 指青黄赤白之色。

color　A common term of Qigong in Buddhism, referring to ① either tangible things, such as the body, the trees and the earth, etc. ; ② or spiritual activity; ③ or green, yellow, red and white colors.

色败【sè bài】　指男女交接过多,损伤肾阳,面色败坏。习练气功提倡节制性欲。

over sexual intercourse　Refers to excessive copulation between man and woman, which injures kidney Yang and corrupts the complexion. In practicing Qigong, libido should be well controlled.

色身【sè shēn】　指躯体,即生命。

physical body　Refers to the human body, which actually means the life.

啬气养神【sè qì yǎng shén】　指爱惜精气,不妄施妄泄,可以补脑养神明。

mild Qi nourishing the spirit　Refers to cherishing the essence and Qi, avoiding absurd execution and discharge. This way of practice can tonify the brain and nourish the spirit.

砂里汞【shā lǐ gǒng】　① 喻心,属火,为正阳之精;② 指神气。

mercury in sand　Refers to ① either the heart that belongs to fire; ② or spiritual Qi.

山根【shān gēn】　指两眼内眦连线之中。

mountain root　Refers to the middle of inner canthus in the eyes.

山头【shān tóu】　喻泥丸宫。

mountain top　Refers to the chamber of the mud bolus [the brain].

山图折脚【shān tú zhé jiǎo】　为动功。其作法为,坐时两脚放伸,治夜梦遗精。

foot kneading A dynamic exercise, marked by stretching the feet in sitting in order to relieve spermatorrhea.

山源【shān yuán】　指鼻下人中,也指鼻部。

mountain origin Refers to the region between the nose and the upper lip, also referring to the nose.

山泽通气法【shān zé tōng qì fǎ】　为动功,即用两手按摩面部,使面部气血流通,有光泽。

mountain and mash ventilation A dynamic exercise, referring to rubbing the face with both hands in order to circulate Qi and the blood in the face and to make the face lustrous.

膻中【shān zhōng】　即胸前正中,相当于男子两乳之间的部位,为宗气所聚之处。也指心包。也属于一个穴位。这一穴位为气功运行的一个常见部位。

thoracic center Refers to the center of the chest, similar to the region between the breasts in men, where thoracic Qi concentrates. It also refers to pericardium and an acupoint. This acupoint is a region usually used for moving essential Qi in practicing Qigong.

闪挫治法【shǎn cuò zhì fǎ】　为动功。凡一切闪挫疼痛,不可护其疼处,将身直立,双手如托千斤,上升放下,缓缓而行,二十四次止。

exercise for sprain A dynamic exercise, marked by standing up with both hands that raise up like holding one thousand Jin (a unit of weight) and then slowly put down for twenty-four times in order to relieve sprain, not to protect the location of sprain.

疝瘕候导引法【shàn jiǎ hòu dǎo yǐn fǎ】　为动功,方法多样,如用手拉两足趾,呼吸五次止,导引腹中之气。祛除疝瘕,通利孔窍。

exercise of Daoyin for abdominal mass Mass is a dynamic exercise with various methods, such as pulling the toes of both feet with both hands, breathing for five times, leading Qi from the abdomen in order to eliminate abdominal mass and to normalize the orifices.

疝气治法【shàn qì zhì fǎ】　动静相兼功,方法多样,如手拉两足趾,行气五息,引气达腹中。

treatment of hernia An exercise combined with dynamic exercise and static exercise with various methods, such as pulling the toes of both feet with both hands, moving Qi with five respirations and leading Qi to the abdominal center.

善【shàn】　① 指美好的精神活动; ② 指大多;③ 指符合事理,为佛家气功习用语。

goodness Refers to ① either fine activity of the spirit; ② or mostly; ③ or agreeing with the principles, which is a common term of Qigong in Buddhism.

善建善抱【shàn jiàn shàn bào】　指建德抱德。建德者外物不能动摇,故情绪稳定不拔;抱德者,专心一志,故意识活动集中而不间断。

improving virtue and keeping virtue Refers to improvement of virtue without any vacillation, indicating that emotion must be stabilized; and keeping virtue with concentration, indicating that the activity of consciousness should be concentrated and should not be interrupted.

S

善人【shàn rén】 指完美之人。

philanthropist Refers to a perfect person.

善摄生【shàn shè shēng】 指善于养生延年的人。

fine regimen Refers to those who are excellent in cultivating health and prolong life.

善忘【shàn wàng】 气功适应证,多因上气不足,下气有余,肠胃实而心肺虚所致。

amnesia An indication of Qigong, usually caused by insufficiency of Qi in the upper and excess of Qi in the lower, excess of the intestines and the stomach as well as deficiency of the heart and the lung.

善为士说【shàn wéi shì shuō】 源自气功专论,阐述习练气功之人出现的景象。

to be excellent in talking with others Collected from a monograph of Qigong, mainly describing the scene of Qigong practice.

缮性【shàn xìng】 指调节精神意识,修治本性。

cultivating nature Refers to regulation of the spirit and consciousness in order to cultivate and control the original nature.

伤风导引法【shāng fēng dǎo yǐn fǎ】 为动功。其作法为,平身坐正,双手擦掌,抚摸阴囊,两肘靠膝,身势向前,先躬而后仰,如此用力四十五遍,则汗透全身,即感觉身体轻松而愈。

exercise of Daoyin for wind damage A dynamic exercise, marked by sitting right, rubbing the palms, fondling the scrotum, putting the elbows on the knees, stretching the body forwards, bending forward first and then raising backward. After practicing for forty-five times, there is sweating all over the body, eventually relaxing the body and healing the body.

伤寒【shāng hán】 气功适应证,指感受寒邪所患之伤寒病证。

cold damage An indication of Qigong, referring to cold damage disease caused by pathogenic cold.

伤寒候导引法【shāng hán hòu dǎo yǐn fǎ】 为动功。其作法为,一般为正坐伸腰,用鼻缓缓吸气,用右手捏鼻,闭目吐气,解表散寒,治伤寒头痛,洒淅恶寒。

exercise of Daoyin for cold damage A dynamic exercise, usually marked by sitting upright, stretching the waist, slowly inhaling with the nose, pinching the nose with the right hand and closing the eyes to exhale in order to release the exterior to dissipate cold, to relieve cold damage, to cure headache and to expel chills with aversion to cold.

伤寒伤风导引法【shāng hán shāng fēng dǎo yǐn fǎ】 为动功,先饮热茶或热汤,颈项要直,舌卷抵上腭,两手握拳,两足趾缩紧,自然汗出而愈。

exercise of Daoyin for cold damage and wind damage A dynamic exercise, marked by drinking hot tea or hot water first, straightening the neck, holding the fists and tightening the toes. Such a dynamic exercise will impel sweating and cure disease caused by cold damage and wind damage.

伤寒伤风症治法【shāng hán shāng fēng zhèng zhì fǎ】 为动静相兼功。凡感冒伤寒,正身盘坐,闭气,反手以两中指插入鼻孔内,摇头数十回,以汗出为度。

treatment of cold damage and wind damage An exercise combined with dynamic exercise and static exercise, marked by sitting with crossed legs when there is common cold, suspending respiration, inserting the middle fingers into the nostrils with backhands and shaking the head for ten times till appearing of sweating.

伤精【shāng jīng】 ① 指损伤肝；② 指损伤津液。

essence damage Refers to ① either impairing the liver; ② or impairing fluid and humor in the body.

伤食导引法【shāng shí dǎo yǐn fǎ】为动功。其作法为，寅卯时辰（三时至七时），披衣起床不食，先正身直立，然后曲肘、前臂着地，脚尖落地，脚跟离地，做倒立姿势十八次。治伤食呕吐。

exercise of Daoyin for apepsia A dynamic exercise, marked by getting up in Yin (the period of a day from 3 a.m. to 5 a.m. in the morning) and Mao (the period of a day from 5 a.m. to 7 a.m. in the morning) every day, standing up, bending the elbows, putting the forearms on the ground, keeping the tiptoes on the ground and leaving the heel from the ground. All this practice is continued for eighteen times in order to relieve apepsia and vomiting.

商曲【shāng qǔ】 足少阴肾经中的一个穴位，位于脐上 2 寸，为气功中常用的意守部位。

Shangqu（KI 17） An acupoint in the kidney meridian of foot Shaoyin, located 2 Cun above the navel, which is the region for concentrating consciousness in practicing Qigong.

商阳【shāng yáng】 手阳明大肠经中的一个穴位，位于食指桡侧指甲角旁 0.1 寸，为气功中常用的意守部位。

Shangyang（LI 1） An acpuoint in the large intestine meridian of hand Yangming, located 0.1 Cun lateral to radialis of the forefinger, which is the region for concentrating consciousness in practicing Qigong.

晌晦入晏息【shǎng huì rù yàn xī】 为静功。其作法为，古之至人，有息无睡，故曰晌晦入晏息。晏息之法当晌晦时，耳无闻，目无见，四体无动，心无思虑，如种火相似，先天元神元气停育相抱，真意绵绵，开合自然，与虚空同体。

respiration without sleep A static exercise, marked by closing the ears and the eyes, inactivating the four limbs, tranquilizing the heart like increasing fire, coordinating the original spirit and original Qi, purifying the mind, opening and closing naturally, and equaling with vacuum.

上闭【shàng bì】 指练习气功，闭塞目、口、耳三关。

upper closure Refers to closure of the eyes, the ears and the mouth in practicing Qigong.

上补混丸下壮元气【shàng bǔ hún wán xià zhuàng yuán qì】 指补脑神于上，壮肾精于下。

nourishing the brain and fortifying the kidney Refers to tonifying the brain spirit in the upper and strengthening the kidney spirit in the lower.

上不闭药不凝【shàng bù bì yào bù níng】 指塞兑（闭口）、垂帘（微闭眼）、逆听才能凝神。

no retention of medicinal and no contem-

S

plation　Refers to no seeing, no speaking and no hearing in order to agglomerate the spirit.

上部八景【shàng bù bā jǐng】　指发神、脑神、眼神、鼻神、耳神、口神、舌神、齿神。

eight upper spirits　Refers to the the brain spirit, the eye spirit, the nose spirit, the ear spirit, the mouth spirit, the tongue spirit and the tooth spirit.

上乘修真三要【shàng chéng xiū zhēn sān yào】　《上乘修真三要》为气功专著,介绍了气功的基本理论和方法,分析了气功习练的要求和希望。作者不详。

Shangcheng Xiuzhen Sanyao(*Cultivation of Three Principal Essentials*)　A monograph of Qigong entitled *Cultivation of Three Principal Essentials*, describing the basic theory and exercises of Qigong, analyzing the principles and requirements of Qigong practice. The author was unknown.

上丹田【shàng dān tián】　两眉间称为上丹田,异名甚多。

upper Dantian(**the region between the eyes**)　Refers to the region between the eyes with various difficult names.

上岛【shàng dǎo】　指上丹田。丹田分为上丹田、中丹田和下丹田。

upper island　Refers to the upper Dantian (the region between the eyes). Dantian is divided into three levels, the first level is called upper Dantian, referring to the region between the eyes; the second level is called middle Dantian, referring to the region below the heart; the third level is called lower Dantian, referring to the region below the navel, similar to the upper pubic region.

上德不德【shàng dé bù dé】　指精神内守,意识不外散。

mental concentration　Refers to keeping the spirit inside and avoiding dispersion of consciousness outside.

上关【shàng guān】　足少阳胆经中的一个穴位,位于颧弓上缘,距耳郭前缘约1寸处,为气功常用意守部位。

Shangguan(**GB 3**)　An acupoint in the gallbladder of foot Shaoyang, located on the upper of the zygoma and about 1 Cun to the upper of the auricle. This acupoint is a region usually used in practice of Qigong.

上焦【shàng jiāo】　三焦之一。将横膈以上的胸部,包括心、肺两脏和头面部称作上焦。

upper energizer　Refers to the region between the upper side of the stomach and the lower side of the throat.

上髎【shàng liáo】　足太阳膀胱经的一个穴位,位第一骶候孔中。这一穴位为气功运行的一个常见部位。

Shangliao(**BL 31**)　An acupoint in the bladder meridian of foot Taiyang, located in the first sacral bone. This acupoint is a region usually used for moving essential Qi in practice of Qigong.

上气海【shàng qì hǎi】　指膻中,即胸前正中,相当于男子两乳之间的部位,为宗气所聚之处。也指心包。也属于一个穴位。这一穴位为气功运行的一个常见部位。

upper Qi sea　A synonym of Danzhong (CV 17), referring to the center of the chest, similar to the region between the breasts in men, where thoracic Qi concentrates. It also refers to pericardium and an acupoint. This acupoint is a region usually used for moving essential

Qi in practice of Qigong.

上气海穴【shàng qì hǎi xué】　膻中的另外一个称谓，是人体的穴位，在前正中线上，两乳头连线的中点。此穴位为气功习练之处。

Shangqihaixue　A synonym of Danzhong (CV 17), an acupoint located in the front midline between the breasts. This acupoint is a region usually used in practice of Qigong.

上气候导引法【shàng qì hòu dǎo yǐn fǎ】　为动功。其作法为，站立两手向后托腰，尽力向上，前后振摇臂肘七次。手不移动，肩臂上下动十四次。可宽胸理气；正坐，两膝足并拢，两足趾相对，足跟向外；两足趾相对，呼吸五次，引心肺元气下降。

exercise of Daoyin for raising Qi　A dynamic exercise, marked by standing up with both hands holding the waist, raising the elbows for seven times, ascending and descending the shoulders for fourteen times in order to soothe the chest; sitting with both knees crossed and both feet corresponding with each other; corresponding both feet with five times of respiration in order to descend original Qi in the heart and the lung.

上清【shàng qīng】　指天上清净之境，喻脑，说明脑在人体之高巅。

upper tranquility　Refers to the clear and quiet state in the sky, indicating the brain that is the peak of the human body.

上清法【shàng qīng fǎ】　为静功。其作法为，先正站立，拳手，漱津液满口，朝食阳，暮食阴；然后倚壁正站立，拳两手，使一足朝前抬高；用舌搅口中，至津液满口，即想气咽入脐，至脚为度。功效为益精养神、补脑。

exercise for clearing the upper　A static exercise, marked by standing up, holding the fists, rinsing fluid and humor in the whole mouth, taking Yang in the daytime and taking Yin in the nighttime; then standing up against the wall, holding the fists, raising one foot forwards; then stirring the mouth, enriching fluid and humor in the mouth, imagining to take Qi into the navel and the feet. Such a static exercise can replenish the essence, nourish the spirit and tonify the brain.

上清黄庭内景经【shàng qīng huáng tíng nèi jǐng jīng】　《上清黄庭内景经》为气功学专著，相传为太上老君所作，阐述气功修炼原理。

Shangqing Huangting Nei jing Jing（*Canon About Upper Clearity and Internal Essence of Imperial Palace*）　A monograph entitled *Canon About Upper Clearity and Internal Essence of Imperial Palace*, legendarily compiled by the Lord Lao Zi, mainly describing the principles of Qigong practice.

上清黄庭外景经【shàng qīng huáng tíng wài jǐng jīng】　《上清黄庭外景经》为气功学专著，世传为东晋魏华存所传，强调"黄庭"为人身根本，修炼时须精至黄庭，神入黄庭，气归黄庭。精、气、神固守于黄庭则病邪自出。

Shangqing Huangting Waijing Jing（*External Scene About the Root of Body in Qigong Practice*）　A monograph of Qigong entitled *External Scene About the Root of Body in Qigong Practice*, written by Wei Huacun in the East Jin Dynasty（217 AD - 420 AD）, emphasizing Huangting（the region below the

S

navel) as the root of the body, suggesting to enter the essence, the spirit and Qi into Huangting (the region below the navel) in practicing Qigong. Only when the essence, Qi and the spirit are kept in Huangting (the region below the navel) can pathogenic factors be expelled.

上清气秘法【shàng qīng qì mì fǎ**】**为静功,方法多样。其作法以夜半子时、寅时为好。服食五脏真气,可延年益寿。**secret method for raising clear Qi** A static exercise with various methods. Practice of Qigong is usually done in Zi (the period of a day from 11 p. m. to 1 a. m.) and Yin (the period of a day from 3 a. m. to 5 a. m. in the morning) for taking the genuine Qi in the five Zang-organs (including the heart, the liver, the spleen, the lung and the kidney) in order to prolong life.

上清司命茅君修行指迷诀 【shàng qīng sī mìng máo jūn xiū xíng zhǐ mí jué**】**《上清司命茅君修行指迷诀》为气功专著,作者不详。**Shangqing Siming Maojun Xiuxing Zhimi Jue** (*Essentials for Sincere Gentlemen to Practice Qigong*) A monograph of Qigong entitled *Essentials for Sincere Gentlemen to Practice Qigong*. The author was unknown.

上清太玄九阳图 【shàng qīng tài xuán jiǔ yáng tú**】**《上清太玄九阳图》为气功学专著,由宋代俟善渊所撰,总结分析了气功的理论和方法。**Shangqing Taixuan Jiuyang Tu** (*Pictures About Upper Clearity and Nine Celestial Yang*) A monograph of Qigong entitled *Pictures About Upper Clearity and Nine Celestial Yang*, written by Si Sh-

anyuan in the Song Dynasty (960 AD - 1279 AD), mainly concluding and analyzing the basic theory and practice of Qigong.

上清握中诀【shàng qīng wò zhōng jué**】**《上清握中诀》为气功专著,成书于南北朝时期,阐述气功的基本理论、方法和功效。作者不详。**Shangqing Wozhong Jue** (*Discussion About Clearing the Upper and Controlling the Middle*) A monograph entitled *Discussion About Clearing the Upper and Controlling the Middle*, compiled in the Northern and Southern Dynasties (420 AD - 589 AD), describing the basic theory, practice and effects of Qigong. The author was unknown.

上清无英真童合游内变玉经【shàng qīng wú yīng zhēn tóng hé yóu nèi biàn yù jīng**】**《上清无英真童合游内变玉经》为气功专著,作者不详。该书以心目内视,精魂交接,上通日月之光,内想外来神气,密会神招,气接日月融光,丹田自生之英玉。**Shangqing Wuying Zhentong Heyou Neibian Yujing** (*Essential Canon About Communication Between the Internal and External, Spirit and Essence*) A monograph of Qigong entitled *Essential Canon About Communication Between the Internal and External, Spirit and Essence*, mainly describing internal view of the heart, combination of the essence and ethereal soul, communicating with the sunshine and the moonshine, imagining to breathe in external spiritual Qi, silently beckoning the spirit, connecting Qi with the sunshine and the moonshine, and producing great jade in Dantian. The author was unknown. Dantian is divided into the upper Dantian (the region between the eyes), the middle Dantian (the region below the heart) and the lower Dantian (the region below the navel).

上鹊桥下鹊桥【shàng què qiáo xià què qiáo】 指练功时,舌舐上腭,有沟通阴阳之作用。

upper bridge of magpies and lower bridge of magpies Refers to the tongue raising at the palate in order to coordinate Yin and Yang.

上天关【shàng tiān guān】 指上丹田。

upper celestial col Refers to the upper Dantian (the region between the eyes).

上天梯【shàng tiān tī】 指脊髓,也指督脉。

upper high ladder Refers to the spinal cord and governor meridian.

上土釜【shàng tǔ fǔ】 指上丹田。

upper cauldron Refers to the upper Dantian (the region between the eyes).

上脘【shàng wǎn】 任脉中的一个穴位,位于脐上 5 寸。这一穴位为气功运行的一个常见部位,为气功常用意守部位。

Shangwan (**CV 13**) An acupoint in the conception meridian, located five Cun above the navel. This acupoint is a region usually used in practice of Qigong.

上弦下弦【shàng xián xià xián】 上弦指初七、初八日之月象,下弦指二十二、二十三日之月象。

upper and lower quarters The upper quarter refers to phase of the moon in the seventh day and the eighth day in any month; and the over quarter refers to the phase of the moon in twenty-second day and twenty-third day in any month.

上星【shàng xīng】 督脉中的一个穴位,位于头正中线,入前发际 1 寸,为气功常用意守部位。

Shangxing (**GV 23**) An acupoint in the governor meridian, located in the midline of the head, about 1 Cun to the anterior hairline. This acupoint is a region usually used in practice of Qigong.

上虚下实【shàng xū xià shí】 上指心,下指腹;指病理状况,即正气虚于上邪气虚于下的证候。

upper deficiency and lower excess Refers to the heart in the upper and the abdomen in the lower. It also refers to pathological condition, indicating deficiency of healthy Qi in the upper and excess of pathogenic Qi in the lower.

上阳子【shàng yáng zǐ】 元代气功学家陈致虚的另外一个称谓,其撰写了多部气功专著,对后世气功学的发展有较大的贡献。

Shang Yangzi Another name of Chen Zhixu, a great master of Qigong in the Yuan Dynasty (1271 AD – 1368 AD) who wrote several monographs of Qigong, making certain contribution to the development of Qigong in the later generations.

上阳子金丹大要【shàng yáng zǐ jīn dān dà yào】《上阳子金丹大要》为气功学专著,由陈致虚所撰,阐述了气功的基本理论和方法,说明了具体习练的原则和要求。

Shangyang Zi Jindan Dayao (***Shangyangzi's Gist About Golden Dan***) A monograph of Qigong entitled *Shangyangzi's Gist About Golden Dan* (*Pills of Immortality*), written by Chen Zhixu, describing the basic theory and exercises of Qigong, introducing

S

the principles and requirements of Qigong practice.

上阳子金丹大要图【shàng yáng zǐ jīn dān dà yào tú】《上阳子金丹大要图》为气功专著,为陈致虚所著,介绍了十三种要图。

Shangyangzi Jindan Dayao Tu(*Pictures of Shangyangzi's Gist About Golden Dan*) A monograph of Qigong entitled *Pictures of Shangyangzi's Gist About Golden Dan*(*Pills of Immortality*), written by Chen Zhixu, introducing thirteen pictures about Qigong practice.

上药三品神与气精【shàng yào sān pǐn shén yǔ qì jīng】《上药三品神与气精》为气功专著,主要阐述精气神三者的关系。作者不详。

Shangyao Sanpin Shenyu Qijing(*Three Essential Medicinals With Spirit*, *Qi and Essence*) A monograph of Qigong entitled *Three Essential Medicinals With Spirit*, *Qi and Essence*, mainly describing the relation between essence, Qi and spirit. The author was unknown.

上元六合之府【shàng yuán liù hé zhī fǔ】 指眉后小穴。

upper primordial mansion among the six directions Refers to a small acupoint behind the eyes.

上致明霞日烟里【shàng zhì míng xiá rì yān lǐ】 指肾气充足,耳目聪明,阴阳平秘,形体健康。

increasing and enriching in the sun rays and the sun mist Refers enrichment of kidney Qi, brightness of the eyesight, balance of Yin and Yang and cultivation of the body.

上杼【shàng zhù】 大椎的一个别名,

是督脉的一个穴位,位于后正中线,第七颈椎棘突下凹陷中。为气功学重要体表标志之一。此穴位为气功习练之处。

Shangzhu A synonym of Dazhui(GV 14), an acupoint in the governor meridian, located in the back midline and in the depression of spinous process in the seventh cervical vertebra, which is the important symbol in Qigong. This acupoint is a region usually used in practice of Qigong.

烧丹【shāo dān】 指神运精气至丹田,一意不散。

burning Dan(**pills of immortality**) Means that the spirit moves the essential Qi to Dantian without any change. Dantian is divided into the upper Dantian(the region between the eyes), the middle Dantian(the region below the heart) and the lower Dantian(the region below the navel).

少思寡欲【shǎo sī guǎ yù】 指习练气功养生法,平素应提高自制力,减少欲望,去掉私心,排除杂念。

less selfishness and little desire Refers to increasing self-control, decreasing desires, eliminating selfishness and relieving distracting thoughts in practicing Qigong.

少思虑养神【shǎo sī lù yǎng shén】 指思虑过度,神气暗耗。减少思虑,神不外驰即养神。

cultivation of the spirit without contemplation Refers to decreasing contemplation in order to avoid egression of the spirit in practicing Qigong.

少冲【shào chōng】 手少阴心经中的一个穴位,位于小指桡侧,为气功常用意守部位。

Shaochong(**HT 9**) An acupoint in the

heart meridian of hand Shaoyin, located in the radialis side of the little finger, which is a region usually used to keep essential Qi in practicing Qigong.

少火【shào huǒ】 指正常的、能充养人体元气的火,能维持人体生命活动的阳气。

normal fire Refers to either normal fire that can cultivate and enrich the original Qi; or Yang Qi that can maintain life activities.

少商【shào shāng】 手太阴肺经的一个穴位,位于拇指桡侧,为气功常用意守部位。

Shaoshang (LU 11) An acupoint in the lung meridian of hand Taiyin, located in the radialis side of the thumb, which is a region usually used to keep essential Qi in practicing Qigong.

少阳之阳【shào yáng zhī yáng】 指少阴经之阳络。

yang in Shaoyang Refers to Yang collaterals in Shaoyang meridian

少阴之阴【shào yīn zhī yīn】 指少阴经之阴络。

yin in Shaoyin Refers to Yin collaterals in Shaoyin meridian

少泽【shào zé】 手太阳小肠经中的一个穴位,位于小指尺侧,为气功常用意守部位。

Shaoze (SI 1) An acupoint in the small intestine meridian of hand Taiyang, located in the ulnar side of the little finger, which is a region usually used to keep essential Qi in practicing Qigong.

少年中年宜练功【shào nián zhōng nián yí liàn gōng】 源自气功专论,主要阐述少年练功根元完固,容易收效。

practice of Qigong in juvenile and midlife Collected from a monograph about

Qigong practice, mainly describing the importance and effect of practicing Qigong in boyhood.

少女【shào nǚ】 指八卦中的兑卦。

young girl Refers to Dui Trigram in the Eight Trigrams.

舌功【shé gōng】 为动功,可灌溉增强五脏的功能。

tongue exercise A dynamic exercise for increasing the functions of the five Zang-organs (including the heart, the liver, the spleen, the lung and the kidney).

蛇行气【shé xíng qì】 为动功。其作法为,先曲身侧卧,再正身,复起坐,闭目随气之所在,闭气不息,少食使肠通畅,咽气作为进食,舌舔出唾液作为水喝,起居适应四时变化,如春出冬藏,心神安静,恬淡虚无,不追求荣华富贵。

snake moving Qi A dynamic exercise, marked by bending the body and lying on one side first, then sitting upright, closing the eyes according to the flow of Qi, stopping respiration, abandoning to take food for dredging the intestines, inhaling Qi as taking food, licking saliva with the tongue as drinking water, following the climatic changes in the four seasons for getting up and sleeping like walking in spring and staying in winter, tranquilizing the heart and spirit, keeping the mind free from avarice and caring less about glory, splendor, wealth and rank.

舍【shě】 佛家气功习用语,指意识活动和平或平等的精神活动,神形维持相对稳定状态。

peace A common term of Qigong in Buddhism, referring to peaceful activity of consciousness or equal activity of the spirit as well as the stability of the spirit and body.

舍椤驮【shě luó tuó】 为静功。其作法为,结跏趺坐,明见是理,意识宽舒,无有疑虑,逐渐达到精神稳定。

exercise for rational trance A static exercise, marked by sitting in lotus position, defining the truth, clearing consciousness without any doubt and eventually stabilizing the spirit.

摄虎兵【shè hǔ bīng】 指胆神勇壮,力能摄虎御兵。

controlling tiger and withstanding solider Indicates that the gallbladder spirit is courageous and strong and can control the tiger and withstand any solider.

摄魂法【shè hún fǎ】 为静功。其作法为,仰卧,去枕,伸足,交手于心上,瞑目,闭气三息,叩齿三边。

exercise for controlling the ethereal soul A static exercise, marked by lying on the back without a pillow, stretching the feet, crossing the hands over the heart, closing the eyes, stopping breathing for three times and clicking the teeth for three ways.

摄魂还魄【shè hún huán pò】 指调整肝肺功能,使其相互作用,维持稳定状态。摄指肝,魄指肺。

controlling the ethereal soul and stabilizing the corporeal soul Refers to the functions of the liver and the lung for keeping the effects and stability of these two organs. In this term, the Chinese characters She (controlling) refers to the liver and Huan (stabilizing) refers to the lung.

摄境从心【shè jìng cóng xīn】 佛家气功习用语,指统摄各种情志而从归于脑神。此为气功中的一种守神方法。

controlling the state to enter the heart A common term of Qigong in Budhism, referring to controlling various emotions and keeping them in the brain spirit. This is a way to keep the spirit in Qigong.

摄三归一【shè sān guī yī】 三指精、气、神;摄精、气、神而为一,可炼成丹。

integration of three and one Refers to integration of essence, Qi and spirit into one for refining Dan (pills of immortality) in practice of Qigong.

摄生服气法【shè shēng fú qì fǎ】 为静功。其作法为,常以生气时(从夜半至日中为生气),正仰卧,瞑目握固,闭气不息于心中,默数至二百,乃口吐气出之,并日增息其数。久行之,神形和调,五脏安和,耳目聪明,举身无病。

exercise for improving life and taking Qi A static exercise, marked by lying on the back from midnight to the noon, closing the eyes, holding the body, silently stopping respiration in the heart for two hundred times, then exhaling it through the mouth and increasing the times. After a long period of practice, the spirit and body will be regulated, the five Zang-organs (including the heart, the liver, the spleen, the lung and the kidney) will be stabilized, the ears and eyes will be improved and the body will be healthy without any disease.

摄生和气法【shè shēng hé qì fǎ】 为静功。其作法为,端坐安稳身体,调和呼吸,无与意争,若不安和即止,调和后再作。久行此法,五脏安而气和,饮食美,百病去,身体轻健。

exercise for improving life and harmoni-

zing Qi A static exercise, marked by sitting upright, stabilizing the body, regulating respiration and avoiding any mental struggle. If the mind is not stable, practice should be stopped and measures should be taken to regulate emotion and tranquilize the mind. After a long period of practice, the five Zang-organs (including the heart, the liver, the spleen, the lung and the kidney) will be stabilized, Qi will be harmonized, diet will be delicious, all diseases will be cured and the body will be cultivated.

摄生集览【shè shēng jí lǎn】《摄生集览》为气功养生专著，论述养生、惜气、堤疾。作者不详。

Shesheng Jilan(*Collection and View of Regimen*)　A monograph of Qigong and life cultivation entitled *Collection and View of Regimen*, describing cultivating life, keeping Qi and nourishing health. The author was unknown.

摄生炼气法【shè shēng liàn qì fǎ】为静功。其作法为，仰卧，徐漱玉泉而咽之，因行气，口但吐气，鼻但吸气，连作三百零六息。

exercise for improving life and refining Qi A static exercise, marked by lying on the back, mildly rinsing saliva and swallowing, moving Qi, exhaling Qi and inhaling Qi through the nose altogether for three hundreds and six times.

摄生三要【shè shēng sān yào】《摄生三要》为气功养生专著，由明代袁坤仪所著，主要论述了气功养生的三个主要方面，即聚精、养气、存神，以及三者之间的相互关系。

Shesheng Sanyao(*Three Essentials for Regimen*)　A monograph of Qigong and life cultivation entitled *Three Essentials for Regimen*, written by Yuan Kunyi in the Ming Dynasty (1368 AD - 1644 AD), mainly describing the three important aspects of Qigong and life cultivation. The three aspects refer to concentration of the essence, cultivation of Qi and stability of the spirit with their interrelations.

摄生消息论【shè shēng xiāo xī lùn】《摄生消息论》为气功学专著，由元代丘处机所著，提倡叩齿、咽津、摩眼等功法，可以延年益寿。

Shesheng Xiaoxi Lun(*Discussion about Improving Life and Regulating Respiration*)　A monograph of Qigong entitled *Discussion about Improving Life and Regulating Respiration*, written by Qiu Chuji in the Yuan Dynasty (1271 AD - 1368 AD), suggesting the exercises of clicking the teeth, swallowing fluid and kneading the eyes for prolonging life and cultivating health.

摄生要录【shè shēng yào lù】《摄生要录》为气功养生专著，由明代沈士著，论述了喜怒哀乐，也阐述了气功理论和方法。

Shesheng Yaolu(*Collection of the Importance of Regimen*)　A monograph of Qigong and life cultivation entitled *Three Essentials for Regimen*, written by Shen Shi in the Ming Dynasty (1368 AD - 1644 AD), discussing various pleasure, anger, sorrow and joy, also describing the theory and practice of Qigong.

摄生纂录【shè shēng zuǎn lù】《摄生纂录》为气功学专著，收录了气功学的基本理论和方法，作者不详。

Shesheng Zuanlu（*Compilation and Collection of Regimen*） A monograph of Qigong entitled *Compilation and Collection of Regimen*，introducing the basic theory and practice of Qigong. The author was unknown.

摄生纂要二十八条【shè shēng zuǎn yào èr shí bā tiáo】 源自气功学专论，主要阐述气功养神炼气及饮食调理之道。

twenty-eight sections for improving life and compiling importance Collected from a monograph of Qigong, mainly describing the ways to nourish the spirit, to refine Qi and to take food in practicing Qigong.

摄心至要【shè xīn zhì yào】 指意念与呼吸相依，是气功调神的关键。

key to regulating the heart Refers to interdependence of consciousness and respiration，which is the key to regulation of the spirit.

摄志褫情【shè zhì chǐ qíng】 即行功中应内守精神（摄志），排除杂念（褫情）。

controlling will and eliminating emotion Refers to concentrating the spirit and eliminating distracting thought.

申天师服气要诀【shēn tiān shī fú qì yào jué】 为静功。半夜之后，睡后以水漱口，仰卧伸手足。徐徐吐气一二十度，候谷气消尽，心静定。

immortal exercise for taking Qi A static exercise，marked by washing the mouth with water after waking up at midnight，lying on the back，stretching the hands and feet，normally exhaling for one to twenty degrees in order to relieve Guqi (gastric Qi or cereal Qi) and to tranquilize the heart.

伸宦【shēn huàn】 指为追逐名利而产生的精神负担，乃气功之大忌。伸，言屈伸之情；宦，言名利之争。

extending eunuch Refers to mental burden due to seeking distinction，which is taboo in practicing Qigong. In this term，extending means emotion of submission and eunuch means dispute of fame and wealth.

身宝【shēn bǎo】 指精与神为人体之宝。

body treasure Refers to the essence and the spirit as the treasure of human body.

身病【shēn bìng】 指由身心保养失宜，散失元气，耗散其气所致。

body disease Caused by failure to cultivate health and dispersion of original Qi and other kinds of Qi.

身不动而心自安，心不动而神自守【shēn bù dòng ér xīn zì ān xīn bù dòng ér shén zì shǒu】 指练功中要身体舒适安静，身静则心安，心安则神守。

Tranquility of the body ensures comfort of the heart，quietness of the heart ensures protection of the spirit. Refers to comforting and tranquilizing the body in practicing Qigong. Only when the body is tranquilized can the heart is stable and only when the heart is stabilized can the spirit be protected.

身城【shēn chéng】 指人之形体是精、气、神的城郭。

body city Means that the human body is the manor of the essence，Qi and the spirit.

身功【shēn gōng】 为静功。其作法为，盘足坐，以一足跟抵住肾囊根下，令精气无漏。

body exercise A static exercise，marked by sitting with crossed legs and holding the scrotum with a foot to prevent leakage of essential Qi.

身解【shēn jiě**】**　指气功中的斋戒、安处、存想和坐忘。斋戒称信解,安处称闲解,存想称慧解,坐忘称定解。

body freedom　Refers to fast, tranquility, contemplation and quiet sitting. Fast means sincerity, tranquility means leisure, contemplation means wisdom and quiet sitting means stability.

身空【shēn kōng**】**　指习练气功,返观内照,形体与意念融为一体,而入无人、无我境界谓之身空。

body vacuum　Refers to retrospection and internal observation in practicing Qigong, indicating integration of the body and the mind. In practice of Qigong, arrival into the state without other people and oneself means vacuum.

身门【shēn mén**】**　指耳、目、口为身之门。

body gate　Refers to the ears, the eyes and the mouth.

身全【shēn quán**】**　指神形合一,身体健康。

entirety of body　Refers to integration of the body and the spirit and cultivation of health.

身室【shēn shì**】**　指气穴。

body chamber　Refers to Qixue (the region below the navel).

身堂【shēn táng**】**　指心。

body hall　Refers to the heart.

身心混沌【shēn xīn hùn dùn**】**　指精神形体,浑然一体,统一协调。混沌为不分解的状态。

inseparability of the body and the heart　Refers to integration of the spirit and body that have never separated from each other.

身中午时【shēn zhōng wǔ shí**】**　即身中一阴产生之时,谓身中午时。

yin generation in the body　Refers to the time that a kind of Yin begins to appear in the body.

深禅定乐【shēn chán dìng lè**】**　佛家气功功法。其作法为,端身正坐,远离世俗喜妙乐,意想神形和合的"纯一妙乐"。

deep dhyana and fixed happiness　The exercise of Qigong in Buddhism, marked by sitting upright, keeping far away from secular happiness, and imagining to integrate the spirit and body as the pure joy.

深根固柢【shēn gēn gù dǐ**】**　指补脑安神,敛肺益气。

deep root and fixed foundation　Refers to tonifying the brain and stabilizing the spirit, astringing the lung and promoting Qi.

深深息【shēn shēn xī**】**　指深长的呼吸。

deep respiration　Refers to deep and long breath.

神【shén**】**　指脑精深细微的物质结构及脑意识思维活动。

spirit　Refers to the profound structure of the brain and the activities of consciousness and thinking in the brain.

神安气宽【shén ān qì kuān**】**　指习练气功,安神而呼吸平和。

stable spirit and spacious Qi　Refers to stabilizing the spirit and balancing respiration in practicing Qigong.

神必清【shén bì qīng**】**　指习练气功,精神意识活动宜清朗、有序、明敏、自然。

spirit requiring purification　Indicates that the activities of the spirit and consciousness should be clear, procedural,

S

bright，quick and natural in practicing Qigong.

神长三寸衣玄黄【shén cháng sān cùn yī xuán huáng】 指脑神的长度、色泽并具阴神、阳神之象。

When the spirit grows three Cun, it will become supreme and yellow. Indicates that the length and color of the spirit in the brain reflect the manifestations of Yin spirit and Yang spirit.

神朝【shén cháo】 指精神的指向和集中。

spiritual direction Refers to the direction and concentration of the spirit.

神驰【shén chí】 指精神意识向外驰散。

spiritual gallop Refers to external dispersion of the spirit and consciousness.

神丹【shén dān】 ① 指气功养生法；② 指金丹，为五金八石烧炼而成。

Spiritual Dan（pills of immortality） Refers to ① either the methods for cultivating life in Qigong；② or golden Dan（pills of immortality）produced by burning five kinds of gold and eight kinds of stones.

神道【shén dào】 ① 指自然变化规律；② 指气功养生法。

spiritual way Refers to ① either principles of natural changes；② or exercises of Qigong and life cultivation.

神动【shén dòng】 指重阳之人，识神情欲躁动，不安其居而外出。

spiritual activity Refers to a person with dysphoria who only paid great attention to Yang, disliking his residence and going to other places.

神盖【shén gài】 指眉。

spiritual lid Refers to the brows.

神根【shén gēn】 指精神意识思维活

动之根，即性，为人的自然本性。

spiritual root Refers to the root of the activities of the spirit，consciousness and thinking, which is human nature.

神功【shén gōng】 ① 指调神为主的功法；② 指神奇的功夫。

spiritual function Refers to ① either the function of regulating the spirit；② or magical skills.

神宫【shén gōng】 指神所居之宫。

spiritual palace Refers to the palace where the spirit is located.

神宫太室说【shén gōng tài shì shuō】 源自气功专论，阐述脑神的结构与五脏神的关系。

idea about spirit palace and supreme chamber Collected from a monograph of Qigong，describing the structure of the spirit in the brain and its relation with the spirit from the five Zang-organs（including the heart，the liver，the spleen，the lung and the kidney）.

神光【shén guāng】 ① 指精神；② 指两眼之精光；③ 指功法。

spiritual light Refers to ① either the spirit；② or the brightness of the eyes；③ or exercises of Qigong practice.

神光无上虚澄内景【shén guāng wú shàng xū chéng nèi jǐng】 为静功。其作法为，于夏历每月十八日在清净的室内坐定，入静后意想自己身在"月宫"之中，月光皎洁明亮，默念道家某一符咒九遍，咽津九口，叩齿九通。

supreme spiritual light in the internal state A static exercise，marked by sitting in a clear and quiet room on 18th in every month in summer，imagining to enter the moon palace with bright moonlight after tranquilization，silently reading a charm in the Daoism for nine times，swallowing fluid for nine times and clicking the teeth for nine times.

神归虚无【shén guī xū wú】　指精神意识活动归于寂寞稳定。

spiritual entrance of vacuum　Refers to silence and stability of the activities of the spirit and consciousness.

神归于毗卢性海【shén guī yú pí lú xìng hǎi】　指习练气功，炼神还虚时，神归于脑中泥丸。

The spirit belongs to genuine sea in Bharhut.　Indicates that the spirit belongs to the mud bolus（brain）in the brain in practicing Qigong.

神和【shén hé】　指精神意识活动喜欢平和稳定。

spiritual harmony　Refers to liking harmony and stability in the activities of the spirit and consciousness.

神化【shén huà】　指神妙的变化。

spirit transformation　Refers to mystical changes.

神机【shén jī】　根源于事物内部的生命活动表现和机转，有如神之发机。

mysterious mechanism　Refers to the activity，manifestation and changes of life from the internal region，like the transformation of the spirit.

神即形【shén jí xíng】　指神为形的细微结构，神是形体的一部分。

The spirit as the body.　Indicates that the spirit is the subtle structure of the body and is part of the body.

神迹【shén jì】　指气功后出现的功能变化。

mysterious manifestation　Refers to the special function after practicing Qigong.

神解【shén jiě】　指调节精神，提高智慧，稳定神形，达到气功的理想境界。

spiritual explanation　Refers to regulating the spirit，increasing wisdom，stabilizing the spirit and body and reaching the ideal state of Qigong.

神经【shén jīng】　指气功学中意识、思维活动所经过的道路。

spiritual path　Refers to the ways along which the activities of consciousness and thinking move in Qigong.

神精【shén jīng】　指神中之精。

spiritual essence　Refers to essence in the spirit.

神精还归【shén jīng huán guī】　指神还身内，精归旧所，神形合一，老复丁壮。

integration of the spirit and essence　Indicates that the spirit enters the body，the essence returns to the original region，the spirit and the body integrate with each other in order to strengthen each other.

神境通【shén jìng tōng】　指习练气功出现的功能变化。

smooth state of the spirit　Refers to the special function in practicing Qigong.

神境智证通【shén jìng zhì zhèng tōng】　佛家气功习用语，指习练佛家气功，可以获得特异功能。

regulation of the spirit and wisdom at the ideal state　A term of Qigong，indicating that practice of Qigong in Buddhism can obtain special functions.

神居窍而千智生【shén jū qiào ér qiān zhì shēng】　指精神意识思维居脑窍之中，智慧生成，化育存焉。

When the spirit has occupied the orifice，thousands of wisdom are produced.　Indicates that when the spirit，consciousness and thinking are kept in the orifice of the brain，wisdom will be produced，and transformation and development

S

will be made.

神立【shén lì】 指神的主宰作用。

spiritual power Refers to the dominant function of the spirit.

神灵【shén líng】 指脑神明净,聪颖目敏;或指特殊功能。

spiritual soul Refers to either the brightness, tranquility and intelligence of the brain spirit; or special functions.

神灵至意【shén líng zhì yì】 指事物对立的双方,虽然相反,但有互相依赖。

interdependence of the spirit and con-sciousness Refers to things that oppose to each other but also depend on each other.

神卢【shén lú】 指脑及脑神。

spiritual chamber Refers to the brain and the brain spirit.

神门【shén mén】 手少阴心经中的一个穴位,位在腕横纹尺侧凹陷处。这一穴位为气功运行的一个常见部位。

Shenmen(HT 7) An acupoint in the heart meridian of hand Shaoyin, loca-ted at the ulnar end of the crease of the wrist and in the depression of the radial side of the tendon of the ulnar flexor, muscle of the wrist. This acupoint is a region usually used for keeping the es-sential Qi in practice of Qigong.

神灭论【shén miè lùn】 《神灭论》为气功学专著,由南北朝范缜缤所撰,阐述形神之间的关系,认为有形才有神。

Shenmie Lun(*Discussion of Spirit Ex-tinction*) A monograph of Qigong en-titled *Discussion of Spirit Extinction*, written by Fan Zhenbin in the South and North Dynasty(420 AD – 589 AD), describing the relation between the body and spirit, indicating that it is the body that produces the spirit.

神明【shén míng】 ① 指事物发生运动变化的内在力量;② 指精神意识思维活动;③ 指日月星辰;④ 指日神。

deities Refers to ① either the internal power of the movement and changes of anything; ② or the activities of the spirit, consciousness and thinking; ③ or the sun, the moon and the stars; ④ or the solar spirit.

神宁则气住【shén níng zé qì zhù】 即神气相合为一。

stabilized spirit keeping Qi Refers to integration of the spirit and Qi.

神凝【shén níng】 指神凝聚于脑而不散漫出身外。

concentration of the spirit Refers to concentrating the spirit in the brain without any external dispersion.

神气【shén qì】 ① 指精神、气魄;② 指自然之气;③ 指阴阳,神为阳,气为阴。

Spiritual Qi Refers to ① either the spirit and ambition; ② or natural Qi; ③ or Yin and Yang, in which the spirit refers to Yang while Qi refers to Yin.

神气和合说【shén qì hé hé shuō】 源自气功专论,主要阐述神气和合的方法。

idea about harmony of the spirit and Qi Collected from a monograph of Qigong, mainly describing the methods for harmonizing the spirit and Qi.

神气舍心【shén qì shě xīn】 指神气舍藏于心。

location of the spirit and Qi in the heart Indicates that it is the heart that stores the spirit.

神气是性命【shén qì shì xìng mìng】 源自气功专论,主要阐述炼内丹就是养气全神的道理。

The spirit and Qi are the foundation of

life. This sentence is collected from a monograph of Qigong, mainly describing the fact that refining the internal Dan (pills of immortality) is the total spirit for nourishing Qi.

神气同体精髓一源【shén qì tóng tǐ jīng suǐ yī yuán】 指"神"与"气","精"与"髓"的密切关系。

The spirit and Qi are of the same physique while the essence and marrow are of the same origin. Refers the close relation between the spirit and Qi as well as the essence and marrow.

神气相抱【shén qì xiāng bào】 指精神活动与机体功能相和谐。

mutual holding of the spirit and Qi Refers to balance between the spirit activity and the physiological functions.

神气养形论【shén qì yǎng xíng lùn】 《神气养形论》为气功学专著,说明神气养形的道理。作者不详。

Shenqi Yangxing Lun (*Discussion of Life Cultivation with the Spirit and Qi*) A monograph of Qigong entitled *Discussion of Life Cultivation with the Spirit and Qi*, describing the principles of the spirit and Qi for cultivating the body. The author was unknown.

神迁【shén qiān】 指妄念引起的精神失调。

spiritual disorder Refers to disorder of the spirit caused by distracting thought.

神清观【shén qīng guàn】 位于山东省,为宋代王重阳开烟霞洞处。

Shenqing Temple In the Shandong Province, where Wang Chongyang in the Song Dynasty (960 AD - 1279 AD) opened a cave for mist and clouds.

神去离形【shén qù lí xíng】 指精神意识活动从身体中消亡。

depletion of the spirit and abandonment of the body Refers to loss of the activities of the spirit and consciousness in the body.

神阙【shén què】 ① 任脉的一个经穴名;② 为人体部位名,即脐;③ 为气功意守部位。

Shenque Refers to ① either the acupoint of Shenque (CV 8) in the conception meridian; ② or the navel; ③ or the place where the consciousness is concentrated in practicing Qigong.

神人【shén rén】 ① 指古代气功学家;② 指行功时,意想出现的人像。

immortal Refers to ① either the masters of Qigong in ancient China; ② or the imagined figure in practicing Qigong.

神舍【shén shě】 即肺神居肺,心神居心,肝神居肝,肾神居肾。

spirit location Means that the lung spirit is located in the lung, the heart spirit is located in the heart, the liver spirit is located in the liver and the kidney spirit is located in the kidney.

神室【shén shì】 指身体中一室,为神所居之处,为内丹生成之处。

spiritual chamber Refers to a chamber of the spirit in the human body where the internal Dan (pills of immortality) is produced.

神守【shén shǒu】 ① 指神情专一,精神内守;② 指鳖。

spiritual concentration Refers to ① either integration of the spirit and emotion and internal concentration of the spirit; ② or turtle.

神术【shén shù】 指古代气功养生术。

spiritual technique Referring to the techniques for cultivating life in ancient

S

China.

神水【shén shuǐ】 ① 指唾液；② 指心之液。

spiritual water Refers to ① either saliva；② or humor in the heart.

神髓【shén suǐ】 指肾神及肾精。

spiritual marrow Refers to kidney spirit and kidney essence.

神体精【shén tǐ jīng】 指五脏、六腑实体与神用清澄、精通，是内丹成就的基础。

spirit manifesting essence Refers to the combination of the five Zang-organs (including the heart, the liver, the spleen, the lung and the kidney) and the six Fu-organs (including the gallbladder, the stomach, the small intestine, the large intestine, the bladder and the triple energizer) with the spirit, which is the foundation for producing the internal Dan (pills of immortality).

神庭【shén tíng】 督脉中的一个穴位，位于头正中线，如前发际 0.5 寸。也指面。这一穴位为气功运行的一个常见部位。

Shenting（**GV 24**） An acupoint in the governor meridian, located in the middle line of the head, 0.5 Cun before hairline. This acupoint is a region usually used for keeping the essential Qi in practice of Qigong.

神通【shén tōng】 指神妙通达。

spiritual opening Refers to marvelous understanding.

神息【shén xī】 指文火安神定息，任其自如。

spiritual respiration Refers to mild fire that stabilizes the spirit and concentrates breath naturally.

神息任天然【shén xī rèn tiān rán】 指神息合于一而任其自然，或谓真意与真息相依。

natural condition of the spirit and respiration Refers to either integration of the spirit and respiration that are acting naturally; or dependence between genuine consciousness and genuine respiration.

神仙【shén xiān】 ① 指习练气功的人；② 指应用气功养生，并且气度不凡，神采清丽洒脱者。

immortal Refers to ① either the practitioners of Qigong; ② or application of Qigong and life cultivation with laudable spirit.

神仙传【shén xiān zhuàn】《神仙传》由东晋葛洪撰，叙述古代传说中的八十四位仙人的事迹。

Shenxian Chuan（*Legend of Immortal*） A book entitled *Legend of Immortal*, written by Ge Hong in the East Jin Dynasty（317 AD - 420 AD）, describing the stories of eighty-four immortals in ancient China.

神仙大药【shén xiān dà yào】 泛指气功。

spiritual large medicinal Usually refers to Qigong.

神仙绝谷炼气法【shén xiān jué gǔ liàn qì fǎ】 为静功。其作法为，安身和体，选择舒适的体位，心无杂念，戒忿怒愁忧，然后仰卧，先缓缓嗽口中津液，并下咽，以鼻微微纳气，徐引之，莫令大极满。

immortal's exercise of stopping diet for refining Qi A static exercise, marked by stabilizing the body, selecting a suitable room, eliminating distracting thought, avoiding any annoyance and anxiety，then lying on the back，mildly rinsing the mouth and swallowing fluid and humor，slowly inhaling Qi through the nose for normal cultivation of the body.

神仙绝谷十二时食气法【shén xiān jué gǔ shí èr shí shí qì fǎ】为静功。其作法为,食气始于夜半,八十一咽;日出,三十六咽;日中,八十二咽;日入,三十六咽;鸡鸣,六十四咽;食时,二十五咽;日昳,六十四咽;黄昏,二十五咽;平旦,四十九咽;禺中,十六咽;哺时,四十九咽;人定,十六咽。

immortal's exercise for stopping diet and inhaling Qi for twelve hours A static exercise，marked by inhaling Qi at midnight，swallowing for eighty-one times；at sunrise，swallowing for thirty-six times；at noon，swallowing for eighty-two times；at sunset，swallowing for thirty-six times；at the time of crow，swallowing for sixty-four times；at the time of taking food，swallowing twenty-five times；at late afternoon，swallowing for sixty-four times；at dusk，swallowing twenty-five times；at dawn，swallowing forty-nine times；at the time near noon，swallowing sixteen times；at night，swallowing for forty-nine times；at the time when all people are sleeping，swallowing for sixteen times.

神仙绝谷食气法【shén xiān jué gǔ shí qì fǎ】为静功。其作法为,常以春二月、三月,九日、十八日、二十七日,起室于山林之中隐静处,近甘泉东流水,向阳之地。香汤沐浴,精念玉房(乳房),内视中丹田,纳气致之于下丹田,又先去鼻中毛,偃卧两足,相去五寸,两臂去身亦五寸。可调和阴阳,增强体质,除体内浊气。

immortal's exercise for stopping diet and inhaling Qi A static exercise，marked by staying in the room in the quiet and secluded mountain near sweet spring on the 9th，18th and 27th in February and March，bathing with scented water with imagination of the jade room (breast)，internally observing the middle Dantian (the region below the heart) and inhaling Qi into the lower Dantian (the region below the navel)，cutting hair in the nose，lying supine with 5 Cun between two feet and 5 Cun between the shoulders and body. Such a static exercise can regulate Yin and yang，strengthen the body and eliminate turbid Qi.

神仙绝谷食五行气法【shén xiān jué gǔ shí wǔ xíng qì fǎ】为静功。其作法为,服食东方青牙,饮以朝华,祝已,舌撩上齿表舐唇,漱口咽之三,以养肝;服食南方朱丹,饮以丹池,祝已,舌撩下齿表,漱口咽之三,以养心;服食西方明石,饮以灵液,祝已,琢齿七,漱口咽之三,以养肺;服食北方元滋,饮以玉饴,祝已,以鼻纳气而咽之三,以养肾;服食中央精气,饮以醴泉,祝已,眩目而咽之三,以养脾。食五行气,内附五脏。

immortal's exercise for stopping diet and inhaling Qi from five directions A static exercise，marked by taking tender shoot from the east，drinking flower blooming in the morning，blessing baby，lifting the tongue to the teeth to lick the lips，rinsing the mouth and swallowing for three times for nourishing the liver；taking red Dan (pills of immortality) from the south，drinking water from Danchi (pool with pills of immortality), lowering the tongue to the inferior teeth, rinsing the mouth and swallowing three times for nourishing the heart; taking bright stone from the west, drinking spiritual humor, blessing baby, clicking the teeth for seven times, rinsing the mouth and swallowing for three times for nourishing the lung; taking the food with original taste from the north, drinking pure sugar, blessing baby, inhaling Qi through the nose and swallowing for three times for nourishing the kidney; taking essential Qi from the center, drinking sweet spring water, blessing baby, closing the eyes and swallowing three times for nourishing the spleen; taking Qi from the five directions connected with the five Zang-organs (including the heart, the liver, the spleen, the lung and the kidney).

神仙起居法【shén xiān qǐ jū fǎ**】** 为动功。其作法为，"行住坐卧处，手摩腹与肚。心腹通快时，两手肠下踞。踞之彻彻膀腰，背拳摩肾部"。

immortal's exercise for daily life A dynamic exercise, marked by "rubbing the abdomen with the hands in the walking, staying, sitting and lying place, lowering the hands to the intestines when the heart and abdomen are clear, squatting with stretched waist and spine, and rubbing the back and kidney region with the fists".

神仙日用导引法【shén xiān rì yòng dǎo yǐn fǎ**】** 动静相兼功。其作法为，每日凌晨或五更初(可不拘早晚)，调神，澄心静虑，握固存神，端坐，屏绝缘务，寂无思念，想身于无身之中，存心于无为之境，便叩齿七通，咽液七数，咽时每度想液直下至丹田。其功效为筋软骨壮气和，有疾除疾，无疾爽神，消食止饥，除身中疾。

immortal's daily exercise of Daoyin An exercise combined with dynamic exercise and static exercise, marked by regulating the spirit in the early morning or at any time, stabilizing the heart, tranquilizing the mind, concentrating the spirit, sitting upright, avoiding any contemplation, thinking the body in the state without the body, keeping the heart in the inactivity state, clicking the teeth for seven times, swallowing saliva for seven times and imagining to swallow saliva into Dantian. Dantian is divided into the upper Dantian (the region between the eyes), the middle Dantian (the region below the heart) and the lower Dantian (the region below the navel). Such an exercise combined with dynamic exercise and static exercise can relax the sinews, strengthen the bones, harmonize Qi, eliminate disease, straighten the spirit if there is no disease, digest food, reduce hunger and expel any disorders in the body.

神仙食气辟谷法【shén xiān shí qì bì gǔ fǎ**】** 为静功。其作法为，先合口引，纳气咽之，满三百六十已上，不得减。多咽益善，咽至千为好。咽而食，日减一餐，十日后能不食。

immortal's exercise for taking Qi and stopping diet A static exercise, marked by closing the mouth first, inhaling Qi and swallowing it for three hundred and sixty times without any reduction, swallowing Qi for thousands of times, reducing one meal each day and stopping taking food after ten days.

神仙食气金匮妙录【shén xiān shí qì jīn kuì miào lù】《神仙食气金匮妙录》为气功养生专著,阐述了辟谷法、行气法、治病法等。作者不详。

Shenxian Shiqi Jingui Miaolu(*Secret Records of Immortal's Taking Qi from Golden Chamber*) A monograph of Qigong and life cultivation entitled *Secret Records of Immortal's Taking Qi from Golden Chamber*, describing the exercises for inedia, moving Qi and curing diseases. The author was unknown.

神形相涵【shén xíng xiāng hán】 指习练气功进入理想境界,神形相互涵育,和调而有固密。

mutual promotion between the spirit and body Indicates that practicing of Qigong reaches the ideal state, during which the spirit and body promote, balance and straighten each other.

神仙行气法【shén xiān xíng qì fǎ】为静功。其作法为,正偃卧,两手握固,两足相去四五寸,两臂距身四五寸,去枕,调节呼吸,三百六十息。

immortal's exercise for moving Qi A static exercise, marked by lying supine, holding both hands, keeping 4 to 5 Cun distance between the feet, keeping the shoulders 4 to 5 Cun toward the body, removing pillow, regulating respiration for three hundred and sixty times.

神仙行气服气法【shén xiān xíng qì fú qì fǎ】 为静功。其作法为,选择清静密室,闭户安床,暖厚席褥。枕高二寸半,方与身平。正偃卧,瞑目闭气,自止于胸膈。以鸿毛放鼻上,毛不动,经三百息。无所闻,目无所视,心无所思,当渐除之。

exercise for immortal moving Qi and re-spiring Qi A static exercise, marked by selecting a quiet and secret room, closing the gate, pacifying the bed, warming and deepening the mattress, keeping a pillow with two Cun height, lying supine, closing the eyes, stopping respiration in the chest and diaphragm, fixing a goose feather on the nose through three hundred periods of respiration, avoiding listening and seeing, and eliminating any ideas in the heart.

神隐书【shén yǐn shū】《神隐书》为气功养生专著,由明代臞仙所著,对精气神的理论阐述颇深,强调精气神对养生的重要性。

Shenyin Shu(*A Book about Hidden Spirit*) A monograph of Qigong and life cultivation entitled *A Book about Hidden Spirit*, written by Qu Xian in the Ming Dynasty(1368 AD – 1644 AD), describing the theory of essence, Qi and spirit, emphasizing the importance of essence, Qi and spirit for life cultivation.

神用形质【shén yòng xíng zhì】 指神是行之用、形之质。

spirit with body and quality Indicates that the spirit is the function of movement and the quality of the body.

神游【shén yóu】 指形体不动,神已动而外至其处。

spiritual travel Refers to immobility of the body and external movement of the spirit.

神与气【shén yǔ qì】 指身体内阴阳两个方面,即气功产药、作丹的基本物质。

Spirit and Qi Refers to Yin and Yang in the body, which is the basic substance for producing medicinal and Dan(pills of immortality)in practicing

S

Qigong.

神宰【shén zǎi】 指神主宰万物。

spiritual domination Indicates that the spirit controls all the things.

神脏【shén zàng】 指藏神的五脏,即心藏神,肝藏魂,脾藏意,肺藏魄,肾藏志。

spiritual viscera Refers to the five Zang-organs (including the heart, the liver, the spleen, the lung and the kidney) that store the spirit, such as the heart storing the spirit, the liver storing the ethereal soul, the spleen storing consciousness, the lung storing the corporeal soul and the kidney storing the will.

神宅【shén zhái】 ① 指脑为神宅; ② 指五脏为神宅; ③ 指全身各部均为神宅。

spiritual residence Refers to ① either the brain; ② or the five Zang-organs (including the heart, the liver, the spleen, the lung and the kidney); ③ or all parts of the body.

神者生之制【shén zhě shēng zhī zhì】 指气功中,神调节意识思维活动,能协调脏腑功能。

spirit controlling life Indicates that the spirit can regulate the activities of consciousness and thinking and coordinate the functions of the five Zang-organs (including the heart, the liver, the spleen, the lung and the kidney) and the six Fu-organs (including the gallbladder, the stomach, the small intestine, the large intestine, the bladder and the triple energizer) in practicing Qigong.

神智【shén zhì】 泛指精神智慧、意识、思维活动。

spiritual wisdom Refers to the activities of the spirit, wisdom, consciousness and thinking.

神自在身一往一来【shén zì zài shēn yì wǎng yì lái】 指脑神在身,发出信息,收回信息,往来不绝。

The spirit exists repeatedly inside the human body. Indicates that the brain spirit inside the body sends information and reclaims inform without any cease.

沈存中【shěn cún zhōng】 北宋科学家沈括的另外一个称谓。沈括不仅是北宋科学家,而且也精于气功养生学研究,与苏轼合著《苏沈良方》,其中论述气功养生法防治疾病,提倡闭息内视五脏,认为静坐专一即能成功。

Shen Cunzhong Another name of Shen Kuo, a great scientist in the North Song Dynasty (960 AD - 1127 AD). He was also proficient in studying Qigong and life cultivation. Shen Kuo was not only a great scientist in the North Song Dynasty (960 AD - 1127 AD), but also proficient in study of Qigong and life cultivation. He worked together with Su Shi, a great official, poet and master of Qigong in the Song Dynasty (960 AD - 1279 AD), to write a important monograph entitled Excellent Formulae of Su Shi and Shen Kuo, describing prevention and treatment of diseases by Qigong and life cultivation, suggesting to stopping respiration for observing the five Zang-organs (including the heart, the liver, the spleen, the lung and the kidney), holding that only quiet sitting can succeed the practice of Qigong.

沈芊绿【shěn gǎn lù】 清代中医学家沈金鳌的另外一个称谓,其精通气功养生,对后世医学气功的推广产生了一定的影响。

Shen Ganlu Another name of Shen Jin'ao, a scientist of traditional Chinese medicine in the Qing Dynasty（1636 AD‑1912 AD）. He was also proficient in studying Qigong and life cultivation, influencing the later generations in a certain extent.

沈金鳌【shěn jīn áo】 清代中医学家,精通气功养生,对后世医学气功的推广产生了一定的影响。

Shen Jin'ao A scientist of traditional Chinese medicine in the Qing Dynasty （1636 AD‑1912 AD）. He was also proficient in studying Qigong and life cultivation, influencing the later generations in a certain extent.

沈括【shěn kuò】 北宋科学家,精于气功养生学研究,与苏轼合著《苏沈良方》,其中论述气功养生法防治疾病,提倡闭息内视五脏,认为静坐专一即能成功。

Shen Kuo A great scientist in the North Song Dynasty（960 AD‑1127 AD）, proficient in study of Qigong and life cultivation. He worked together with Su Shi, a great official, poet and master of Qigong in the Song Dynasty （960 AD‑1279 AD）, to write a important monograph entitled Excellent Formulae of Su Shi and Shen Kuo, describing prevention and treatment of diseases by Qigong and life cultivation, suggesting to stopping respiration for observing the five Zang-organs（including the heart, the liver, the spleen, the lung and the kidney）, holding that only quiet sitting can succeed the practice of Qigong.

沈时誉聚精法【shěn shí yù jù jīng fǎ】

为功法,其作法为:"半夜子时即披衣起坐,两手搓极热,以一手将外肾兜住,以一手掩脐而凝神于内肾。久久习之而精旺也矣。"

exercise for renal essence invigoration A dynamic exercise, marked by getting up and sitting in Zi（the period of the day from 11 p.m. to 1 a.m. in the noon）at midnight, rubbing the hands warm, holding the external kidney with one hand, covering the navel with the other hand and concentrating the spirit in the internal kidney. After practice for a long time, the essence will be enriched.

审视瑶函【shěn shì yáo hán】 《审视瑶函》为中医眼科专著,兼论气功,由明代傅仁宇所著。

Shenshi Yaohan (*A Great Book about Examination of the Eyes*) A monograph of ophthalmology in traditional Chinese medicine entitled *A Great Book about Examination of the Eyes*, written by Fu Renyu in the Ming Dynasty（1368 AD‑1644 AD）. This monograph also describes the theory and practice of Qigong.

肾【shèn】 五脏之一,为元气生发之地。

kidney One of the five Zang-organs（including the heart, the liver, the spleen, the lung and the kidney）and is the foundation of the original Qi.

肾痹【shèn bì】 气功适应证,症见腰背偻曲不能伸、下肢挛曲、腰痛、遗精等。

kidney impediment An indication of Qigong, usually caused by difficulty to stretch the waist and back, twisted legs, lumbago and spermatorrhea.

肾病【shèn bìng】 气功适应证,泛指

S

肾脏发生的多种疾病。

kidney disease An indication of Qigong, referring to various diseases occurring in the kidney.

肾病导引【shèn bìng dǎo yǐn】 为动功,方法多样。如正面坐,双手从两耳左右上举,做三至五次。

exercise of Daoyin for kidney disease A dynamic exercise with various methods, such as sitting upright, raising the hands from the sides of the ears for three to five times.

肾病候导引法【shèn bìng hòu dǎo yǐn fǎ】 为动功。其作法为,无声用呬字出气。温肾纳气,治咽喉窒塞,腹满耳聋。两脚交叉而坐,用手握住脚腕部,头向后仰,尽力牵引,作七次。温阳散寒,治肾气壅塞。

exercise of Daoyin for kidney disease A dynamic exercise, marked by exhaling without any sound, warming the kidney and inhaling Qi in order to relieve throat stagnation, abdominal fullness and deafness; siting with crossed feet, holding the ankles with hands, turning the head backwards for seven times, warming Yang and expelling cold in order to cure stagnation of kidney Qi.

肾藏精【shèn cáng jīng】 指藏本脏之精,即先天之精;指五脏六腑之精,即后天之精。

kidney storing essence Refers to either storage of the kidney essence which is the innate essence; or essence of the five Zang-organs (including the heart, the liver, the spleen, the lung and the kidney) and the six Fu-organs (including the gallbladder, the stomach, the small intestine, the large intestine, the bladder and the triple energizer) which

is the postnatal essence.

肾功【shèn gōng】 为动功。其作法为,用手兜裹外肾两子,一手擦下丹田,左右换手,各八十一遍。

kidney exercise A dynamic exercise, marked by wrapping the external sides of the kidneys with one hand and rubbing the lower Dantian (the region below the navel) with the other hand and vice versa for eighty-one times respectively.

肾精导引法【shèn jīng dǎo yǐn fǎ】 为静功,作法为嘘吸偃仰,久则节欲养生,固护真元,早卧晚起,必待日光。

exercise of Daoyin for invigorating kidney essence A static exercise, marked by mild respiration without looking up. Such a way of practice will expel desires in order to cultivate life and to protect genuine origin. Practitioners should sleep early and get up late till the sun rises.

肾气【shèn qì】 指肾脏的功能活动,为肾精所化。肾气也是大横的一个别称,是足太阴脾经中的一个穴位,位于脐中旁开 3.5 寸处,为气功常用意守部位。

kidney Qi Refers to the functional activity of the kidney and the transformation of the kidney essence. Kidney Qi is also a synonym of Daheng (SP 15), which is an acupoint in the spleen meridian of foot Taiyin, located 3.5 Cun lateral to the navel. This acupoint is a region usually used in practice of Qigong.

肾神【shèn shén】 肾的物质精微结构和功能作用的聚合。位于肾,出于肾,藏之于肾。

kidney spirit Refers to the aggregation of the structure and function of nutrient substance, which is located in the kidney and starts from the kidney.

肾神去【shèn shén qù】　与七神去相同，指损伤五脏六腑的情况。肝神损伤于魂散失目不明，心神损伤于神散失唇见青白，肺神损伤于魄不在身鼻不通，肾神损伤于意出身外食不甘味，头神损伤于神出泥丸头目眩晕，腹神损伤于胃肠神散，四肢神损伤于骨关节重滞不动。

loss of kidney spirit　The same as loss of seven spirits, refers to different ways to damage the spirit from the five Zang-organs (including the heart, the liver, the spleen, the lung and the kidney) and the six Fu-organs (including the gallbladder, the stomach, the small intestine, the large intestine, the bladder and the triple energizer). The spirit in the liver is damaged by dispersion of the ethereal soul; the spirit in the heart is damaged by loss of the spirit and change of the lips; the spirit in the lung is damaged by dispersion of the corporeal soul and obstructed nose; the spirit in the kidney is damaged by no pure emotion and no good food; the spirit in the brain is damaged by dispersion of the spirit from the mud bolus (the brain) and dizziness; the spirit in the abdomen is damaged by dispersion of the spirit in the stomach and intestines; the spirit in the four limbs is damaged by stagnation of the joints.

肾为一体之宗【shèn wéi yì tǐ zhī zōng】　指肾中含有阴阳二气；指肾藏精，为生命的根本。

kidney as the origin of the body　Refers to the fact that the kidney contains Yin and Yang and that the kidney stores the essence and is the root of life.

肾阳【shèn yáng】　人体阳气的根本，对各脏腑有温煦和推动的作用。

kidney Yang　The origin of Yang Qi in the human body, which warms and promotes the five Zang-organs (including the heart, the liver, the spleen, the lung and the kidney) and the six Fu-organs (including the gallbladder, the stomach, the small intestine, the large intestine, the bladder and the triple energizer).

肾液【shèn yè】　指习练气功时通过含气漱口、叩齿所化生的津液。

kidney humor　Refers to fluid and humor produced by containing Qi, rinsing the mouth and clicking teeth in practicing Qigong.

肾阴【shèn yīn】　肾脏之精液是人体阴液的根本，对各脏腑起着濡润、滋养作用。

kidney Yin　The essential humor in the kidney, is the origin of Yin humor in the human body, which moistens and nourishes the five Zang-organs (including the heart, the liver, the spleen, the lung and the kidney) and the six Fu-organs (including the gallbladder, the stomach, the small intestine, the large intestine, the bladder and the triple energizer).

肾俞【shèn yú】　足太阳膀胱经的一个穴位，位于第二腰椎刺突下旁开1.5寸。这一穴位为气功运行的一个常见部位。

Shenshu（BL 23）　An acupoint in the bladder meridian of foot Taiyang, located 1.5 Cun lateral to the lower region of furcella in the second lumbar vertebra. This acupoint is a region usually used for keeping the essential Qi in practice of Qigong.

S

肾脏导引法【shèn zàng dǎo yǐn fǎ】为动功,即正坐,以两手上从耳左右引胁,三五度。

exercise of Daoyin for the kidney A dynamic exercise, marked by sitting upright, stretching the flanks with both hands rising towards the ears for three to five degrees.

肾脏修养法【shèn zàng xiū yǎng fǎ】为静功,常以十月、十一月、十二月,北面坐,鸣金梁,食饮玉泉三次后讫。

exercise for cultivating the kidney A static exercise, marked by sitting to the north side in October, November and December every year, sounding with golden beam and taking food three times in Yuquan (CV 3), which is an acupoint in the conception meridian.

肾着【shèn zhuó】 气功适应证,多由肾虚寒湿内着所致。

kidney stagnation An indication of Qigong, usually caused by kidney deficiency with coldness and dampness.

肾主骨【shèn zhǔ gǔ】 是因为肾主藏精,精生髓,髓充骨则健。

kidney governing bones Means that the kidney governs and stores essence, in which the essence produces marrow and the marrow enriches the bones. That is why the kidney governs the bones.

肾子【shèn zǐ】 即睾丸。习练气功时,可平坐,膝不可低,睾丸不可着在所坐处。

testis A special organ in the male body. In practicing Qigong, practitioners can sit quietly, avoiding to lower the knees and keep the testis over the sitting region.

肾子【shèn zǐ】 为睾丸的另外一个别称。

kidney seed A synonym of scrotum.

甚深法界【shèn shēn fǎ jiè】 为祖窍的异名,位于心与脐之正中。

deep region A synonym of Zuqiao, referring to the region between the heart and the navel.

胂【shèn】 ① 指夹脊肉,即骶棘肌;② 指髂嵴以下的肌肉,即臀大肌。

shen Refers to ① either sacrospinous muscle; ② or crest of ilium.

慎独【shèn dú】 指内守精神,审查自己的意识,排除杂念,以稳定情绪。

inner concentration Refers to concentrating the spirit inside the body, examining oneself consciousness, eliminating distracting thought and stabilizing emotion.

升观【shēng guān】 两眼上视泥丸之意。

ascending view Refers to the eyes observing the chamber of the mud bolus (the brain).

升观鬓不斑法【shēng guān bìn bù bān fǎ】 为静功。子午时,握固端坐,凝神绝念,两眼令光上视泥丸。

ascending view and blackening hair exercise A static exercise, marked by sitting quietly, concentrating the spirit, eliminating ideas and observing the mud bolus (the brain) with the brightness of the eyes.

升降【shēng jiàng】 指习练小周功法,由督脉上升,通三关,进阳火;自任脉下降,复返坤腹,退阴符。

ascent and descent Refers to the fact that the governor meridian ascends through three passes and enters Yang fire while the conception meridian descends and returns to the abdomen.

升降进退【shēng jiàng jìn tuì】 指人

体内阴阳二气的相互作用，运动变化，升
降浮沉。

**ascent and descent，entrance and re-
treat** Refers to interaction and changes of Yin Qi and Yang Qi in the body.

升明【shēng míng】 指火象夏气，其平
气上升而光明显露，使万物得繁华外露。

ascent with brightness Refers to normal Qi flowing upwards，appearing
brightness and enabling all things to develop prosperously.

升腾【shēng téng】 据载为古代气功，
通过锻炼，可以使身体轻灵飞腾。

rise up Refers to the body appearing
light and like flying through exercise
and practice of Qigong.

升天【shēng tiān】 即真气运行至
头部。

ascending to the sky Refers to genuine
Qi flowing to the top of the head.

生门【shēng mén】 指前七窍，也
指脐。

life gate Refers to either seven ori-
fices；or the navel.

生门死户【shēng mén sǐ hù】 指天地
之根，即脑。

life door Refers to the root of the sky
and the earth，indicating the brain in
Qigong.

生气【shēng qì】 ① 指自然之气；
② 指六阳为生气；③ 指人体的生命
活动。

life Qi Refers to ① either natural Qi；
② or six Yang；③ or life activities.

生气时【shēng qì shí】 指夜半子时，
一阳初生之时。

life Qi period Refers to midnight during which Yang begins to grow.

生气通天论【shēng qì tōng tiān lùn】
《黄帝内经·素问》的篇名。生气，指人

的生命活动。天，指自然界。主要讨论
人的生命活动与自然界的变化有着息息
相通的联系。

**discussion about life Qi communicating
with the sky** Life Qi refers to life activity and the sky refers to the natural
world. This chapter describes the close
relationship between life activity and
natural changes.

生身处【shēng shēn chù】 指丹田
或脐。

body origin Body origin refers to Dantian or navel. Dantian is divided into
upper Dantian（the region between the
eyes），the middle Dantian（the region
below the heart）and the lower Dantian
（the region below the navel）.

生死穴【shēng sǐ xué】 精气聚散常在
此处，水火发端也在此处，阴阳变化也在
此处，有无出入也在此处。

life and death acupoint Refers to the
region where the essential Qi concentrates and disperses there，water and
fire appear there，Yin and Yang
change there，exit and entrance exist
there.

生死在泥丸【shēng sǐ zài ní wán】
强调脑在气功锻炼中至关重要。

**Life and death are related to the mud bo-
lus（the brain）.** Emphasizes the importance of the brain in practicing
Qigong.

生在坤，种在乾【shēng zài kūn zhòng
zài qián】 源自气功专论。主要阐述下
丹田为生药之处，然后将此药搬运入脑，
加以锻炼。

life in Kun and origin in Qian Collected from a monograph about Qigong.
Kun refers to the earth and Qian refers
to the sky. It describes that medicine

S

for life is produced in the lower Dantian (the region below the navel) and transferred to the brain for Qigong practice.

省眠【shěng mián**】** 指道家气功习练中，要省眠，以免睡梦中神意驰走。

seldom sleeping Refers to sleeping less in practicing Qigong in order to prevent dispersion of the spirit and consciousness in sleeping.

圣度【shèng dù**】** 指圣人和调阴阳的法度。

sacred standard Refers to the moral standard, depending on which Shengren (sage) harmonized Yin and Yang.

圣济闭气法【shèng jì bì qì fǎ**】** 为静功。其作法为，以鼻微微引气纳之，数满于口中微吐之，如此再三，可长吐之，饥取食止。

sacred deep breathing exercise A static exercise, marked by mildly inhaling through the nose and mildly exhaling for three times or for a long time when the mouth is full without taking any food.

圣济闭气却病法【shèng jì bì qì què bìng fǎ**】** 为静功。其作法为，闭气之时，当苦体中满，发烦闭，以意推排，令气周布四肢，上至头中，遍行一身，意得之者，手足皆热常汗出。

exercise of sacred holding the breath for relieving disease A static exercise, marked by holding the breath, eliminating annoyance, promoting communication of all parts, spreading Qi to the four limbs, the head and the whole body in order to warm the hands and to increase sweating normally.

圣济导引按蹻【shèng jì dǎo yǐn àn qiāo**】** 为动功。其作法为，正坐，身体挺直，两手交叉，置于项后，托定后脑，面微向上仰，头左右摇动，项与手相对用力，然后两手离开颈项，仍交叉，抱住一只脚心，用力抱紧，腰膝弯曲，脚心用力向前蹬。令人精和血通，邪气不入，久行之无病。

exercise of Daoyin for sacred pressing and raising A dynamic exercise, marked by sitting upright, straightening the body, crossing the hands to hold the back of the head, slightly raising the face, shaking the head from the left to the right and vice versa, holding the neck with the hands, then crossing the hands to hold one sole, bending the waist and knees and thrusting the soles in order to normalize the flow of essence and blood, to prevent invasion of pathogenic factors and to avoid occurrence of any diseases.

圣济服气法【shèng jì fú qì fǎ**】** 为静功。正脚卧，叩齿三十六下，吐去浊恶气，即上下卷肚七下，左右亦如之，各七次，即闭气，鼓腹令气满，及微闭三五咽以下为一歇，咽多为佳。

exercise for sacred breath A static exercise, marked by lying with raised feet, clicking the teeth for thirty-six times, vomiting turbid Qi, moving the abdomen upward and downward for seven times as well as left and right for seven times in order to hold the breath, beating the abdomen to enrich Qi, slightly swallowing for three to five times and more swallowing for strengthening the body.

圣济神仙服气法【shèng jì shén xiān fú qì fǎ**】** 为静功。其作法为，存心如婴儿在母胎，十月成就，筋骨柔和，以心息念，和气自至，呼吸如法，咽之不饥，百毛孔开，息无塞滞。

exercise of sacred and immortal breath　A static exercise，marked by keeping the heart like an embryo in the mother's body for ten months，softening the sinews and bones with heart breathing，harmonizing Qi，normalizing respiration，swallowing without any anger，opening all the orifices and preventing any stagnation.

圣济总录【shèng jì zǒng lù】《圣济总录》为宋代问世的医学专著，其中也收录有气功养生之法。作者不详。

Shengji Zonglu（*General Collection of Sage Studies*）　A monograph about Qigong entitled *General Collection of Sage Studies*，compiled in the Song Dynasty（960 AD - 1279 AD），which has collected some theory and methods of Qigong practice. The author was unknown.

圣济总录论子时【shèng jì zǒng lù lùn zǐ shí】《圣济总录论子时》为气功专论，论述颇为简明而有特色。作者不详。

sacred and general collection about the discussion of Zi（**the period of the day from 11 p. m. to 1 a. m.**）　Collected from a monograph of Qigong，mainly describing the conciseness and characteristics of Qigong practice. The author was unknown.

圣人【shèng rén】① 指古代德高望重的人，包括医家和气功家；② 佛家气功习用，泛指习练气功断惑证理的人。

Shengren（**Sage**）　Refers to ① either the important men with noble character and high prestige，such as great doctors and great masters of Qigong；② or the practitioners who can relieve puzzles and prove rules in practicing Qigong in Buddhism.

圣胎【shèng tāi】① 指胎息气功；② 指习练佛家气功；③ 指神气凝结而作丹。

sacred embryo　Refers to ① either fetal respiration in practicing Qigong；② or Qigong practice in Buddhism；③ or concentration of the spirit and Qi developing into Dan（pills of immortality）.

盛神法【shèng shén fǎ】　源自气功专论，阐述盛神的方法，提出养气存神的盛神之道。

exercise for exuberating the spirit　Collected from a monograph of Qigong，mainly describing the method to exuberate the spirit and suggesting the right way to nourish Qi and keep the spirit.

失神者亡【shī shén zhě wáng】　指神气涣散，阴阳不平衡，脏腑功能失调，无神气则衰亡。强调神的重要。

no spirit no life　Refers to the fact that dispersion of the spiritual Qi causes disorder of Yin and Yang and malfunction of the viscera，suggesting the importance of the spirit.

失声导引法【shī shēng dǎo yǐn fǎ】为静功。其作法为，意想肾水升至肺润之，呼吸归丹田，调息息。治失声。

exercise of Daoyin for aphasia　A static exercise，imagining to promote kidney water to moisten the lung and to return breath to Dantian for regulating respiration. Such a static exercise can cure aphasia. Dantian is divided into the upper Dantian（the region between the eyes），the middle Dantian（the region below the heart）and the lower Dantian（the region below the navel）.

S

施肩吾【shī jiān wú】　唐代气功学家，著有多部气功专著，提倡习练气功应明四时、阴阳、五行。

Shi Jianwu　A master of Qigong in the Tang Dynasty (618 AD - 907 AD). He wrote several monographs of Qigong, suggesting to pay attention to the four seasons, Yin and Yang, and five elements (including wood, fire, earth, metal and water) in practicing Qigong.

施希圣【shī xī shèng】　唐代气功学家施肩吾的另外一个称谓，其著有多部气功专著，提倡习练气功应明四时、阴阳、五行。

Shi Xisheng　Another name of Shi Jianwu, a master of Qigong in the Tang Dynasty (618 AD - 907 AD). He wrote several monographs of Qigong, suggesting to pay attention to the four seasons, Yin and Yang, and five elements (including wood, fire, earth, metal and water) in practicing Qigong.

十缠【shí chán】　佛家气功习用语，指十种损伤情志的精神活动，如无惭、无愧、嫉、悔、昏沉等。

ten harmful activities　Refers ten activities of the spirit that damage emotions, such as proudness, hatred, regret and drowsiness, etc.

十二地支【shí èr dì zhī】　即子、丑、寅、卯、辰、巳、午、未、申、酉、戌、亥。

twelve earthly branches　Refers to the earthly branches of Zi, Chou, Yin, Mao, Chen, Si, Wu, Wei, Shen, You, Xu and Hai.

十二多【shí èr duō】　指多思、多念、多欲、多事、多语、多笑、多愁、多乐、多喜、多怒、多好、多恶十二多。

twelve overdoings　Refers to excessive thought, ideas, desire, matter, talk, laugh, anxiety, happiness, joy, anger, fancy and nausea.

十二经脉【shí èr jīng mài】　指与脏腑有络属关系的手三阴经、手三阳经、足三阴经、足三阳经。

twelve meridians　Refers to three meridians of hand Yin, three meridians of hand Yang, three meridians of foot Yin and three meridians of foot Yang, all of which are connected with the five Zang-organs (including the heart, the liver, the spleen, the lung and the kidney) and six Fu-organs (including the gallbladder, the stomach, the small intestine, the large intestine, the bladder and the triple energizer).

十二经脉起止【shí èr jīng mài qǐ zhǐ】　十二经脉即手三阴经脉、手三阳经脉、足三阴经脉、足三阳经脉，共十二条。每一条经脉又与脏腑相联系。

beginning and ending of the twelve meridians　The twelve meridians include three Yin meridians of hand, three Yang meridians of hand, three Yin meridians of foot and three Yang meridians of foot. Each meridian is connected with five Zang-organs (including the heart, the liver, the spleen, the lung and the kidney) and the six Fu-organs (the gallbladder, stomach, small intestine, large intestine, bladder and triple energizer).

十二经脉之海【shí èr jīng mài zhī hǎi】　指冲脉。冲脉为气血之海。

sea of the twelve meridians　Refers to the thoroughfare meridian which is the sea of Qi and blood.

十二经终【shí èr jīng zhōng】　指十二经脉之气终绝的症状。

exhaustion of twelve meridians　Refers

to the disease caused by exhaustion of Qi in the twelve meridians.

十二科法【shí èr kē fǎ**】** 即练功的十二个层次。

twelve stages Refers to twelve levels in practice of Qigong.

十二律【shí èr lǜ**】** 即用十二个长度不同的律音,吹出十二个长度不同的标准音,叫十二律。

twelve tonalities Refers to using twelve different pitch pipes to blow twelve standard sounds.

十二辟卦【shí èr pì guà**】** 气功文献借用为阴阳消长的说理工具,指《易经》中的六卦象征阴息阳消。

twelve monarch Trigrams Refers to six Trigrams that symbolize the growth of Yang and the decline of Yin, and the other six Trigrams that symbolize the growth of Yin and the decline of Yang.

十二伤【shí èr shāng**】** 指久视伤血,久卧伤气,久立伤骨,久行伤筋,久坐伤肉,远思强健伤人,忧恚悲哀伤人,喜乐过差伤人,汲汲所愿伤人,戚戚所患伤人,寒暖失节伤人,阴阳不交伤人。

twelve impairments Refers to the fact that watching for a long time damages the blood, sleeping for a long time damages Qi, standing for a long time damages bones, walking for a long time damages sinews, sitting for a long time damages muscles, strengthening the body for a long time damages health, sorrow for a long time damages life, happiness for a long time damages life, desiring for a long time damages life, anxiety for a long time damages life, deviation coldness and hotness damages life and non-combination of Yin and Yang damages life.

十二少【shí èr shǎo**】** 指减少意识思维活动及不合自然的行为。

twelve reductions Refers to reducing the activities of consciousness and thinking and unnatural behavior.

十二神女【shí èr shén nǚ**】** 指睫毛,为目之卫。

twelve goddesses Refers to eyelash that protects the eyes.

十二时【shí èr shí**】** 指一日的十二时辰,因为古代将每日分为十二个时辰。

twelve periods Refers to the time of a whole day because in ancient China one day was divided into twelve periods, the same as twenty-four hours at the present.

十二时辰【shí èr shí chen**】** 指一日的十二时辰,因为古代将每日分为十二个时辰。

twelve hours Refers to the time of a whole day because in ancient China one day was divided into twelve periods.

十二息【shí èr xī**】** 指十二种呼吸治病的方法,即十二种命功。

twelve respirations Refers to the methods to treat diseases through twelve ways of respiration.

十二象【shí èr xiàng**】** 即《易经》中的两卦一共有十二爻。

twelve symbols Refers to twelve lines in two Trigrams in *Yijing*. In *Yijing*, the Chinese character of Yi means simplification, change and no change, not just change.

十二消息卦【shí èr xiāo xi guà**】** 即气功文献借用为阴阳消长的说理工具,指《易经》中的六卦象征阴息阳消。

twelve fluctuated Trigrams Refers to six Trigrams that symbolize the growth of Yang and the decline of Yin，and the other six Trigrams that symbolize the growth of Yin and the decline of Yang.

十二消息说【shí èr xiāo xi shuō**】** 源自气功专论，主要阐述阴极阳生，阳极阴生，阴阳之间的气化作用。

twelve fluctuating elaborations Collected from a monograph of Qigong, mainly describing twelve ways for discussing the situation during which Yang grows when Yin is extreme and Yin grows when Yang is extreme.

十二月【shí èr yuè**】** 指一年十二个月都应自然练好气功。

twelve months Refers to the whole year during which the practice of Qigong must be done naturally.

十二月服气法【shí èr yuè fú qì fǎ**】** 为静功。其作法为，每年每月采取必要措施，白日取阳，晚上取阴。正月朝食阳气一百八十，暮食阴气二百。二月朝食阳气一百八十，暮食阴气一百八十。三月朝食阳气二百，暮食阴气一百六十。四月朝食阳气二百二十，暮食阴气一百四十。五月朝食阳气二百四十，暮食阴气一百二十。五月朝食阳气二百四十，暮食阴气一百四十。六月朝食阳气二百二十，暮食阴气一百四十。七月朝食阳气二百，暮食阴气一百六十。八月朝食阳气一百八十，暮食阴气一百八十。九月朝食阳气一百六十，暮食阴气二百。十月朝食阳气一百四十，暮食阴气二百二十。十一月朝食阳气一百二十，暮食阴气二百四十。十二月朝食阳气一百四十，暮食阴气二百六十。

taking Qi in twelve months A static exercise, referring to the fact that every month there are measures for taking Yang in the daytime and Yin in the nighttime. In January, Yang Qi is taken one hundred and eighty times in daytime and Yin Qi is taken two hundred times in dusk；in February, Yang qi is taken one hundred and eighty times in daytime and Yin Qi is taken one hundred and eighty times in dusk；in March, Yang qi is taken two hundred times in daytime and Yin Qi is taken one hundred and sixty times in dusk；in April, Yang qi is taken two hundred and twenty times in daytime and Yin Qi is taken one hundred and forty times in dusk；in May, Yang qi is taken two hundred and forty times in daytime and Yin Qi is taken one hundred and twenty times in dusk；in June, Yang Qi is taken two hundred and twenty times in daytime and Yin Qi is taken one hundred and forty times in dusk；in July Yang Qi is taken two hundred times in daytime and Yin Qi is taken one hundred and sixty times in dusk；in August, Yang qi is taken one hundred and eighty times in daytime and Yin Qi is taken two hundred times in dusk；in October, Yang Qi is taken one hundred and forty times in daytime and Yin Qi is taken two hundred and twenty times in dusk；in November, Yang Qi is taken one hundred and twenty times in daytime and Yin Qi is taken two hundred and forty times in dusk；in December, Yang Qi is taken one hundred and forty times in daytime and Yin Qi is taken two hundred and sixty times in dusk.

十二月节后导引法【shí èr yuè jié hòu dǎo yǐn fǎ**】** 为动功。其作法为，十二月节后每日子丑时，正坐，神入静。一手抱阴囊,一手在肚脐部旋转按摩。其功效为强身。

exercise of Daoyin after fest days of December A dynamic exercise, marked by quietly sitting upright in Zi (the period of the day from 11 p.m. to 1 a.m.) and Chou (1 a.m. to 3 a.m. in the morning) every day in December for practicing Qigong, tranquilizing the spirit, holding the scrotum with one hand and kneading the navel with the other hand. Such a dynamic exercise can strengthen the body.

十二月中导引法【shí èr yuè zhōng dǎo yǐn fǎ**】** 为动功。其作法为,指十二月中每日子丑时,侧卧,两膊屈置于胸前,调息,呼吸三次,咽唾液。其功效有疏通经络,延年益寿之效。

exercise of Daoyin in the middle of December A dynamic exercise, marked by lying on one side in Zi (the period of the day from 11 p.m. to 1 a.m.) and Chou (the period of the day from 1 a.m. to 3 a.m. in the morning) every day in December for practicing Qigong, bending the arms to the chest, regulating respiration, breathing for three times, and swallowing saliva. Such a dynamic exercise can unlock the meridians and prolong life.

十三伤【shí sān shāng**】** 指十三种损伤精神的意识思维活动,为引起形体精神受伤的原因。

thirteen impairments Refers to thirteen activities of consciousness and thinking that damage the spirit, eventually injuring the body and the spirit.

十力【shí lì**】** 指十种认识自然与社会的精神思维活动。

ten activities Refers to the ten ways for knowing the activities of the spirit and thinking in the natural world and society.

十六锭金【shí liù dìng jīn**】** 保健身体和治疗疾病的一些重要方法,用中文的十六个字表达。同十六字诀,为静功。一吸便提,气气归脐;一提便咽,水火相见。

sixteen ingot gold Refers to some important ways for nourishing health and treating disease, which are described with sixteen special Chinese characters. It is the same as formula of sixteen-characters, which is a static exercise, referring to sixteen important ways for strengthening health and treating any disease which are described with sixteen special Chinese characters. In practice, after inhalation, it must be enhanced. When any Qi is inhaled, it should be returned to the navel. When it is enhanced, it must be swallowed in order to coordinate water and fire.

十六段锦法【shí liù duàn jǐn fǎ**】** 为动功,为调身、调气和调神。其作法为,自然坐或盘膝坐式;或站式,姿势定后,平和呼吸,闭口握固,冥心安神,叩齿三十六通。其功效为治各种疾病,强壮身体,保持健康。

sixteen paragraph brocade methods A dynamic exercise for regulating the body, Qi and the spirit, marked by naturally sitting or sitting with crossed knees, or standing up, pacifying respiration after decision of posture, closing the mouth, tranquilizing the heart, stabilizing the spirit and clicking the teeth for thirty-six times. Such a dynamic exercise can cure various diseases, strengthen the body and improve health

S

care.

十六字诀法【shí liù zì jué fǎ**】** 为静功。一吸便提，气气归脐；一提便咽，水火相见。

formula of sixteen-characters A static exercise, referring to sixteen important ways for strengthening health and treating any disease which are described with sixteen special Chinese characters. In practice, after inhalation, it must be enhanced. When any Qi is inhaled, it should be returned to the navel. When it is enhanced, it must be swallowed in order to coordinate water and fire.

十七种净土【shí qī zhǒng jìng tǔ**】** 佛家气功习用语，指十七种调和神形的意识、行为活动。

seventeen kinds of Sukhavati A common term of Qigong in Buddhism, referring to seventeen ways for regulating mental activities and physical movements.

十三虚无【shí sān xū wú**】** 源自气功专论，阐述道家倡导的以虚为道的十三条气功养生要点。

thirteen nihilities Collected from a monograph of Qigong, mainly describing the thirteen important ways for practicing Qigong and cultivating life suggested by Daoism, among which mentality, tranquility, concentration and quietness always are lost while avarice, greed and confusion always exist.

十使【shí shǐ**】** 指精神失调后引起的十种损伤情志的行为，如贪欲、嗔恚、无明、慢、疑等。

ten harmful behaviors Refers to ten damages after psychataxia, such as greed, anger, dimness, slowness and

suspection, etc.

十天干【shí tiān gān**】** 即甲、乙、丙、丁、戊、己、庚、辛、壬、癸。

ten heavenly stems Refers to the heavenly stems of Jia, Yi, Bing, Ding, Wu, Ji, Geng, Xin, Ren and Gui.

十一月节导引法【shí yī yuè jié dǎo yǐn fǎ**】** 为动功。其作法为，十一月节每日子丑时，站立身体，两足靠拢，两手由下向上伸，吸气五次，周而复始七次。功效为令人神清气爽。

exercise of Daoyin in feast days of November A dynamic exercise, marked by standing up in Zi (the period of the day from 11 p.m. to 1 a.m.) and Chou (1 a.m. to 3 a.m. in the morning) every day in November for practicing Qigong, closing up the feet, raising the hands, inhaling five times and moving in cycle for seven times. Such a dynamic exercise can purify the spirit and clear Qi.

十一月中导引法【shí yī yuè zhōng dǎo yǐn fǎ**】** 为动功。其作法为，十一月中每日子丑时，平坐伸足，两手交叉向上，引下腹部气到口中会合，咽下唾液二次。功效为胸中阳气充盈，身体强健。

exercise of Daoyin in the middle of November A dynamic exercise, marked by sitting upright with stretching foot in Zi (the period of the day from 11 p.m. to 1 a.m.) and Chou (from 1 a.m. to 3 a.m. in the morning) every day in November for practicing Qigong, crossing hands upwards, leading Qi in the lower abdomen to the mouth, and swallowing saliva twice, the effect of which is to enrich Yang Qi in the chest and strengthen the body.

十月【shí yuè**】** 属亥月，是月阳气衰，阴气渐盛。

october October of traditional Chinese calendar is similar to November in Christian calendar. During this period Yang Qi is declined and Yin Qi is exuberant.

十月而生【shí yuè ér shēng**】** 指人体从胚胎形成到出生为十个月。

birth after ten month Refers to the fact that only after ten months of conception can a baby be born.

十月怀胎【shí yuè huái tāi**】** 指人体从胚胎形成到出生为十个月。

conception in ten months Refers to the fact that only after ten months of conception can a baby be born.

十月圣胎完【shí yuè shèng tāi wán**】** 指练功十月，"知白守黑，一年之内，九转功成也"。

important practice of ten months Refers to success in a year with nine transformations with the knowledge of the white and the black after practice of Qigong for ten months.

十月中导引法【shí yuè zhōng dǎo yǐn fǎ**】** 为动功。其作法为，十月中每日丑寅时，正坐，排除杂念，气息绵绵，同时吞咽口中唾液。其作用是身心安适，强健身体。

exercise of Daoyin in the middle of October A dynamic exercise，marked by sitting upright in Chou (the period of a day from 1 a. m. to 3 a. m. in the morning) and Yin (the period of a day from 3 a. m. to 5 a. m. in the morning) every day in October for practicing Qigong， eliminating distracting thought，mildly breathing and swallowing saliva in the mouth. Such a dynamic exercise can balance the body and heart and strengthen health.

石得之【shí dé zhī**】** 宋代杰出气功学家石泰的另外一个称谓，也是著名的医学家。

Shi Dezi Another name of Shi Tai，a great master of Qigong in the Song Dynasty（960 AD - 1279 AD），who was also a doctor of traditional Chinese medicine.

石关【shí guān**】** 足少阴肾经，位于脐下 3 寸。此穴位为气功习练之处。

Shiguan（KI 18） An acupoint in the kidney meridian of foot Shaoyin，located 3 Cun below the navel. This acupoint is a region usually used in practice of Qigong.

石涧道人【shí jiàn dào rén**】** 元代气功理论家俞琰的另外一个称谓。

Shijian Daoren Another name of Yu Yan，a great master of Qigong theory in the Yuan Dynasty（1271 AD - 1368 AD）.

石淋【shí lín**】** 气功适应证，多因湿热下注，煎熬尿液，结为砂石所致。

stony stranguria An indication of Qigong，usually caused by downward flow of damp-heat that fries urine and changes into stone.

石淋候导引法【shí lín hòu dǎo yǐn fǎ**】** 为静功。其作法为，仰卧，两手放膝头，脚跟放臀下，口吸气鼓腹，待气充满腹部时，用鼻呼出。

exercise of Daoyin for calculus stranguria A static exercise，marked by lying on the back，pressing on the knees with the hands，turning the feet to the buttocks，breathing in through the mouth to protect the abdomen，and breathing out through the nose when there is sufficient Qi in the abdomen.

S

石室【shí shì】 指气功家隐居山中，修习气功的房屋。

stone chamber Refers to the house in a mountain where the masters of Qigong earnestly practiced and developed Qigong.

石水【shí shuǐ】 气功适应证，指水肿病之一；指单腹胀。

stone water An indication of Qigong, referring to edema and abdominal distension.

石泰【shí tài】 宋代的一位杰出的气功学家，也是著名的医学家。

Shi Tai A great master of Qigong in the Song Dynasty（960 AD - 1279 AD），who was also a doctor of traditional Chinese medicine.

石杏林【shí xìng lín】 宋代杰出气功学家石泰的另外一个称谓，也是著名的医学家。

Shi Xinglin Another name of Shi Tai, a great master of Qigong in the Song Dynasty（960 AD - 1279 AD），who was also a doctor of traditional Chinese medicine.

时病【shí bìng】 指因于劳、逸、饥、饱引起脏腑失调而感受风、寒、暑、湿等四时之邪所生之病。

seasonal epidemics Refers to the disease caused by disorders of the five Zang-organs（including the heart, the liver, the spleen, the lung and the kidney）and six Fu-organs（including the gallbladder, the stomach, the small intestine, the large intestine, the bladder and the triple energizer）due to labor, rest, hunger and overeating as well as the pathogenic factors in the four seasons due to wind, cold, summer-heat and dampness.

时气候导引法【shí qì hòu dǎo yǐn fǎ】 为动功。其作法为，早晨刚起床时，用手从头上拉耳向上，并牵拉鬓发，左右手交替，活血通络，养发聪耳。

seasonal exercise of Daoyin A dynamic exercise, marked by pulling the ears upwards with both hands after getting up in the morning and pulling the hair on the temples, crossing the hands in order to activate the blood, unblock the collaterals, nourish hair and improve the ears.

时思太仓不饥渴【shí sī tài cāng bù jī kě】 为静功。其作法为，经常咀嚼太和之气，意想着胃，念着"我有长生之道，不食自饱"。功效为解饥止渴。

thinking stomach without hunger A static exercise, marked by always chewing harmonized Qi, imagining the stomach, reading the concept that "I know the way to prolong life and are always completely full without taking food". The effect of such a practice is to relieve hunger and thirst.

时照图【shí zhào tú】 人身元气，运行于任、督二脉，子时到尾闾（十二消息卦用复卦表示，下同），丑时到肾堂（临卦），寅时到玄枢（泰卦），卯时到夹脊（大壮卦），辰时到陶道（夬卦），巳时到玉枕（乾卦），午时到泥丸（姤卦），未时到明堂（遁卦），申时到膻中（否卦），酉时到中脘（观卦），戌时到神阙（剥卦），亥时气归于气海（坤卦）。

procedure picture Refers to the original Qi in the human body that moves through the conception meridian and the governor meridian, reaching coccyx in Zi（the period of the day from 11 p.m. to 1 a.m.）（twelve kinds of information are related to the Trigrams

and mentioned later on), reaching the
kidney (Lin Trigram) in Chou (the period of a day from 1 a.m to 3 a. m. in
the early morning), reaching the pivot
(Tai Trigram) in Yin (thee period of a
day from 3 a.m. to 5 a.m. in the early
morning), reaching the acupoint of
Jiaji (Strong Trigram) located on the
back in Mao (the period of a day from
5 a. m. to 7 a. m. in the morning),
reaching an acupoint of Taodao (Guai
Trigram) located on the governor meridian in Chen (the period of a day
from 7 a.m. to 9 a.m in the morning),
reaching the acupoint of Yuzhen (BL
9) (Qian Trigram) in Si (the period of
a day from 9 a.m to 11 a.m in the
morning), reaching the mud bolus (the
brain) (Gou Trigram) in Wu (the period of a day from 11 a.m. to 1 p.m. in
the noon), reaching the nose (Dun
Trigram) in Wei (the period of a day
from 1 p.m. to 3 p.m. in the afternoon), reaching Danzhong (CV 17)
(Pi Trigram) in Shen (the period of a
day from 3 p.m. to 5 p.m. in the afternoon), reaching Zhongwan (CV
12) (Guan Trigram) in You (the period of a day from 5 p.m. to 7 p.m. in
the afternoon), reaching Shenque (CV
8) (Bao Trigram) in Xu (the period of
a day from 7 p. m. to 9 p. m. in the
evening) and reaching Qihai (CV 6)
(Kun Trigram) in Hai (the period of a
day from 21 p. m. to 23 p. m. at
night).

时中【shí zhōng**】**　同允执厥中,指不
偏不倚,两在其中。

center of time　The same as neutrality,
referring to balance and the center.

利【shí**】**　指应用气功治疗疾病的良好
效果。

benefit　Refers to the good effect of
Qigong in curing diseases.

识【shí**】**　佛家气功习用语,① 指心意;
② 指一切精神现象。

cognition　A common term of Qigong
in Buddhism, referring to ① either
consciousness; ② or all the manifestations of the essence and the spirit.

识垢【shí gòu**】**　指妄念、杂念。

whim　Refers to wild fancy and distracting thought.

食后将息法【shí hòu jiāng xī fǎ**】**　为
动功。其作法为,平旦点点讫,即自以热
手摩腹,出门庭行五六十步消息之。中
食后,还以热手摩腹,行一二百步、缓缓
行,勿令气急,行讫,偃卧。

exercise of respiration after meal　A dynamic exercise, marked by rubbing the
abdomen with hot hands at dawn, going out to walk for fifty or sixty steps;
rubbing the abdomen with hot hands
after lunch, walking slowly for one
hundred or two hundred steps and lying
supine after walking.

食气【shí qì**】**　① 指习练气功,纳气于
内以气为食;② 指调节呼吸。

taking Qi　Refers to ① either inhaling
Qi like food in practicing Qigong; ② or
regulation of respiration.

食气补泻【shí qì bǔ xiè**】**　气功专论
原则。

taking Qi for tonification and purgation
The principle of treatment in Qigong.

食日月精法【shí rì yuè jīng fǎ**】**　为静
功。其作法为,日初、日中、或日入之时,
正立向日,展两手,闭气九遍,仰天噙日
光,咽之九度可益精气,令人强壮不老。
以月初、月正中、或月入之时,正立向月,

展两手,闭气九遍,仰天噏月光,咽之九度。令人阴气盛,妇人有子。

exercise for taking essence from the sun and the moon A static exercise, marked by standing up to the sun in the morning, or at the noon, or at dusk, stretching the hands, closing respiration for nine times, raising head to absorb sunlight for nine times to enrich the essential Qi and strengthen the body; or marked by standing upright to the moon at the beginning of a month, or the middle of a month, or the end of a month, stretching the hands, closing respiration for nine times, raising the head to absorb the moonlight for nine degrees. Such an exercise of practicing Qigong can exuberating Yin Qi and enable women to conceive baby.

食伤饱【shí shāng bǎo】 气功适应证,指食过于饱,脾气受伤,致气急烦闷,不能安卧。

damage due to supersaturation An indication of Qigong, referring to damage of spleen Qi, irritancy, dyspnea and difficulty to sleep caused by supersaturation.

食伤饱候导引法【shí shāng bǎo hòu dǎo yǐn fǎ】 为静功。其作法为,正坐、伸直腰,用口吸气数十次,吸满则吐出,以腹满消除为止,不消再行此法。

exercise of Daoyin for indigestion A static exercise, marked by sitting upright, unbending the waist, inhaling through the mouth for dozens of times and exhaling after sufficient inhaling. When abdominal distension is relieved, the practice of Qigong with static exercise can be stopped. If abdominal distension is not relieved, the practice of Qigong with static exercise cannot be stopped.

食十二时气法【shí shí èr shí qì fǎ】 为静功。其作法为,坐势,或站势。从夜半子时开始,服食十二时之气,意引自然清气入丹田。

exercise for inhaling twelve hours after meal A static exercise, marked by sitting or standing from midnight, taking Qi for twelve hours from the midnight and leading clear Qi into Dantian with consciousness. Dantian is divided into the upper Dantian (the region between the eyes), the middle Dantian (the region below the heart) and the lower Dantian (the region below the navel).

使【shǐ】 ① 指引起精神失调;② 指人无尽的烦恼。

disturbance Referring to ① either imbalance of the spirit; ② or secular annoyance.

使气【shǐ qì】 指神御气,神行气行,神宁气住。

driving Qi Refers to the fact that the spirit controls Qi; or the spirit moves and Qi moves; or the spirit is quiet and Qi is stabilized.

使者车【shǐ zhě chē】 指"凡聚火而心行意,使以攻疾病,而曰使者车"。

attack cart Refers to "attack disease with accumulation of fire and concentration of consciousness".

始觉【shǐ jué】 佛家气功习用语,指依气功之功,而显术体之觉性,即提高觉悟。

deep consciousness A term of Qigong, referring to improving consciousness according to the exercise of Qigong practice.

世间安得有无体独知之精【shì jiān

ān dé yǒu wú tǐ dú zhī zhī jīng】 指精
神藏于形体之内，没有形体，便没有精神
意识思维活动。

**How to understand original essence in the
human body in this world**? Refers to
the fact that the essence and spirit are
conserved inside the body and that
there will be no activities of the spirit，
consciousness and thinking if there is
no physique.

事林广记【shì lín guǎng jì】《事林广
记》为综合性类书，兼收养生气功，成书
于宋元，由陈元靓著写，兼有不少气功养
生学的记述。

Shilin Guangji（*General Records of All
Things*） A comprehensive monograph
with Qigong and life cultivation entitled
General Records of All Things，written
by Chen Yuanliang in the late Song Dy-
nasty（960 AD－1279 AD）and early
Yuan Dynasty（1271 AD－1368 AD），
collecting a lot of literature about
Qigong and life cultivation.

拭摩神庭【shì mó shén tíng】 为动
功，即用两手按摩面部，使面部气血流
通，有光泽。

rubbing face A dynamic exercise，re-
ferring to rubbing the face with both
hands in order to circulate Qi and blood
in the face and make the face lustrous.

拭目【shì mù】 熨目的另外一个称谓，
为动功，指经常按摩腹部，能健脾胃，帮
助消化，防治水谷积滞不化。为内伤调
中之法。

wiping the eyes A synonym of rubbing
the abdomen，is a dynamic exercise，
marked by rubbing the abdomen for
fortifying the spleen and stomach，di-
gesting food，preventing and curing indigestion. Such a dynamic exercise is

for curing internal damage and regulating the middle.

释迦牟尼佛【shì jiā móu ní fó】 印度
佛教创始人，开佛家气功之先河。生于
公元前 565，卒于公元前 485 年。

Sakyamuni Buddha Sakyamuni Buddha
（565 BC－485 BC）was the creator of
Buddhism in the India.

释家功【shì jiā gōng】 指源于佛家的
功法。

Buddhist exercise Refers to the exercise for practicing Qigong in Buddhism.

嗜眠候导引法【shì mián hòu dǎo yǐn
fǎ】 为动功。其作法为，屈膝张腿盘脚
而坐，两手从脚弯内伸进握住两脚，尽力
牵拉两次。提神醒脑，治嗜睡，精神
不振。

exercise of Daoyin for prolonged sleep
A dynamic exercise，marked by sitting
with bending the knees，stretching the
legs and crossing the feet，holding the
feet with both hands along the internal
bend of the foot，and pulling the feet
forcefully for twice. Such a dynamic
exercise can improve the spirit，refresh
the brain，and relieve prolonged sleep
and lassitude.

嗜卧【shì wò】 气功适应证，指不论昼
夜，时时欲睡，呼之能醒，醒后复睡。多
因脾虚湿胜所致。

prolonged sleep An indication of
Qigong，referring to sleep day and
night and continuing to sleep after waking up when being called. Such a disorder is caused by deficiency of the
spleen and exuberance of dampness.

嗜欲【shì yù】 指不正当的嗜好和欲
念，难获气功的成功。

abnormal desire Refers to hobby and
wishes，making it difficult to practice

S

Qigong.

嗜欲不能劳其目, 淫邪不能惑其心
【shì yù bù néng láo qí mù yín xié bù néng huò qí xīn】 练气功之人依此而行, 才能容易获得成功。
Improper addiction and avarice could not distract the eyes and ears, obscenity and fallacy could not tempt the heart. Those who practice Qigong in such a way can certainly succeed.

收神【shōu shén】 指习练气功到了神化之际, 有遥视、遥感力。
spirit control Means remote vision and remote emotion at the state of spirit transformation in practicing Qigong.

收神论【shōu shén lùn】 源自气功专论, 主要阐述收神与产丹的关系。
Discussion of spirit control Collected from a monograph of Qigong, mainly describing the relationship between spirit control and Dan production.

收视返听【shōu shì fǎn tīng】 指练功时视而不见、听而不闻的内守状态。
supreme inward contemplation Refers to the state of internal concentration marked by vision without listening and listening without any vision in practicing Qigong.

收拾身心【shōu shi shēn xīn】 指调节形神。
somatic and cardiac regulation Refers to regulating the body and the spirit.

收心【shōu xīn】 指学练气功, 首先要排除外界富贵声色的诱惑和干扰, 不胡思乱想, 要把思想意念集中到练功上来。这是对初学气功者的基本要求。
heart concentration Refers to study about how to practice Qigong. To practice Qigong, temptation and disturbance of external world as well as disor-derly conjecture and fancy should be eliminated first. Thought and consciousness should be concentrated on Qigong practice. This is the basic requirement for the beginners to study Qigong.

收在一处【shōu zài yī chù】 指精神意识活动高度集中统一。
unity of concentration Refers to great centralization and unity of the spirit and consciousness activities.

手朝三元【shǒu cháo sān yuán】 指头顶部, 经常用于从前额向头顶部抚摩如梳状, 能固脑坚发。
hand fondling three origins Refers to kneading from the forehead to the top of the head in order to protect the brain and the hair.

手功【shǒu gōng】 为动功。其作法为, 除胸脯邪, 除臂液邪, 治四肢, 除心胸风邪。
hand exercise A dynamic exercise, marked clenching the hands to eliminate pathogenic factors in the chest and arms in order to relieve pathogenic wind in the heart and to harmonize the body.

手厥阴经别【shǒu jué yīn jīng bié】 十二经别之一, 为气功习练之处。从腋窝前下三寸处手厥阴心包经渊腋穴分出, 进入胸腔内, 分别归属于上、中、下三焦。
branch of hand Jueyin Refers to one of the twelve branches of meridians, which separates from the pericardium meridian of hand Jueyin in the posterior part of the armpit and enters the thorax, separately connected with the upper energizer, the middle energizer and the lower energizer. This branch is

the region usually used in practice of Qigong.

手厥阴络脉【shǒu jué yīn luò mài**】**十五络脉之一,为气功习练之处。从腕上二寸内关穴处分出,出于两筋之间,沿着本经上行,联系心包,络于心系。

collateral of hand Jueyin Refers to one of the fifteen collaterals of meridians, which starts from the acupoint Neiguan (PC 6) located from the wrist, coming out from the middle of two sinews, ascending along the pericardium meridian of hand Jueyin, connecting with the pericardium and returning to the heart system. This collateral is the region usually used in practice of Qigong.

手厥阴心包经【shǒu jué yīn xīn bāo jīng**】**十二经脉之一,为气功习练之处。起于胸中,出属于心包络,向下穿过膈肌,从胸至腹依次联络上、中、下三焦。

pericardium meridian of hand Jueyin One of the twelve meridians that starts from the chest, entering the pericardium, and connected with the upper triple energizer, the middle energizer and the lower energizer along the chest and the abdomen through the diaphragm. This meridian is the region usually used in practice of Qigong.

手三阳经【shǒu sān yáng jīng**】**指手阳明大肠经,手太阳小肠经和手少阳三焦经,为气功习练之处。

three Yang meridians of the hand Refers to the large intestine meridian of hand Yangming, the small intestine meridian of hand Taiyang and the triple energizer meridian of hand Shaoyang. These meridians are the regions usually used in practice of Qigong.

手三阴经【shǒu sān yīn jīng**】**指手太阴肺经、手少阴心经和手厥阴心包经,为气功习练之处。

three Yin meridians of the hand Refers to the lung meridian of hand Taiyin, the heart meridian of hand Shaoyin and the pericardium meridian of hand Jueyin. These meridians are the regions usually used in practice of Qigong.

手少阳经别【shǒu shào yáng jīng bié**】**十二经别之一,为气功习练之处。在头之顶巅部从手少阳三焦经分出,下入缺盆(锁骨上窝),经过上、中、下三焦,散布于胸中。

branch of hand Yaoyang Refers to one of the twelve branches of meridians, which separates from the triple energizer meridian of hand Shaoyang on the top of the head, descends to supraclavicular fossa and spreads in the chest through the upper energizer, middle energizer and lower energizer. This branch is the region usually used in practice of Qigong.

手少阳络脉【shǒu shào yáng luò mài**】**十二经脉之一,为气功习练之处。起始于中焦,向下联络大肠,环循胃上口,横行出于胸壁外上方,向下沿上臂内侧前缘,行于手少阴心经和手厥阴心包经外侧。

collateral of hand Yaoyang Refers to one of the fifteen collaterals of meridians, which starts from the middle energizer to connect with the large intestine and the upper part of the stomach, transversely moving the lateral side of the chest, flowing along the internal side of the upper limb, and moving along the external sides of the heart meridian of hand Shaoyin and the pericardium meridian of hand Jueyin. This

S

collateral is the region usually used in practice of Qigong.

手少阳三焦经【shǒu shào yáng sān jiāo jīng】 十二经脉之一，为气功习练之处。从无名指尺侧指甲角旁（关冲）起始，沿无名指尺侧缘上行，入缺盆，向下穿越膈肌，统属上、中、下三焦。

triple energizer meridian of hand Shaoyang One of the twelve meridians that starts from Guanchong（TE 1）and ascends to the supraclavicular fossae from the third finger, finally descending through the diaphragm to connect with the triple energizer. This meridian is the region usually used in practice of Qigong.

手少阴经别【shǒu shào yīn jīng bié】 十二经别之一，为气功习练之处。从手少阴心经分出后，在腋窝前下方（渊腋）两筋之间进入胸腔，属于心，向上走到喉咙，浅出面部，与太阳小肠经在目内眦处会合。

branch of hand Shaoyin Refers to one of the twelve branches of meridians, which separates from the heart meridian of hand Shaoyin to the chest along the center of the two sinews in the armpit, flowing upwards to the throat and complexion, and finally connecting with the small intestine meridian of hand Taiyang in the inner canthus. This branch is the region usually used in practice of Qigong.

手少阴络脉【shǒu shào yīn luò mài】 十五络脉之一，为气功习练之处。从通里穴处分出，别走手太阳小肠经，在腕后一寸半处别而上行，沿着本经进入心中，向上联系舌根，归属于目系（眼球后联系于脑的组织）。

collateral of hand Shaoyin Refers to one of the fifteen collaterals of meridians, which starts from Tongli（HT 5）and separates from the small intestine meridian of hand Taiyang, flowing upwards from the posterior part of the wrist to the tongue root, finally returning to the eyes. This collateral is the region usually used in practice of Qigong.

手少阴心经【shǒu shào yīn xīn jīng】 十二经脉之一，起于心中，为气功习练之处。

hand Shaoyin heart meridian One of the twelve meridians, starting from the heart. This meridian is the region usually used in practice of Qigong.

手太阳经别【shǒu tài yáng jīng bié】 十二经别之一，为气功习练之处，于肩关节部从手太阳小肠经分出，向下入腋窝，入胸腔络心脏，向下联系小肠。

branch of hand Taiyang Refers to one of the twelve branches of meridians, which separates from the small intestine meridian of hand Taiyang on the shoulder joint and descends to the armpit, entering thorax and into the heart, finally connecting with the small intestine. This branch is the region usually used in practice of Qigong.

手太阳络脉【shǒu tài yáng luò mài】 指十五络脉之一，为气功习练之处。从腕上五寸支正穴处分出，与手少阴心经汇合。

collateral of hand Taiyang Refers to one of the fifteen collaterals of meridians, which starts from the anterior part of the wrist and connects with the heart meridian of hand Shaoyin. This collateral is the region usually used in practice of Qigong.

手太阳小肠经【shǒu tài yáng xiǎo cháng jīng】 为十二经脉之一,为气功习练之处。起于小指尺侧指甲角旁(少泽),沿手掌尺侧缘上行,沿前臂背面尺侧缘上行,交会督脉于大椎穴,向前下入缺盆(锁骨上窝),深入胸腔,联络心脏,沿食管下行,穿隔到胃,入属小肠。

small intestine meridian of hand Taiyang One of the twelve meridians, which starts from Shaoze (SI 1) beside the ulnaris of the little finger, ascending along the ulnar side and the back of forearm, connecting with the governor meridian in Dazhui (GV 14), descending along the supraclavicular fossae into the chest to connect with the heart, and moving downwards along the esophagus into the stomach, and finally connected with the small intestine. This meridians the region usually used in practice of Qigong.

手太阳之别【shǒu tài yáng zhī bié】 指十五络脉之一,为气功习练之处。从腕上五寸支正穴处分出,与手少阴心经汇合。

collateral of hand Taiyang Refers to one of the fifteen collaterals of meridians, which starts from the anterior part of the wrist and connects with the heart meridian of hand Shaoyin. This collateral is the region usually used in practice of Qigong.

手太阴经别【shǒu tài yīn jīng bié】 十二经别之一,为气功习练之处。从手太阴肺经分出,进入腋窝前下方渊腋处,行于手少阴经别之前,进入胸中,走向肺,散布联络大肠,向上浅出缺盆(锁骨上窝),沿着喉咙,合入于子阳明大肠经。

branch of hand Taiyin Refers to one of the twelve branches of meridians, which separates from the lung meridian of hand Taiyin to the armpit and before the heart meridian of hand Shaoyin, then entering the chest, flowing to the lung, spreading to the large intestine, leaving the supraclavicular fossa, and connecting with the large intestine meridian of hand Yangming along the throat. This branch is the region usually used in practice of Qigong.

手太阴络脉【shǒu tài yīn luò mài】 十五络脉之一,为气功习练之处。脉从腕关节上方列缺穴处分出,与手太阴经并行,直入掌中,于大鱼际。

collateral of hand Taiyin Refers to one of the fifteen collaterals of meridians, which starts from Quexue (ST 12) on the upper part of the wrist and flows together with the lung meridian of hand Taiyin, directing entering the palms and spreading to the large thenar eminence. This collateral is the region usually used in practice of Qigong.

手太阴心经【shǒu tài yīn xīn jīng】 为十二经脉之一,为气功习练之处。起始于中焦,向下联络大肠,环循胃上口,穿过踊肌,入属肺脏,从肺系(气管、喉部)横行出于胸壁外上方,行于手少阴心经和手厥阴心包经外侧。

hand Taiyin heart meridian Refers to one of the twelve branches of meridians, which starts from the middle energizer and connects downwards with the large intestine, surrounding the top of the stomach, passing through diaphragm, entering the lung system to move transversely to the lateral side of the chest, finally connecting with the heart meridian of hand Shaoyin and the large intestine meridian of hand Jueyin. This meridian is the region usually used in practice of Qigong.

手太阴之别【shǒu tài yīn zhī bié】 十五络脉之一，为气功习练之处。脉从腕关节上方列缺穴处分出，与手太阴经并行，直入掌中，于大鱼际。

collateral of hand Taiyin Refers to one of the fifteen collaterals of meridians, which starts from Quexue（ST 12）on the upper part of the wrist and flows together with the lung meridian of hand Taiyin, directing entering the palms and spreading to the large thenar eminence. This collateral is the region usually used in practice of Qigong.

手心热【shǒu xīn rè】 气功适应证，指手足心热、咽干、烦渴，多是精液之损。

feverish palms An indication of Qigong, refers to damage of semen that causes heart heat, dry throat and polydipsia.

手阳明大肠经【shǒu yáng míng dà cháng jīng】 十二经脉之一，为气功习练之处。从示指桡侧指甲角旁（商阳）起始，络于肺，向下贯穿膈肌，入属大肠。

large intestine meridian of hand Yangming One of the twelve meridians that starts from Shangyang（LI 1）, ascending upwards to the lung, descending through the diaphragm, and connected with the large intestine. This meridian is the region usually used in practice of Qigong.

手阳明经别【shǒu yáng míng jīng bié】 十二经别之一，为气功习练之处。从于阳明大肠经手部分出后，沿着臂、肘、臑、肩部分，分布于胸膺乳房等部位。

branch of hand Yangming Refers to one of the twelve branches of meridians, which separates from the large in-

testine meridian of hand Yangming, flowing along the arm, elbow, forelimb and shoulder, finally distributing in the chest and breasts. This collateral is the region usually used in practice of Qigong.

手阳明络脉【shǒu yáng míng luò mài】 十五络脉之一，为气功习练之处。从偏历穴处分出，在腕上三寸处别走手太阴肺经；其支络，从偏历向上沿臂，遍布于牙齿；另一条支络，从下颌角入耳。

collateral of hand Yangming Refers to one of the fifteen collaterals of meridians, which starts from acupoint Pianli（LI 16）and separates from the lung meridian of hand Taiyin at 3 Cun on the wrist, one collateral flowing upwards from Pianli（LI 16）along the shoulder to the teeth, the other collateral entering the ears from the lower jaw. This collateral is the region usually used in practice of Qigong.

手足不遂候导引法【shǒu zú bù suì hòu dǎo yǐn fǎ】 为静功。① 指极力左右踢动两脚，闭气不息，两做九遍；② 指仰卧，两脚舒展，腰伸直，两膝靠拢，用口吸气，连做七遍；③ 正身仰卧，松解衣服，两手各用四指握住拇指，舒展两臂。

exercise of Daoyin for hand and foot reverse movement A static exercise, marked by ① kicking the feet and suspending respiration for nine times; ② lying on the back, extending both feet, stretching the waist, crossing the knees, breathing in through the mouth for seven times; ③ lying on the back, loosening the clothes, holding the thumbs in both hands with the four fingers on each hand in order to unfold the arms.

守诚【shǒu chéng】 指调神与调气,使之神凝而精气聚。

defending honesty Refers to regulation of the spirit and Qi in order to condense the spirit and to accumulate the essence and Qi.

守寸【shǒu cùn】 指意念不离上丹田。

defending Cun Means that thought should not leave the upper Dantian (the region between the eyes).

守道安乐法【shǒu dào ān lè fǎ】 为静功,指调气、调神,使精神意识和言语行为适应自然和社会变化规律。

exercise of peace and happiness in defending Dao A static exercise, referring to regulation of Qi and the spirit in order to enable the spirit, thought, speech and action to adapt to the changes of social rules.

守庚申【shǒu gēng shēn】 指练气功时,于庚申日通夕静坐不眠,叫做守庚申。

defending Gengshen Refers to tranquilly sitting without sleep on the days of Gengshen which means 57th year of the sexagenary cycle.

守规中【shǒu guī zhōng】 指练气功,意识活动集中于丹田或身体之中。

defending mind concentration Refers to concentration of mental activity in Dantian or the body in practicing Qigong. Dantian is divided into the upper Dantian (the region between the eyes), the middle Dantian (the region below the heart) and the lower Dantian (the region below the navel).

守静笃【shǒu jìng dǔ】 指练功中,精神意识活动处于高度清静的状态。

supreme tranquilization Refers to perfect and tranquil state of the spirit and consciousness activities in practicing Qigong.

守灵【shǒu líng】 指心。

defending soul Refers to the heart.

守明堂法【shǒu míng táng fǎ】 为静功。其作法为,身正坐,二目先守明堂,少时明堂发暖,似有蠕动,即从门户而入,将此正念收归土釜,若存若亡,静六根(眼、耳、鼻、舌、身、意),却万虚。久行之,功成健身益寿延年。

exercise for defending nose A static exercise, marked by sitting upright, defending the nose with the eyes that immediately makes the nose warm and seemingly moving like entering from the door, transmitting it to Tufu (the region below the heart), tranquilizing the six roots (the eyes, the ears, the nose, the tongue, the body and the mind) and relaxing all the body. To practice Qigong in such a way will successfully nourish the body and prolong life.

守默【shǒu mò】 即习练气功的养心法,精神处于静止状态。

defending silence Refers to the method to nourish the heart in practicing Qigong in order to tranquilize the essence and the spirit.

守三一【shǒu sān yī】 指气功锻炼中使精、气、神融合。

defending three and one Refers to combination of the essence, Qi and the spirit in practicing Qigong.

守身【shǒu shēn】 即气功引申为指内守精神,外养形体。

defending the body Refers to internal concentration of the essence and spirit for nourishing the body in practicing

S

Qigong.

守身炼形【shǒu shēn liàn xíng】 指意守身神，炼养形体。

defending life and refining body Refers to mentally concentrating the spirit in the body and essentially nourishing the body in practicing Qigong.

守身炼形作丹说【shǒu shēn liàn xíng zuò dān shuō】 源自气功专论，阐述习练气功，形体阴平阳秘出现的景象。

idea about defending the life and refining the body Collected from a monograph, describing the scene of stable Yin and compact Yang in practicing Qigong.

守神【shǒu shén】 指排除外界事物的干扰。

defending spirit Refers to eliminating disturbance of anything in the external world.

守五神【shǒu wǔ shén】 指意守心、肝、肾、脾、肺五脏之神。

defending five spirits Refers to mentally concentrating the spirit from the heart, the liver, the kidney, the spleen and the lung.

守虚无【shǒu xū wú】 指意念内守脑神，虚静恬淡，寂寞无为。

defending nothingness Refers to internal concentration of the spirit in the brain in order to ensure tranquility, calmness, silence and inaction.

守玄白法【shǒu xuán bái fǎ】 为静功。其作法为，清晨或坐，或卧均可。存想泥丸中有黑气，心中有白气，脐中有黄气，三气俱生，如云气覆身。

exercise for concentrating imagination A static exercise, referring to sitting or lying in the morning, imagining black Qi in the mud bolus (the brain), white Qi in the heart and yellow Qi in the navel. These three kinds of Qi in the body are just like cloudy Qi covering the body.

守一【shǒu yī】 ① 指精思固守，与形相抱，形神合一；② 指习练气功之根基；③ 指法于自然；④ 指意识思维活动集中于一；⑤ 指阴阳协调，精神乃治，身体健康。

defending one Refers to ① either defending the essence and thought, interconnection with the body, integration of the body and spirit；② or the foundation for practicing Qigong；③ or following the natural law；④ or concentration of the activities of consciousness and thought；⑤ or regulation of Yin and Yang in order to maintain the essence and spirit as well as to cultivate health.

守一处和【shǒu yī chù hé】 指守住一处真元，使其调达和谐。

defending integration and keeping balance Refers to concentrating genuine origin in order to regulate and to harmonize it.

守一法【shǒu yī fǎ】 为静功。其作法为，避免精神刺激，不喜不怒，认真实践；作法为守身体的一部分，如守丹田，守形体，守精神。功效为稳定精神。

exercise of tranquilization A static exercise, referring to avoidance of stimulating the essence and spirit with serious practice and without pleasure and anger. The practice mainly focuses on defending a special part of the body, such as Dantian, physical region, essence and spirit. The effect of such a practice is to stabilize the essence and the spirit. Dantian is divided into the upper Dantian（the region between the eyes），the middle Dantian（the region below the heart）and the lower Dantian（the region below the navel）.

守一明法【shǒu yī míng fǎ】 为静功。其作法为，守一精明之时，面向日方，意想日之精明，始正赤，终正白，久久正青。守一光明法时，意想日光之光，日中之明。守之无懈，百病除去，身体和柔，得天地之气而延寿。

defending integration and clearing formula A static exercise. In concentrating essential brilliance，the face turns to the sunshine to imagine the essence and brightness of the sun which is red at the beginning and white at the end. In concentrating brightness，imagination should focus on the brightness of the sunshine. Continuous practice in such a way will relieve any diseases，relax the body and prolong life.

守一坛【shǒu yī tán】 指守规中。规中指黄庭，即下丹田。

defending altar Refers to defending the yellow chamber which refers to the lower Dantian（the region below the navel）.

守一要领论【shǒu yī yào lǐng lùn】 源自气功专论，主要阐述练功的姿势虽有行住立坐卧睡的不同，但全在意念上下功夫。

idea about defending the importance Collected from a monograph，mainly describing different ways to practice Qigong like walking，staying，standing up，sitting，lying and sleeping which all depend on the important functions of thought.

守一之宜【shǒu yī zhī yí】 指固精守肾，不妄泄漏，不喜不怒，情志安和，"百

日为小静，二百日为中静，三百日为大静"。

caution for concentration Refers to concentrating the spirit and protecting the kidney without any dispersion，quietness without any pleasure and anger，harmonizing the emotion and mentality. Such a way of practicing Qigong will make "mild quietness after one hundred days，well quietness after two hundred days and great quietness after three hundred days".

守一子【shǒu yī zǐ】 清代气功学家闵一得的另外一个称谓。

Shou Yizi Another name of Min Yide，a great master of Qigong in the Qing Dynasty（1636 AD‐1912 AD）.

守于内息【shǒu yú nèi xī】 即意识活动与呼吸相结合。意识活动集中于呼吸，不使其分散。

defending the internal respiration Refers to combination of consciousness activity and respiration，indicating concentration of consciousness activity on respiration without any dispersion.

守玉关【shǒu yù guān】 为动静相兼功。其作法为，行住坐卧，一意不散，固守丹田，默运神气。

defending immortal pass An exercise combined with dynamic exercise and static exercise，referring to concentration of the mind in walking，sitting，staying and lying in order to defend Dantian and quietly transmit the spirit and Qi. Dantian is divided into the upper Dantian（the region between the eyes），the middle Dantian（the region below the heart）and the lower Dantian（the region below the navel）.

守真【shǒu zhēn】 指内守精神，调合

S

形神,使之达到神形高度稳定的状态。

defending genuineness Refers to internal concentration of the essence and the spirit as well as combination of the body and the spirit in order to enable the spirit and the body to reach the stable state.

守真一【shǒu zhēn yī】 指意守真一之道,即意识思维活动集中统一之意。

defending genuine one Refers to concentrating mind on the genuine way, indicating concentration and unity of the activities of consciousness and thought.

守中【shǒu zhōng】 ① 指习练气功,意识思维活动意守身体中的脏腑,或其他部位;② 指习练气功,意守身体体表正中线的部位;③ 指意守黄庭。

defending the center Refers to ① either concentrating the activities of consciousness and thought in the five Zang-organs (including the heart, the liver, the spleen, the lung and the kidney) and the six Fu-organs (including the gallbladder, the stomach, the small intestine, the large intestine, the bladder and the triple energizer) or other regions in the body; ② or concentrating the mind on the midline of the body; ③ or concentrating the mind on the Yellow Chamber (the region below the navel).

守中抱一【shǒu zhōng bào yī】 即强调气功锻炼中精神内守,形神协调的重要性。

defending center and embracing one Refers to the importance of internal concentration of the essence and spirit as well as regulation of the body and the spirit in practicing Qigong.

守中道【shǒu zhōng dào】 指内壮功的三要则,① 其一为"在乎含其眼光,凝其耳韵,匀其鼻息,缄其口气";② 其二为用手轻揉胃部;③ 其三为"气积而力自积,气充而力自周"。

defending the central way Refers to three principles in strengthening the internal regions. ① The first is "to keep the vision, to concentrate the charm of the ears, to uniform the nasal respiration and to seal oral respiration". ② The second is to mildly knead the stomach region. ③ The third is "to accumulate Qi in order to promote self-accumulation and to enrich Qi in order to promote self-circulation".

首功【shǒu gōng】 为动功。其作法为,两手掩耳,即以第二指压中指上,用第二指弹脑后两骨作响声,谓之鸣天鼓,两手扭项左右反顾,肩膊随转。二十四次,两手交叉,抱项后面仰视,使手与项争力。

head exercise A dynamic exercise, marked by covering the ears with both hands, pressing the middle finger with the second finger, flicking and the two bones behind the brain with sounding by the second finger, turning the hands and scapulae from the left to the right and vice versa for twenty-four times respectively, crossing the hands to hold the neck to observe the back and making the hands and neck to force each other.

首甲定运【shǒu jiǎ dìng yùn】 指从甲子年开始定六十年之运。

decision to move from the first Jia Refers to the movement of sixty years from the first year of Jiazi. The ten heavenly stems and twelve earthly stems are combined with each other to form sixty years, the first of which is Jiazi year.

寿府【shòu fǔ**】** ① 指黄庭；② 亦说指肾。

longevity mansion Refers to ① either the yellow chamber (the region below the navel); ② or the kidney.

寿亲养老新书【shòu qīn yǎng lǎo xīn shū**】** 《寿亲养老新书》为老年医学专著，兼述气功养生法，为元代邹铉所著。

Shouqin Yanglao Xinshu (*New Book about Longevity for Nourishing Old People***)** A monograph of gereology with discussion of Qigong and life cultivation entitled *New Book about Longevity for Nourishing Old People*, written by Zou Xuan in the Yuan Dynasty(1271 AD – 1368 AD).

寿人经【shòu rén jīng**】** 《寿人经》为气功养生专著，由清代气功学家汪晟编辑，主要内容为理脾土诀，理肺金诀、理肾水诀、理肝木诀、理心火诀、坐功诀、长揖诀、导引诀。

Shouren Jing (*Longevity Cano***)** A monograph of Qigong and life cultivation entitled *Longevity Canon*, compiled by Wang Zheng in the Qing Dynasty (1636 AD – 1912 AD), mainly describing the formula of the spleen-earth, the formula of the lung-metal, the formula of the kidney-water, the formula of the liver-wood, the formula of the heart-fire, the formula of sitting practice, formula of long practice and formula of Daoyin.

寿人经长揖法【shòu rén jīng cháng yī fǎ**】** 为动功。其作法为，叉两手，托天当面，作揖伏于地九次，叉两手，左右揖伏于地各五次。功效为疏通四肢腰背筋脉，关节灵通。

exercise of longevity for long salute A dynamic exercise, marked by raising the folded hands to the chin for saluting the sky and the earth for nine times; raising the folded hands to the chin for saluting the earth to the left and right for five times respectively. The effect of such a practice of Qigong is to unobstruct the four limbs, the waist, the back, the sinews, the meridians and the joints.

寿人经理五脏诀【shòu rén jīng lǐ wǔ zàng jué**】** 为动静相兼功口诀，指理脾土诀、理肺金诀、理肾水诀、理肝木诀和理心火诀。

formula for longevity and regulation of the five Zang-organs A formula combined with static exercise and dynamic exercise, referring to regulating the formula of the spleen-earth, the formula of the lung-metal, the formula of the kidney-water, the formula of the liver-wood and the formula of the heart-fire.

寿人经坐功法【shòu rén jīng zuò gōng fǎ**】** 为静功。其作法为，两足曲膝而盘，气由尾闾上达泥丸，下注丹田九次，气由左右两臂，达于手指者七次，气又由左右两股，达足趾七次。功效为疏通周身血脉，调和五脏。

exercise of longevity for sitting practice A static exercise, marked by hunkering with bending the knees. In such a way of practice, Qi flows from coccyx to the mud bolus (the brain) and descends to Dantian for nine times; Qi reaches the fingers from the shoulders for seven times; Qi reaches the toes from the thighs for seven times. The effect of such a way of practice will unobstruct

S

blood vessels in the whole body and balance the five Zang-organs (including the heart, the liver, the spleen, the lung and the kidney). Dantian is divided into the upper Dantian (the region between the eyes), the middle Dantian (the region below the heart) and the lower Dantian (the region below the navel).

寿世保元【shòu shì bǎo yuán】《寿世保元》为医学专著,兼论气功,由明代龚廷贤著,除医论之外,重点介绍"呼吸静功"和"六字气诀"(吹、呼、嘻、呵、嘘、呬),有具体方法和应用主治。

Shoushi Baoyuan (*Protection of the Origin in the Longevity World*)   A monograph of traditional Chinese medicine and Qigong entitled *Protection of the Origin in the Longevity World*, written by Gong Tingxian in the Qing Dynasty (1636 AD‐1912 AD). Apart from traditional Chinese medicine, it also introduces static exercise of respiration and Qi formula with six Chinese characters as well as the methods, application and treatment. The six Chinese characters include Chui (blowing), Hu (exhaling), Xi (sighing), Ke (breathing out), Xu (breathing out slowly) and Xi (panting).

寿世传真【shòu shì chuán zhēn】《寿世传真》为气功养生专著,由清代徐文弼所编,提倡综合调摄,主张应用气功预防调摄,祛邪治病。

Shoushi Chuanzhen (*Transmission of Truth in the Longevity World*)   A monograph of Qigong and life cultivation entitled *Transmission of Truth in the Longevity World*, compiled by Xu Wenbi in the Qing Dynasty (1636 AD‐

1912 AD), suggesting to comprehensively nursing and defending the body with Qigong in order to expel pathogenic factors and prevent diseases.

寿世传真分行外功法【shòu shì chuán zhēn fēn xíng wài gōng fǎ】为动功,指心功、首功、面功、耳功、目功、口功、舌功、齿功、鼻功、手功、足功、肩功、背功、腹功、腰功、肾功。

exercise of longevity for transmitting genuineness and separating external dynamic exercise   A dynamic exercise, referring to the heart exercise, the head exercise, the face exercise, the ear exercise, the eye exercise, the mouth exercise, the tongue exercise, the tooth exercise, the nose exercise, the hand exercise, the foot exercise, the shoulder exercise, the back exercise, the abdomen exercise, the waist exercise and the kidney exercise.

寿世青编【shòu shì qīng biān】《寿世青编》为气功养生专著,由清代龙乘辑,广泛收集了养生却病之道、练功导引之法。

Shoushi Qingbian (*Green Compilation of Longevity World*)   A monograph of Qigong and life cultivation entitled *Green Compilation of Longevity World*, written by Long Cheng in the Qing Dynasty (1636 AD‐1912 AD), entirely collecting the ways to cultivating health, preventing disease and practicing Qigong.

寿世青编导引十六势【shòu shì qīng biān dǎo yǐn shí liù shì】为动功,行动时间为每日子后寅前,两目垂帘,披衣端坐,两手握固跌坐,以左足后跟曲顶肾茎根下动处,不令精窍漏泄。

sixteen ways of longevity for arranging

Daoyin A dynamic exercise, marked by practicing after Zi (the period of the day from 11 p.m. to 1 a.m. in the noon) and before Yin (the period of the day from 3 a.m. to 5 a.m. in the morning), lowering the eyes behind a screen, sitting with throwing on the clothes, holding the insteps with both hands, twisting the left heel to the lower region of the kidney to prevent leakage of male urethra.

寿世青编十二段功【shòu shì qīng biān shí èr duàn gōng】 为动功,即叩齿、咽津、浴面、鸣天鼓、运膏肓、托天、左右开弓、摩丹田、擦内肾、擦涌泉穴、摩夹脊穴、提腿。

exercise of twelve courses for longevity A dynamic exercise, referring to clicking the teeth, swallowing fluid, washing the face, sounding the celestial drum (rubbing the occipital), moving Gaohuang (BL 43), raising the fists upwards, stretching the hands from the left to the right and vice versa, rubbing Dantian, wiping the internal kidney, wiping acupoint Yongquan (KI 1), rubbing acupoint Jiaji (EX‐B2) and lifting the legs.

寿世新编【shòu shì xīn biān】 《寿世新编》为中医专著,兼论气功养生,由清代万潜斋编,书中列举养生要论,强调清心寡欲,调息保精等气功方法。

Shoushi Xinbian (*New Compilation of Longevity*) A monograph of traditional Chinese medicine, also including Qigong and life cultivation, entitled *New Compilation of Longevity*, compiled by Wan Jianzhai in the Qing Dynasty (1636 AD‐1912 AD). It lists the main ideas of life cultivation and em-phasizing the importance of purifying the heart and reducing the desires as well as regulating respiration and stabilizing the essence in practicing Qigong.

受【shòu】 佛家气功习用语,① 指身体受外界影响引起的感受,如痛痒、喜乐、忧悲等;② 指接受而后选择环境,导引入静的精神境界。

reception A common term of Qigong in Buddhism, referring to ① either feeling of the influence from the external world, such as painful itching, happiness and anxiety and sorrow; ② or selection of the state after reception and entering the tranquil state of the essence and the spirit.

梳发【shū fà】 为动功,使头部气血流畅,头脑清醒,疏风、散火、祛邪。

combing exercise A dynamic exercise that can smooth Qi and the blood in the head, sober the brain, dredge wind, disperse fire and eliminate evils.

俞府【shū fǔ】 足少阴肾经中的一个穴位,位于锁骨下缘。这一穴位为气功运行的一个常见部位。

Shufu (**KI 27**) An acupoint in the kidney meridian of foot Shaoyin, located below the clavicle. This acupoint is a region usually used for keeping the essential Qi in practice of Qigong.

疏食【shū shí】 即素食,无油荤之食。

vegetarian diet Refers to food without oil and meat.

熟摩尺宅【shú mó chǐ zhái】 指两手摩面,静心安神以习练气功。

rubbing face An exercise for tranquilizing the heart and stabilizing the spirit in practicing Qigong.

黍米珠【shǔ mǐ zhū】 ① 指内丹,为体内阴阳两方面的相互作用而成;② 指大

S

丹之象。

millet and rice pearls Refers to ① either the internal Dan（pills of immortality）achieved by the mutual activity of Yin and Yang；② or the scene of large Dan（pills of immortality）。

蜀王乔【shǔ wáng qiáo**】** 为动功。其作法为，正坐，伸直腰，两上肢向上伸展，两手掌上仰，用鼻吸气后闭气不息，至极限为止，反复作七次。

king Shu's style A dynamic exercise，marked by sitting upright，stretching the waist，spreading the upper limbs，raising the both fists，stopping breath after breathing in through the nose to the extreme for seven times repeatedly.

蜀王台【shǔ wáng tái**】** 为动功。其作法为，端坐，生腰，直上展两臂，仰两手掌，以鼻纳气，闭之，自极，七息。功效为除胁下积聚。

king Shu's stage A dynamic exercise，marked by sitting upright，stretching the waist，spreading the arms，raising both fists，breathing in through the nose and stopping breath to the extreme for seven times. Such a dynamic exercise can relieve abdominal mass below the rib-sides.

术数【shù shù**】** 即气功。

magical calculation Refers to Qigong，a special explanation of Qigong in ancient China.

束之太紧【shù zhī tài jǐn**】** 指初学气功的人，意守过于紧张，即可引起烦躁火炎之患。

tense mind Indicates that the beginners of Qigong study seem very nervous and are fidgety.

数度【shù dù**】** 指意念从头至足导引，先内后外，反复若干次。

number degree Indicates that consciousness leads Qi from the head to the feet and from the internal first and then to the external for several times.

数息观【shù xī guān**】** 为静功。其作法为，计数呼吸次数，以停止散乱的意识活动。注意计数时形体放松，缓和自然。

idea about timed respiration A static exercise，marked by counting the numbers of respiration to stop dispersion of consciousness activity，and naturally relaxing the body when counting the numbers of respiration.

数息思神【shù xī sī shén**】** 指调节呼吸与调节精神相结合的一种习练方法。

counting respiration and considering the spirit Refers to regulating respiration combined with the regulation of the spirit，which is one method for practicing Qigong.

漱齿【shù chǐ**】** 指经常漱口刷牙，能使牙齿坚固以防虫蛀。

brushing teeth Refers to rinsing the mouth and the teeth in order to strengthen the teeth and prevent being bitten by insects.

漱为醴泉【shù wéi lǐ quán**】** 指鼓漱唾液后滋生的津液，有润泽身体各部之功。

rinsing with sweet spring A term of Qigong，referring to fluid and humor produced after rinsing the mouth for swallowing saliva，which is effective for moistening the whole body.

漱咽灵液【shù yàn líng yè**】** ① 指增强身体抵抗力；② 指体生光滑气香兰；③ 指却灭百邪玉炼颜；④ 指养阴清热，平秘阴阳。

rinsing and swallowing spiritual humor Refers to ① either strengthening the body；② or smoothness of the body like Chinese cymbidium；③ or eliminating all pathogenic factors to refine the face；④ or nourishing Yin，clearing heat and balancing Yin and Yang.

霜降九月中坐功 【shuāng jiàng jiǔ yuè zhōng zuò gōng】 为动功。其作法为，每日丑寅时（一至五时），平坐，舒两手攀两足，随用足间力，纵而复收五七次，叩齿、吐纳、咽液。

sitting exercise in September with frost descent A dynamic exercise，marked by sitting in Chou（the period of a day from 1 a.m. to 3 a.m. in the morning）and Yin（the period of a day from 3 a.m. to 5 a.m. in the morning），relaxing the hands to hold the feet，releasing and turning with the sole energy for five to seven times，clicking the teeth，breathing in and out，and swallowing humor.

水不胜火【shuǐ bù shèng huǒ】 水为阴，火为阳。指中年以上之人，多阴虚阳亢，上热下寒。

water failing to control fire Water refers to Yin and fire refers to Yang. Among those more than mid-aged people，Yin is often deficient while Yang is always hyperactive；the upper part of the body is often hot while the lower part of the body is always cold.

水朝元【shuǐ cháo yuán】 指五脏之气上朝天元。

water turning to origin Refers to Qi from the five Zang-organs（including the heart，the liver，the spleen，the lung and the kidney）flowing up to the celestial origin.

水潮【shuǐ cháo】 喻增加口腔内的唾液。

torrent Refers to increasing saliva in the mouth.

水潮除后患法 【shuǐ cháo chú hòu huàn fǎ】 动静相兼功。平明睡时，即起端坐，凝神息虑，舌舐上腭，闭口调息，津液自生，渐至满口，分作三次，以意送下。

method for increasing saliva to eliminate disease An exercise combined with dynamic exercise and static exercise，marked by sitting after lying in the daybreak，concentrating the spirit，stabilizing respiration，raising the tongue to the upper jaw，closing the mouth to regulate breath，naturally producing fluid and humor fully into the mouth for three times in order to push it downwards.

水道【shuǐ dào】 ① 指水液运行的通道；② 指足阳明胃经中的一个穴位。这一穴位为气功运行的一个常见部位。

water way Refers to ① either passageway of water and fluid；② or an acupoint point located in the stomach meridian of foot Yangming，known as Shuidao（ST 28）. This acupoint is a region usually used for keeping the essential Qi in practice of Qigong.

水沟【shuǐ gōu】 督脉的一个穴位，位于人中之中。这一穴位为气功运行的一个常见部位。

Shuigou（GV 26） An acupoint in the governor meridian，located in the center of Renzhong（the region between the nose and the mouth）. This acupoint is a region usually used for keeping the essential Qi in practice of Qigong.

水谷之海【shuǐ gǔ zhī hǎi】 指的是胃，胃主受纳，腐熟水谷。

water and cereal sea Refers to the

S

stomach that receives and digests water and food.

水观法【shuǐ guān fǎ】 为静功。其作法为，盘膝坐势，自然呼吸，任其自然。

water inspecting exercise A static exercise, marked by sitting quietly, crossing the legs, breathing naturally and staying naturally.

水火【shuǐ huǒ】 水为阴，火为阳。以水火变化来比喻阴阳协调变化。

water and fire Water refers to Yin and fire refers to Yang. Usually the changes of water and fire are used to describe the changes of Yin and Yang.

水火半斤【shuǐ huǒ bàn jīn】 水指元精，火指元神。水火半斤指水火相当，调和运炼。

water and fire in equilibrium In this term, water refers to the original essence and fire refers to the original spirit, indicating that water and fire coordinate and regulate with each other in practicing Qigong.

水火发端处【shuǐ huǒ fā duān chù】 指精气聚散之处。

location of water and fire Refers to the place where essence and Qi are concentrated and also dispersed.

水火既济【shuǐ huǒ jì jì】 指心肾相交。

balance of water and fire Refers to combination of the heart and the kidney.

水火交【shuǐ huǒ jiāo】 精属水，神属火。

combination of water and fire The essence belongs to water and the spirit belongs to fire.

水火交，永不老【shuǐ huǒ jiāo yǒng bù lǎo】 水，即真水；火，即真火。水上

火下，借戊己真土之枢机，逐真火上升，真水下降，同归土釜，水火既济，结成金丹。

combination of water and fire ensuring longevity In this term, water refers to genuine water, fire refers to genuine fire. Based on the earth foundation, water ascends and fire descends, eventually enabling genuine fire to ascend and genuine water to descend, finally all entering Dantian. Combination of water and fire ensures the formation of golden Dan (pills of immortality). Dantian is divided into the upper Dantian (the region between the eyes), the middle Dantian (the region below the heart) and the lower Dantian (the region below the navel).

水火全功【shuǐ huǒ quán gōng】 指水火既济，心肾相交。

full effect of water and fire Refers to harmonization of water and fire as well as combination between the heart and the kidney.

水火调节法【shuǐ huǒ tiáo jié fǎ】 为静功，主要调身、调气、调神。其作法为，自然坐式或自然站式均可。安神调气，使呼吸平和后，可不注意呼吸。

exercise for regulating water and fire A static exercise for regulating the body, Qi and spirit, marked by naturally sitting or standing up, stabilizing the spirit, regulating Qi, and paying less attention to respiration when respiration is pacified and balanced.

水火相求【shuǐ huǒ xiāng qiú】 源自气功专论，说明水火相求，合二而一是维持身体各部稳定的基础。

mutual demand of water and fire Mutual demand of water and fire is collected from a monograph，describing that water and fire mutually depend on each other to stabilize the body.

水瘕痹【shuǐ jiǎ bì】 气功适应证，指水结成形而小便不适之病症。

dysuria An indication of Qigong，usually caused by stagnation of water and retention of urine.

水晶塔【shuǐ jīng tǎ】 即洁净透明。喻习练气功出现的景象，形体如冰雕玉砌，内外澄洁。

crystal pagoda Refers to cleanness and transparency，describing the image of Qigong practice like ice sculpture and jadeware.

水炼法【shuǐ liàn fǎ】 为静功。先想两肾中间有一点极明，注视良久，水火交媾，玉池水生。

water exercise technique A static exercise，marked by imagining a little brightness in between the two kidneys，integrating water and fire with each other and producing water in the mouth after long period of fixed observation.

水轮【shuǐ lún】 眼科五轮之一，指瞳孔。

water wheel One of the five kinds of wheels in the ophthalmology，referring to the pupila.

水气【shuǐ qì】 气功适应证，① 指水肿；② 指水饮、痰饮。

water Qi An indication of Qigong，refers to ① edema，② retained fluid and phlegmatic rheuma.

水泉【shuǐ quán】 大敦的一个别称，是足厥阴肝经的一个穴位，位于踇趾外侧，为气功常用意守部位。

Shuiquan A synonym of Dadun（LR 1），an acupoint in the liver meridian of foot Jueyin，located lateral to the big toe. This acupoint is a region usually used in practice of Qigong.

水仙赋【shuǐ xiān fù】 《水仙赋》为气功专著，为南梁陶弘景所著。

Shuixian Fu（*Narcissus Composition*） A monograph of Qigong entitled *Narcissus Composition*，written by Tao Hongjing in the South Liang Dynasty（502 AD - 557 AD）.

水相观【shuǐ xiāng guān】 为静功。其作法为，意想水澄清、明洁，精神集中于水而不分散。

water image inspection A static exercise，marked by clarifying the mind with water and concentrating the spirit on water without any dispersion.

水泻导引法【shuǐ xiè dǎo yǐn fǎ】 为动功。其作法为，心静神定，并双目，交双足站立，紧缩肛门，两手握拳垂直，缩腹耸肩，运气上提，使督脉气上升，治腹泻。

exercise of Daoyin for diarrhea A dynamic exercise，marked by tranquilizing the heart and stabilizing the spirit，closing the eyes，standing with crossed feet，tightening the anus，holding both hands，contracting the abdomen，shrugging shoulders，raising up Qi for moving，and ascending Qi in the governor meridian in order to treat diarrhea.

水脏【shuǐ zàng】 指肾，肾主水，调节人体水液代谢。

water viscus Refers to the kidney that regulates water metabolism in the body.

水真水，火真火【shuǐ zhēn shuǐ huǒ zhēn huǒ】 人心中一点真液，即真水；肾中一点真阳，即真火。

Water with genuine water and fire with genuine fire. The genuine fluid in the heart belongs to genuine water, the genuine Yang in the kidney belongs to genuine fire.

水之功效【shuǐ zhī gōng xiào】 说明水的重要意义,即神水生于气中,金液降于天上。

effect of water Refers to the importance of water in life. Traditionally it is believed that spiritual water originates from Qi and golden fluid descends from the sky.

水之精为志,火之精为神【shuǐ zhī jīng wéi zhì huǒ zhī jīng wéi shén】 指神、志由心火和肾水所主。

The essence in water is will while the essence in the fire is spirit. This is a celebrated dictum in Qigong classics. The so-called spirit and will are controlled by heart fire and kidney water.

水中火发【shuǐ zhōng huǒ fā】 水为阴,水中为阴之极,火为阳,火发为阳生。火发于水中,即阴极一阳生。

fire appearing in water Water pertains to Yin and the central part of water reflects the extreme stage of Yin; fire pertains to Yang and hyperactivity of fire indicates the production of Yang. That is why fire occurs in water, indicating that extreme Yin produces Yang.

水中银【shuǐ zhōng yín】 喻心,属火,为正阳之精;指神气。

silver in water Refers to the heart that belongs to fire; or spiritual Qi.

水肿【shuǐ zhǒng】 气功适应证,指体内水湿停留,面目、四肢、胸腹甚至全身浮肿的一种疾病。

edema An indication of Qigong, marked by retention of water dampness and dropsy of the face, the eyes, the four limbs, the chest and the abdomen.

水肿候导引法【shuǐ zhǒng hòu dǎo yǐn fǎ】 为静功。其作法为,正坐,摆动两臂,闭气不息十二遍。可利水通络,调和五脏气血,治五劳,水肿。

exercise of Daoyin for edema A static exercise, marked by sitting quietly, swinging the shoulders, closing breath for twelve times in order to promote water, to relax collaterals, to regulate Qi and the blood in the five Zang-organs (including the heart, the liver, the spleen, the lung and the kidney), and to treat five kinds of consumption and edema.

睡不厌缩,觉不厌伸【shuì bù yàn suō jué bù yàn shēn】 指人睡觉时姿式宜侧卧如弓,以使精气不走失;醒时舒伸两脚,以使经脉气血流畅。此亦为养生之道,属动静相兼功。

Sleep should not avoid stooping and waking up should not avoid stretching. This is a celebrated dictum, indicating that in sleep one should lie on one side like a bow in order to prevent dispersion of the essential Qi; and that in waking up one should stretching the feet in order to promote flow of Qi and the blood in the meridians and vessels. This is also an exercise combined with dynamic exercise and static exercise for cultivating life.

睡功玄诀【shuì gōng xuán jué】 指睡功中深奥的道理。

supreme formula for lying practice Supreme formula for lying practice is a term of Qigong, referring to the principle of exercise for lying practice.

睡如猫,精不逃;睡如狗,精不走【shuì rú māo jīng bù táo shuì rú gǒu

jīng bù zǒu】　主要强调睡的姿势，若如此法，能养真元之气而固精。

Sleep in the way of a cat, the essence will not dissipate; sleep in the way of a dog, the essence will not disappear.　This is a celebrated dictum, emphasizing the style of sleep. In such a way of sleep will nourish the genuine and original Qi and protect the essence.

顺逆【shùn nì】　① 顺指一生二，二生三，三生万物，逆为合三归一；② 指五行相生为顺，相克为逆；③ 指还精补脑。

smoothness and converse　① Smoothness refers to one producing two, two producing three and three producing all the things in the universe; ② while converse refers to integration of three into one. Among the five elements (including wood, fire, earth, metal and water), smoothness refers to promotion while converse refers to restriction; ③ smoothness and converse also refer to concentrating the essence in order to tonify the brain.

顺逆三关【shùn nì sān guān】　指炼精化气，炼气化神，炼神还虚。

three joints in smoothness and converse　Refers to refining the essence to transform Qi, refining Qi to transform the spirit and refining the spirit to improve deficiency.

司马承祯【sī mǎ chéng zhēn】　唐代气功学家，著有气功学专著。

Sima Chengzhen　A great master of Qigong in the Tang Dynasty (618 AD – 907 AD), writing several monographs about Qigong.

司马承祯导引存想【sī mǎ chéng zhēn dǎo yǐn cún xiǎng】　为动静相兼功。每日自夜半子时至日中午时，先平

卧舒展四肢，次起身导引，喘息均定。久作身体轻和，健康延年。

Sima Chengzhen's contemplation of Daoyin　An exercise combined with static exercise and dynamic exercise, marked by practice from Zi (the period of the day from 11 p.m. to 1 a.m.) and Wu (the period of the day from 11 a.m. to 1 p.m.), lying on the back first to stretch the four limbs, then standing up to activate Daoyin with normal respiration in order to relax the body, to cultivate health and to prolong life.

司马承祯导引术【sī mǎ chéng zhēn dǎo yǐn shù】　指选择天气清和晴朗的日子，于卯时进行，先解散头发，用于从前额向上至头顶梳理三百六十五下，将头发散放于背后。面向东平坐，两手握固，闭目集中精神，叩齿三百六十下，放松身体，调匀呼吸。

Sima Chengzhen's exercise of Daoyin　Refers to practice of Qigong in Mao (the period of a day from 5 a.m. to 7 a.m. in the morning) when the weather is fine, marked by releasing hair first with the hands combining hair from the forehead to the top of the head for 365 times, then sitting in the east with hands holding strictly, closing the eyes to concentrate the spirit and clicking the teeth for 360 times in order to relax the body and to regulate respiration.

司马子微【sī mǎ zǐ wēi】　唐代气功学家司马承祯的另外一个称谓，著有气功学专著。

Sima Ziwei　Another name of Sima Chengzhen, a great master of Qigong in the Tang Dynasty (618 AD – 907 AD) who wrote several monographs about Qigong.

丝竹空【sī zhú kōng】 手少阳三焦经的一个穴位，位于眉毛外侧段凹陷处。这一穴位为气功运行的一个常见部位。

Sizhukong（**TE 23**） An acupoint in the triple energizer meridian of hand Shaoyang, also called Juliao or Muliao, located in the lateral depression of the eyebrow. This acupoint is a region usually used for keeping the essential Qi in practice of Qigong.

思【sī】 ① 指思想、意志等精神活动；② 指思考功德过失而决定行为；③ 指人体七情之一，思虑过度，引起神形失调而致病。

thinking Refers to ① either the activities of thought, consciousness and spirit; ② or thinking about how to solve the problems of negligence of virtue; ③ or one of the seven emotions, indicating excessive contemplation that has imbalanced the spirit and body and caused various diseases.

思虑之神【sī lǜ zhī shén】 指自然、社会因素引起的意识思维活动。

spirit of thinking and considering Refers to the activities of thought and consciousness related to natural factors and social factors.

思其身洞白【sī qí shēn dòng bái】 为静功，指存思自己身中纯白无杂，冰晶玉洁，为古代存想功法之一。

pure white imagination of the body A static exercise, referring to purity and flawlessness in the mind and body, which is one way of inward contemplation in ancient China.

思三台厌恶法【sī sān tái yàn wù fǎ】 为动静相兼功。其作法为，在清净房中，正坐，想三台遮盖头部，意念两肾气从胸中出与三台相接，稍过，叩齿十四遍，用鼻轻微吸气，然后闭气，待津液满口时咽下。

exercise of three stages for contemplating averseness An exercise combined with dynamic exercise and static exercise, marked by sitting upright in the clean and quiet room, imagining that the three stages cover the head and kidney Qi from the chest connects with the three stages, then clicking the teeth for fourteen times, inhaling mildly through the nose and reducing respiration for swallowing saliva when fluid and humor are full in the mouth.

思身神【sī shēn shén】 指思维意识活动集中于身中之神，以稳定情绪。

thinking the body and the spirit Refers to concentrating the activities of thought and consciousness in the spirit in order to stabilize the mood.

思维修【sī wéi xiū】 佛家气功习用语，指佛家静坐凝神，专注一境的习练方法。

thinking cultivation A common term of Qigong in Buddhism, referring to sitting quietly and concentrating the spirit in practicing Qigong in Buddhism.

死灰【sǐ huī】 指心既然不动，如枯木一般。

dead ash Refers to tranquility of the heart, just like withered tree.

死气【sǐ qì】 指六阴时之气。

dead Qi Refers to the Qi in the time controlled by six kinds of Yin.

四不【sì bù】 指不视、不听、不言、不虑，避免外界刺激，而稳定情绪、养气、养形、全性。

four kinds of no Refers to no vision, no listening, no speech and no consideration in order to prevent irritation by external world and to stabilize the mind for cultivating Qi, nourishing the body and perfecting the property.

四不得【sì bù dé】 即道家对练功者在道德修养、意识修养上的四点要求。

four undesirables Refers to four requirements of moral cultivation and emotional cultivation for practicing Qigong in Daoism,

四禅定【sì chán dìng】 佛家气功方法,指处禅定、二禅定、三禅定、四禅定。

four dhyana A method for Qigong practice in Buddhism, including first dhyana, second dhyana, third dhyana and fourth dhyana.

四大【sì dà】 指道大、天大、地大、人大。

four kinds of greatness Refers to great Dao, great sky, great earth and great man.

四大不调【sì dà bù tiáo】 指代身体的四种不适现状。

four major incoordinate ways Refers to four disorders in the body.

四得【sì dé】 指练功达到某种理度时,人体阴、阳、神、气得到高度结合和统一的景况。

four states Refers to the level of Qigong practice, indicating coordination and unification of Yin, Yang, the spirit and Qi.

四德【sì dé】 指行四德,与社会相适应,才能维持精神意识活动的有序化运动。

four moralities Refers to keeping the four moralities in doing anything in order to adapt to the social conditions and to maintain the normal activities of spirit and consciousness.

四定【sì dìng】 指心定、力定、神定、息定。

four tranquilizations Refers to tranquilizing the heart, the energy, the spirit and the respiration.

四段锦【sì duàn jǐn】 为动功。其作法为,站立,双脚平拉开以肩相齐,调匀呼吸,双眼平视前方,排除杂念,为预备式。

four sectional exercise A dynamic exercise, marked by standing up with both feet stretched to correspond to the shoulders, regulating respiration and observing the front with the eyes in order to eliminate distracting thought and to prepare for practicing Qigong.

四根结【sì gēn jié】 指经脉之气的起始和归结之所,为气功意守部位。

four starts and ends Refers to the region where Qi in the meridians starts and ends, which is the region for concentration in practicing Qigong.

四关【sì guān】 ① 指耳、目、心、口;② 指四肢肘、膝四大关节;③ 指肘、膝关节的五俞。

four cols Refers to ① either the ears, the eyes, the heart and the mouth; ② or the four elbows and the four joints in the knees; ③ or the five acupoints located in the elbows and the joints of the knees.

四关三部【sì guān sān bù】 四关三部中的四关指四肢的肘膝关节;三部指诊脉的人迎、寸口、跗阳三个部位。

four joints and three regions In this term, the so-called four joints and three regions refers to the joints in the knees and elbows; the so-called three regions refers to Renying (ST 9), Cunkou (radial artery pulsation) and

Fuyang（BL 59）.

四官【sì guān】 指目、舌、鼻、耳。

four orifices Refers to the eyes, tongue, nose and ears.

四合【sì hé】 指气功过程中神形合一的状态。

four integrations Refer to the manifestations of the spirit and boy integrated with each other in practicing Qigong.

四极【sì jí】 ① 四肢的别称；② 也指四方。

four extremities Four extremities refer to ① either the synonym of the four limbs；② or the four directions.

四季摄养法【sì jì shè yǎng fǎ】 为静功。其作法为，先春养阳法，先夏养阳法，先秋养阴法，先冬养阳法。

exercise for seasonal life cultivation Exercise for seasonal life cultivation is a static exercise，referring to nourishing Yang in spring；nourishing Yang in summer；nourishing Yin in autumn；and nourishing Yang in winter.

四街【sì jiē】 指经脉之气汇聚和流通的四大通道，称谓气街。

four streets Refers to the four great ways through which Qi from the meridians coordinates with each other.

四灵【sì líng】 指肝魂、肺魄、心神、肾志。

four souls Refers to the ethereal soul in the liver，the corporeal soul in the lung，the spirit in the heart and the will in the kidney.

四六【sì liù】 指二十四种损坏情志的精神活动。

four-six Refers to twenty-four kinds of spiritual activities that damage emotion.

四配五气【sì pèi wǔ qì】 指练功时将五脏之精气凝聚于中宫，为"结丹"做好准备。

compatibility of Qi in the five Zang-organs Refers to concentration of the spiritual Qi from the five Zang-organs to the middle chamber for construction of Dan（pills of immortality）.

四配阴阳【sì pèi yīn yáng】 源自气功专论，说明乾坤作用在于调节自然阴阳。

compatibility of Yin and Yang Collected from a monograph of Qigong，explaining that the function of Qian Trigram and Kun Trigram is to regulate natural Yin and Yang.

四气诀【sì qì jué】 为静功。其作法为，春肝气盛者，调嘘气以利之；夏心气盛者，调呵气以疏之；秋肺气盛者，调咽气以泻之；冬肾气盛者，调吹气以平之。

formula for seasonal Qi A static exercise. Exuberance of liver Qi in spring can promote slow respiration；exuberance of heart Qi in summer can dredge abused Qi；exuberance of lung Qi in autumn can pour laryngeal Qi；exuberance of kidney Qi in winter can regulate respiration.

四气摄生图【sì qì shè shēng tú】 《四气摄生图》为养生学专著，兼收气功论述，作者和成书年代不详。

Siqi Shesheng Tu（*Pictures About Regimen in the Four Seasons*） A monograph about life cultivation and Qigong entitled *Pictures About Regimen in the Four Seasons*. The author and the concerned dynasty were unknown.

四气调神【sì qì tiáo shén】 动静相兼功，阐述人体顺应春温、夏热、秋凉、冬寒四时气候的变化来调摄精神活动。

seasonal regulation of Qi An exercise

combined with dynamic exercise and static exercise, describing the fact that human body should conform to warm spring, hot summer, cool autumn and cold winter in order to regulate the spiritual activity.

四气调神大论【sì qì tiáo shén dà lùn】《一黄帝内经·素问》的一个篇名。主要论述了春夏秋冬四时气候的变化规律和人应该如何去顺时养生的方法。

great discussion about regulating spirit with four kinds of Qi The title of a chapter in *Plain Conversation* in Huangdi Neijing（entitled *Yellow Emperor's Internal Canon of Medicine*）, mainly describing about the changing rules of Qi in spring, summer, autumn and winter as well as about how to follow the changes of Qi in the four seasons in order to cultivate life.

四神【sì shén】 指朱砂、水银、铅、硝。

four spirits Refer to cinnabar, mercury, lead and saltpeter.

四慎【sì shèn】 指习练气功,一慎口舌,二慎舌利,三慎处闹,四慎力斗。常思过多,即可安时处和,和调神形。

four cautions The practice of Qigong, referring to being cautious about the mouth and the tongue, lingual function, disturbance and combating. Such ways of caution can ensure balance and harmony and regulate the spirit and the body.

四时【sì shí】 ①指身中之四时,即一岁至三十、三十至六十、六十至九十、九十至百岁或百二十岁;②指年中的四时,即春温、夏热、秋凉、冬寒;③指月中之四时;④指日中之四时;⑤佛家指晨朝、日中、黄昏、夜半为四时。

four periods Refers to ① either the four times in a life, including one year to thirty years, thirty years to sixty years, sixty years to ninety years, and ninety years to one hundred year or one hundred and twenty years; ② or four seasons in a year, i. e. spring, summer, autumn and winter; ③ or four periods in a month; ④ or four periods in a day; ⑤ or morning, noon, dusk and midnight in Buddhism.

四太【sì tài】 指道有太易、太初、太始、太素。

four kinds of supremeness Refers to the fact that Dao contains supreme in simplicity, origin, initialization and plainness.

四威仪【sì wēi yí】 指佛家气功中的行、住、坐、卧四种功法。

four behavioral modes Refers to four methods of Qigong practice in Buddhism, including moving, staying, sitting and lying.

四相【sì xiàng】 指佛家中的四种呼吸状态,也就是调息的功夫。

four demonstrations Refers to the four ways of respiration in Buddhism, indicating the skills of regulating respiration.

四象【sì xiàng】 ①指伏羲八卦,一分为二,二分为四;②指金、木、水、火;③指太阴、少阴、太阳、少阳。

four images Refers to ① ether the Eight Trigrams created by Fu Xi, among which one develops into two and two develops into four; ② or four elements, i. e. metal, wood, water and fire; ③ or Taiyin, Shaoyin, Taiyang and Shaoyang.

四形【sì xíng】 指形和、形逸、形刚、

S

形骸。

four physiques Refers to harmony, leisure, firmness and pressure of the body.

四远【sì yuǎn】 指习练气功,一当远嫌疑,二当远小人,三当远苟得,四当远行止。依此四远,可避免精神刺激,稳定情绪。

four ways of leaving Refers to practicing Qigong, characterized by relieving suspicion, parting villain, avoiding irregularity and refusing to run far away, which can prevent irritating the spirit and stabilize the emotion.

四月中导引法【sì yuè zhōng dǎo yǐn fǎ】 为功法。四月中每日寅卯时,坐定一刻,左手朝天,右手按住胸部,引气上升入到咽喉处十五次,使咽部津液下降。调和阴阳,发散肺、脐之积滞,疏达气机。

exercise of Daoyin in the middle of April A dynamic exercise, marked by sitting a while in Yin (the period of a day from 3 a. m. to 5 a. m. in the morning) and Mao (the period of a day from 5 a. m. to 7 a. m. in the morning), rising up the left hand, pressing the chest with the right hand, promoting Qi to enter the throat for fifteen times and descending fluid from the throat in order to harmonize Yin and Yang, to disperse stagnation in the lung and navel, and to soothe the functional activity of Qi.

四诊【sì zhěn】 指望诊、闻诊、问诊、切诊。

four diagnostic methods Refers to inspection, listening and smelling, inquiry and taking pulse.

四正【sì zhèng】 ① 指子、午、卯、酉四时;② 指东、西、南、北四个正方向。

four kinds of righteousness Refers to ① either four periods, i. e. Zi (the period of a day from 11 p. m. to 1 a. m.), Wu (the period of a day from 11 a. m. to 1 p. m.), Mao (the period of a day from 5 a. m. to 7 a. m. in the morning) and You (the period of a day from 5 p. m. to 7 p. m. in the afternoon); ② or four directions, i. e. the east, the west, the south and the north.

四政【sì zhèng】 即四方之政,指土运主岁平气之年的正常情况。

four ways of governing Refers to governing in the four directions, indicating the normal function of earth reign governing a normal year.

四肢拘挛不得屈伸【sì zhī jū luán bù dé qū shēn】 气功适应证,指由于人体虚弱,皮肤汗孔开疏、风邪乘虚而入,损伤于筋所引起的四肢拘挛不得屈伸之症。

inability to flex and stretch due to spasm of the limbs An indication of Qigong, caused by opening of sweat pores and invasion of pathogenic wind due to weakness of the body.

四肢拘挛不得屈伸导引法【sì zhī jū luán bù dé qū shēn dǎo yǐn fǎ】 为动功,方法多样。如坐,两手抱左膝,伸直腰,用鼻深吸气七次,展右脚,再如两手抱右膝至胸部。强腰脚,补肝肾。

exercise of Daoyin for inability to flex and stretch due to spasm of the limbs A dynamic exercise with various methods, such as sitting with both hands holding the knees, straightening the waist, breathing through the nose for seven times and stretching the right foot; holing the right knee with both hands to the chest in order to strengthen the waist and the feet as well as to tonify the liver and the kidney.

四肢神去【sì zhī shén qù】 指四肢神损伤于骨关节重滞不动。

loss of spirit in the four limbs Refers to the spirit in the four limbs is damaged by stagnation of the joints.

四肢之一【sì zhī zhī yī】 指手足心，为气功锻炼中四肢的守意部位。

one of the parts in the four limbs Refers to the palms and soles, which are the regions for concentrating the mind in practicing Qigong.

嵩山【sōng shān】 位于山东登封，唐代著名气功家司马承祯曾在此进行气功实践活动。

Songshan Mountain Located in the Dengfeng County in Shandong Province, where Sima Chengzhen, a great master of Qigong in the Tang Dynasty (618 AD – 907 AD), practiced Qigong.

嵩山服气法【sōng shān fú qì fǎ】 为静功。其作法为，每日常卧，摄心绝想，闭气握固，鼻引口吐，无令耳闻，唯是细微。

exercise for taking Qi in Songshan Mountain A static exercise, marked by lying every day, controlling the heart to eliminate any thought, stopping respiration forcefully, inhaling through the nose and exhaling through the mouth, avoiding to hear about anything and acting mildly.

嵩山太无先生气经【sōng shān tài wú xiān shēng qì jīng】 《嵩山太无先生气经》为气功专著，重点阐述形与气的关系。作者不详。

Songshan Taiwu Xiansheng Qijing (*Mr. Tai Wu's Canon of Qi in Songshan Mountain*) Songshan Taiwu Xiansheng Qijing is a monongraph of Qigong entitled *Mr. Tai Wu's Canon of Qi in Songshan Mountain*, mainly describing the interrelation of the body and Qi. The author was unknown.

宋玄白卧雷【sòng xuán bái wò léi】 为动功，即仰面正卧，两手从胸口到肚脐周围往来按摩，翻江搅海，运气九口。

Song Xuan lying on snow A dynamic exercise, marked by lying upright, kneading from the chest to the abdomen and navel with both hands like turning in the river and rotating in the sea, and finally moving Qi from nine times.

送归土釜【sòng guī tǔ fǔ】 指凝神入气后产药。土釜指丹田。

delivering into cauldron Refers to production of medicinal by concentration of the spirit in Qi. In this term, cauldron refers to Dantian which is divided into the upper Dantian (the region between the eyes), the middle Dantian (the region below the heart) and the lower Dantian (the region below the navel).

送气【sòng qì】 指意念导引自然之气。

delivering Qi Refers to leading natural Qi with consciousness.

送气法【sòng qì fǎ】 为静功。其作法为，每清朝初，面向午，展两手于膝上，心眼观气入项下达涌泉，朝朝如此。

exercise for delivering Qi A static exercise, marked by imagining to face the noon at early morning, putting the hands on the knees, observing Qi with the eyes in the heart to lead it into Yongquan (KI 1) repeatedly every morning.

送神之地【sòng shén zhī dì】　指耳。
the place for delivering the spirit　Refers to the ears.

苏沈良方【sū shěn liáng fāng】　《苏沈良方》为中医专著,兼论气功,刊于公元 1075 年,以临床验方为主,兼及医理、医案、本草、灸法等。作者不详。
Sushen Liangfang (*Su Shen's Best Formula*)　A monograph of traditional Chinese medicine with discussion of Qigong entitled *Su Shen's Best Formula* published in 1075, mainly describing the clinical experience in dealing with any diseases, also mentioning the theory of medicine, medical records, materia medica, acupuncture and moxibustion. The author was unknown.

苏轼【sū shì】　宋代著名的文学家和诗人,精于气功研究,注重气功实践,善于静功。
Su Shi　A great litterateur and poet in the Song Dynasty (960 AD – 1279 AD). He was skillful in studying Qigong, paying great attention to Qigong practice and emphasizing static exercise.

苏轼气功术【sū shì qì gōng shù】　为静功。其作法为,每夜子时以后披衣起,面东偏南,盘足,叩齿三十六通。意想内观五脏:肺色白、肝色青、脾色黄、心色赤、肾色黑。随后意想心为火,光明洞彻照耀入下丹田中。
Su Shi's exercise of Qigong　A static exercise, marked by getting up in Zi (the period of the day from 11 p. m. to 1 a. m.), turning to the east and near the south, crossing the feet, clicking the teeth for thirty-six times, imagining to observe the colors of the five Zang-organs (white color of the lung, green color of the liver, yellow color of the spleen, red color of the heart and black color of the kidney) and finally imagining fire in the heart that brightens the lower Dantian (the region below the navel).

苏玄朗【sū xuán lǎng】　晋隋时期著名的气功学家苏元朗的另外一个称谓。苏元朗曾著有三部气功专著,据说活了三百多年。
Su Xuanlang　Another name of Su Yuanlang, a great master of Qigong in the Jin Dynasty (266 AD – 420 AD) and Sui Dynasty (581 AD – 618 AD) who wrote three monographs of Qigong. It was said that he lived for three hundred years.

苏元朗【sū yuán lǎng】　晋隋时期的一位著名的气功学家,著有三部气功专著,据说活了三百多年。
Su Yuanlang　A great master of Qigong in the Jin Dynasty (266 AD – 420 AD) and Sui Dynasty (581 AD – 618 AD) and wrote three monographs of Qigong. It was said that he lived for three hundred years.

苏子瞻【sū zǐ zhān】　宋代著名的文学家和诗人苏轼的另外一个称谓。苏轼精于气功研究,注重气功实践,善于静功。
Su Zizhan　Another name of Su Shi, a great litterateur and poet in the Song Dynasty (960 AD – 1279 AD). Su Shi was skillful in studying Qigong, paying great attention to Qigong practice and emphasizing static exercise.

素华始玄初元内景【sù huá shǐ xuán chū yuán nèi jǐng】　其作法为,于夏历每月初一日夜间,在清净的室内坐定入静,意想自己坐于昆仑上顶,下为大海,烟波浩渺，无边无际，自水底透起一月轮，有微光。

internal scene with pure magnificence and supreme origin A static exercise，marked by sitting quietly in a clear room at night on the first day of every month in summer，imagining to have reached the Kunlun Mountain peak，entered the large sea without any limit and observed glimmer in the sea.

素锦衣裳黄云带【sù jǐn yī shang huáng yún dài】 指肺的外象和结构。

silk clothes with yellow cloud belt A celebrated dictum，referring to the manifestation and structure of the lung.

素髎【sù liáo】 督脉中的一个穴位，位于鼻尖正中。这一穴位为气功运行的一个常见部位。

Suliao（GV 25） An acupoint in the governor meridian，located in the middle of nose tip. This acupoint is a region usually used for keeping the essential Qi in practice of Qigong.

素履往【sù lǚ wǎng】 指人行为坦白，意识纯朴，即可稳定情绪，行其所愿。

open-hearted Refers to frank and honest behavior that can stabilize the mind and realize the desire.

素朴散人【sù pǔ sǎn rén】 指清代气功学家刘一明，其撰写了多部专著，介绍了气功的基本理论和方法。

frank and honest man Refers to Liu Yiming who was a great master of Qigong in the Qing Dynasty（1636 AD - 1912 AD）and wrote several monographs about Qigong to introduce the basic theory and practice of Qigong.

宿食不消【sù shí bù xiāo】 气功适应证，本病多由于脏气虚弱，脾胃有寒，阳气不运，致食入不易消化。

dyspepsia An indication of Qigong，usually caused by deficiency of visceral Qi，coldness of the spleen and stomach，and inactivation of Yang Qi.

宿食不消候导引法【sù shí bù xiāo hòu dǎo yǐn fǎ】 为动功，方法多样。如正坐，伸直腰，右手上举仰掌，左手托左胁，用鼻尽力吸气七次。温中散寒，消食导滞，治胃中寒气，食不消化。

exercise of Daoyin for dyspepsia A dynamic exercise with various methods，such as sitting upright，stretching the waist，raising the right hand to lift the fist，supporting the left flank with the left hand，and inhaling Qi through the nose for seven times for warming the center to disperse cold and digesting food to solve stagnation. Such a dynamic exercise can cure cold Qi in the stomach and dyspepsia.

塑锁梳法【sù suǒ shū fǎ】 静功三法，① 指塑法，即习练气功时调身的方法；② 指锁法，即练气功时，闭其口，若以锁锁住，不得开；③ 指梳发，即塑锁皆是制外之法，梳则由外而内。

exercise for sculpturing locking and combing Refers to three static exercises，referring to ① either sculpturing exercise，which is the way to regulate the body in practicing Qigong；② or locking exercise，which is the way to close the mouth in practicing Qigong，not locking with the lock，otherwise the mouth cannot be opened；③ or combing exercise，which is a way to control the external and combs from the external to the internal.

随【suí】 ① 指卦名，为人有贞正之德，余皆效仿、学习；② 指精神紧张、惊惧后，

S

应调节精神，入内室（不受干扰）休息。

following Refers to ① either the name of Trigram in the Eight Trigrams from Yijing (*Canon of Simplification*, *Change and No Change*), indicating that loyal morality of human beings must be followed and studied; ② or regulating the spirit and resting in the room when the spirit is nervous and frightened.

随分觉【suí fēn jué】 佛家气功习用语，即习练气功后而得。

acquired sense A common term of Qigong Buddhism, referring to achievement after practicing Qigong.

髓海【suǐ hǎi】 ① 指脑；② 指脊髓。

sea of marrow Refers to ① either the brain; ② or spinal marrow.

岁会【suì huì】 指中运的五行之气，与年支方位的五行之气相同，为运气和平之年。

yearly confluence Refers to Qi in the five elements (including wood, fire, earth, metal and water) during central movement, similar to that in yearly position which is a harmonized year in moving Qi.

岁立【suì lì】 指天干与地支配合，推演五运六气的运转，便可确立每岁之气候变化。

yearly determination Refers to combination of the Heavenly Stems and Earthly Branches and promoting the revolving of five motions and six Qi in order to establish the changes of climate every year.

岁主【suì zhǔ】 指六气司天在泉各主持一岁之气。

yearly dominator (**the principal part of the yearly Qi**) Refers to the fact that

the six kinds of Qi govern the sky and control a yearly Qi in the earth.

孙不二【sūn bù èr】 宋代气功学家，为全真清净派创始人。

Sun Bu'er A master of Qigong in the Song Dynasty (960 AD - 1279 AD), also the founder of Tranquil School in Acme Genuine Dao.

孙富春【sūn fù chūn】 宋代气功学家孙不二的另外一个称谓，他也是全真清净派创始人。

Sun Fuchun Another name of Sun Bu'er, a master of Qigong in the Song Dynasty (960 AD - 1279 AD), also the founder of entire genuine tranquil school.

孙敬远【sūn jìng yuǎn】 东晋气功学家孙泰为的另外一个称谓。

Sun Jingyuan Another name of Sun Tai, a master of Qigong in the East Jin Dynasty (317 AD - 420 AD).

孙思邈【sūn sī miǎo】 唐代大医药家、气功养生家。

Sun Simiao A great doctor and a great master of Qigong for nourishing life in the Tang Dynasty (618 AD - 907 AD).

孙思邈摩腹法【sūn sī miǎo mó fù fǎ】 即早上吃饭后，用热手摩腹，出门走五六十步。中饭后，还用热手摩腹，缓行一二百步。

Sun Simiao's exercise for rubbing abdomen A way to cultivate health. After taking breakfast, measures should be taken to rub the abdomen with warm hands and walk for fifty to sixty steps. After taking lunch, measures should be taken to rub the abdomen with warm hands and amble for one hundred or two hundred steps.

孙泰【sūn tài】 东晋气功学家。

Sun Tai A master of Qigong in the East Jin Dynasty（317 AD－420 AD）.

孙真人铭【sūn zhēn rén míng】　源自气功专论,主要阐述调神惜气对延年益寿的重要意义。

Sun Zhenren's inscription Collected from a monograph of Qigong，mainly describing the importance of regulating the spirit and cherishing Qi for prolonging life and cultivating health.

孙真人四季行功养生歌【sūn zhēn rén sì jì xíng gōng yǎng shēng gē】　源自气功专论,主要介绍春嘘、夏呵、秋呬、冬吹、四季长呼、嘻的健身作用。

Sun Zhenren's song for practicing Qigong and nourishing life in the four seasons Collected from a monograph of Qigong，mainly introducing the effect of breathing out slowly in the spring，breathing out in the summer，panting in the autumn and blowing in the winter as well as exhaling and joying in the four seasons for fortifying the body.

孙真人卫生歌【sūn zhēn rén wèi shēng gē】　源自气功专论,主要阐述养生长寿之道及气功方法,重点论述调神养气的重要性。

Sun Zhenren's hygiene song Collected from a monograph of Qigong，mainly describing the ways for cultivating health，prolong life and practicing Qigong，emphasizing the importance of regulating Qi and nourishing Qi.

飧霞服气【sūn xiá fú qì】　指习练气功时,意引云霞,并气送归丹田。

taking Qi from meal and cloud Refers to imagining cloud and sending Qi to Dantian in practicing Qigong. Dantian is divided into the upper Dantian（the region between the eyes），the middle Dantian（the region below the heart）and the lower Dantian（the region below the navel）.

损益【sǔn yì】　源自专论,阐述习练气功要明损益,然后由浅入深,积少成大。

loss and profit Collected from a monograph of Qigong，describing that loss and profit must be clear in practicing Qigong，and trials must be done from the elementary to the profound and from small increments to abundance.

损有余补不足论【sǔn yǒu yú bǔ bù zú lùn】　源自文化专论,论述损有余,补不足,维持事物之间的平衡以喻气功调节身体各部,保持神形稳定的道理。

discussion about reducing sufficiency and enriching insufficiency Collected from a monograph of traditional Chinese culture，describing that reducing sufficiency and enriching of insufficiency can balance different things，indicating that Qigong regulates all parts of the body in order to stabilize the spirit and body.

损之又损【sǔn zhī yòu sǔn】　指习练五阴神祝法,可少食食物,从少食逐渐到不食食物。

loss and loss Refers to practice of Qigong based on immortal's exercise with five Yin，indicating gradual reduction of diet.

缩身【suō shēn】　导引姿势,指蜷起或收缩身体。

twisting posture The style of Daoyin，referring to curling up or shrinking the body.

S

T

他心通【tā xīn tōng】 指练气功出现的潜能。

potentiality Refers to the potentiality in practicing Qigong.

胎藏【tāi cáng】 佛家气功习用语,指人体具有神形平衡的作用,其作用发生发展,犹如子在母胎,逐渐生长发育。

fetal growth A common term of Qigong in Buddhism, referring to balance between the spirit and the body, the effect of which is similar to the growth of embryo in mother's uterus.

胎食胎息法【tāi shí tāi xī fǎ】 为静功。其作法为,常须闭其心,去其思,微其息,息以鼻而不以口,使气常有储,名之曰胎息,漱其舌下泉,咽之,数十息之间相继咽之,名之曰胎食。为之者不息,可以不饥,可以不病。

exercise for fetal taking and fetal respiration A static exercise, marked by always stabilizing the heart, eliminating ideas, mildly breathing, breathing through the nose not through the mouth in order to concentrate Qi, which means fetal respiration; rinsing the tongue below and swallowing saliva for dozens of time, which means fetal respiration. Those who insist on practicing Qigong never feel hungry and never contract diseases.

胎息【tāi xī】 ① 指丹田呼吸;② 指深长呼吸;③ 指守真一之道;④ 指如婴儿在母胎之息;⑤ 指调节自身阴阳。

fetal respiration Refers to ① either respiration in Dantian; ② or deep and long respiration; ③ or concentrating the genuine essence, Qi and spirit; ④ or respiration like embryo in mother's uterus; ⑤ or regulating Yin and Yang in the body. Dantian is divided into the upper Dantian (the region between the eyes), the middle Dantian (the region below the heart) and the lower Dantian (the region below the navel).

胎息抱一歌【tāi xī bào yī gē】 《胎息抱一歌》为气功专论,主要论述胎息与抱一,保持一身阴阳和平。作者不详。

Taixi Baoyi Ge (*Song about Integration of Fetal Respiration*) A monograph of Qigong entitled *Song about Integration of Fetal Respiration*, mainly describing fetal respiration and integration as well as harmonization of Yin and Yang in the human body. The author was unknown.

胎息法【tāi xī fǎ】 为静功,主要作用为调身、调神、调气。其作法为,自然坐,盘膝坐,或仰卧均可,握拳如婴儿,唇齿相著,鼻吸鼻呼,闭息合眼,口不嘘吸。

exercise of fetal respiration A static exercise for regulating the body, the spirit and Qi; marked by naturally sitting or sitting with crossed knees or lying on the back, holding the fists as that of a baby, interacting with the lips and teeth, breathing in and out through the nose, suspending respiration, closing the eyes and avoiding exhalation through the mouth.

胎息经【tāi xī jīng】《胎息经》为气功专著，阐述胎息的含义、行胎息气功的方法，说明神气合一是健康长寿之路。作者和年代不详。

Taixi Jing(*Canon of Fetal Respiration*) A monograph of Qigong entitled *Canon of Fetal Respiration*, describing the meaning of fetal respiration, the methods for practicing fetal respiration in Qigong and integration of the spirit and Qi as the way for cultivating health and prolonging life. The author and the related dynasty were unknown.

胎息经疏略【tāi xī jīng shū lüè】《胎息经疏略》为气功养生专著，由明代王文禄所著，主要论述胎息法的主要理论和方法。

Taixijing Shulüè(*Sketchiness of Fetal Respiration Canon*) A monograph of Qigong entitled *Sketchiness of Fetal Respiration Canon*, written by Wang Wenlu in the Ming Dynasty (1368 AD - 1644 AD), mainly describing the theory and methods for practicing Qigong with fetal respiration.

胎息精微论【tāi xī jīng wēi lùn】《胎息精微论》为气功专著，论述身体阴阳平秘对抵抗早老，增进健康的作用及气功功法。作者不详。

Taixi Jing Weilun(*Particular Discussion of Fetal Respiration with Essence*) A monograph of Qigong entitled *Particular Discussion of Fetal Respiration with Essence*, mainly describing the effect of stable and compact Yin and Yin in preventing senility and increasing health as well as the exercises for practicing Qigong. The author was unknown.

胎息秘要歌诀【tāi xī mì yào gē jué】《胎息秘要歌诀》为气功专著，集气功胎息法精深秘要之论编著成歌。作者不详。

Taixi Miyao Geque(*Secret Songs for Fetal Respiration*) A monograph of Qigong entitled Formula with *Secret Songs for Fetal Respiration*, compiled with secret songs to describe the profound exercises for practicing Qigong with fetal respiration. The author was unknown.

胎息铭【tāi xī míng】 源自气功专论，提出胎息气功的呼吸出入之气，宜均匀、细缓、深长。

inscription of fetal respiration Collected from a monograph of Qigong, suggesting that Qi with breath in practicing Qigong with fetal respiration should be equal, mild and deep.

胎息铭解【tāi xī míng jiě】 源自气功专论，主要阐述气功的具体实施方法及注意事项。

inscriptive explanation of fetal respiration Collected from a monograph of Qigong, mainly describing the methods and matters needing attention in practicing Qigong.

胎息守五脏气至骨成仙【tāi xī shǒu wǔ zàng qì zhì gǔ chéng xiān】 指气功练到一定的程度，可以达到延年益寿，甚至具有特异功能的"仙人"境界。

Fetal respiration protects the five Zang-organs and Qi reaches the bones and becomes immortal. This is a celebrated dictum, referring to the fact that practice of Qigong into a certain degree can prolong life and reach a special state like immortal.

胎息赞【tāi xī zàn】 源自气功专论，

T

主要阐述气功可以保养元气,抗老防衰。

praising fetal respiration Collected from a monograph of Qigong, mainly describing that Qigong can protect and nourish the original Qi, resist senility and prevent decline.

胎仙【tāi xiān】 指习练胎息法,延年益寿的人。

fetal immortal Refers to the exercise for fetal respiration and the people with prolonged life.

胎圆【tāi yuán】 指经过一定时间的气功锻炼,力到功深,神形和调,达到某种理想境界。

fetal circle Refers to great merit of practice, regulation of the spirit and body and reaching the ideal state after practicing Qigong for a certain period of time.

太仓【tài cāng】 指胃。

supreme store Refers to the stomach.

太冲【tài chōng】 足厥阴肝经的一个穴位,为气功排毒之处。这一穴位为气功运行的一个常见部位。

Taichong(LR 3) An acupoint located in the liver meridian of foot Jueyin, through which toxin is expelled in practicing Qigong. This acupoint is a region usually used for keeping the essential Qi in practice of Qigong.

太初【tài chū】 ① 指形成天地的元气;② 指道的本源。

initialization Refers to ① either the original Qi that has formed the sky and earth; ② or the origin of Dao.

太定【tài dìng】 指习练气功时,思想意识活动保持稳定静止的姿态。

supreme tranquilization Refers to stabilizing and tranquilizing the activities of thinking and consciousness in practicing Qigong.

太和【tài hé】 ① 指阴阳和平;② 指太阴、太阳、中和三气和合为一。

supreme harmony Supreme harmony refers to ① either harmony between Yin and Yang; ② or integration of Qi from Taiyin, Taiyang and central harmony.

太和精气【tài hé jīng qì】 指阴阳合一。

integration of essence and Qi Refers to integration of Yin and Yang.

太极【tài jí】 ① 指阴阳两方面的原始混沌之气;② 指含运动与静寂于内;③ 指太和之气;④ 指天地万物之根。

supreme tally Refers to either original Qi containing Yin and Yang; or integration of movement and tranquility; or unity of opportunities in Qi; or harmonized Qi; or the root of all things in the universe.

太极拳【tài jí quán】 动功功法之一,在练习时要求精神专一,呼吸和动作配合。

taijiquan One of the methods used in dynamic exercise, referring to shadow boxing. In practice of Taijiquan, the spirit must be concentrated, respiration and movement must be coordinated with each other.

太极真人法【tài jí zhēn rén fǎ】 为静功,即五阴神祝法。其作法为,以鸡鸣平旦之时,卧式或坐式均可,叩齿九通,然后行五法之神祝。

supreme immortal exercise A static exercise, referring to supreme immortal exercise, marked by lying or sitting at dawn, clicking the teeth for nine times and then moving in the spiritual ways of the five elements (including wood, fire，earth，metal and water）.

太极之蒂【tài jí zhī dì**】**　为祖窍异名。

pedicel in the supreme pole　The synonym of Zuqiao which is an acupoint located in the region between the heart and the navel.

太怒伤身【tài nù shāng shēn**】**　指过度愤怒，情志失调而伤害生活人体。

rage impairing body　A celebrated dictum，referring to rage and emotional disorder that damage the body.

太平观【tài píng guàn**】**　在茅山侧，即晋代气功学家陶弘景华阳馆。

supreme Mansion　Located in Maoshan Mountain and is the Huayang Museum of Tao Hongjing who was a great master of Qigong in the Jin Dynasty（266 AD－420 AD）.

太平经【tài píng jīng**】**　《太平经》为道家早期经典著作，其中保存了一些道家气功的文献资料。

Tai Ping Jing（*Canon of Supreme Peace*）　A monograph of Daoism entitled *Canon of Supreme Peace*，which was compiled early in ancient China and collected some literature about Qigong in Daoism.

太平经圣君秘旨【tài píng jīng shèng jūn mì zhǐ**】**　《太平经圣君秘旨》为气功专著，作者不详，主要论述的是精气神的关系。

Taiping Jingsheng Junmi Zhi（*Secret Decree of Holy Immortal*）　A monograph of Qigong entitled *Secret Decree of Holy Immortal*，mainly discussing the relationship between essence，Qi and spirit. The author was unknown.

太平气【tài píng qì**】**　指阴阳之气的高度协调稳定。喻身体阴平阳秘，则形神和调，形体轻健。

supreme stability　Refers to high coordination and stability of Yin Qi and Yang Qi，indicating stability of Yin and compactness of Yang，coordination of the body and the spirit as well as health of the body.

太平清领书【tài píng qīng lǐng shū**】**　即太平经，为道家早期经典著作，其中保存了一些道家气功的文献资料。

Taiping Qing Lingshu（*Canon of Supreme Peace*）　A monograph of Daoism entitled *Canon of Supreme Peace* which was compiled early and collected some literature about Qigong in Daoism.

太平御览【tài píng yù lǎn**】**　《太平御览》为气功专著，为宋代李昉等十四人所编撰。

Taiping Yulan（*Emperor's Inspection in the Taiping Reign Title*）　A monograph of Qigong entitled *Emperor's Inspection in the Taiping Reign Title*，compiled by Li Fang and other thirteen scholars in the Song Dynasty（960 AD－1279 AD）.

太平御览存泥丸法【tài píng yù lǎn cún ní wán fǎ**】**　为动功。其作法为，早起东向坐，以两手相摩令热，以手摩额上至顶上，满二九止，名曰存泥丸法。

exercise for rubbing mud bolus（the brain）　A dynamic exercise，marked by sitting eastward in the morning，rubbing both hands warm and then scraping the forehead and the top of the head for eighteen times，known as protection of the mud bolus（the brain）.

太清存想法【tài qīng cún xiǎng fǎ**】**　为静功。其作法为，闭气九十息，一咽腹

T

丰满,强筋骨。

supreme meditation A static exercise, marked by suspending respiration for ninety times and enriching the abdomen through just one inhalation for strengthening the sinews and the bones.

太清导引养生法【tài qīng dǎo yǐn yǎng shēng fǎ】 为动功。其作法为,晨起,面向东方,吸气至丹田盈满后呼,呼气出丹田至虚时吸,如此五次。

supreme Daoyin and life cultivation A dynamic exercise, marked by facing to the east in the early morning, breathing in deep into Dantian, breathing out all from Dantian. Such a dynamic exercise should be done for five times. Dantian is divided into the upper Dantian (the region between the eyes), the middle Dantian (the region below the heart) and the lower Dantian (the region below the navel).

太清导引养生经【tài qīng dǎo yǐn yǎng shēng jīng】《太清导引养生经》为气功专著,作者不详,主要阐述行气导引法。

Taiqing Daoyin Yangsheng Jing (*Canon of Supreme Cultivation of Life*) A monograph of Qigong entitled *Canon of Supreme Cultivation of Life*, mainly describing the methods for promoting Qi and practicing Qigong. The author was unknown.

太清调气服气法【tài qīng tiáo qì fú qì fǎ】 为动静相兼功。其作法为,夜半及五更后,漱咽灵液,仰卧,展手及足,头着枕,心定无绝念。

supreme exercise for regulating and taking Qi An exercise combined with dynamic exercise and static exercise, marked by gargling and swallowing humor in the midnight or early morning, lying on the back with pillow under the head, stretching the hands to the feet, and tranquilizing the heart without any avarice.

太清调气经【tài qīng tiáo qì jīng】《太清调气经》为气功专著,作者姓名、成书年代不详。

Taiqing Tiaoqi Jing (*Canon of Supreme Regulation of Qi*) A monograph of Qigong entitled *Canon of Supreme Regulation of Qi*. The author and the related dynasty were unknown.

太清服气法【tài qīng fú qì fǎ】 为静功。其作法为,出服气、入息即住,气息少时,似闭气满,可强身健脑延年。

supreme taking of Qi A static exercise, marked by keeping inhalation after exhalation in order to enrich Qi, to strengthen the body, to improve the brain and to prolong life.

太清服气口诀【tài qīng fú qì kǒu jué】《太清服气口诀》为气功专著。作者姓名、成书年代不详。主要论述内服元气的方法。

Taiqing Fuqi Koujue (*Supreme Pithy Formula For Taking Qi*) A monograph of Qigong entitled *Supreme Pithy Formula For Taking Qi*, mainly describing the methods of inhaling the original Qi. The author and compiling time were unknown.

太清经断谷方【tài qīng jīng duàn gǔ fāng】《太清经断谷方》为气功养生专著,作者不详。内容主要介绍辟谷诸方及欲还食谷解药。

Taiqing Jingduan Gufang (*Supreme Formulae For Inedia*) A monograph of Qigong entitled *Supreme Formulae For*

Inedia, mainly describing the ways to suspend diet and antidote. The author was unknown.

太清王老口传服气法【tài qīng wáng lǎo kǒu chuán fú qì fǎ】 为静功。其作法为，朝暮子午四时初学服气，觉心下胃中满，但少食即可，久作自觉通下到脐下丹田中，后觉鸠中气出即可，熟练后，行坐卧皆可行功。可健身延年，疗治百病。

supreme technique for intake of Qi A static exercise, marked by inhaling in Zi (the period of the day from 11 p.m. to 1 a.m.) and Wu (the period of the day from 11 a.m. to 1 p.m.), feeling that there is sufficient Qi in the heart and stomach with a bit of diet, flowing Qi downwards to the lower Dantian (the region below the navel) after a long period of practice, finishing moving Qi after feeling that Qi flows out of the throat, and sitting or lying after sufficient practice. Such a static exercise can cultivate health, prolong life and treat all diseases.

太清咽液法【tài qīng yàn yè fǎ】 为静功。其作法为，行住坐卧均可，习练时当绝思念念，存心于无为之境，委形于无为之身。

supreme taking of saliva A static exercise, marked by walking or staying or sitting or lying, avoiding any ideas in practicing Qigong in order to tranquilize the heart and to harmonize the body.

太清咽气法【tài qīng yàn qì fǎ】 为静功。其作法为，即服气，日夜要须四度，仰卧、缩两脚，伸两手著两胁边，咽气十口气即满丹田。

supreme swallowing of Qi A static exercise, marked by taking Qi in the day-time or nighttime in four ways, then lying on the back, shrinking the feet, stretching the hands to the rib-sides and swallowing Qi for ten times for enriching Dantian. Dantian is divided into the upper Dantian (the region between the eyes), the middle Dantian (the region below the heart) and the lower Dantian (the region below the navel).

太清运气法【tài qīng yùn qì fǎ】 为静功。其作法为，若先运阳气，觉脚先冷后热，可调和身之阴阳，疗四肢疾，延年健美。

supreme transportation of Qi A static exercise, marked by moving Yang Qi first in order to make the foot warm and then cold, to regulate Yin and Yang in the body, to cure disorders in the four limbs, to cultivate health and to prolong life.

太清运元气法【tài qīng yùn yuán qì fǎ】 为静功。其作法为，元气与外气都不相杂，若咽生气入，须臾即从下泄出去，不得停肠中。

supreme transportation of original Qi A static exercise, referring to no mixture of the original Qi and external Qi. If Qi is inhaled deep into the body, it should be excreted from the lower region and cannot be maintained in the intestines.

太清真人络明诀【tài qīng zhēn rén luò míng jué】 《太清真人络明诀》为气功专著，作者不详，成书于宋代，强调存想在练功中的作用。

Taiqing Zhenren Luoming Jue (*Immortal's Supreme Formula for Regulating Collaterals*) A monograph of Qigong entitled *Immortal's Supreme Formula for Regulating Collaterals*,

T

compiled in the Song Dynasty（960 AD‐1279 AD）, mainly describing the effect of inward contemplation in practicing Qigong. The author was unknown.

太清治身法【tài qīng zhì shēn fǎ】为动功。其作法为，晨起先嘘，两手掌摩，令热，按额上二七，名为存泥丸，令人身神具。

supreme treatment of body　A dynamic exercise, marked by breathing out slowly in the early morning with both hands rubbing warm over the forehead or the mud bolus（the brain）for fourteen times in order to clarify the spirit.

太清中黄胎藏论略【tài qīng zhōng huáng tāi cáng lùn lüè】《太清中黄胎藏论略》为气功专论，主要阐述胎息方法及强身却病，返老还童，延年益寿的道理。作者不详。

Taiqing Zhonghuang Taicang Lunlüe（*Supreme Discussion About Prolonging Life*）　A monograph about Qigong entitled *Supreme Discussion About Prolonging Life*, mainly describing the principles of fetal respiration for strengthening the body, expelling disease, rejuvenating, and prolonging life.

太清中黄真经【tài qīng zhōng huáng zhēn jīng】《太清中黄真经》为气功养生专著，作者名为九仙君，中黄真君注，成书年代不详。

Taiqing Zhonghuang Zhenjing（*Canon of Supreme Analysis and Explanation*）　A monograph of Qigong entitled *Canon of Supreme Analysis and Explanation*, compiled by Jiu Xianjun and explained by Huang Zhenjun. The time of compilation was unclear.

太上纯阳真君了三得一论【tài shàng chún yáng zhēn jūn liǎo sān dé yī lùn】《太上纯阳真君了三得一论》为气功专论，指出养神、养精、养气是气功锻炼的基础。作者不详。

Taishang Chunyang Zhenjun Liaosan Deyi Lun（*Discussion About Supreme and Pure Immortal's Clearness of Three and Achievement of One*）　A monograph about Qigong entitled *Discussion About Supreme and Pure Immortal's Clearness of Three and Achievement of One*, describing that the foundation of practicing Qigong depends on nourishing the spirit, the essence and Qi.

太上洞房内经注【tài shàng dòng fáng nèi jīng zhù】《太上洞房内经注》为气功专著，由宋代周真人撰，认为习练气功应以存想意守为主。

Taishang Dongfang Neijing Zhu（*Supreme Exercise for Regulating Internal Essence in Nuptial Chamber*）　A monograph entitled *Supreme Exercise for Regulating Internal Essence in Nuptial Chamber*, written by Zhou Zhenren in the Song Dynasty（960 AD‐1279 AD）, describing the importance of keeping consciousness in practicing Qigong.

太上黄庭外景玉经【tài shàng huáng tíng wài jǐng yù jīng】《太上黄庭外景玉经》为气功学专著，世传为东晋魏华存所传。

Taishang Huangtinhg Waijing Yujing（*External Scene About the Root of Body in Qigong Practice*）　A monograph about Qigong entitled *External Scene About the Root of Body in Qigong Practice*, written by Wei Huacun in the East Jin Dynasty（317 AD‐420 AD）.

太上混元按摩法【tài shàng hún yuán àn mó fǎ】为动功。其作法为，通过按肌、提肩、抱头、扭腰、托膝、伸脚等方法，除以痼疾，延年益寿，适合老年人习练。

Tuina exercise for supreme somatic training A dynamic exercise for old people, characterized by pressing the muscles, raising the shoulders, holding the head, wrenching the waist, supporting the knees and stretching the feet, effective in treating chronic disease, prolonging life and cultivating health.

太上九要印妙经【tài shàng jiǔ yào yìn miào jīng】《太上九要印妙经》为气功专著，由唐代张果老所著，全面深入地分析和阐述了气功的基本理论和方法。

Taishang Jiuyao Yinmiao Jing (*Canon of Nine Supreme Essentials*) A monograph of Qigong entitled *Canon of Nine Supreme Essentials*, written by Zhang Guolao in the Tang Dynasty (618 AD – 907 AD), thoroughly analyzing and describing the basic theory and practice of Qigong.

太上老君【tài shàng lǎo jūn】对老子的尊称。

Supeme Great Immortal A celebration of Lao Zi who was the founder of the important Chinese thought known as Dao.

太上老君说常清静妙经【tài shàng lǎo jūn shuō cháng qīng jìng miào jīng】《太上老君说常清静妙经》为气功专著，作者不详。主要从清心除欲谈气功养神，认为人心本自清净，常为物欲干扰而不得清静。

Taishang Laojun Shuo Changqing Jingmiao Jing (*Immortal's Explanation About Lustration and Tranquilization*) A monograph about Qigong entitled *Immortal's Explanation About Lustration and Tranquilization*, mainly describing that only when the heart is tranquilized and desires are eliminated can the spirit be nourished through practicing Qigong, and that only when the heart is tranquilized can disturbance be avoided. The author was unknown.

太上老君虚无自然本起经【tài shàng lǎo jūn xū wú zì rán běn qǐ jīng】《太上老君虚无自然本起经》为气功专著，作者不详。从天地之生成讲到人体之修炼。

Taishang Laojun Xuwu Ziran Benqi Jing (*Canon About Immortal's Supreme Approach of Nothingness and Naturalness*) A monograph of Qigong entitled *Canon About Immortal's Supreme Approach of Nothingness and Naturalness*, describing from the formation of the sky and the earth to the practice of Qigong for cultivating health.

太上老君养生诀【tài shàng lǎo jūn yǎng shēng jué】《太上老君养生诀》为气功专著，作者不详，主要论述气功养生的基本知识，各种习练方法及防治效用。

Tianshang Laojun Yangsheng Jue (*Supreme Great Immortal's Exercise for Cultivating Health*) A monograph of Qigong entitled *Supreme Great Immortal's Exercise for Cultivating Health*, mainly describing the basic knowledge of Qigong and life cultivation as well as the exercises of Qigong practice and the effects of prevention and treatment of diseases. The author was unknown.

太上太清天童护命妙经注【tài shàng tài qīng tiān tóng hù mìng miào jīng

zhù】《太上太清天童护命妙经注》为气功专著,为宋代候善渊所著,强调护命养生。

Taishang Taiqing Tiantong Huming Miaojing Zhu(*Explanation About Supreme Protection and Cultivation of Life*) A monograph about Qigong entitled *Explanation About Supreme Protection and Cultivation of Life*, written by Hou Shanyuan in the Song Dynasty(960 AD‐1279 AD), emphasizing the importance of protecting life and nourishing the body in practicing Qigong.

太上修真原章【tài shàng xiū zhēn yuán zhāng】《太上修真原章》为气功学专著,作者不详。

Taishang Xiuzhen Yuanzhang(*Original Cultivation of Health*) A monograph of Qigong entitled *Original Cultivation of Health*. The author was unknown.

太上玄元皇帝【tài shàng xuán yuán huáng dì】 指老子。

Supreme Abstruse Emperor Refers to Lao Zi, who was the founder of the most important Chinese thought known as Dao.

太上养神【tài shàng yǎng shén】 指最后的方法是养神,意识思维活动的平静,全身各部系统和合。

supreme cultivation of spirit Refers to the fact that the best method is to cultivate the spirit, to tranquilize the activities of consciousness and thinking and to harmonize all the parts in the body.

太上养生胎息气经【tài shàng yǎng shēng tāi xī qì jīng】《太上养生胎息气经》为气功专著,作者不详,主要阐述胎息养。

Taishang Yangsheng Taixi Qijing(*Qi Canon of Life Cultivation and Fetal Respiration*) A monograph about Qigong entitled *Qi Canon of Life Cultivation and Fetal Respiration*, mainly describing fetal respiration. The author was unknown.

太上玉轴进取法【tài shàng yù zhóu jìn qǔ fǎ】 为静功。每至半夜后生气时或五更睡醒之初,先吹出腹中浊恶之气一九口,闭目叩齿三十六下,以警身神。

supreme enterprising exercise A static exercise. When breathing in midnight or just before dawn, it is necessary to blow foul smell for one to nine times and to click the teeth for thirty-six times with closure of the eyes in order to invigorate the spirit in the body.

太上玉轴六字气诀【tài shàng yù zhóu liù zì qì jué】 为动静相兼功。其作法为,以呼而自泻出脏腑之毒气,以吸而自采天地之清气以补之。当日小验,旬日大验。年后万病不生,延年益寿。

supreme six characters formula exercise An exercise combined with static one and dynastic one, marked by purging toxic Qi in the five Zang-organs(including the heart, the liver, the spleen, the lung and the kidney) and the six Fu-organs(including the gallbladder, the stomach, the small intestine, the large intestine, the bladder and the triple energizer) through exhalation, and taking pure Qi from the sky and the earth through inhalation. The practice is a little test in one day and a great test in ten days. A year of practice will prevent any disease and prolong life.

太上玉轴咽气法【tài shàng yù zhóu yàn qì fǎ】 为静功。其作法为,气海中气随吐而上，直至喉中，候吐极之际，闭口连鼓而咽之，使内外气相应。

supreme exercise for swallowing Qi A static exercise. In practicing Qigong, Qi from the sea of Qi flows up to the throat through vomiting, making it possible for the mouth to swallow and the internal Qi and external Qi to coordinate with each other.

太上玉轴转气诀【tài shàng yù zhóu zhuǎn qì jué】 为静功。其作法为，闭目握固仰卧，倚两拳于乳间，竖膝举背及尻，以调和五脏，强身健体，防病。

supreme exercise for regulating Qi A static exercise. In practicing Qigong, the practitioner should close the eyes and lie on the back with the hands pressing over the breasts and the knees turning to the back and buttocks in order to regulate the five Zang-organs (including the heart, the liver, the spleen, the lung and the kidney), to strengthen the body and to prevent diseases.

太始【tài shǐ】 ①指形成天地的元气；②指道的本源。

initialization Refers to ① either the original Qi that has formed the sky and earth; ② or the origin of Dao.

太始氏胎息诀【tài shǐ shì tāi xī jué】 静功口诀，指示练气功可达到人与自然高度的协调统一。

Mr. Tai Shi's formula for fetal respiration A static exercise, referring to coordination and unification of man with the natural world in practicing Qigong.

太思虑则伤乎气【tài sī lù zé shāng hū qì】 思虑过度可以损伤人体的气，忧虑思虑过度可影响肺气的升降及脾的运化，最终导致气机失调和气的不足。

excessive contemplation damaging Qi A celebrated dictum, referring to the fact that excessive contemplation will damage Qi in the human body and excessive anxiety will affect the ascent and descent of lung Qi as well as the movement and transformation of the spleen, eventually resulting in disorder of Qi activity and insufficiency of Qi.

太素【tài sù】 ①指形成生命的纯洁物质；②书名，为中医经典著作。

supreme purity Refers to ① either pure substance that has conceived life; ② or the title of a classic canon in traditional Chinese medicine.

太素经摩面法【tài sù jīng mó miàn fǎ】 为动功。其作法为，两手摩切令热摩面，又摩切两掌令热以拭两目，又两手摩切令热以摩发理栉，又两于摩切令热以互摩两臂。

facial rubbing exercise A dynamic exercise, marked by rubbing the hands hot to knead the face, the eyes, the hair and the shoulders.

太微宫【tài wēi gōng】 指脑神所居之宫，亦指脑。

supreme tiny palace Refers to either the chamber of brain spirit; or the brain.

太喜伤神【tài xǐ shāng shén】 指言喜过度而损失精神。

overjoy impairing spirit A celebrated dictum, referring to great rejoicing in speaking that damages the spirit.

太虚【tài xū】 即空虚寂无之境界。

supreme vacuum Refers to the state of void.

太虚本动【tài xū běn dòng】 指宇宙自然不断运动变化。

dynamic universe A celebrated dictum,

T

referring to the constant and natural movement of the universe.

太虚宫【tài xū gōng】 在山东栖霞，为气功家丘处机得道处。

Supreme Void Palace Refers to the place in Xixia County in Shandong Province where Qiu Chuji, a great master of Qigong in the Jin Dynasty（1115 AD－1234 AD），achieved Dao.

太玄【tài xuán】 指谷道。

supreme abstruseness Refers to grain trail（the anus）.

太玄关【tài xuán guān】 指虚仓穴。精气聚散常在此处，水火发端也在此处，阴阳变化也在此处，有无出入也在此处。

supreme abstruse col Refers to Xuwei Acupoint where the essential Qi concentrates and disperses there，water and fire appear there，Yin and Yang change there，exit and entrance exist there.

太玄朗然子进道诗【tài xuán lǎng rán zǐ jìn dào shī】《太玄朗然子进道诗》为气功专著，由宋代希岳述所著。本书为诗文体裁，描述了练气功的方法和气功境界。

Taixuan Langran Zijin Daojing（*Poets Related to Supreme Description About the Techniques and states of Qigong*） A monograph about Qigong entitled *Poets Related to Supreme Description About the Techniques and states of Qigong*，written by Xi Yueshu in the Song Dynasty（960 AD－1279 AD），mainly describing the methods and states of Qigong in poems.

太阳【tài yáng】 足少阳胆经中的一个穴位瞳子髎的另外一个称谓，位于目外眦外侧0.5寸。

Taiyang A synonym of Tongziliao（GB 1）which is an acupoint in the gallbladder meridian of foot Shaoyang，located 0.5 Cun lateral to the outer canthus.

太阳移在月明中【tài yáng yí zài yuè míng zhōng】 指的是阴阳合璧，即阴中有阳，阳中有阴，阴阳和调。

mediation of Taiyang and Taiyin A celebrated dictum，referring to combination of Yin and Yang，indicating Yin within Yang，Yang within Yin，and regulation of Yin and Yang.

太阳之气【tài yáng zhī qì】 指元神。

Qi of Taiyang Refers to the original spirit.

太一【tài yī】 ① 指合二为一；② 指太极。

supreme one Refers to ① either integration of two；② or Taiji, which means Supreme Pole.

太一含真【tài yī hán zhēn】 指运动中形神和谐，可练形养神。

supreme truth Refers to integration of the spirit and the body that can exercise the body and nourish the spirit.

太一山【tài yī shān】 即陕西中南山。

Supreme Mountain A synonym of Zhongnan Mountain in Shaanxi Province.

太一游宫【tài yī yóu gōng】 指北极星恒居北方。

supreme travel mansion Refers to Polaris in the north.

太一元气【tài yī yuán qì】 指形体生成之初。

supreme original Qi Refers to initiative of body.

太乙【tài yǐ】 ① 指北极星；② 指大脑。

supreme Yi Refers to ① either Polaris；② or the brain.

太乙天符【tài yǐ tiān fú】　即司天之气、中运之气合岁支之气三者会合。

supreme year position　Refers to integration of Qi of Sitian，Qi of Zhongyun and Qi of Suizhi.

太一流珠【tài yì liú zhū】　指内丹。神运精气谓之丹。

supreme flow of pearl　Refers to the internal Dan（pills of immortality）which means integration of the essence，Qi and the spirit.

太易【tài yì】　指尚未形成生命之先。

prebiotic phase　Refers to the time when embryo is not conceived.

太阴【tài yīn】　① 指手太阴肺经、足太阴脾经；② 指月；③ 指阴之盛极。

Taiyin　Refers to ① either hand Taiyin meridian and foot Taiyin meridian；② or the moon；③ or supreme Yin.

太阴炼形书【tài yīn liàn xíng shū】源自气功专著，阐述女子习练气功之法。

somatic exercise of supreme Yin　Connected from a monograph of Qigong，mainly describing the methods for women to practice Qigong.

太阴之精【tài yīn zhī jīng】　指元精。

essence of Taiyin　Refers to the original essence.

太元【tài yuán】　指泥丸宫。

supreme origin　Refers to the chamber of the mud bolus（the brain）.

太真【tài zhēn】　为金的别名。

supreme truth　A synonym of Jin（metal）.

泰【tài】　泰为乾卦、坤卦组成，乾为阳，坤为阴。阴阳和合，在天地则是自然之泰。

Tai　Refers to combination of Qian（sky）Trigram and Kun（earth）Trigram. In the Eight Trigrams，Qian（sky）refers to Yang while Kun（earth）refers to Yin. Integration of Yin and Yang is the natural environment in the sky and the earth.

泰定【tài dìng】　指神息相依，阴平阳秘，神形和泰而稳定的状态。

harmony　Refers to the conditions of dependence between the spirit and respiration，coordination of Yin and Yang，and stability of the spirit and body.

泰和【tài hé】　指天地之气，交合为一。喻身体阴平阳秘。

natural coordination　Refers to integration of Qi from the sky and the earth，comparing to coordination of Yin and Yang in the human body.

泰氏法【tài shì fǎ】　为静功。其作法为，行住坐卧，安闲自得，内守精神，不受社会的影响和外物的牵累。

Tai's exercise　A static exercise，marked by quietly and naturally walking，staying，sitting and lying，internally concentrating the essence and spirit，avoiding being affected by social world and hampered by external world.

贪【tān】　佛家气功习用语，即不舍之意，如贪欲、贪爱，是引起精神活动紊乱的原因之一。

Greed　A common term of Qigong in Buddhism，referring to the causes of disorders in the spirit activity.

贪浊【tān zhuó】　佛家气功习用语，指贪欲引起情志损伤，神形失调。

greed impairment　A common term of Qigong in Buddhism，referring to greedy desires that have damaged emotional activities and disharmonized the spirit and the body.

T

瘫痪治法功【tān huàn zhì fǎ gōng】动静相兼功。其作法为，立定，用右手指右，以目视左，运气二十四口，左脚前指。左依此行。

exercise for curing paralysis An exercise combined with dynamic exercise and static exercise, marked by standing up, stretching the right hand toward the right direction, seeing the left side with the eyes, moving Qi for twenty-four times, and stretching the left foot forwards; then stretching the left hand toward the left direction, seeing the right side with the eyes, moving Qi for twenty-four times, and stretching the right foot forwards.

昙峦【tán luán】 南北朝时期的僧人兼医生，对气功学亦有研究和实践。

Tan Luan A Buddhist and doctor in the South and North Dynasties (420 AD - 589 AD), who also well studied and practiced.

昙鸾【tán luán】 南北朝时期的僧人兼医生昙峦的另外一个称谓，其对气功学亦有研究和实践。

Tan Luan Another name of Tan Luan, a Buddhist and doctor in the South and North Dynasties (420 AD - 589 AD), who also well studied and practiced.

谈玄【tán xuán】 源自气功专论，说明人与天地相应。

talking supremeness Collected from a monograph of Qigong, indicating correspondence between man and the sky and the earth.

痰火治法【tán huǒ zhì fǎ】 为静功。其作法为，以舌舐上腭，取赤龙水吞下至丹田，以意送出大便去，连吞四五口。

exercise for curing phlegm fire A static exercise, marked by lapping the palate with the tongue, swallowing water in the mouth into Dantian, imagining to defecate and to swallow for four or five times. Dantian is divided into the upper Dantian (the region between the eyes), the middle Dantian (the region below the heart) and the lower Dantian (the region below the navel).

痰饮候导引法【tán yǐn hòu dǎo yǐn fǎ】 为静功。其作法为，左侧或右侧而卧，闭气不息，至极限时慢慢呼出，十四遍，消痰饮，右病卧右，左病卧左。以念引气，以祛除痰饮。

exercise of Daoyin for phlegm detention A static exercise, marked by lying on the left side or right side, stopping respiration, slowly exhaling for fourteen times after maximum of stopping breath for relieving phlegm detention; lying on the right side if the disease is located in the right side, lying on the left side if the disease is located in the left side, leading Qi with consciousness to eliminate phlegm distention.

谭伯玉【tán bó yù】 金元时期著名的气功家谭处端的另外一个称谓，其著有气功专著，介绍了气功的基本理论与方法。

Tan Boyu Another name of Tan Chuduan, a master of Qigong in the Jin Dynasty (1115 AD - 1234 AD) and Yuan Dynasty (1271 AD - 1368 AD) who wrote a monograph of Qigong, introducing the basic theory and practice of Qigong.

谭处端【tán chù duān】 金元时期著名的气功家，著有气功专著，介绍了气功的基本理论与方法。

Tan Chuduan A master of Qigong in

the Jin Dynasty（1115 AD – 1234 AD）and Yuan Dynasty（1271 AD – 1368 AD）who wrote a monograph of Qigong，introducing the basic theory and practice of Qigong.

谭玉【tán yù】　金元时期著名的气功家谭处端的另外一个称谓,其著有气功专著,介绍了气功的基本理论与方法。

Tan Yu　Another name of Tan Chuduan，a master of Qigong in the Jin Dynasty（1115 AD – 1234 AD）and Yuan Dynasty（1271 AD – 1368 AD）who wrote a monograph of Qigong，introducing the basic theory and practice of Qigong.

谭自然廓然灵通【tán zì rán kuò rán líng tōng】　为静功。其作法为,侧卧,以悟性调神为主。强调调神时灵活、不执著、不拘泥。

tan's exercise for natural regulation of the spirit　A static exercise，marked by lying on one side and regulating the spirit according to savvy. Such a static exercise emphasizes the intelligence for regulating the spirit without any rigidity and stiffness.

潭底日红【tán dǐ rì hóng】　指练功时肾中一阳之气升,犹如红日由下而上。

red sun in deep pool　Refers to rising up of Yang in the kidney in practicing Qigong，just like sunrise.

韬光尚志真仙【tāo guāng shàng zhì zhēn xiān】　是对明代气功学家张三丰的赞美,其深入系统地研究和发展了气功的理论和方法。

genuine immortal with hidden talents and high aspirations　Celebration of Zhang Tong，a great master of Qigong in the Ming Dynasty（1368 AD – 1644 AD），thoroughly and systematically studied

and developed the theory and practice of Qigong.

桃康【táo kāng】　即九灵铁鼓,精气聚散常在此处,水火发端也在此处,阴阳变化也在此处,有无出入也在此处。

peach health　The same as nine genius-fire drums，refers to the region where the essential Qi concentrates and disperses there，water and fire appear there，Yin and Yang change there，exit and entrance exist there.

陶成公骑龙【táo chéng gōng qí lóng】　为动功。其作法为,盘膝而坐,双手轻握拳,手向左甩,头扭向右侧。反之手向右甩,头扭向左侧,同时各运气九口。

Tao Chenggong riding Loong　A dynamic exercise，marked by sitting with crossed the legs，mildly holding the fists with both hands，swinging the hands to the left and turning the head to the right，then swinging the hands to the right and turning the head to the left，and moving Qi for nine times respectively.

陶道【táo dào】　督脉中的一个穴位,位于后正中线,第一腰椎刺突下凹陷中,为气功中常用的意守部位。

taodao（GV 13）　An acupoint in the governor meridian，located in the depression of spinous process in the thoracic vertebra on the middle line over the back，which is the region for concentrating consciousness in practicing Qigong.

陶弘景【táo hóng jǐng】　梁代著名医学家和气功养生家,著作丰厚,成为后世气功家所宗。

Tao Hongjing　A great doctor of traditional Chinese medicine and a great master of Qigong and life cultivation in

T

the Liang Dynasty (502 AD - 557 AD). He wrote several important monographs that greatly influenced the masters of Qigong in the later generations.

陶弘景导引按摩法 【táo hóng jǐng dǎo yǐn àn mó fǎ】 为动功。其作法为,清旦未起,啄齿二七,闭目握固,漱漏唾三咽,气寻闭而不息,自极,极乃徐徐出气,满三止,便起。

Tao Hongjing's exercise for kneading A dynamic exercise, marked by pecking the teeth for two to seven times in the early morning, rinsing, leaking, spitting and swallowing for three times, closing Qi without stopping respiration, and starting moving Qi after slowly exhaling Qi for three times.

陶弘景炼魂魄法 【táo hóng jǐng liàn hún pò fǎ】 为静功。其作法为,常以本命之日,向其方面,叩齿三通,心存再拜而微祝曰:太一镇生,三气合真。生我五脏,摄我精神。

Tao Hongjing's exercise for refining the ethereal soul and corporeal soul A static exercise, marked by paying attention to every day, clicking the teeth for three times, purifying the heart and worshiping the Taiyi (the origin of everything in the universe) and the concentrated three kinds of Qi that have produced the five Zang-organs (including the heart, the liver, the spleen, the lung and the kidney) and the spirit.

陶弘景头面五官按摩法 【táo hóng jǐng tóu miàn wǔ guān àn mó fǎ】 为动功,方法多样。如常每旦啄齿三十六通,能至三百弥佳,令人齿坚不痛。次则以舌漱液,满口中津液,咽之三过止。

Tao Hongjing's exercise of tuina for the head, face and five sense organs A dynamic exercise with various methods, such as rinsing the teeth every morning for thirty-six times or even for three hundred times in order to straighten the teeth and relieve pain, then rinsing humor with the tongue, enriching fluid and humor in the month and swallowing for three times.

陶弘景运日月法 【táo hóng jǐng yùn rì yuè fǎ】 为静功。其作法为,习练时,意想自己的形象在对面前方,并意想面上有日月之光芒,洞照一形,使日在左,月在右,离面前约九寸。存毕,啄齿三通。

Tao Hongjing's exercise for moving the sun and the moon A static exercise, marked by imagining that the image is in the front, the sunlight and the moonlight are in the surface, the sun is in the left side and the moon is in the right side, about nine Cun to the front. After imagination, the teeth are pecked in three ways.

陶弘景杂病导引法 【táo hóng jǐng zá bìng dǎo yǐn fǎ】 为动功,方法多样。如静坐,以左手托头,仰右手南上,尽势托以身,并手振动三。右托头振动亦三,除人睡闷。

Tao Hongjing's exercise of Daoyin for miscellaneous diseases A dynamic exercise with various methods, such as sitting quietly, holding up the head with the left hand, raising the right hand to the south, stretching the body, and vibrating the body with the hands for three times, holding up the head with the right hand to vibrate the body also for three times in order to relieve depressed sleep.

陶山丹室 【táo shān dān shì】 位于浙

江瑞安，为梁朝陶弘景习练气功之处。

Dan（pills of immortality）chamber in Taoshan Mountain Used to be located in the Rui'an County in Zhejiang Province, was the place where Tao Hongjing, a great doctor of traditional Chinese medicine and a great master of Qigong and life cultivation in the Liang Dynasty（502 AD – 557 AD）, practiced, studied and developed Qigong there.

陶通明【táo tōng míng】 梁朝著名医学家和气功养生家陶弘景的另外一个称谓，其著作丰厚，成为后世气功家所宗。

Tao Tongming Another name of Tao Hongjing, a great doctor of traditional Chinese medicine and a great master of Qigong and life cultivation in the Liang Dynasty（502 AD – 557 AD）. He wrote several important monographs that greatly influenced the masters of Qigong in the later generations.

淘气诀【táo qì jué】 为动功。其作法为，夜卧闭息，觉后欲服气者，先则掏转令宿食气得出，然后调服其法，闭目握固，仰倚两拳于乳间，两膝举背及尻内，闭气鼓气，海中气便自出，斡而转之，呵而出之，九或十八次止，是淘气毕，则调之导引，东向坐，不息，四通，啄齿，十四次，愈龋齿痛。

formula for exchanging respiration A dynamic exercise, marked by lying at night, stopping respiration, exhaling food Qi before inhaling Qi, then regulating respiration, closing the eyes, putting the fists over the region between the breasts, raising the back with the knees to the buttocks, closing Qi and promoting Qi to flow naturally from the sea, rotating Qi and breathing out Qi for nine or eighteen times; then sitting to the east, stopping respiration, dredging the four directions, pecking the teeth for fourteen times after rinsing Qi and regulating Daoyin. Such a dynamic exercise can cure pain in dental caries.

醍醐【tí hú】 ① 指乳路之精品；② 指味中第一，药中第一。

cream Refers to ① either essential element in the breast; ② or the first taste and the first medicinal.

醍醐灌顶【tí hú guàn dǐng】 指通过智慧、启迪，除却疑虑，而心地清凉。

enlightenment Refers to eliminating doubt through wisdom and enlightenment in order to eliminate doubt as well as to cool and to refresh the heart.

体本抱神【tǐ běn bào shén】 指形神合一。

holding the spirit with the body Means to integrate the body and the spirit.

体内运天经【tǐ nèi yùn tiān jīng】 指五脏六腑之神，各有其体，各有其用，同天地，顺阴阳，适社会，自然而然。

moving celestial meridians in the body Refers to the spirit of the five Zang-organs（including the heart, the liver, the spleen, the lung and the kidney）and the six Fu-organs（including the gallbladder, the stomach, the small intestine, the large intestine, the bladder and the triple energizer）, each of which all has its form and function, naturally integrating with the sky and the earth, following Yin and Yang, and adapting to the society.

体臭【tǐ xiù】 气功适应证，即体内向外散臭气，多因气血不和，湿热内畜所致。

T

physical odour An indication of Qigong, usually caused by external dispersion of odour, disharmony of Qi and blood and internal accumulation of dampness and heat.

天【tiān】 ①指自然界；②佛家气功习用语,指光明；③指大脑。

sky Refers to ① either natural world; ② or brightness, which is a term of Qigong in Buddhism; ③ or the brain.

天仓【tiān cāng】 指口。

celestial warehouse Refers to the mouth.

天常【tiān cháng】 指天的正常变化。

normal environment Refers to normal climate changes.

天池【tiān chí】 ①指脑；②为手厥阴心包经中的一个穴位,位于乳头外侧1寸处。

celestial pool Refers to ① either a term of Qigong, indicating the brain; ② or Tianchi（PC 1）which is an acupoint in the pericardium meridian of hand Jueyin, located 1 Cun lateral to the breast.

天冲【tiān chōng】 足少阳胆经的穴位,位于耳郭后上方。这一穴位为气功运行的一个常见部位。

Tianchong（GB 9） An acupoint in the gallbladder meridian of foot Shaoyang, located above the auricle. This acupoint is a region usually used for keeping the essential Qi in practice of Qigong.

天出其精【tiān chū qí jīng】 指阳精及生长之气。

natural formation of essence Refers to the essence of Yang and exuberance of Qi.

天道【tiān dào】 ①指大道；②指易之道；③指即天之理。

celestial Dao Refers to ① either the great Dao; ② or the principles of Yijing, in which Yi means simplification, change and no change; ③ or the natural law.

天地储精【tiān dì chǔ jīng】 指人得天地之精英而生。

acquirement of essence from the sky and earth Refers to the fact that human beings are alive, depending on the essence from the sky and earth.

天地媾其精【tiān dì gòu qí jīng】 指阴阳相交,天地为阴阳,去类比象之意。

convergence of essence in the sky and earth Refers to coordination of Yin and Yang because the sky and earth also belong to Yin and Yang.

天地合精【tiān dì hé jīng】 指阴阳和合而为一。

integration of essence in the sky and earth Refers to integration and combination of Yin and Yang.

天地交合时【tiān dì jiāo hé shí】 指子时,即夜间十一时至一时。

time for the communication of the sky and earth Refers to midnight, i.e. 11 p.m - 1 a.m.

天地镜【tiān dì jìng】 佛家气功习用语,指认识世界的精神活动。

universal mirror A term of Qigong in Buddhism, refers to universal recognition in the spirit activity.

天地灵根【tiān dì líng gēn】 指脑。

spiritual root in the sky and earth Refers to the brain.

天地日月【tiān dì rì yuè】 指人体内阴阳两个方面。

sky-earth-sun-moon Refers to Yin and Yang in human body.

天地袭精【tiān dì xí jīng】　指"天地之袭精为阴阳,阴阳专精为四时,散精为万物,则至精之气,周遍于天地之间,而物物得其所受"。

interaction of essence between the sky and earth　Refers to the fact that the factors interacting the essence in the sky and earth are Yin and Yang which concentrate the essence in the four seasons and transfer the essence to all the things in the universe.

天地之精【tiān dì zhī jīng】　指天地之精气,指人体。

spirit in the sky and earth　Refers to natural essential Qi and human body.

天地之元【tiān dì zhī yuán】　指神。

origin of the sky and earth　Refers to the spirit.

天地至精【tiān dì zhì jīng】　指阴阳合璧,神形和一。

perfect essence in the sky and earth　Refers to either harmony of Yin and Yang, or integration of the spirit and the body.

天度【tiān dù】　日月之行。《黄帝内经》把周天定位三百六十五度,气功依次来阐述人体精气的运动。

natural measurement　Refers to the movement of the sun and the moon. The universe was decided into three hundreds and sixty-five degrees in Huangdi Neijing (entitled *Yellow Emperor's Internal Canon of Medicine*), which was the right way to analyze the movement of the essence and Qi in Qigong.

天耳【tiān ěr】　佛家气功习用语,指听力的特别功能。

celestial ear　A term of Qigong in Buddhism, referring to superior listening ability.

天耳通【tiān ěr tōng】　指习练气功后出现的功能变化。

extensive hearing　Refers to extensive hearing ability after practice of Qigong.

天耳智证通【tiān ěr zhì zhèng tōng】佛家气功习用语,指习练气功,得色界天耳根,听闻无碍的境界。

extensive hearing ability　A term of Qigong in Buddhism, referring to acquirement of special function in practicing Qigong, the manifestation of which is the ability to listen the sounds from all directions.

天符【tiān fú】　指人体最上部位,即头。

celestial top　Refers to highest part of the body, i.e. the head.

天府【tiān fǔ】　指胸襟浩大广远,也指肺经中的一个穴位。这一穴位为气功运行的一个常见部位。

celestial mansion　Refers to broad minded, or an acupoint in the lung meridian. This acupoint is a region usually used for keeping the essential Qi in practice of Qigong.

天根【tiān gēn】　①指元阳;②指人的禀赋;③为佛家气功习用语,指自然标志。

natural root　Refers to ① either origin of Yang; ② or human quantities; ③ or a term of Qigong in Buddhism, referring to natural symbol.

天功【tiān gōng】　指顺应自然,安时处和。

celestial function　Refers to conforming to the natural environment.

天宫【tiān gōng】　指脑神所居之宫,亦指脑。

T

celestial palace Refers to either the chamber that stores the spirit in the brain or the brain.

天谷【tiān gǔ】 指上丹田。

Tiangu Refers to upper Dantian（the region between the eyes）.

天谷山【tiān gǔ shān】 青城山的另外一个称谓。

celestial Mountain Valley A synonym of Qingcheng Mountain in Sichuan Province.

天鼓【tiān gǔ】 指耳。

celestial drum Refers to the ears.

天官【tiān guān】 指人体的耳、目、鼻、口、形。

celestial official Refers to the ears, the eyes, the nose, the mouth and the body.

天癸【tiān guǐ】 指肾中精气充盛，或元阴，或月经。

tiangui Refers to either exuberance of spiritual Qi in the kidney; or original Yin; or menstruation.

天果【tiān guǒ】 泛为佛家气功习用语，指学习气功，自控精神与形体，维持神形稳定的安适状态。

celestial fruit A common term of Qigong in Buddhism，referring to somatic and spiritual integration by control the spirit and body.

天和【tiān hé】 ① 指天地之和气；② 指元气。

natural harmony Refers to ① either harmonization of Qi from the sky and earth; ② or the original Qi.

天河【tiān hé】 指人与天相应，宇宙有天河，人亦有天河。

celestial river Refers to correspondence between man and the sky. It was believed that celestial river was not on-ly in the universe, but also in the world of human beings.

天河水逆流【tiān hé shuǐ nì liú】 指神运精气，从督脉逆上入泥丸为天河水逆流，亦指练功过程中吞咽口中的津液。

reverse flow of celestial river Refers to the movement of the essence of Qi with the function of the spirit，indicating that the governor meridian runs upwards into the mud bolus（the brain）or saliva is swallowed during the procedure of Qigong practice.

天魂【tiān hún】 ① 指火中之水；② 亦指汞。

celestial soul Refers to ① either wood in fire; ② or mercury.

天机【tiān jī】 ① 指自然升降之机及天赋灵机；② 指灵性；③ 指天意。

celestial way Refers to ① either natural mechanism，endowment and secret; ② or intelligence; ③ or providence.

天机潮候篇【tiān jī cháo hòu piān】 源自气功专论，按一月中的日期和时辰，列出练功最佳时间表。

discussion about celestial tide Collected from a monograph of Qigong，listing the best time for practicing Qigong according to the days and times in every month.

天交于地【tiān jiāo yú dì】 指通过伏羲创建的八卦解读阴阳。

communication of the sky with the earth Refers to explanation of Yin and Yang through exposition of the Eight Trigrams created by Fu Xi，the ancestor of Chinese civilization.

天精【tiān jīng】 指天空中的精气。

celestial essence Refers to pure air in the universe.

天君【tiān jūn】 指脑及脑神。

celestial monarch Refers to the brain or the brain spirit.

天乐【tiān lè】 指调节阴阳之意、意识活动稳定、精神意识专一。

celestial pleasure Refers to either regulation of Yin and Yang; or stabilized activity of consciousness; or concentration of the spirit and consciousness.

天理【tiān lǐ】 指自然之理，为习练气功避免精神刺激，守神于身内，稳定神形之意。

natural law Refers to perfect law in Qigong practice for avoiding stimulation of the spirit, concentrating the spirit inside the body and stabilizing the spirit and body.

天髎【tiān liáo】 手少阳三焦经中的一个穴位，位于背外上方，为气功常用意守部位。

Tianliao（TE 15） An acupoint in the triple energizer meridian of hand Shaoyang, located above the lateral side of the back. This acupoint is a region usually used in practice of Qigong.

天满【tiān mǎn】 指百会穴，为气功学重要体表标志之一。

celestial fullness Refers to an acupoint called Baihui（GV 20）, a region usually used in practicing Qigong and the place for all spirits to coordinate.

天门【tiān mén】 指鼻孔、精神意识活动、脑中之枢机。

celestial gate Refers to either nostrils; or activities of the spirit and consciousness; or chamber of the brain.

天命【tiān mìng】 ① 指人的气质；② 指自然规律。

destiny Refers to ① either temperament of man; ② or natural law.

天魔【tiān mó】 指习练气功中的幻象。

celestial ghost Refers to illusion in practicing Qigong.

天目【tiān mù】 指明堂下，两眉连线中点上方。

celestial vision Refers to the upper point between the brows.

天年【tiān nián】 指天赋之年。

celestial year Refers to span of life.

天七地三【tiān qī dì sān】 指阴阳配合，合二为一。

celestial seven and earthly three Refers to combination between Yang and Yin.

天窍【tiān qiào】 指头之五官。

upper orifices Refers to the five organs in the brain.

天情【tiān qíng】 指人自然具有的性情。

natural temperament Refers to natural human qualities.

天然真火【tiān rán zhēn huǒ】 指调节呼吸，绵绵若存，任其自然。

natural true fire Refers to regulating respiration with natural style.

天人发机景象【tiān rén fā jī jǐng xiàng】 源自气功专论，指天人合发机，取天地之气以养身体之阳气。

scenery of integration between the sky and man Collected from a monograph of Qigong, referring to obtaining Qi from the sky and earth to nourish Yang Qi in the body.

天人合发机【tiān rén hé fā jī】 源自气功专论，指子时为天人合发之实际真机。

natural and human convergence Collected from a monograph of Qigong, referring to the ideal time for the correspondence between human beings and the universe in Zi（the period of the day from 11 p.m. to 1 a.m.）.

天人合发,万物定基【tiān rén hé fā wàn wù dìng jī】 指人天相应,万物定基而人安和。

Correspondence between man and the universe lays the foundation for the development of things in the world. This celebrated dictum means that only when human beings communicate with the sky and earth can all the things in the world develop naturally and all the people live a peaceful and harmonious life.

天人合发至机【tiān rén hé fā zhì jī】 指任督脉交接之处。

opportunity for the sky and man to integrate with each other Refers to the region where the conception meridian and the governor meridian communicate with each other.

天日不行【tiān rì bù xíng】 指天不运行,日月星不移,天之气不调,则天道宇宙毁灭。

no movement of the sky Refers to failure of man to correspond to the sky. If the sky does not move, the sun, the moon and the stars will not change, and celestial Qi will not regulate, eventually causing destroy of the universe.

天容【tiān róng】 手太阳小肠经的一个穴位,位于平下颌角,为气功学重要体表标志之一。

Tianrong（SI 17） An acupoint located in the small intestine meridian of hand Taiyang, one of the important symbols in Qigong practice. This acupoint is a region usually used in practice of Qigong.

天使【tiān shǐ】 佛家气功习用语,指自然和社会对人的损害。

natural impairment A common term of Qigong in Buddhism, referring to natural damage or social damage.

天寿【tiān shòu】 指先天赋给的寿命限度。

celestial span of life Refers to natural longevity.

天枢【tiān shū】 足阳明胃经中的一个穴位,位于脐旁开 2 寸。这一穴位为气功运行的一个常见部位。

Tianshu（ST 25） An acupoint in the stomach meridian of foot Yangming, located 2 Cun beside the navel. This acupoint is a region usually used for keeping the essential Qi in practice of Qigong.

天台【tiān tái】 指鼻。

celestial platform Refers to the nose.

天台白云子【tiān tái bái yún zǐ】 指唐代气功学家司马承祯,赞美其对气功学的特别贡献。

white Cloud in the Celestial Mountain A celebration of Sima Chengzhen, a great master of Qigong in the Tang Dynasty（618 AD – 907 AD）.

天台道者胎息诀【tiān tái dào zhě tāi xī jué】 为静功口诀,指习练保持心气平和,避免不正常的意念活动。

daoist's fetal respiration formula in celestial mansion A static exercise, referring to harmonization of heart Qi for avoiding abnormal activity of emotion.

天台山【tiān tái shān】 位于浙江省东部,为佛家天台宗的发源地。

Celestial High Mountain Refers to the mountain in the east of Zhejian Province, which is the origin of Tiantai Sect in Buddhism.

天堂【tiān táng】 指脑神所居之处。

paradise Refers to the location of

spirit in the brain.

天庭【tiān tíng】 指两眉之间。

natural courtyard Refers to the point between the brows.

天庭地关列斧斤【tiān tíng dì guān liè fǔ jīn】 指开通天庭,调节阴阳,使人健康长寿。

The celestial paradises and the terrestrial all maintain axes. This celebrated dictum means to dredge the forehead and to regulate Yin and Yang in order to nourish the body and to prolong the life.

天文【tiān wén】 指日、月、星、辰、风、云、露、霜、雪等在宇宙自然中分布运行的现象。

celestial movement Refers to the manifestations of the sun, the moon, the stars, the wind, the cloud, the rain, the dew, the frost and the snow.

天下无二道,圣人无两心【tiān xià wú èr dào shèng rén wú liǎng xīn】 指道、儒、释三家均以习练性命双修功为法,专心一志,修身养性。

In the earth, there are no two Dao; in Shengren (sage) s, there are no two hearts. This celebrated dictum means that Daoism, Confucianism and Buddhism all take refining life with Qigong as the principle for concentrating the heart and mind in order to cultivate the body and to nourish the life.

天仙【tiān xiān】 ① 指神通,即有精深气功术的人;② 佛家气功习用语,指具有特异功能的人。

celestial immortal Refers to ① either theurgy, great master of Qigong; ② or a term of Qigong in Buddhism, referring to a person with special ability.

天仙地仙【tiān xiān dì xiān】 指具有

高深气功理论和实践的气功家。

celestial immoral and earthly immoral Refers to the excellent master of Qigong with great theory and practice of Qigong.

天仙金丹心法【tiān xiān jīn dān xīn fǎ】 《天仙金丹心法》为气功专著,论述最好的气功文献,作者不详。

Tian Xian Jin Dan Xin Fa (*Mental Cultivation Methods of Celestial Immortals with Golden Dan*) A monograph about Qigong entitled *Mental Cultivation Methods of Celestial Immortals with Golden Dan (Pills of Immortality)*, thoroughly discussing the literature of Qigong. The author was unknown.

天仙正理直论【tiān xiān zhèng lǐ zhí lùn】 《天仙正理直论》为气功专著,为明代伍守阳撰,伍守虚注。

Tian Xian Zheng Li Zhi Lun (*Direct Discussion About the Natural Theory of Celestial Immortals*) A monograph of Qigong entitled *Direct Discussion About the Natural Theory of Celestial Immortals*, written by Wu Shouyang and explained by Wu Shouxu in the Ming Dynasty (1368 AD - 1644 AD).

天心【tiān xīn】 指天空的正中。

celestial center Refers to the celestial center.

天星和气【tiān xīng hé qì】 指脑神稳定,和气内生。

stability of celestial Qi Refers to harmonious Qi in the brain.

天行【tiān xíng】 ① 指天体的运行;② 指传染病的流行;③ 佛家气功习用语,为五行之一。

celestial movement Refers to ① either celestial movement; ② or epidemic disease spreading; ③ or a term of Qigong in Buddhism, which is one of the five elements (including wood, fire, earth, metal and water).

天行健【tiān xíng jiàn】 指自然界无灾害,正常运行。

normal celestial movement Refers to normal celestial movement.

天修子【tiān xiū zǐ】 清代气功学家,撰有一部特别的气功专著。

Tian Xiuzi A great scholar and master of Qigong in the Qing Dynasty (1636 AD - 1912 AD), who wrote a special monograph of Qigong.

天眼【tiān yǎn】 佛家气功习用语,指能知人的现在和未来精神思维活动,能视世间一切物。

celestial eyes A term of Qigong, referring to the extensive eyesight of all the things in the world through the activities of the spirit and consciousness at the present and in the future.

天眼通【tiān yǎn tōng】 指习练气功后能看到天下之物。

extensive eyesight Refers to the ability to see things behind the sky after practice of Qigong.

天眼智证通【tiān yǎn zhì zhèng tōng】 佛家气功习用语,指习练气功,得色界天眼根,自在清净,照久无碍的境界。

extensive movement of eyesight A term of Qigong in Buddhism, referring to acquirement of special function in practice of Qigong, indicating perfect observation of the universe, tranquilization of the mind and no disorders in the body.

天一【tiān yī】 指人与自然合二为一,为顺应自然之意。

celestial one Refers to the integration of man and nature, similar to the idea

of correspondence between human beings and the universe.

天隐子导引术【tiān yǐn zǐ dǎo yǐn shù】 为静功。其作法为,将意守、吐纳、咽津与导引相结合的一种功法。

Tian Yinzi's Daoyin technique A static exercise, referring to a special method in practicing Qigong, which is connected with consciousness concentration, expiration, inspiration and swallowing saliva.

天隐子养生书【tiān yǐn zǐ yǎng shēng shū】 《天隐子养生书》为气功专著,为唐代气功学家司马承祯所撰。

Tianyinzi Yangsheng Shu (*Tian Yinzi's Book About Health Cultivation*) A monograph of Qigong entitled *Tian Yinzi's Book About Health Cultivation*, written by Sima Chengzhen, a great master of Qigong in the Tang Dynasty (618 AD - 907 AD).

天应星,地应潮【tiān yìng xīng dì yìng cháo】 指人天相应,乾坤日月星辰之阴阳升降、交会。

The sky responding to stars and the earth responding to tides Refers to correspondence between human beings and the sky as well as the ascent, descent and combination of Yin and Yang in the sun, the moon and the stars.

天元【tiān yuán】 ① 指周历火;② 指自然变化之本。

celestial origin Refers to ① either week calendar; ② or the root for natural changes.

天元先生服气法【tiān yuán xiān shēng fú qì fǎ】 为静功。其作法为,每日常卧,摄心绝想,闭气握固,鼻引口吐,无令耳闻,有益于健康长寿,除却嗜欲。

Mr. Taiyuan's exercise for taking Qi　A static exercise, marked by lying every day, tranquilizing the heart, suspending respiration, breathing in through the nose, breathing out through the mouth, and avoiding listening anything. Such a static exercise can cultivate health, prolong life and eliminate indulgence.

天则【tiān zé】　指自然法则，自然之理。

celestial law　Refers to natural law and natural principles.

天真【tiān zhēn】　指人的自然本性或天然真理。

natural truth　Refers to human inherent quality or natural truth.

天中【tiān zhōng】　① 指鼻；② 指天之正中央。

celestial middle　Refers to ① either the nose; ② or the celestial center.

天中之天【tiān zhōng zhī tiān】　即玄中之玄，指脑。

sky in sky　Refers to the brain.

天中之岳【tiān zhōng zhī yuè】　指鼻。

high mountain in the sky　Refers to the nose.

天周二十八宿【tiān zhōu èr shí bā xiù】　指天体运行环周于二十八宿之间。二十八宿是古代天文学的星座名称，周天之星分四方，每方各有七宿。

twenty-eight celestial mansions　The title of constellation used in ancient times. The constellations in the sky are divided into four directions, each direction contains seven constellations.

天竺【tiān zhú】　指古代印度国。古代中国和东亚的一些国家将印度称为天竺。

tianzhu　Refers to ancient India. In ancient times, China and other countries in the East Asia called Indian Tianzhu. China first called India Sindhu in Shiji (Historical Records).

天竺按摩十八势【tiān zhú àn mó shí bā shì】　为动功。其作法为，两手相握，扭转翻动如洗手样；两手轻轻相叉，翻动反复向胸来回运动，每日坚持习练三遍，强身除疾，延年益寿。

ancient India's eighteen postures of tuina　A dynamic exercise, marked by shaking the hands, turning round the hands like washing, gently interacting the hands, turning round the hands to the chest to move and constantly practicing for three times every day. Such a dynamic exercise can strengthen the body and prolong life.

天竺三时【tiān zhú sān shí】　指热时为正月十六日至五月十六日之间，雨时为五月十六日至九月十六日之间，寒时为九月十六日至正月十五日之间。

triple periods　Refer to heat time from January sixteenth to May sixteenth, rain time from May sixteenth to September sixteenth, and cold time from September sixteenth to January fifteenth.

天柱【tiān zhù】　足太阳膀胱经的一个穴位。也指颈。这一穴位为气功运行的一个常见部位。

Tianzhu（BL 10）　Refers to an acupoint in the gallbladder meridian of foot Taiyang, or the neck. This acupoint is a region usually used for keeping the essential Qi in practice of Qigong.

天宗【tiān zōng】　指日月星。

T

celestial ancestor Refers to the sun, the moon and the stars.

添油【tiān yóu】 指习练气功,荣养真阴。

increasing oil Refers to sincerely nourishing Yin in practicing Qigong.

田伯油【tián bó tián】 清代气功家、养生家田绵淮的另外一个称谓。

Tian Botian Another name of Tian Jinhuai, a great master of Qigong and life cultivation in the Qing Dynasty (1636 AD－1912 AD).

田绵淮【tián mián huái】 清代气功家、养生家。

Tian Jinhuai A great master of Qigong and life cultivation in the Qing Dynasty (1636 AD－1912 AD).

恬淡虚无【tián dàn xū wú】 ① 指凝神入静;② 指意识思维活动的相对静止;③ 指淡泊,不慕荣利。

tranquilized mind Refers to ① either concentration and tranquilization of the spirit; ② or quiet activities of consciousness and thinking; ③ or not seeking fame and wealth.

恬和养神【tián hé yǎng shén】 指意识思维活动清和安静,才能保养精神。

quietly and gently nourishing the spirit Indicates that only when the activities of consciousness and thinking are stable and tranquil can the essence and the spirit be protected and nourished.

填离取坎【tián lí qǔ kǎn】 指练功中取肾阳(即坎中之阳)与心阴(即离中之阴)结合而产金丹。

stuffing Li Trigram and taking Kan Trigram Refers to combination of kidney Yang (Yang in the Kan Diagram) and hear Yin (Yin in the Li Diagram) that has produced golden Dan (pills of im-

mortality). In this term Kan Trigram is in the Eight Trigrams from Yijing (*Canon of Simplification*, *Change and No Change*).

调伏法【tiáo fú fǎ】 佛家功法。其作法为,取黑月日中,亦夜半起首,不论善恶日行之。行者面向南方蹲居,以右足蹈左足上,即观自身遍法界。

exercise for mental regulation An exercise in Buddhism, marked by raising the head when there is no moon and no sun, practicing Qigong at any time no matter it is good or evil, squatting to the south, treading the left foot with the right food and consciously observing all parts of the body.

调气【tiáo qì】 指行功中,调节呼吸有而至无,无而至有。

regulating Qi Refers to regulating respiration from abundance to vacuum and from vacuum to abundance in practicing Qigong.

调气导引法【tiáo qì dǎo yǐn fǎ】 为动功。其作法为,两手相捉如洗手,两手相叉,翻覆向胸前,两手相重共按髀,徐徐掖身,两手抱头,两手据地,锁身曲脊三度。

exercise of Daoyin for regulating Qi A dynamic exercise, marked by holding the hands like washing, overlapping the hands toward the chest, strongly pressing the thighs with both hands, mildly turning the body, holding the head with the hands, pressing the ground with the hands, straightening the body and bending the spine for three degrees.

调气法【tiáo qì fǎ】 指夜半至第二日中午为调气时间,古人认为这段时间为生气之时。

exercise for regulating Qi Refers to regulating Qi from the midnight to the noon which was believed to be the time for producing Qi in ancient China.

调气液法【tiáo qì yè fǎ**】**为静功。其作法为,大张口呵之,十呵、二十呵即鸣天鼓七或九,用舌撩华池而咽津,复咽令口中热气退止。

exercise for regulating Qi and humor A static exercise, marked by opening the mouth to breathe out for ten times or twenty times that is similar to sounding the celestial drum (rubbing the occipital) for seven or nine times, raising the mouth with the tongue for swallowing fluid in order to eliminate hot Qi in the mouth.

调停火候托阴阳【tiáo tíng huǒ hòu tuō yīn yáng**】**揭示了火候的实质,就是阴阳的应用。

regulating and stopping fire in order to support Yin and Yang A celebrated dictum, referring to the essence of fire duration, indicating the application of Yin and Yang.

调息法【tiáo xī fǎ**】**为静功。其作法为,"调息之法,不拘时候。随便而坐,纵任其体,不倚不曲,解衣缓带,务令调适。口中舌搅数遍,微微呵出浊气,鼻中微微纳之,或三、五遍,或一、二遍"。

exercise for regulating respiration A static exercise, marked by "regulating respiration at any time, sitting at any place in any way without any strict requirement, disrobing clothes naturally, stirring the tongue for several times, mildly exhaling turbid Qi and slowly inhaling Qi for three to five times or one to two times".

调息偈【tiáo xī jì**】**源自气功专论,形象地阐述了调息的一般要求。

regulating respiration with Gatha Collected from a monograph of Qigong, vividly describing the normal requirement for regulating respiration.

调息四相【tiáo xī sì xiāng**】**即调息要以自然、均匀、细致、深长为基础。

four ways for regulating respiration Means that respiration should be regulated naturally, fairly, meticulously and deeply.

调息与数息【tiáo xī yǔ shù xī**】**指调节呼吸,任其自然,并有种种意念呼吸。

regulating respiration with various ways Refers to naturally regulating respiration with various ways of imagining respiration.

调血【tiáo xuè**】**指心的作用是调理血脉。

regulating the blood Means that the function of the heart is to regulate the blood vessels.

调引筋骨有偃仰之方【tiáo yǐn jīn gǔ yǒu yǎn yǎng zhī fāng**】**指气功调身能锻炼肢体,活动筋骨,使身体强健。

exercise for regulating and leading sinews and bones with descent and ascent A celebrated dictum, referring to exercising the limbs and trunk by regulating the body, and activating the sinews and bone in order to strengthen the body.

调真息【tiáo zhēn xī**】**指意念调节呼吸。

regulating genuine respiration Means to regulate respiration with consciousness.

调肢体法【tiáo zhī tǐ fǎ**】**为动功。其作法为,两臂左挽右挽,左右前后轻摆,头项左右顾,腰胯左右转,时俯时仰,两手相提如洗手,掩目摩面,每个动作十数次。

T

Exercise for regulating the body A dynamic exercise, marked by pulling and swaying the shoulders from the left to the right and from the front to the back, turning the head and neck from the left to the right and vice versa, turning the waist from the left to the right for raising and lowering and vice versa, holding the hands like washing, closing the eyes and kneading the face for ten times respectively.

铁裆功【tiě dāng gōng】 同两颗梨，指睾丸。

exercise for the strong crotch The same as two pears, refers to the testicles.

铁拐仙指路法【tiě guǎi xiān zhǐ lù fǎ】 为动功。其作法为，正站立，右手指右，左脚前踏。以目左视，运气二十四口。少顷，左手指左，右脚前踏，以目右视，运气二十四口，可重复数次。

fire crutch immortal's exercise for leading road A dynamic exercise, marked by standing up, directing the right with the right hand, treading forward with the left foot, seeing the left with the eyes, moving Qi for twenty-four times and continuing repeatedly, then directing the left with the left hand, treading forward with the right foot, seeing the right with the eyes, moving Qi for twenty-four times and continuing repeatedly.

铁脚道人【tiě jiǎo dào rén】 气功养生家，著有气功专著，提倡清心寡欲，炼气以养生防病。其姓名与年代不详。

tiejiao Daoren（Daoist with iron feet） A master of Qigong and life cultivation, who wrote a monograph of Qigong, suggesting to purify the heart and eliminate desires, describing that practice of Qigong can cultivate life and prevent disease. The name of the author and the related dynasty were unknown.

听宫【tīng gōng】 为手太阳小肠经中的一个穴位，位耳屏与下颌关节之间。这一穴位为气功运行的一个常见部位。

Tinggong（SI 19） An acupoint in the small intestine meridian of hand Taiang, located in between the tragus and mandibular condyloid process. This acupoint is a region usually used for keeping the essential Qi in practice of Qigong.

听会【tīng huì】 为足少阳胆经中的一个穴位，位于耳屏间切迹的前方。这一穴位为气功运行的一个常见部位。

Tinghui（GB 2） An acupoint in the gallbladder meridian of foot Shaoyang, located anterior to the intertragic notch. This acupoint is a region usually used for keeping the essential Qi in practice of Qigong.

通【tōng】 为佛家气功习用语，指神形作用自在无碍，人有神通和智慧。

unobstruction A term of Qigong, indicating that the spirit and body are comfortable and unimpeded and human beings are of remarkable ability and intelligent wisdom.

通关法【tōng guān fǎ】 为静功。其作法为，取自然坐式，或盘膝坐式。坐定之后，意引气于心脐上三寸不前不后，不左不右之中，引气到脐下，心脐下分开两路，脐下两腿之前，至足背转足底，向足跟绕腿后，上行至命门，会合后从右转左，从右旋而上，升至右背到心，复由心向前入肾，旋转三遍后，再到命门，上至大椎，分两路到两肩，经肘后外关达掌心，循内关过肩井，由项后透泥丸，行明堂，入双瞳，自面部入胸膈，复到脐上三寸处，复旋转三遍。

exercise for penetration　A static exercise，marked by naturally sitting or sitting with crossed legs，mentally leading Qi to the region about 3 Cun between the heart and the navel and finally to the region below the navel；then promoting Qi to flow in two ways below the heart and the navel to the region before the legs；then promoting Qi to flow from the acrotarsium to the sole，from the heel to the back of the leg，and from the back of the leg to the life gate；then promoting Qi to turn from the right to the left，to return from the right to the upper，to raise from the right side of the back to the heart，to turn from the heart to the kidney，and finally to reach the life gate after three times of rotation；then promoting Qi to flow from the life gate to Dazhui（GV 14）and the shoulders in two ways and from the elbows to the palms；then promoting Qi to flow from Neiguan（PC 6）to Jianjing（GB 21）and from the back of neck to the mud bolus（the brain）；then promoting Qi to flow from the nose to the pupils，from the face to the chest and diaphragm and from the diaphragm to the region 3 Cun above the navel for three times respectively.

通利道路无终休【tōng lì dào lù wú zhōng xiū】　指两手按摩面部，高下随形不休息，以通利耳、目、口、鼻之经脉。

unobstructed way without termination　Means to knead the face with both hands，and to move upwards and downwards without any rest in order to open the meridians related to the ears，the eyes，the mouth and the nose.

通妙【tōng miào】　金代气功学家刘处玄的另外一个称谓，其为全真随山派创始人。

tong Miao　Another name of Liu Chuxuan，a great master of Qigong in the Jin Dynasty（1120 - 1203）and the founder of Suishan Mountain School in Acme Genuine Dao.

通命【tōng mìng】　指舌神之名。

unobstructed life　Refers to the spirit in the tongue.

通天下一气耳【tōng tiān xià yī qì ěr】指天下万事万物都生于一气，一气含有阴阳两个方面，为"一气生万物"之意。

opening up one kind of Qi in the whole world　Means that all the things in this world are produced by one kind of Qi which contains Yin and Yang.

通微显化真人【tōng wēi xiǎn huà zhēn rén】　明代英宗皇帝对张三丰的封号。张三丰为明代的气功学家，深入系统地研究和发展了气功的理论和方法。

supernatural Immortal　A great master of Qigong in the Ming Dynasty（1368 AD - 1644 AD），thoroughly and systematically studied and developed the theory and practice of Qigong，was conferred Supernatural Immortal by Yingzong Emperor in the Ming Dynasty（1368 AD - 1644 AD）.

通玄子【tōng xuán zǐ】　金代气功学家刘志渊的另外一个称谓，其撰有气功专著。

tong Xuanzi　Tong Xuanzi was another name of Liu Zhiyuan，a master of Qigong in the Jin Dynasty（1120 - 1203）and wrote an important monograph of Qigong.

同类【tóng lèi】　气功文献中指一类形质的阴阳,谓之同类,同类阴阳才能交感。

Similarity　In the literature of Qigong, it refers the same nature of Yin and Yang and that only the same Yin and Yang can integrate with each other.

桐柏观【tóng bǎi guàn】　位于浙江桐柏山上,为东晋道家葛洪炼丹之处。

tongbai Temple　Located in the Tongbai Mountain in Zhejiang Province, where Ge Hong, a great Daoist in the East Jin Dynasty（317 AD – 420 AD）studied and developed alchemy.

童子【tóng zǐ】　指目珠。

Pupil　Refers to eyeball.

瞳子髎【tóng zǐ liáo】　足少阳胆经中的一个穴位,位于目外眦外侧 0.5 寸。此穴位为气功习练之处。

Tongziliao（GB 1）　An acupoint in the gallbladder meridian of foot Shaoyang, located 0.5 Cun lateral to the outer canthus. This acupoint is a region usually used in practice of Qigong.

痛痹【tòng bì】　气功适应证,指寒痹,由风寒湿邪侵袭肢节、经络所致。

pain impediment　An indication of Qigong, referring to cold impediment caused by invasion of pathogenic cold and dampness into the limb joints, meridians and collaterals.

痛风【tòng fēng】　气功适应证,疼痛剧烈。

Gout　An indication of Qigong, which means severe pain.

头北面西【tóu běi miàn xī】　指应用头北西面身法习练气功,易于入静。

head in the north and face in the west　Refers to the way to maintain the body in practicing Qigong, marked by turning the head and face to the north and west to tranquilize the mind in practicing Qigong.

头冲【tóu chōng】　手阳明大肠经中的一个穴位臂臑的另外一个称谓,位于曲池和肩髃的连线上。此穴位为气功习练之处。

Touchong　A synonym of Binao（LI 14）which is an acupoint in the large intestine meridian of hand Taiyang, located above the line between Quchi（LI 11）and Jianyu（LI 15）. This acupoint is a region usually used in practice of Qigong.

头戴天神【tóu dài tiān shén】　指脑为神宅,主精神意识思维活动。

head wearing celestial spirit　Refers to the spiritual chamber in the brain which controls the activity of the spirit, consciousness and emotion.

头临泣【tóu lín qì】　足少阳胆经的一个穴位,位于眉上发际 0.5 寸。这一穴位为气功运行的一个常见部位。

Toulinqi（GB 15）　An acupoint in the gallbladder meridian of foot Shaoyang, located 0.5 Cun above the eyes and toward the hairline. This acupoint is a region usually used for keeping the essential Qi in practice of Qigong.

头面风【tóu miàn fēng】　气功适应证,指身体虚弱,复受风寒或风热侵袭所致经久不愈之头痛证。

wind in the head and face　An indication of Qigong, which refers to headache difficult to relieve due to deficiency of the body with invasion of wind cold or wind heat.

头面风候导引法【tóu miàn fēng hòu dǎo yǐn fǎ】　为动功,方法多样。如正

坐,伸腰拔背,头向左右侧活动,然后闭目,用鼻吸气,至极限时慢慢呼出,作七息,治头风疼痛。

exercise of Daoyin for facial wind　A dynamic exercise with various methods, such as sitting with stretching the waist and back, turning the head to the left and right, closing the eyes, breathing through the nose and slowly exhaling for seven times in order to treat migraine and headache.

头面观【tóu miàn guān】　指头面的内部结构及其外象。

manifestations of the head and face　Refers to the internal structure and external images of the head and face.

头神去【tóu shén qù】　指七神去。七神去指损伤五脏六腑的情况。肝神损伤于魂散失目不明,心神损伤于神散失唇见青白,肺神损伤于魄不在身鼻不通,肾神损伤于意出身外食不甘味,头神损伤于神出泥丸头目眩晕,腹神损伤于胃肠神散,四肢神损伤于骨关节重滞不动。

loss of head spirit　Refers to different ways to damage the spirit from the five Zang-organs (including the heart, the liver, the spleen, the lung and the kidney) and six Fu-organs (including the gallbladder, the stomach, the small intestine, the large intestine, the bladder and the triple energizer). The spirit in the liver is damaged by dispersion of the ethereal soul; the spirit in the heart is damaged by loss of the spirit and change of the lips; the spirit in the lung is damaged by dispersion of the corporeal soul and the obstructed nose; the spirit in the kidney is damaged by no pure emotion and no good food; the spirit in the brain is damaged by disper-sion of the spirit from the mud bolus (the brain) and dizziness; the spirit in the abdomen is damaged by dispersion of the spirit in the stomach and intestines; the spirit in the four limbs is damaged by stagnation of the joints.

头痛【tóu tòng】　气功适应证,指头的某些部位或全头疼痛的疾病。

headache　An indication of Qigong, referring to pain in some other places or in the whole head.

头痛治法【tóu tòng zhì fǎ】　为静功。其作法为,盘膝端坐,用两手大拇指和示指掐住左右两侧耳门,闭住眼耳口鼻,送丹田七孔之气上升顶门,日行数次,以愈为度。

treatment of headache　A static exercise, marked by sitting with crossed legs, pressing the left and right ears with the thumbs and forefingers, closing the eyes, ears, mouth and nose, transmitting Qi from the seven orifices in Dantian to the top for several times every day in order to cure the disease. Dantian is divided into the upper Dantian (the region between the eyes), the middle Dantian (the region below the heart) and the lower Dantian (the region below the navel).

头为天象【tóu wéi tiān xiàng】　指头在身体的最高部位而象天。

head as the celestial phenomena　Refers to the head which is the highest position of the body, just like the sky.

头围【tóu wéi】　指头的左右前后周长。

head regions　Refers to the left side, the right side, the anterior side and the posterior side of the head.

头维【tóu wéi】　足阳明胃经的一个穴

T

位,位头部额角入发际 0.5 寸,距头正中线 4.5 寸处。这一穴位为气功运行的一个常见部位。

Touwei(ST 8) An acupoint in the stomach meridian of foot Yangming, located 0.5 Cun from the frontal angle to the hairline and 4.5 Cun toward the midline in the head. This acupoint is a region usually used for keeping the essential Qi in practice of Qigong.

头有九宫【tóu yǒu jiǔ gōng】 指脑内结构,谓脑中有九室。

nine chambers in the head Refers to the structure of the brain, existing nine kinds of chambers.

头之一【tóu zhī yī】 指顶。"头之一者,顶也;七正之一者,目也;腹之一者,脐也;脉之一者,气也;五脏之一者,心也;四肢之一者,手足心也;骨之一者,脊也;肉之一者,肠胃也。"

top of head Refers to the top of the head. "The first in the head is the top; the first among the seven orifices are the eyes; the first in the abdomen is the navel; the first in the meridians is Qi; the first among the five Zang-organs (including the heart, the liver, the spleen, the lung and the kidney) is the heart; the first among the four limbs are the palms and soles; the first in the bones is spine; and the first among the muscles are the intestines and stomach."

土朝元【tǔ cháo yuán】 与"五气朝元"含义一致。

earthly archaeus Refers to Qi from the five Zang-organs (including the heart, the liver, the spleen, the lung and the kidney) that flows up to the celestial origin.

土釜【tǔ fǔ】 指气海,指下丹田。

tufu Refers to Qi sea and the lower Dantian (the region below the navel).

土宫黄气【tǔ gōng huáng qì】 指中央之气。

yellow Qi in the earthly palace Refers to the central Qi.

吐故纳新调气法【tǔ gù nà xīn tiáo qì fǎ】 为动静功。其作法为,平明面向午,展两手于膝上,徐徐按捺支节,口吐浊气,鼻引清气,即所谓吐故纳新。

regulating Qi through exhaling the old and inhaling the new A dynamic and static exercise, marked by starting practicing in the morning and facing the noon, putting the hands on the knees, mildly pressing the joints, exhaling turbid Qi through the mouth and inhaling pure Qi through the nose.

吐纳【tǔ nà】 习练气功的一种方法,主要是习练呼吸,使腹中恶浊之气随呼而出,清新太和之气由鼻而入。

exhaling the old and inhaling the new Refers to a way of practicing Qigong, marked by practicing respiration in order to expel turbid Qi in the abdomen and to inhale pure Qi from the nose.

吐纳以炼五脏【tǔ nà yǐ liàn wǔ zàng】 指习练气功,调节五脏功能,提高健康水平。

Refine the five Zang-organs through exhaling the old and inhaling the new. Refers to regulating the functions of the five Zang-organs (including the heart, the liver, the spleen, the lung and the kidney) and improving health in practicing Qigong.

吐气【tǔ qì】 指呼气,呼时念吹、呼、唏、呵、嘘、呬六字。

exhaling Qi Refers to exhalation, during which six Chinese characters must be read, i. e. Chui (blowing), Hu (exhaling), Xi (sighing), Ke (breathing out), Xu (breathing out slowly) and Xi (panting).

吐去浊气须知【tǔ qù zhuó qì xū zhī】源自专论,主要阐述吐去浊气的不同作法。

attention about exhaling turbid Qi Connected from a monograph, mainly describing different ways to exhale turbid Qi.

吐酸导引法【tǔ suān dǎo yǐn fǎ】为静功。其作法为,静心、调息,意念守背,运行至肾,从肾处引水上顶门,从上滴下心头以灌溉之。

exercise of Daoyin for sour regurgitation A static exercise, marked by tranquilizing the heart, regulating respiration, keeping consciousness on the back and to the kidney, conducting water from the kidney to the top and from the top to the heart in order to irrigate all parts of the body.

吐血【tù xiě】气功适应证,多由虚损及饮酒、劳损所致。

hematemesis An indication of Qigong, usually caused by deficiency, detriment and sprain.

瘭【tuí】气功适应证,指睾丸肿大的疾病。

severe swelling An indication of Qigong, referring to a disease due to severe swelling of the testicles.

瘭瘘候导引法【tuí lòu hòu dǎo yǐn fǎ】为静功。其作法为,正身仰卧,四肢伸直,静心存想天上的月亮又红又圆。消肿散结,治睾丸肿痛。

exercise of Daoyin for swollen scrotum A static exercise, marked by lying on

the back, stretching the four limbs, tranquilizing the heart, and imagining the red and round moon. Such a static exercise can subside swelling to dissipate indurated mass and cure swelling and pain of scrotum.

腿脚疼痛治法【tuǐ jiǎo téng tòng zhì fǎ】为动功,其作法为,立定,左手舒指,右手捏肚,闭气一口,左右相同。行三五转,坐定,令人摩腿数百止,日行三度。

exercise for curing leg and foot pain A dynamic exercise, marked by standing up, relaxing the fingers in the left hand and pinching the abdomen with the right hand and vice versa, stopping respiration for a while, returning for three to five times, sitting quietly, rubbing the legs for several hundreds of times, and practicing for three degrees everyday.

退藏沐浴【tuì cáng mù yù】指初练气功之时容易产生急躁情绪(如急于求成之类),这时要清除烦躁火炎,犹如借水以熄火。

quitting bath Indicates that irritable emotion is easy to appear in early practice of Qigong and measures should be taken to eliminate irritable emotion just like to extinguish fire with water.

退藏于密【tuì cáng yú mì】指意守下丹田。下丹田则指气海,指脐下。

quitting dense storage Refers to concentrating consciousness in the lower Dantian (the region below the navel). Lower Dantian (the region below the navel) refers to either Qihai (CV 6) located below the navel; or the region below the navel.

退阴符候【tuì yīn fú hòu】指从午时开始,阴气逐时而生。

T

yin receding　Refers to Yin Qi that begins to grow from Wu (the period of the day from 11 a. m. to 1 p. m. in the noon).

吞景咽液【tūn jǐng yàn yè】　指习练气功,采日月之光华并津液咽之。

absorbing natural profit and taking saliva　Refers to practice of Qigong, marked by collecting sunshine and moonshine as well as swallowing fluid and humor.

吞气【tūn qì】　指把气从口中咽入腹中,亦即服气、食气。

taking Qi　Refers to swallow Qi from the mouth into the abdomen, also called taking Qi and feeding Qi.

吞吐之术【tūn tǔ zhī shù】　即调节呼吸,为命功之一。

exercise of inhalation and exhalation　Refers to regulation of respiration, which is one of the life activities.

屯蒙【tún méng】　① 指调节阴阳工气;② 指屯卦、蒙。

tun and Meng　Refers to ① either Yin Qi and Yang Qi; ② or Tun Trigram and Meng Trigram.

屯蒙水火抽添论【tún méng shuǐ huǒ chōu tiān lùn】　源自气功专论,主要用八卦知识阐述温养、抽添、进火、退符之理。

discussion about lifting and pressing water and fire according to the law of Tun Trigram and Meng Trigram　Collected from a monograph of Qigong, mainly describing warm nourishment, ascent and descent, importing and exporting fire with the knowledge of the Eight Trigrams.

屯蒙之理【tún méng zhī lǐ】　指一天之内,阴阳之间的变化作用。

law of Tun Trigram and Meng Trigram　Refers to daily variation of Yin and Yang.

托踏法【tuō tà fǎ】　为动功。其作法为,两手上托,如举千斤之重,两脚踏地,如竖石柱之直,尽力上托,闭气不出。

raising and treading exercise　A dynamic exercise, marked by raising the hands like holding up a thousand kilograms of a pole and treading the feet on the ground like erecting a stone pillar without exhalation.

托踏轻骨法【tuō tà qīng gǔ fǎ】　为动功。其作法为,两手上托,如举大石,两脚前踏,如履平地,存想神气,依按四时,嘘、呵十四次。

exercise for raising and treading bones　A dynamic exercise, marked by raising the hands like holding up a large stone, treading the hands forward like walking on the flat, contemplating the spirit and Qi in the four seasons, breathing out slowly and naturally for about fourteen times.

橐籥【tuó yuè】　① 指呼吸自然之气,在丹田内交换,有如橐籥之鼓风;② 指心肾。

bellow　Refers to ① either breathing with natural Qi that exchanges in Dantian like airing in bellow; ② or the heart and kidney. Dantian is divided into the upper Dantian (the region between the eyes), the middle Dantian (the region below the heart) and the lower Dantian (the region below the navel).

拓天【tuò tiān】　为动功,指两手翻掌心向上用力向上举或向上推。

expanding the sky　A dynamic exercise, referring to turning the palms and forcibly raising upwards or pushing upwards.

T

唾血候导引法【tuò xuè hòu dǎo yǐn fǎ**】** 为动功。其作法为，正坐，伸展下肢，两手指放在两足趾上。舒展腰部筋脉治腰扭伤不能前俯，唾血久病。久炼，身体弯曲灵便。

exercise of Daoyin for hemoptysis　A dynamic exercise，marked by sitting upright，stretching the legs，putting the fingers in both hands on the toes in two feet， extending the sinews and meridians in the waist for curing sprained waist and chronic hemoptysis. Long period of practice will relax the body and make the body nimble.

W

外奔二景法【wài bēn èr jǐng fǎ】 为静功。其作法为，于寂静的夜晚，在清净的室内静坐，断绝一切杂念，微闭目，意想从自己心中放出一团赤色气体，赤气又结成周围绕有云气的车，自己登车冉冉直上天空。

exercise for reaching to the two external sceneries A static exercise, marked by sitting quietly in a clean and peaceful room at night, expelling all distracting thought, subtly closing the eyes, imagining to emit a group of red Qi from the heart which eventually concentrates and forms a cart of cloudy Qi. The practitioners can climb up to the sky with this cart of cloudy Qi.

外丹【wài dān】 ① 指在鼎炉中烧炼矿石药物以制丹药；② 指习练气功。

external Dan（pills of immortality） Refers to ① either baking minerals in the cauldron to produce medicinals; ② or Qigong practice.

外丹内丹论【wài dān nèi dān lùn】源自气功学专论，主要阐述了外丹、内丹的简要含义。

discussion about external Dan and internal Dan Collected from a monograph about Qigong, mainly describing the meaning of external Dan（pills of immortality）and internal Dan（pills of immortality）.

外鼎内鼎【wài dǐng nèi dǐng】 外鼎即丹田之形，内鼎指丹田中之气。

external cauldron and internal cauldron External cauldron refers to the form of Dantian and the internal cauldron refers to Qi in Dantian. Dantian is divided into the upper Dantian（the region between the eyes），the middle Dantian（the region below the heart）and the lower Dantian（the region below the navel）.

外固三要【wài gù sān yào】 三要即三宝，耳、目、口。外固三要即指垂帘、反听、闭口。

three external strengthening points A term of Qigong, referring to sitting behind a screen, concentration of respiration and closing the mouth. The so-called three strengthening points refers to the ears, the eyes and the mouth.

外观【wài guān】 手少阳三焦经的一个穴位，位于腕背横纹上 2 寸。这一穴位为气功运行的一个常见部位。

waiguan（TE 5） An acupoint in the triple energizer meridian of hand Shaoyang, located 2 Cun above the transverse line on the back of the wrist. This acupoint is a region usually used for keeping the essential Qi in practice of Qigong.

外呼吸【wài hū xī】 指口鼻之呼吸，浅而不接续。

external respiration Refers to respiration through the mouth and the nose which cannot be continued if it is weak.

外金丹【wài jīn dān】 指炼精、气、神，

使神形合一,动静适宜。

external golden Dan（pills of immortality） Refers to the essence，Qi and the spirit，indicating integration of the spirit and the body as well as suitability of dynamics and statics.

外其身而身存【wài qí shēn ér shēn cún**】** 指不以生命为念,而反身体健康,益寿延年。

External cultivation protects the body. Refers to the fact that only when consciousness is not just related to life can health be maintained and life be prolonged.

外气【wài qì**】** 指呼吸自然太和之气。

external Qi Refers to Qi related to natural and harmonious respiration.

外三宝【wài sān bǎo**】** 指耳、目、口。

three external treasures Refers to the ears，the eyes and the mouth.

外三要【wài sān yào**】** ① 指口、鼻两孔；② 指玄牝之门。玄牝指天与地、鼻与口、上与下等。

three external orifices Refers to ① either the mouth and the nostrils；② or the gate of Xuanpin which refers to the sky and the earth，the nose and the mouth，the upper and the lower，etc.

外象【wài xiàng**】** 指日、月、星辰、云雾之象。

external images Refers to the images of the sun，the moon，the stars and cloud and mist.

外药【wài yào**】** 指精、气、神，即交感之精、呼吸之气、思虑之神。

external medicinal Refers to the essence，Qi and the spirit，indicating essence in communication，Qi in respiration and the spirit in consciousness.

外药火候【wài yào huǒ hòu**】** 源自气功专论,主要阐述身心不动,呼吸自然,神气入于其根。

external medicinal and smelting Collected from a monograph of Qigong，mainly describing the importance of quietness of the body and the heart，natural respiration and existence of the spirit and Qi in the root.

外应尺宅【wài yìng chǐ zhái**】** 指脾运健,水谷精微充养形体,面部芳华有光彩。

external response to complexion Refers to active movement of the spleen，nourishing the body with nutrients of food and water and splendor of complexion.

外应眼童鼻柱间【wài yìng yǎn tóng bí zhù jiān**】** 指胆外应眼、眉。

external relationship between the eyes and brows Refers to the gallbladder that corresponds to the eyes and brows.

完骨【wán gǔ**】** ① 指颞骨乳突；② 指足少阳胆经的一个穴位；③ 鸣天鼓时叩击的一个部位。这一穴位为气功运行的一个常见部位。

mastoid process Refers to ① either mastoid process of temporal bone；② or an acupoint in the gallbladder meridian of foot Shaoyang，known as Wangu（SI 4）；③ or the clicking position for occipital-knocking therapy. This acupoint is a region usually used for keeping the essential Qi in practice of Qigong.

顽石产玉【wán shí chǎn yù**】** 喻人在气功状态下,吸日月精华之气而作丹,与自然相应。

hard rock producing jade Compares to inhalation of Qi from solar and lunar essence in order to produce Dan（pills of immortality) and correspond to the natural world in practicing Qigong.

挽弓势【wǎn gōng shì】 导引姿势,指两手作牵拉弓箭的姿态。

bow drawing posture Refers to the posture of Daoyin, indicating the posture of hands pulling the bow and arrow.

万法【wàn fǎ】 即宇宙万物生成变化之法,亦指各种气功功法的道理,都相同。

all methods Refers to the ways that all the things in the universe grow and develop. It also refers to various methods in practicing Qigong.

万古丹中王【wàn gǔ dān zhōng wáng】 指丹经之祖。

king of vanguard in antiquity Refers to the original classic of Qigong.

万类【wàn lèi】 即宇宙中一切生物。气功文献中用指人类。

all races Refers to all the biology in the universe or human beings according to the literature of Qigong.

万虑皆遣【wàn lù jiē qiǎn】 指练功时要做到排除一切杂念,意识高度集中。

eliminating all distracting thoughts Refers to elimination of all avarices and concentration of emotion and consciousness in practicing Qigong.

万虑俱忘【wàn lù jù wàng】 指练气功,忘却各种各样的念头。

forgetting all distracting thoughts Refers to forgetting any ideas in practicing Qigong.

万物【wàn wù】 宇宙一切物体的统称。

all things Refers to all the things in the universe.

万象主宰【wàn xiàng zhǔ zǎi】 指心与脐之间。

domination of all phenomena Refers to the region between the heart and navel.

腕【wàn】 指手臂与手掌相连接的部位。

wrist Refers to the region between the arm and palm.

汪昂【wāng áng】 清代中医学家,也通气功,自幼坚持练功,年虽过八十但依然体魄健壮。

Wang Ang A scientist of traditional Chinese medicine in the Qing Dynasty (1636 AD - 1912 AD), who was very proficient in Qigong. He began to insist on practicing Qigong when he was young. When he was over eighty years old, he was still quite healthy and strong.

汪讱庵【wāng rèn ān】 清代中医学家并通气功的汪昂的另外一个称谓,其自幼坚持练功,年虽过八十但依然体魄健壮。

Wang Ren'an Another name of Wang Ang, a scientist of traditional Chinese medicine in the Qing Dynasty (1636 AD - 1912 AD), who was very proficient in Qigong. He began to insist on practicing Qigong when he was young. When he was over eighty years old, he was still quite healthy and strong.

汪昙【wāng zhěng】 清代气功养生家,撰有气功专著。

Wang Zheng An important master of Qigong and life cultivation in the Qing Dynasty (1636 AD - 1912 AD). He wrote a monograph of Qigong to introduce the theory and practice of Qigong.

王弼【wáng bì】 三国时期的气功学家,撰有气功专论,从本末、动静、自然、无为等方面阐述气功。

Wang Bi A great scholar and master of Qigong in the Three Kingdoms Period（220 AD - 280 AD）, who wrote several monographs of Qigong, describing the principles and practice of Qigong according to the beginning and ending, activity and tranquility, nature and inactivity.

王充【wáng chōng】 东汉思想家、文学理论家和气功学家。

Wang Chong A great thinker, theorist of literature and master of Qigong in the East Han Dynasty（25 AD - 220 AD）.

王重阳【wáng chóng yáng】 金代气功学家,撰有多部气功专著,为全真道的创始人。

Wang Zhongyang A great master of Qigong in the Jin Dynasty（1142 - 1217）who wrote several monographs of Qigong, the founder of Acme Genunine Dao.

王重阳养寿法 【wáng chóng yáng yǎng shòu fǎ】 为静功,主要阐述老人于十二时中行住坐卧,不动不摇,精神内守,延年益寿。

Wang Zhongyang's exercise for longevity A static exercise, referring to the fact that old people should walk, sit and lie quietly without any disturbance in order to concentrate the spirit and Qi for cultivating health and prolonging life.

王处一【wáng chù yī】 金代气功学家,为全真道嵛山派的创始人。

Wang Chuyi A great master of Qigong in the Jin Dynasty（1142 - 1217）, who was the founder of Yushan school in Acme Genuine Dao.

王船山【wáng chuán shān】 明清时期思想家和气功学家,撰有气功专著,在气功学方面有突出贡献。

Wang Chuanshan A great thinker and master of Qigong in the late Ming Dynasty（1368 AD - 1644 AD）and the early Qing Dynasty（1636 AD - 1912 AD）, who wrote a monograph of Qigong, contributing a great deal to the development of Qigong.

王德威【wáng dé wēi】 金代气功学家王重阳的另一称谓,撰有多部气功专著,为全真道的创始人。

Wang Dewei Another name of Wang Zhongyang who was a great master of Qigong in the Jin Dynasty（1142 - 1217）who wrote several monographs of Qigong, the founder of Acme Genunine Dao.

王而农【wáng ér nóng】 明清时期思想家和气功学家王船山的另一称谓。

Wang Ernong Another name of Wang Chuanshan who was a great thinker and master of Qigong in the late Ming Dynasty（1368 AD - 1644 AD）and the early Qing Dynasty（1636 AD - 1912 AD）.

王方平胎息诀【wáng fāng píng tāi xī jué】 为静功,主要阐述神凝则心安的理法。

Wang Fangping's fetal respiration formula A static exercise, referring to the theory and methods for concentration of the spirit and tranquilization of the heart.

王夫子【wáng fū zǐ】 明清时期思想家和气功学家王船山的另一称谓。

Wang Fuzi Another name of Wang Chuanshan who was a great thinker and master of Qigong in the Ming Dynasty（1368 AD - 1644 AD）and Qing Dynas-

W

ty（1636 AD‐1912 AD）.

王辅嗣【wáng fǔ sì】 三国时期气功学家王弼的另一称谓,撰有气功专论,从本末、动静、自然、无为等方面阐述气功。

Wang Fusi Another name of Wang Bi who was a great master of Qigong in the Three Kingdoms Period（220 AD‐280 AD）, who wrote several monographs of Qigong, describing the principles and practice of Qigong according to the beginning and ending, activity and tranquility, nature and inactivity.

王晖【wáng huī】 唐代气功学家王玄览的另外一个称谓,撰有多部气功专著,主张气功入静。

Wang Hui Another name of Wang Xuanlan, a great master of Qigong in the Tang Dynasty（618 AD‐907 AD）, who wrote several monographs of Qigong, emphasizing tranquility in Qigong.

王姜斋【wáng jiāng zhāi】 明清时期思想家和气功学家王船山的另一称谓,撰有气功专著,在气功学方面有突出贡献。

Wang Jiangzhai Another name of Wang Chuanshan who was a great thinker and master of Qigong in the late Ming Dynasty（1368 AD‐1644 AD）and the early Qing Dynasty（1636 AD‐1912 AD）, who wrote a monograph of Qigong, contributing a great deal to the development of Qigong.

王荩臣【wáng jìn chén】 明代学者和气功学家王象晋的另外一个称谓,其撰有多部气功专著,强调元气在气功养生中的重要性。

Wang Jinchen Another name of Wang Xiangjin, a great scholar and master of Qigong in the Ming Dynasty（1368

AD‐1644 AD）who wrote several monographs of Qigong, emphasizing the importance of original Qi in Qigong and life cultivation.

王晋【wáng jìn】 先秦时期的气功学家王乔的另外一个称谓。

Wang Jin Another name of Wang Qiao who was a great master of Qigong before the Qin Dynasty（475 BC‐221 BC）.

王康宇【wáng kāng yǔ】 明代学者和气功学家王象晋的另外一个称谓,其撰有多部气功专著,强调元气在气功养生中的重要性。

Wang Kangyu Another name of Wang Xiangjin, a great scholar and master of Qigong in the Ming Dynasty（1368 AD‐1644 AD）who wrote several monographs of Qigong, emphasizing the importance of original Qi in Qigong and life cultivation.

王龙图静养火候【wáng lóng tú jìng yǎng huǒ hòu】 为静功。其作法为,右侧卧式睡法,治失眠、多梦、梦游等。

Wang Longtu's exercise for nourishing duration of heating A static exercise, marked by lying on the right side for treating insomnia, dreaminess and sleepwalk.

王乔【wáng qiáo】 先秦时期的气功学家。

Wang Qiao A great master of Qigong before the Qin Dynasty（475 BC‐221 BC）.

王世廉【wáng shì lián】 明代气功学家王文禄的另一称谓,其研究气功养生,著有多部气功专著。

Wang Shilian Another name of Wang Wenlu, a great master of Qigong in the Ming Dynasty（1368 AD‐1644 AD）, who studied Qigong and life cultivation and wrote several monographs.

王世雄【wáng shì xióng】 金代气功学家王重阳的另一称谓,为全真道的创始人。

Wang Shixiong Another name of Wang Chongyang who was a great master of Qigong before the Jin Dynasty (1142 – 1217), the founder of Acme Genuine Dao.

王说山人服气说【wáng shuō shān rén fú qì shuō】 源自气功专论,主要阐述服气的方法、注意事项、功效主治。

Wang Shuoshan's method for inhalation of Qi Collected from a monograph of Qigong, referring to paying attention to any matters and the effect of Qigong practice in treating any diseases.

王焘【wáng tāo】 唐代医学家和气功学家,著有气功养生专著。

Wang Tao A great doctor and master of Qigong in the Tang Dynasty (618 AD – 907 AD), who wrote a monograph of Qigong and life cultivation.

王惟一【wáng wéi yī】 宋末元初的针灸学家和气功学家,撰有针灸专著,其中也论述了气功养生。

Wang Weiyi Wang Weiyi was a great master of acupuncture, moxibustion and Qigong in the late Song Dynasty (960 AD – 1279 AD) and early Yuan Dynasty (1271 AD – 1368 AD), who wrote a monograph of acupuncture and moxibustion, including the introduction and discussion of Qigong and life cultivation.

王惟一论丹【wáng wéi yī lùn dān】 源自气功专论,阐述了习练气功的基本方法及要领.

Wang Weiyi's discussion about Dan（pills of immortality） Collected from a monograph of Qigong, referring to discussion about the basic methods and requirements in practicing Qigong.

王文禄【wáng wén lù】 明代气功学家,研究气功养生,著有多部气功专著。

Wang Wenlu A great master of Qigong in the Ming Dynasty （1368 AD – 1644 AD）, who studied Qigong and life cultivation and wrote several monographs.

王文禄胎息法【wáng wén lù tāi xī fǎ】 为静功,指神气相注是习练胎息的关键。

Wang Wenlu's fetal respiration formula A static exercise, referring to concentration of the spirit and Qi which is the key in practicing fetal respiration.

王羲之【wáng xī zhī】 东晋书法家和气功学家。

Wang Xizhi A great calligrapher and master of Qigong in the East Jin Dynasty （317 AD – 420 AD）.

王象晋【wáng xiàng jìn】 明代学者和气功学家,其撰有多部气功专著,强调元气在气功养生中的重要性。

Wang Xiangjin A great scholar and master of Qigong in the Ming Dynasty （1368 AD – 1644 AD） who wrote several monographs of Qigong, emphasizing the importance of original Qi in Qigong and life cultivation.

王玄览【wáng xuán lǎn】 唐代气功家,撰有多部气功专著,主张气功入静。

Wang Xuanlan A great master of Qigong in the Tang Dynasty （618 AD – 907 AD）, who wrote several monographs of Qigong, emphasizing tranquility in Qigong.

王逸少【wáng yì shào】 东晋书法家和气功学家王羲之的另一称谓。

W

Wang Yishao Another name of Wang Xizhi who was a great calligrapher and master of Qigong in the East Jin Dynasty (317 AD - 420 AD).

王玉阳【wáng yù yáng】 金代气功学家王处一的另一称谓,为全真道嵛山派的创始人。

Wang Yuyang Another name of Wang Chuyi who was a great master of Qigong in the Jin Dynasty (1142 - 1217), who was the founder of Yushan school in Acme Genuine Dao.

王远知【wáng yuǎn zhī】 东晋气功学家,撰有气功专著,习练非常成功。

Wang Yuanzhi A great master of Qigong in the East Jin Dynasty (317 AD - 420 AD) who wrote a monograph of Qigong and succeeded in practicing Qigong.

王允卿【wáng yǔn qīng】 金代著名气功学家王重阳的另一称谓,为全真道的创始人。

Wang Yunqing Another name of Wang Chongyang who was a great master of Qigong in the Jin Dynasty (1142 - 1217), contributing a great deal to the development of Qigong.

王嚞【wáng zhé】 王重阳的另外称谓,为宋代的真教创始者,也为气功的发展做出了特殊贡献。

Wang Zhe Another name of Wang Chongyang who was the founder of genuine religion and also a great master of Qigong in the Song Dynasty (960 AD - 1279 AD).

王知明【wáng zhī míng】 金代气功学家王重阳的另一称谓,撰有多部气功专著,为全真道的创始人。

Wang Zhiming Another name of Wang Chongyang who was a great mas-

ter of Qigong in the Jin Dynasty (1115 AD - 1234 AD) who wrote several monographs of Qigong, the founder of Acme Genuine Dao.

王中孚【wáng zhōng fú】 金代著名气功学家王重阳的另一称谓,为气功的发展做出了特殊贡献。

Wang Zhongfu Another name of Wang Chongyang who was a great master of Qigong in the Jin Dynasty (1142 AD - 1217 AD), contributing a great deal to the development of Qigong.

王仲任【wáng zhòng rèn】 东汉思想家、文学家和气功学家王充的另外一个称谓。

Wang Zhongren Another name of Wang Chong who was a great thinker, master of literature and Qigong in the East Han Dynasty (25 AD - 220 AD).

王子晋【wáng zǐ jìn】 王乔的另一个称谓,为先秦时期的气功学家。

Wang Zijin Another name of Wang Qiao who was a great master of Qigong before the Qin Dynasty (475 BC - 221 BC).

王子晋吹笙【wáng zǐ jìn chuī shēng】 为静功。其作法为,身端坐,两手捏拿胸傍二穴。主治通任脉,除百病。

Wang Zijin's flute exercise A static exercise, marked by sitting with both hands kneading two acupoints located on the sides of the chest. Such a static exercise can promote the flow of the conception meridian and treat various diseases.

王子乔【wáng zǐ qiáo】 王乔的另外一个称谓,为先秦时期的气功学家。

Wang Ziqiao Another name of Wang Qiao who was the founder of genuine religion and also a great master of

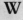

Qigong before the Qin Dynasty（475 BC－221 BC）.

王子乔导引法【wáng zǐ qiáo dǎo yǐn fǎ**】**　为动功，通过各种方式方法以达静安、平宁、和谐和长寿的作用。

Wang Ziqiao's Daoyin method　A dynamic exercise，referring to various ways in practicing Qigong for tranquility，balance，harmonization and longevity.

王子乔导引图【wáng zǐ qiáo dǎo yǐn tú**】**　为动功。其作法为，伸左脚，屈右膝，引脾气，去心腹寒热，胸臆邪胀。

Wang Ziqiao's Daoyin posture　A dynamic exercise，marked by stretching the left foot，bending the right knee and leading spleen Qi. Such a dynamic exercise can expel cold and heat and relieve chest distention caused by pathogenic factors.

王子乔内气法王惟一论丹【wáng zǐ qiáo, nèi qì fǎ wáng wéi yī lùn dān**】**为静功。其作法为，枕当高四寸，解衣拔发，正卧，足相去各五寸半，去身各三寸。可延年益寿，预防病病，除百病。

Wang Ziqiao's inner breathing exercise　A static exercise，marked by lying on the back with the pillow about 4 Cun high，undoing the clothes，draping hair，turning the feet for 5 and a half Cun and moving the body for 3 Cun. Such a static exercise can prolong life，cultivating health，preventing disease and treating various diseases.

王子乔入神导引法【wáng zǐ qiáo rù shén dǎo yǐn fǎ**】**　为静功。其作法为，解衣拔发，正偃卧，枕高四寸，各致五脏所竟而复始，延年益寿除百病。

Wang Ziqiao's mental Daoyin method　A static exercise，marked by lying on a pillow about 4 Cun high with divestiture of clothes and draping hair for the purpose of expiration，inspiration and stability of the five Zang-organs（including the heart，the liver，the spleen，the lung and the kidney）in order to prolong life.

王子乔胎息诀【wáng zǐ qiáo tāi xī jué**】**　指静功口诀。主要阐述练功以静心头、安精气神的理法。

Wang Ziqao's fetal respiration formula　A static exercise，referring to the basic theory and methods of Qigong practice for tranquilizing the heart and the mind，promoting the essence，Qi and the spirit.

王祖源【wáng zǔ yuán**】**　清代气功学家，集录各家气功养生之长并结合自己的实践，撰有气功专著。

Wang Zuyuan　A great master of Qigong in the Qing Dynasty（1636 AD－1912 AD）who wrote a monograph of Qigong according to the advantages of other masters of Qigong and himself experience.

罔象【wǎng xiàng**】**　① 指虚无；②指行动中，意识思维活动的相对静止而忘记自己的存在。

vacuum of image　Refers to ① either nihility；② or forgetting self-existence after practicing Qigong with tranquilized activities of consciousness and thought.

往北接度【wǎng běi jiē dù**】**　指习练小周天功，意守丹田，待丹田精气盈满，往北接引，使到尾间，再导引之，冲关荡窍而行周天火候。

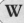

practice of Daoyin in coccyx　Refers to concentration of consciousness in Dantian in practicing small celestial cycle， turning to the coccyx when the essence and Qi in Dantian are exuberant, and finally leading it to rush the marsh orifice and duration of heating in the celestial cycle. Dantian is divided into the upper Dantian (the region between the eyes), the middle Dantian (the region below the heart) and the lower Dantian (the region below the navel).

往来【wǎng lái】　指一日之间阴阳的变化。

going out and coming in Refers to changes of Yin and Yang in a day.

妄见【wàng jiàn】　佛家气功习用语，指迷妄之见识。

avarice A common term of Qigong in Buddhism, referring to the idea about delusion.

妄念【wàng niàn】　指邪念、杂念。

wild fancy Refers to wicked idea and distracting thought.

妄念才兴神即迂【wàng niàn cái xìng shén jí yū】　指排除杂念，意守元神在练功中的重要性。

Elimination of distracting thought will enhance the spirit. Refers to the importance of eliminating delusion and concentrating the spirit in practicing Qigong.

妄情【wàng qíng】　佛家气功习用语，指虚妄不实的情识。

dishonest sentiment A common term of Qigong in Buddhism, referring to false and unreal sentiment and idea.

妄想【wàng xiǎng】　指杂念。

delusion Refers to distracting thought.

妄心【wàng xīn】　指心乱神散。

distracting thought Refers to confusion of the mind and dispersion of the spirit.

妄语【wàng yǔ】　佛家气功学习用语，指妄有所谈，言不当实。

wild talk A common term of Qigong in Buddhism, referring to the talk that is wild and unreal.

忘机【wàng jī】　指减少思虑，乃至灭绝杂念，气功中常用此以调神、养神。

secular oblivion Refers to reducing contemplation and eliminating distracting thought, which is used to regulate and to nourish the spirit in practicing Qigong.

忘机绝虑【wàng jī jué lù】　即气功锻炼中要剔除机心，杜绝谋虑，使神志处于清净无为，淡泊宁静的境界，方才利于调神。

secular oblivion without consideration Means to eliminate any desires, ideas and consideration as well as to stabilize and to tranquilize the mind and consciousness in order to regulate the spirit.

忘气【wàng qì】　指排除了自身形体的存在。

forgetting Qi Refers to eliminating the existence of self-body in practicing Qigong.

忘形【wàng xíng】　即忘记自己的形体。

somatic oblivion Means to have forgotten self-body.

望后三候【wàng hòu sān hòu】　指练功的时间选择。

viewing three periods backward Refers to selection of the time for practicing Qigong.

望前三候【wàng qián sān hòu】　指练功中的时间选择。

viewing the three periods in front Refers to selection of the time for practicing Qigong.

危坐【wēi zuò】　端身正坐。

straight sitting Refers to sitting with upright body.

威光门【wēi guāng mén】　指脑。

mighty bright gate Refers to the brain.

威明【wēi míng】　指胆神勇悍而刚。

mighty brightness Refers to cholic braveness.

威仪行气法【wēi yí xíng qì fǎ】　为静功，主要为调身、调气、调神。

exercise for mighty regulation of Qi A static exercise, mainly for regulating the body, Qi and the spirit.

微明【wēi míng】　指人调节平衡的智慧和深沉的预见。

Twilight Refers to wisdom and prediction in regulating balance.

韦驮献杵【wéi tuó xiàn chǔ】　为动功。其作法为，取立位，两足分开与肩宽，弃除杂念，精神集中，调匀呼吸，两手缓慢上举至胸前，两足趾用力着地，两手分开高举，有调筋骨、和气血作用。

extending exercise A dynamic exercise, marked by standing up, separating both feet, eliminating distracting thought, concentrating the spirit, regulating respiration, slowly raising up to the chest and above the head with the hands, forcefully pressing the ground with the toes in both feet and separately raising both hands. Such a dynamic exercise can regulate sinews and bones as well as harmonize Qi and the blood.

唯心【wéi xīn】　佛家气功习用语，指唯有一心，即意念专一。

concentrating the heart A common term of Qigong in Buddhism, referring to tranquilizing the heart and concen-

trating consciousness.

尾椿【wěi chūn】　指尾骨。

tail toon Refers to coccyx.

尾骶【wěi dǐ】　指骶骨和尾骨，也称为尻骨、尾底骨、尾脊骨。

sacrococcyx Refers to coccyx and sacrum, also called sacral bone, lower buttock bone and buttock and spine bone.

尾骶骨【wěi dǐ gǔ】　骶骨和尾骨的别称。

buttock and sacrum bone A synonym of the coccyx and the sacrum.

尾脊骨【wěi jǐ gǔ】　骶骨和尾骨的别称。

buttock and spine bone A synonym of the coccyx and the sacrum.

尾闾【wěi lǘ】　① 指古代传说中海水归宿之处；② 指尾骶骨之末节；③ 指督脉中的长强穴。

weilǘ Refers to ① either the legendary place that water from the sea returns into it; ② or the end of sacrococcyx; ③ or Changqiang（CV 1），an acupoint in the governor meridian.

尾闾坠气导引法【wěi lǘ zhuì qì dǎo yǐn fǎ】　为动功。其作法为，调息，咬牙闭气，耸肩，双圆睁，左右转动，肛门紧缩上提，气自然升提。

exercise of Daoyin for dropping Qi from coccygeal end A dynamic exercise, marked by regulating respiration, clicking the teeth to stop breath, shrugging the shoulders, opening the eyes and turning from the left to the right and vice versa, shrinking and raising the anus in order to enable Qi to flow upwards naturally.

尾翳【wěi yì】　① 指胸骨剑突；② 指穴位名，为任脉中的一个穴位，位于腹正中线,脐上 7 寸。此穴位为气功习练之处。

weiyi Refers to ① either mucronate cartilage; ② or Jiuwei (CV 15), which is an acupoint in the conception meridian, located in the abdominal middle line, 7 Cun above the navel. This acupoint is a region usually used in practice of Qigong.

委和【wěi hé】 指木运不及,其阳和之气委曲或弃而不用。

entrusting harmony Refers to failure of the wood to move entirely in which Yang Qi is tactful or is not applied.

委气法【wěi qì fǎ】 为静功,指调身、调气、调神。其功效为安神和泰,调节形神,通利气机。

exercise for entrusting Qi A static exercise, referring to regulation of the body, Qi and the spirit. The effect of such a practice of Qigong is to stabilize the spirit, to harmonize the essence, to regulate the body and spirit and to promote the functional activity of Qi.

委身放体【wěi shēn fàng tǐ】 指放松身体,气功中忌讳形体紧张。

relaxation of the body Refers to avoiding intensity of the body in practicing Qigong.

委形【wěi xíng】 指放松身体。

entrusting form Refers to relaxation of the body.

委志虚无【wěi zhì xū wú】 指习练气功,放松形体和精神,使意念活动处于相对静止的状态。

relaxation and tranquilization Refers to relaxing the body and the spirit and relatively tranquilizing the activity of consciousness in practicing Qigong.

委中【wěi zhōng】 足太阳膀胱经的

一个穴位,位于腘窝横纹中央,为行功中精气运行的通道。

Weizhong (BL 40) An acupoint in the bladder meridian of foot Taiyin, located in the center of the transverse line in popliteal space, acting as the passageway of the essence and Qi in Qigong practice.

卫气【wèi qì】 指运行于脉外之气。

defense Qi Refers to Qi defending the skin.

卫生歌【wèi shēng gē】 源自气功专论,介绍诸家气功养生之言,编辑成歌诀。

health song Collected from a monograph of Qigong, referring to compiling the ideas of various masters about Qigong into songs.

卫生之经【wèi shēng zhī jīng】 指习练气功,内守精神,使神形合一;稳定意识思维活动;保持身体的纯和之气而不外散。

theory of health cultivation Refers to the theory and methods for cultivating health, indicating internal concentration of the spirit, integration of the spirit and the body, stabilizing the activities of consciousness and thinking and keeping pure Qi in the body without any dispersion.

未济【wèi jì】 指水火不交。

Disharmony Refers to failure of water and fire to coordinate with each other.

未尽宫真人【wèi jìn gōng zhēn rén】 指大肠所主神名。

genuine man without entering palace Refers the name of the spirit in the large intestine.

未炼还丹先炼性【wèi liàn huán dān xiān liàn xìng】 指学习练气功之先,应

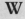

炼性炼神,涵养本性。

practicing property before practicing Huandan（elixir） Refers to refining the property and the spirit in practicing Qigong in order to conserve natural character.

未炼之纯【wèi liàn zhī chún】 指习练气功时,神不静而意识思维活动不稳定,每遇外感而即发。

no honest practice Refers to dishonest and intranquil activities of consciousness and thinking in practicing Qiong which often cause various problems.

未漏者【wèi lòu zhě】 指未婚具童贞之体者。按传统说法,这种人练功易见成效。

no leakage Refers to virginity. Traditionally it is believed that only those who are not married can effectively practice Qigong.

未那识【wèi nà shí】 佛家气功习用语,又称意识,为思维量度之意。

consciousness A common term of Qigong in Buddhism, referring to the degree of consciousness.

未修大药先修心【wèi xiū dà yào xiān xiū xīn】 指精神意识思维活动,能安定精神情绪。

cultivating the heart before cultivating large medicine Refers to the activities of spirit, consciousness and thought in order to stabilize the spirit and emotion.

味于无味【wèi yú wú wèi】 即食而不知其味,以保持味觉的平和,使饮食之味不乱于心。

tasting no taste Means to pay no attention to the taste of food in order to normalize the taste sense and to avoid food taste affecting the heart.

胃气【wèi qì】 ① 指胃受纳与腐熟水谷的生理功能;② 指脉象,即脾胃功能在脉象中的反映。

stomach Qi Refers to ① either the physiological function of the stomach in receiving and digesting food and water; ② or the conditions of pulse which reflect the functions of the spleen and stomach.

胃俞【wèi shū】 足太阳膀胱经中的一个穴位,位第十二胸椎棘突下旁开1.5寸。这一穴位为气功运行的一个常见部位。

Weishu（BL 21） An acupoint in the bladder meridian of foot Taiyang, located 1.5 Cun lateral to the spinous process of the twelfth thoracic vertebra. This acupoint is a region usually used for keeping the essential Qi in practice of Qigong.

胃脘【wèi wǎn】 上脘的一个别称,属于任脉中的一个穴位,位于前正中线,脐上5寸,为气功常用意守部位。

Weiwan A synonym of Shangwan（CV 13）, which is an acupoint in the conception meridian, located on the anterior midline, about 5 Cun above the navel.

魏翱【wèi áo】 东汉著名气功学家魏伯阳的另外一个称谓,其著有气功专著,为气功经典著作。

Wei Ao Another name of Wei Boyang, a famous master of Qigong in the East Han Dynasty（25 AD - 220 AD）, who wrote an important monograph of Qigong.

魏伯阳【wèi bó yáng】 东汉著名气功学家,著有气功专著,为气功经典著作。

Wei Boyang A famous master of Qigong in the East Han Dynasty（25

AD－220 AD），who wrote an important monograph of Qigong.

魏伯阳破风法【wèi bó yáng pò fēng fǎ】 动静相兼功。其作法为，端坐，右手作拳，拄右胁，左手按膝舒拳，存想运气于病处，右左各六口。主治久年瘫痪。

Wei Boyang's exercise for paralysis An exercise combined with dynamic exercise and static exercise, marked by sitting upright, holding the right hand as a fist for pressing the right rib, pressing the knee to relax the left hand, imagining to move Qi to the location of disease from the left to the right and vice versa for six times respectively. Such an exercise combined with dynamic exercise and static exercise can cure chronic paralysis.

魏伯阳谈道【wèi bó yáng tán dào】 为动功。其作法为，身体坐于椅上，椅略比腿高，右腿自然放下，左腿弯搭于椅上，左手平举，右手摩腹，凝神运气十二口。主治肩背疼痛。

Wei Boyang's talking about Dao A dynamic exercise, marked by sitting on the chair which is slightly higher than the leg, naturally laying down the right leg, bending the left leg over the chair, raising the left hand flatly, rubbing the abdomen with the right hand, concentrating the spirit and moving Qi for twelve times respectively. Such a dynamic exercise can cure shoulder pain and back pain.

魏夫人【wèi fū rén】 魏华存，为晋朝道家大师，其所传《黄庭经》为后世内丹修炼之经典著作。

Madam Wei Another name of Wei Boyang, a famous master of Qigong in the East Han Dynasty（25 AD－220 AD），who wrote an important monograph of Qigong.

魏华存【wèi huá cún】 晋朝道家大师，其所传《黄庭经》为后世内丹修炼之经典著作。

Wei Huacun A great master of Daoism in the Jin Dynasty（266 AD－420 AD）. The Huangting Canon disseminated by him was a classical canon for refining the internal Dan（pills of immortality）in the later generations.

温病候导引法【wēn bìng hòu dǎo yǐn fǎ】 为静功。其作法为，静心存想心气色赤，肝气色青，肺气色白，脾气色黄，肾气色黑，五脏气色充满全身，能扶正祛邪。

exercise of Daoyin for warm disease A static exercise, marked by tranquilizing the heart and imagining that Qi in the heart is red, Qi in the liver is green, Qi in the lung is white, Qi in the spleen is yellow and Qi in the kidney is black, indicating Qi from the five Zang-organs（including the heart, the liver, the spleen, the lung and the kidney）in the whole body to reinforce healthy Qi and to dispel pathogenic factors.

温养【wēn yǎng】 ① 指习练气功，导引入静，意识活动逐步处于相对稳定的状态；② 指和调阴阳并两相得配；③ 指调养时ческий纯正火候。

warmly nourishing Refers to ① either gradually stabilizing the activity of consciousness by tranquilization in practicing Qigong；② or regulating and combining Yin and Yang；③ or purifying fire through regulation and cultivation.

温养成丹【wēn yǎng chéng dān】 即温养成丹的方法。

Dan（pills of immortality）formed by

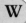

warmly nourishing   Refers to the methods for forming Dan (pills of immortality) by warmly nourishing the body.

温养法【wēn yǎng fǎ】 为静功。其作法为，自然坐式，意守规中，洗心涤虑，六门紧闭，万缘放下，不挂一丝，内想不出，外想不入，十二时中，念兹在兹，回光返照。

exercise for warmly nourishing   A static exercise, marked by sitting naturally, keeping consciousness normally without any change, purifying the heart and mind, closing six portals, putting down all costae without any contemplations and wishes, keeping the present and staying at the present in the twelve periods with sudden spurt of vitality prior to collapse.

温养火候【wēn yǎng huǒ hòu】 指练气功中，圣胎结成，须温温养之，真息往来，绵绵密密，谓之温养火候。

warmly nourishing fire duration   Indicates that when sacred fetal respiration in Qigong practice is formed, it should be warmly, continuously and closely nourished.

瘟疫秘禁法【wēn yì mì jìn fǎ】 为静功。其作法为，思其身为五玉；又思冠金巾，思心如炎火；又思其发散以搜身；又思五脏之气从两目出，周身如云雾，肝青气，肺白气，脾黄气，肾黑气，心赤气，五色纷错。可避疫，预防感染。

exercise for preventing pestilence   A static exercise marked by imagining the body as five kinds of jade, imagining crown scarf and the heart like hot fire; imagining searching the body through diffusion; imagining that Qi in the five Zang-organs (including the heart, the liver, the spleen, the lung and the kidney) originates from the eyes and the whole body is just like cloud and mist, in which the liver Qi is green, the lung Qi is white, the spleen Qi is yellow, the kidney Qi is black and the heart Qi is red. Such a static exercise can prevent pestilence and infection.

文火【wén huǒ】 指意念作用下，呼吸绵绵，不使其间断。

mild fire   Refers to normal respiration without any disturbance.

文始先生【wén shǐ xiān shēng】 古代著名气功学家关尹子的另外一个称谓，著有气功专论，年代不详。

Mr. Wenshi   Another name of Guan Yinzi, a great master of Qigong in ancient China and wrote a monograph about Qigong. The dynasty related was unknown.

文武火【wén wǔ huǒ】 指调节呼吸时武火为意念，呼吸加强；文火为意念，呼吸之气减弱，绵绵若存。

mild and heavy fire   Refers to the fact that, in regulating respiration, the heavy fire refers to consciousness and respiration should be enhanced; and that the mild fire refers consciousness and respiration should be abated and continued.

文逸曹仙姑歌【wén yì cáo xiān gū gē】 源自气功专论，主要论述精气神的关系及对人的重要性。

Wenyi Caoxian's aunt song   Collected from a monograph about Qigong, mainly describing the relation about the essence, Qi and the spirit as well as the importance to human beings.

文子【wén zǐ】 古代气功家辛铏，所处时代不详。

Wen Zi   Another name of Xin Xing, a

W

great master of Qigong in the ancient. The related dynasty was unknown.

我【wǒ】 佛家气功习用语，① 指生命、本体；② 指精神活动。

myself A common term of Qigong in Buddhism，referring to ① either life and body；② or activity of the essence and the spirit.

我命在我不在天【wǒ mìng zài wǒ bù zài tiān】 指生命居于自己，非天命所定，习练气功，即可还精补脑延年。

My life belongs to me，not to the sky. Indicates that life is controlled by myself，not controlled by the sky. Thus practice of Qigong can tonify the brain and prolong the life with the essence.

我心治官乃治【wǒ xīn zhì guān nǎi zhì】 指意识和调，五官聪彻明朗，味和气正。

only when our hearts control ourselves can the officials control themselves Indicates regulation of consciousness，intelligence of the five organs and rectification of stupidity.

卧禅法【wò chán fǎ】 为静功。其作法为，睡时头朝东方，侧身卧，一手曲肘，头枕于手心处，另一手放于肚脐处，着床之腿曲起，上面一只腿伸。

exercise for lying dhyana A dynamic exercise，marked by turning the head towards the east and lying on the right side，bending the elbows，putting the head over the palm，putting the other hand over the navel，bending the leg over the bed and stretching the other leg.

卧法【wò fǎ】 佛家气功功法，即夜卧时，右胁卧，两脚相对，两手相握，不散乱心，心神宁静，然后入睡。

exercise for lying An exercise of Qigong practice in Buddhism，referring to lying at night on the right side，closing two feet and holding two hands，stabilizing the heart and tranquilizing heart spirit for normal sleep.

卧功法【wò gōng fǎ】 为动功。作法为，夜卧醒时，常叩齿九通，咽唾九过，以手按鼻左右上下数十过。

technique for lying A dynamic exercise，marked by waking up at night，clicking the teeth for nine times，swallowing and spitting for nine times，pressing the nose with the hands from the left to the right and from the upper to the lower for ten times.

卧功五段【wò gōng wǔ duàn】 为动功，方法多样。如仰卧，伸两足，竖足趾，伸两臂，伸十指，俱用力向下，左右连身牵动数遍。

five courses of lying exercise A dynamic exercise with several methods，such as lying on the back，stretching the feet，lifting the toes，stretching the arms and ten fingers，forcefully turning downwards，and tugging the body with the left arm and right arm for many times.

卧虎扑食【wò hǔ pū shí】 为动功。其作法为，取弓箭步，弯腰向前，两手撑地，昂头前视，胸向前俯，如虎扑食。

lying tiger pouncing food A dynamic exercise，marked by running like shooting arrow，stooping forwards，pressing the ground with both hands，raising the head to see the front and turning the chest forwards like a tiger pouncing food.

偓佺【wò quán】 古代传说中的神仙，有走马导引势。

Wo Quan An immortal in ancient China who rode on horse to practice Daoyin.

偓佺飞行逐走马【wò quán fēi xíng zhú zǒu mǎ】 为动功。其作法为,两脚自然分开,两手平举与肩平,如托重物姿势。头向左,眼看左手,左手掌心向下,右脚跟提起,右足尖着地,运气九口,转身向右侧,姿势向左,运气九口。治疗赤白痢疾。

immortal Wo Quan flying for chasing and running horse A dynamic exercise, marked by naturally separating the feet, raising the hands to the level of the shoulders like raising heavy things, turning the head to the left side, seeing to the left side, lowering the left palm, lifting the right foot with the toes touching the ground, moving Qi for nine times; then turning the body to the right side, posturing to the left side, and moving Qi for nine times. Such a dynamic exercise can cure multi-coloured dysentery.

握固【wò gù】 ① 指四指握住拇指的姿势;② 指大指掐中指指节;③ 指调节精神。

grasping and solidifying Refers to ① either the four fingers in a hand to grasp the thumb; ② or the thumb pinching the knuckles of the second finger; ③ or regulating the spirit.

兀然放神【wū rán fàng shén】 指精神放松,使心如枯木,身若委衣。

mental relaxation Refers to relaxation of the spirit in order to quiet the heart and to normalize the body.

乌肝兔髓【wū gān tù suǐ】 指日精月华、元神元精。

crow liver and rabbit marrow Refers to solar essence and moonlight as well as the original spirit and the original essence.

邬遇微静坐默持【wū yù wēi jìng zuò mò chí】 为静功。其作法为,盘膝而坐,以两手按膝。凝神存想,闭气,令气周流,运气四十九门。

quiet sitting with silent action A static exercise, marked by sitting with crossed legs, pressing the knees with both hands, silently contemplating, suspending respiration, promoting Qi to flow in the whole body and circulating Qi for forty-nine times.

无【wú】 ① 指静,指与有相对;② 指空,为理想境界。

nothingness Refers to ① either quietness; or non-existence; ② or vacuum, which is a ideal state.

无碍【wú ài】 佛家气功学术语,指神形和一,通体自在通达安适。

no obstacle A common term of Qigong in Buddhism, referring to spiritual and somatic integration.

无常【wú cháng】 佛家气功学术语,指世间一切事物,生天流迁,刹那不住。

indefiniteness A common term of Qigong in Buddhism, referring to the fact that all the things in the world have come out from the sky and turned to all the areas without any prevention.

无方【wú fāng】 指修习佛家气功,达到涅槃境界,无一定之方,无一定之法。

indefinite method Refers to the fact that there are no special methods for practice of Qigong in Buddhism.

无极【wú jí】 ① 指原始的无形无象的本体;② 指极为无形态;③ 指太极未变化之前,阴阳双方不动不发,相对稳定的状态。

endlessness Refers to ① either noumenon without form and image at the

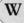

primitive period; ② or nonpolarity without form; ③ or the supreme pole before any change of Yin and Yang, a stable condition.

无极界【wú jí jiè】 即宇宙三界之。在天地未分之前,混沌世界称为无极界。

nonpolar phase Refers to three realms in the universe. Before the sky and the earth were separated from each other, the chaotic world was called nonpolar phase.

无己【wú jǐ】 指人的思想行为有善恶二性之外,还有无记性。

neutral quality Refers to the fact that human beings not only have moral emotion and immoral emotion, but also have no memory.

无己【wú jǐ】 即无我。

disinterestedness Refers to anatta which means no care about oneself.

无疆【wú jiāng】 即无穷尽也。一指广博,一指长久。

infinitude Refers to inexhaustibility, indicating width and longinquity.

无来无去不出不入【wú lái wú qù bù chū bú rù】 指习练气功达到一定的功夫,就能保持身体阴阳相对平衡的状态。

no arrival, no leave, no egress and no entrance Refers to the certain function of Qigong practice that can keep the balance of Yin and Yang in the body.

无量【wú liàng】 即无穷无尽之意。如《尊经玉清经》说,"若诸真人,无量大神"。

immeasurability Refers to endless development in the world. In *Zunjing Yuqing Canon*, it says that "the genuine man is the greatest immortal with all immeasurability".

无明【wú míng】 佛家气功学术语,指

认识事物,分别是非的精神活动。

recognition A common term of Qigong in Buddhism, referring to differentiation of the spiritual activities, which is the way to recognize all the things.

无明病【wú míng bìng】 佛家气功学术语,即不认识佛家稳定神形的方法,神形不调而导致疾病的发生。

non-cognitive disease A common term of Qigong in Buddhism, referring to the method for understanding how Buddhism stabilizes the spirit and body. If the spirit and body are not regulated, disease will occur.

无明惑【wú míng huò】 佛家气功学术语。无明惑指障蔽中道实相理之惑,迷于根本理体,精神意识紊乱、不调,影响神形稳定。

non-cognitive disorder A common term of Qigong in Buddhism, referring to puzzle due to failure in understanding the purity and origin of the theory and practice of Qigong, causing disorder and inability of the spirit and the body.

无念【wú niàn】 ① 指没有念头,即精神思维活动平静,故习练气功,有无念为本之说。② 佛家气功习用语,指无妄念,为正念的异名。

no idea Refers to ① either no intention, indicating that the activities of the spirit and thinking are tranquilized; or no wild fancy in the practice of Qigong; ② or a common term of Qigong in Buddhism, which is a synonym of genuine thought without wild fancy.

无上【wú shàng】 指最佳或最好的习练气功的方法。

best formula Refers to the ideal method used to practice Qigong and to cultivate health.

无上真人【wú shàng zhēn rén】　古代气功学家关尹子的另外一个名称,著有气功专论,年代不详。

Supreme Immortal　Another name of Guan Yinzi, a great master of Qigong in ancient China and wrote a monograph about Qigong. The dynasty related was unknown.

无神无知【wú shén wú zhī】　指习练气功时,精神意识活动处于相对稳定状态,达到忘去一切,使大脑得到充分的安静、休息。

no sense of spirit and knowledge　Relatively tranquilizing the activities of the spirit and consciousness in practicing Qigong, making it possible for people to forget everything and to tranquilize the mind for rest.

无生【wú shēng】　指寂寞和涅槃,意为精神活动稳定安适。

nirvana　Refers to tranquility and stability of the spirit activity.

无树根【wú shù gēn】　源自气功专论。阐述了习练气功的感受,抗老延寿的作用及幻景出现的景象。

no tree root　Collected from a monograph of Qigong, mainly describing professional experience of Qigong, elaborating the effect of prolonging life and manifestation of fairyland in practicing Qigong.

无体性自通【wú tǐ xìng zì tōng】　佛家气功习用语,指习练气功,一窍通百窍通,通达诸法无性之理,神形调和,意识稳定,情绪良好。

natural obtainment of unique passageway　A common term of Qigong in Buddhism, referring to special achievement in practicing Qigong, characterized by smoothness of one thing that ensures smooth flowing of everything, regulation of the spirit and body, stability of the consciousness and favorable emotion.

无头疽【wú tóu jū】　气功适应证,指初起无头,发于骨骼及关节间的疮疡。症以漫肿,皮色不变,疼痛彻骨,难消、难脓、难溃、难敛为特征。

deep abscess　An indication of Qigong, refers to abscess that initially occurs in the region between the skeleton and joint, characterized by diffuse swelling, no change of skin color, serious pain and difficulty in elimination, purulency, ulceration and restraint.

无妄【wú wàng】　① 指无妄念、妄想之意;② 指神形性疾病,不要有忘念、妄想,情绪稳定,安心静养,不吃药也会好转。

no avarice　Refers to ① either no wild fancy and no delusion; ② or disease related to the spirit and body to be treated by stability of emotion, quietness of the heart and tranquility of the mind without any wild fancy and delusion. Such a way to tranquilize and purify the heart and the mind certainly can cure disease without taking any medicinal.

无为【wú wéi】　① 指不妄为;② 指非姻缘和合形成,为佛家气功习用语;③ 指精神稳定。

inaction　Refers to ① either inactivity; ② or absolute existence, which is a common term of Qigong in Buddhism; ③ or stability of the spirit.

无为法【wú wéi fǎ】　即道之真理也,与有为法相对。

inactivity approach　Refers to the truth in Daoism, relative to promising idea.

W

无为之术【wú wéi zhī shù】 为古代气功功法之一，指意识思维活动合乎自然，不妄作劳。

inactive technique Refers to one of the methods for practicing Qigong in ancient times, indicating that the activities of consciousness and thinking should accord with nature.

无我【wú wǒ】 佛家气功习用语，指世界一切事物，都无独立的实体存在。

self-nonexistence A common term of Qigong in Buddhism, refers to no independent entity in all the things in the world.

无物【wú wù】 指目不见物，意不想物。并非客观事物不存在。

invisibility Refers to the eyes that observe nothing and the mind that thinks about nothing in practicing Qigong. But it does not mean that there exists nothing.

无相【wú xiàng】 佛家气功学术语，即众相，指的是常境无相，常智无缘。

alaksana A common term of Qigong in Buddhism, referring to basic knowledge and methods in practicing Qigong.

无象【wú xiàng】 无象即无极，二仪未分，阴中合阳也。

no extremity Refers to the fact that there is Yang in Yin and Yin in Yang.

无心【wú xīn】 ① 佛家气功习用语，指真心离妄念；② 指思维意识活动的相对稳定；③ 指思维意识活动的统一；④ 指与有心相对。

casualness A common term of Qigong in Buddhism, referring to ① either tranquilizing the heart without any avarice；② or stabilizing the activities of thinking and consciousness；③ or unity of the activities of thinking and consciousness；④ or similarity to existence.

无心得大还【wú xīn dé dà huán】 源自气功专论。主要阐述修炼气功而达到养生长寿的境地，关键是去除欲念，保持清静。

non-desire ensuring great achievement Connected from a monograph of Qigong, mainly describing professional discussion about Qigong, mainly describing the ideal state for cultivating health and prolonging life in practicing Qigong in order to eliminate avarice and to keep tranquility and quietness.

无形【wú xíng】 指"大道无形，生育天地飞"，即无形象可求。引申为静之意。

formlessness Refers to the fact that the greatest road is intangible and it is just the intangible road that promotes the development of the sky and the earth, indicating tranquility and quietness.

无学【wú xué】 佛家气功学术语，指学习佛学，泛指学习应用佛家气功，已达身体的稳定状态，不再学习义理、功法。

no need of study A common term of Qigong in Buddhism, referring to application of Qigong in Buddhism and avoidance of studying any theory and methods.

无学道【wú xué dào】 佛家气功学术语，指学习佛家气功戒、定、慧三法，断自然与社会的烦恼，以实现精神世界的理想境界。

avoidance of studying Dao A common term of Qigong in Buddhism, referring to relieving social and natural annoyance when studying the methods of Qigong in Buddhism.

无摇汝精【wú yáo rǔ jīng】 指内守精

神,不动情伤精。

internal concentration of spirit Refers to keeping the essence and the spirit inside and avoiding damage of the essence with excitation.

无英【wú yīng】 指肝神名。如《黄庭内景经》说:"百病所钟存无英。"

liver spirit Refers to the concentration of the spirit in the liver. In *Huangting Neijing Canon*, it says that the existence of the spirit in the liver is due to the relief of all diseases.

无忧普济开微洞明真君【wú yōu pǔ jì kāi wēi dòng míng zhēn jūn】 指无以杂念扰乱神明,大功将自然而至。即是内守精神,调节魂魄,气功将自然获得成效。

immortal without anxiety and desire Refers to the fact that there is no distracting thought to disturb the spirit and that the great merit will be naturally perfected. Even if measures are taken to keep the spirit inside and to regulate the ethereal soul and corporeal soul, the practice of Qigong will certainly be successful.

无忧普济开微洞明真君【wú yōu pǔ jì kāi wēi dòng míng zhēn jūn】 对宋代大道教创始人、气功学家刘德仁的赞美。

entirely helping without any anxiety and opening subtle hole to indicate genuine immortal The celebration of Liu Deren, who the founder of Daoism and a greater master of Qigong.

无忧子【wú yōu zǐ】 即刘德仁,是宋代大道教创始人,也是一位气功专家。

Man Without Anxiety Another name of Liu Deren who was the creator of Daoism and a great master of Qigong in the Song Dynasty（960 AD – 1279 AD）.

无欲观妙【wú yù guān miào】 指意识活动宁静,静而后一阳生,萌发奇妙生机。

marvelous view without desire Refers to tranquilization of consciousness activities in order to promote the development of Yang and to germinate fantastic vitality.

无诤三昧法【wú zhèng sān mèi fǎ】 佛家气功功法。其作法为,盘膝正坐,导引入静,与人群保持良好的关系,自然精神内守,神形和平。

harmonious Samadhi A method of Qigong practice in Buddhism, marked by sitting with crossed knees in order to tranquilize the mind, maintaining good relationship with others, keeping the spirit naturally inside and harmonizing the spirit and body.

无住【wú zhù】 指脑神无丝毫念头留住,为至静至虚的境界。亦指精神意识思维活动不会凝住不变。

absolute tranquility Refers to either no existence of any idea in the brain spirit which is the ideal state of tranquility without any deficiency; or no absolute concentration and no absolute change in the activities of the spirit, consciousness and thinking.

无子候导引法【wú zǐ hòu dǎo yǐn fǎ】 为静功。其作法是,傍晚月初出,日入之时,面向月正立,闭气不息,至极限时慢慢呼出,作八遍。吸入日久使妇女形体健康,还能延年益寿。

Wu Zihou's Daoyin exercise A static exercise, marked by standing up in moonrise and sunset, facing the moon, stopping respiration, then slowly breathing out for eight times. To inhale the moonshine for a long time will cultivate women's health and prolong life.

毋以妄念戕真心，毋以客气伤元气【wú yǐ wàng niàn qiāng zhēn xīn wú yǐ kè qì shāng yuán qì】 练功者要清除妄念，心神才能安宁，要抵御邪气的侵入，元气才不会损伤。

Never destroy the genuine heart with wild fancy, never damage the original Qi with pathogenic factors. In practicing Qigong, measures should be taken to eliminate wild fancy in order to stabilize the heart spirit. Only when invasion of pathogenic factors is resisted can the original Qi be protected.

吾丧我【wú sàng wǒ】 指忘记自我，与自然和社会融为一体的境界，此多指气功的入静。

I forgetting myself Means that anyone should integrate with the natural world in order to tranquilize the mind in practicing Qigong.

吴猛【wú měng】 晋代著名的气功家。
Wu Meng A great master of Qigong in the Jin Dynasty (266 AD–420 AD).

五痹【wǔ bì】 气功适应证，① 指筋痹、脉痹、肌痹、皮痹、骨痹的总称；② 指筋痹、骨痹、血痹、肉痹、气痹的总称；③ 指风痹、寒痹、湿痹、热痹、气痹的总称。

five impediments An indication of Qigong, refer to ① either sinew impediment, meridian impediment, muscle impediment, skin impediment and bone impediment; ② or sinew impediment, bone impediment, blood impediment, flesh impediment, and Qi impediment; ③ or wind impediment, cold impediment, dampness impedi-

ment, heat impediment and Qi impediment.

五并【wǔ bìng】 指五脏精气内虚，为邪气所兼并而出现的精神症状。即"精气并于心则喜，并于肺则悲，并于肝则忧，并于脾则畏，并于肾则恐"。

five mergers Refers to five emotional troubles caused by deficiency of essential Qi in the the five Zang-organs (including the heart, liver, spleen, lung and kidney). The fact is that "happiness is caused by concentration of essential Qi in the heart, sorrow is caused by concentration of essential Qi in the lung, anxiety is caused by concentration of essential Qi in the liver, fear is caused by concentration of essential Qi in the spleen, and terrifying is caused by concentration of essential Qi in the kidney".

五仓【wǔ cāng】 指五脏之神。
five stores Refer to the spirit in the five Zang-organs (including the heart, liver, spleen, lung and kidney).

五藏【wǔ cáng】 指心藏神，肺藏魄，肝藏魂，脾藏意，肾藏精志。

five preservations Refers to the fact that the heart stores the spirit, the lung stores the ethereal soul, the liver stores the corporeal soul, the spleen stores consciousness and the kidney stores the essence and will.

五常【wǔ cháng】 指五行，即木、火、土、金、水。
five normalities Refers to the five elements, i. e. wood, fire, earth, metal and water.

五车【wǔ chē】 ① 指气功功夫不同；② 指气血沿任督运行。
five carts Refers to either ① different

skills in practicing Qigong and movement of Qi; ② or the blood through the conception meridian and governor meridian.

五车三乘【wǔ chē sān chéng】 指羊车小乘、鹿车中乘、牛车大乘、大牛车上乘、大白牛车无上乘。

three classes of five carts A term of Qigong, refers to the fact that the sheep cart is the small class, the deer cart is the middle class, the cow cart is the large class, the big cow cart is the upper class and the big white cow cart is not the upper class.

五尘【wǔ chén】 佛家气功习用语,指色、声、香、味、触等引起精神活动变化的环境。

five dusts A common term of Qigong in Buddhism, refers to the changed conditions of the spirit activity caused by color, sound, fragrance, taste and contact.

五辰行事法【wǔ chén xíng shì fǎ】 为功法,夜半时作功,坐卧均可。

exercise focusing on five times A dynamic exercise, characterized by sitting or lying at midnight to practice Qigong.

五持【wǔ chí】 佛家气功习用语,① 指闻持,即稳定精神;② 法持,即消除烦恼;③ 义持,即内守精神;④ 根持,即排除杂念;⑤ 藏持,即稳定情绪。

five dharani A common term of Qigong in Buddhism, refers to stabilization of the spirit, elimination of annoyance, internal concentration of the spirit, removal of distracting thoughts and stabilization of emotion.

五厨【wǔ chú】 指五脏得自然之气而充满,五神得自然之气而静正。

five vigorous spirits Refers to exuberance of the five Zang-organs (including the heart, the liver, the spleen, the lung and the kidney) with the support of natural Qi; or the quietness of the five kinds of spirit with the support of natural Qi.

五厨经气法【wǔ chú jīng qì fǎ】 源自气功专论,主要阐述调节意识思维活动,使之泰和,则五脏之神静正,五脏之气充满,即可绝五味,除嗜欲,增进健康,延年益寿。

exercise for regulating Qi in the five Zang-organs Collected from a monograph of Qigong, describing the way to regulate the activities of consciousness and thinking for ensuring peace and balance, which will tranquilize the spirit in the five Zang-organs and enrich Qi in the five Zang-organs, eventually eliminating all carnal desires, cultivating health and prolonging life.

五厨经气法注【wǔ chú jīng qì fǎ zhù】 《五厨经气法注》为气功养生专著,作者不详。

Wuchu Jingqifa Zhu (*Explanation of Exercise for Regulating Qi in the Five Zang-Organs*) A monograph of Qigong and life cultivation entitled *Explanation of Exercise for Regulating Qi in the Five Zang- Organs*. The author was unknown.

五大【wǔ dà】 佛家气功习用语,指的是地、水、火、风、空。

five supremacies A common term of Qigong in Buddhism, referring to the earth, water, fire, wind and hollow.

五大观【wǔ dà guān】 佛家气功功法,指意象中的地之白色、水之绿色、火之黄赤色、风之黑色、空静之青色。

W

five mental visions An exercise of Qigong in Buddhism, referring to the imagination of the earth as white, the water as green, the fire as yellow and red, the wind as black and the void quietness as blue.

五毒【wǔ dú】 指酸、苦、甘、辛、咸五味。

five tastes Refers to sourness, bitterness, sweetness, pungency and saltiness.

五夺【wǔ duó】 指气血津液严重耗损。

five exhaustions Refers to prohibition of purgation in five ways due to severe loss of Qi, blood, fluid and humor.

五发【wǔ fā】 指五脏之病。即阴病发于骨,阳病发于血,阴病发于肉,阳病发于冬,阴病发于夏。

five onsets Refer to onset of diseases in the the five Zang-organs (including the heart, liver, spleen, lung and kidney). Usually Yin disease occurs in the bones, Yang disease occurs in the blood, Yin disease occurs in the muscles, Yang disease occurs in winter and Yin disease occurs in summer.

五风【wǔ fēng】 指五脏之风,如肝风、肺风、脾风、肺风、肾风。

five winds Refers wind in the five Zang-organs (including the heart, liver, spleen, lung and kidney), including liver wind, heart wind, spleen wind, lung wind and kidney wind.

五府【wǔ fǔ】 指与五脏配之五腑,即小肠、大肠、胆、胃、膀胱。

five mansions Refers to the small intestine, large intestine, gallbladder, stomach and bladder that are combined with the five Zang-organs (including the heart, the liver, the spleen, the lung and the kidney).

五盖【wǔ gài】 佛家气功习用语,指失调的情志活动损伤人体良好的精神状态。

five lids A common term of Qigong in Buddhism, refers to the disordered activity of emotion that has damaged the body.

五根【wǔ gēn】 佛家气功习用语,① 指信、精进、念、定、慧为五根;② 指眼、耳、鼻、舌、身为五根。

five roots A common term of Qigong in Buddhism, refers to ① either belief, essence, idea, decision and wisdom; ② or the eyes, the ears, the nose, the tongue and the body.

五更【wǔ gēng】 指自昏至晓之一夜分为五刻。

midnight Divided into five periods.

五宫【wǔ gōng】 ① 指东、南、西、北、中五方;② 指中央土位;③ 指五脏。

five palaces Refer to ① either five directions of the east, the south, the west, the north and the center; ② or five central positions; ③ or five Zang-organs (including the heart, the liver, the spleen, the lung and the kidney).

五鼓【wǔ gǔ】 五更的别称,指自昏至晓之一夜分为五刻。

midnight/five drums A synonym of midnight which is divided into five periods.

五关【wǔ guān】 指耳、目、口、鼻、身。

five cols Refer to the ears, the eyes, the mouth, the nose and the body.

五官【wǔ guān】 ① 指眼、耳、鼻、舌、口、唇;② 五色,即青、赤、黄、白、黑;③ 佛家气功习用语,指生、老、病、死、县官。

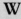

five organs Refers to ① either five orifices such as the eyes, the nose, the ears, the tongue and the lips; ② or five colors such as blue, red, yellow, white and black; ③ or five conditions such as birth, senility, illness, death and county official, which is a common term of Qigong in Buddhism.

五鬼【wǔ guǐ】 指五种浊气,为五尸的别称。道家认为,人体五脏内有五种浊气,会威胁人体的健康,即"青尸、赤尸、黄尸、白尸、黑尸"。

five ghosts A synonym of five foul smells, refers to blue foul smell, red foul smell, yellow foul smell, white foul smell and black foul smell. Daoism believes that there are five kinds of foul Qi in the five Zang-organs (including the heart, the liver, the spleen, the lung and the kidney) that threaten health.

五海【wǔ hǎi】 指脑为髓之海,冲为血海,命门为精海,丹田为气海,胃为水谷之海。

five seas Refers to the brain as the sea of marrow, the thoroughfare meridian as the sea of blood, the life gate as the sea of essence, Dantian as the sea of Qi and the stomach as the sea of water and cereal. Dantian is divided into the upper Dantian (the region between the eyes), the middle Dantian (the region below the heart) and the lower Dantian (the region below the navel).

五湖【wǔ hú】 指各有液所主之位,东西南北中,此是五剧。

five lakes Refers to the five locations of humor in the five Zang-organs (including the heart, the liver, the spleen, the lung and the kidney), similar to the east, the west, the south, the north and the center.

五华【wǔ huá】 指五脏精华。

five essences Refers to the essence in the the five Zang-organs (including the heart, liver, spleen, lung and kidney).

五化【wǔ huà】 指五行的气化。五行之间不断变化发展之生、长、化、收、藏五个生化阶段。

five transformations Refers to Qi transformation in the five elements (including wood, fire, earth, metal and water), including sprouting, growth, transformation, collection and storage.

五化论【wǔ huà lùn】 源自气功专论,阐述五化的含义及其变化。

discussion about five transformations Collected from a monograph of Qigong, including the implication and changes of five transformations.

五荤【wǔ hūn】 指五辛,即以小蒜、大蒜、韭、芸苔、胡荽为五荤。

five flavors Refer to rocambole, garlic, leek, winter rape and coriander.

五火【wǔ huǒ】 指五脏之亢阳。

five fires Refer to Jueyang in the the five Zang-organs (including the heart, liver, spleen, lung and kidney).

五觉【wǔ jué】 佛家气功习用语,指五种精神意识思维活动。

five senses A common term of Qigong in Buddhism, referring to five activities of the spirit, consciousness and thinking.

五戒【wǔ jiè】 指禁除五种影响精神稳定的因素。

five disciplines Refers to elimination of five factors that affect the spirit.

五金八石【wǔ jīn bā shí】 五金包括朱砂、雄黄、雌黄、硫黄、白上黄(一作水

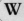

银)；八石包括曾青、空青、石胆、砒霜、白盐、白矾、马牙硝。

five metals and eight minerals In this term, five metals refer to cinnabar, realgar, gamboge, sulfur and mercury; the eight minerals refer to azurite ore, hollow azurite, chalcanthitum, arsenic, white salt, alum and crystalized mirabilite.

五精【wǔ jīng】 指五脏的精气。

five essences Refer to essential Qi in the five Zang-organs (including the heart, the liver, the spleen, the lung and the kidney).

五腊【wǔ là】 指一年中正月一日、五月五日、七月七日、十月一日、十二月正腊日为良辰。

five favorable days Refer to the first day in the January, fifth day in the May, seventh day in the July, the first day in the October, and the eighth day in the December in the traditional Chinese calendar.

五龙棒圣【wǔ lóng bàng shèng】 指五为土之数，龙为性之灵；五龙为五脏，圣为脑神。

five kinds of Loong unifying sage Refers to the fact that five is the number of the earth and Loong is the property of the spirit; or the five kinds of Loong represent the five Zang-organs (including the heart, the liver, the spleen, the lung and the kidney) and Shengren (sage) represents the spirit in the brain.

五龙盘体法【wǔ lóng pán tǐ fǎ】 为静功，指东首而寝，侧身而卧。

kneading the body with five kinds of Loong A static exercise, referring to lying on the east and on one side in practicing Qigong.

五轮观【wǔ lún guān】 佛家气功用语，指观自身腰下、脐轮、心上、额、顶上。

inspection of five wheels A common term of Qigong in Buddhism, referring to inspecting the lower part of the waist, the area of the navel, the upper part of the heart, the forehead and the top of the head.

五脉【wǔ mài】 ① 指五脏五俞穴；② 指五脏脉象。

five pulses Refers to ① either the acupoints located in the meridians of the five Zang-organs (including the heart, the liver, the spleen, the lung and the kidney); ② or the manifestations of the five Zang-organs (including the heart, the liver, the spleen, the lung and the kidney).

五内【wǔ nèi】 指五脏。

five bosoms Refer to the five Zang-organs (including the heart, liver, spleen, lung and kidney).

五气【wǔ qì】 ① 指五脏产生的情志活动，即喜、怒、忧、悲、恐；② 五运之气，即金、木、水、火、土；③ 五种气味，即臊、焦、香、腥、腐；④ 五味所化之气；⑤ 五色之气，即青、白、赤、黑、黄气；⑥ 土气，土位中央，其数为五，故名。

five Qi Refers to ① either five emotions caused by the five Zang-organs (including the heart, liver, spleen, lung and kidney), such as happiness, anger, anxiety, sorrow and fear; ② or Qi from the five elements, including metal, wood, water, fire and earth; ③ or five tastes, such as restlessness, anxiety, fragrance, stench and putridity; ④ or Qi transformed by the five tastes; ⑤ or Qi from the colors, including green Qi, white Qi, red Qi, black Qi and yellow Qi; ⑥ or earth Qi because earth is located in the center and that is why its numbers are five.

五气朝元【wǔ qì cháo yuán】 指五脏之气上朝天元。

five Qi turning to the origin Refers to Qi from the five Zang-organs (including the heart, the liver, the spleen, the lung and the kidney) flowing up to the celestial origin.

五气朝元法【wǔ qì cháo yuán fǎ】 为静功,指调身、调神、调气。其作法为,宽松衣服,放松人体和精神,盘坐,闭目塞兑,舌抵上腭,双手臂下垂,身体沉稳,调匀呼吸,凝神入定。

concentration of five Qi A static exercise for regulating the body, the spirit and Qi, marked by loosening the clothes, relaxing the body and spirit, sitting upright with crossed knees, closing the eyes and oral cavity, holding the upper jaw with the tongue, lower the hands and shoulders, stabilizing the body, regulating respiration and concentrating the spirit.

五气更立【wǔ qì gēng lì】 指术、火、土、金、水五运之气更迭主时。

alteration of the five elements Refers to change of Qi from the five elements, i. e. wood, fire, earth, metal and water.

五气护身法【wǔ qì hù shēn fǎ】 为静功。其作法为,为避五疫毒气的传染,在屋内先要集中神思,觉得自心好像太阳样的光明将要进入病室时,先想象有青气自肝脏发出,向左而运行于东方,化作繁荣的林木,以诱导肝气。

exercise for five Qi to defend the body A static exercise, referring to the fact that the spirit and mind must be concentrated in the room to make the heart felt as bright as the sun in order to avoid invasion of five pathogenic factors. When entering the ward, measures should be taken to imagine that green Qi appears from the liver, flowing to the east from the left and transforming into prosperous forest in order to change liver Qi.

五千言【wǔ qiān yán】 指《老子》的代称。

five thousand characters Refers to the full text of *Lao Zi*, also known as Dao De Jing (Canon of Dao and Morality) which is composed of five thousand characters.

五禽戏【wǔ qín xì】 指一曰虎,二曰鹿,三曰熊,四曰猿,五曰鸟。为东汉名医华佗所创。

five animals exercise Includes tiger, deer, bear, monkey and bird. Five animals exercise is created by Hua Tuo, a great doctor in the East Han Dynasty (25 AD - 220 AD).

五禽戏第二法【wǔ qín xì dì èr fǎ】 为动功,调身、调气、调神。其作法为,羡门虎势戏,闭气低头,拳战如虎发威势,两手如提千斤铁,轻起来,莫放气,平身吞气入腹,使神气之上而复,觉得腹内如雷鸣,或五七次,如此行之。

the second technique of the five animals exercise A dynamic exercise for regulation of the body, Qi and the spirit, marked by suspending breath, lowering the head, holding the hands heavily, raising the arms lightly, inhaling air naturally into the abdomen, ascending and returning spiritual Qi, intensifying

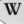

the abdomen like thunder for five or seven times according to the styles of tiger.

五禽戏第一法【wǔ qín xì dì yī fǎ】为动功,其作法为,以虎、鹿、熊、猿、鸟的形式坐、立、卧,并动、静、行。

the first technique of five animals exercise A dynamic exercise, marked by sitting, standing up, lying according to the styles of tiger with active, quiet and stretching activities.

五色【wǔ sè】指青、赤、黄、白、黑,反映五脏病变及各种证候的五种病色。

five colors Refers to blue, yellow, red, white and black colors as well as the manifestations of the diseases related to the the five Zang-organs (including the heart, liver, spleen, lung and kidney).

五色童子【wǔ sè tóng zǐ】指五脏之神,即青童子为肝神,赤童子为心神,白童子为肺神,黑童子为肾神,黄童子为脾神。

five kinds of boys A term of Qigong, refers to the spirit in the five Zang-organs (including the heart, the liver, the spleen, the lung and the kidney), among which the so-called green boy represents the liver spirit, the so-called red boy represents the heart spirit, the so-called white boy represents the lung spirit, the so-called black boy represents the kidney spirit and the so-called yellow boy represents the spleen spirit.

五神【wǔ shén】指五种浊气,是五尸的别称。道家认为,人体五脏内有五种浊气,会威胁人体的健康,即"青尸、赤尸、黄尸、白尸、黑尸"。

five gods A synonym of five foul smells, refers to blue foul smell, red foul smell, yellow foul smell, white foul smell and black foul smell. Daoism believes that there are five kinds of foul Qi in the five Zang-organs (including the heart, the liver, the spleen, the lung and the kidney) that threaten health.

五神【wǔ shén】① 指五脏之神; ② 指无方之神。

five spirits Refer to ① either the spirit in the five Zang-organs; ② or the spirit in five directions.

五尸【wǔ shī】指五种浊气。道家认为,人体五脏内有五种浊气,会威胁人体的健康,即"青尸、赤尸、黄尸、白尸、黑尸"。

five foul smells Refers to blue foul smell, red foul smell, yellow foul smell, white foul smell and black foul smell. Daoism believes that there are five kinds of foul Qi in the five Zang-organs (including the heart, the liver, the spleen, the lung and the kidney) that threaten health.

五十而复大会【wǔ shí ér fù dà huì】指营气与卫气一昼夜各行五十周次之后,便会合一次。

reconvergence after fifty times of circulation Refers to the way of Qigong practice in which nutrient Qi and defense Qi will integrate with each other after fifty times of movement in the daytime and nighttime.

五十营【wǔ shí yíng】指经肺之气在人体内运行,一昼夜循环周身五十次。

fifty circulations Refer to circulation of Qi fifty times in the all the meridians through the whole body.

五石【wǔ shí】指丹砂、雄黄、白矾、曾

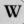

青、磁石五种矿物质药物。

five minerals Refer to five kinds of mineral medicinals, including cinnabar, realgar, alum, azurite ore and magnetite.

五石散【wǔ shí sàn】 指古代气功锻炼中,兼服五石者。

five mineral powders Refer to a formula used in ancient China for practicing Qigong.

五时【wǔ shí】 指一年中的春、夏、长夏、秋、冬。

five seasons Refer to the spring, summer, late summer, autumn and winter in a year.

五时七候【wǔ shí qī hòu】 指学道之人,心有五时,身入气候。

five stages and seven states Refers to the fact that the great scholars have five stages in the heart and reach seven states in physical movement.

五枢【wǔ shū】 足少阳胆经中的一个穴位,位于腹外侧,此穴位为气功习练之处。

Wushu（GB 27） An acupoint in the gallbladder meridian of foot Shaoyang, located lateral to the abdomen. This acupoint is a region usually used in practice of Qigong.

五衰【wǔ shuāi】 佛家气功习用语,指人将死时出现的五种表现。

five collapses A common term of Qigong in Buddhism, referring to five dying symptoms.

五台山【wǔ tái shān】 指山西的清凉山,为佛教的四大名山。

Wutai Mountain Also called Qingliang Mountain in Shanxi Province, one of the four important mountains in Buddhism.

五态【wǔ tài】 指五种不同体质类型的人。根据人的不同形态,筋骨的强弱,气血的盛衰,区分为太阴之人、少阴之人、太阳之人、少阳之人、阳明和平之人。

five shapes Refer to five bodily forms, including Taiyin person, Shaoyin person, Taiyang person, Shaoyang person and Yangming balanced person divided according to different styles and conditions of the sinews, the bones, Qi and the blood.

五停心观【wǔ tíng xīn guān】 佛家气功功法,指不净观、慈悲观、因缘观、界分别观、数息观。

five mental observations An exercise of Qigong in Buddhism, refers to repeated view (patikulamanasikara), mercy view, karma view, separate view and constant view.

五位【wǔ wèi】 指东西南北中五方的定位。

five directions Refer to the east, the west, the south, the north and the center.

五位相得【wǔ wèi xiāng dé】 指洛书,是阴阳五行术数之源。在古代传说中有神龟出于洛水,其甲壳上有此图像。

achievement among the five elements Refers to Luo Shu which is the origin of Yin-Yang and five elements. In antiquity there was a legendary story about supernatural tortoise that appeared from Luo River with the image of five elements on its carapace.

五仙观【wǔ xiān guān】 相传为五仙人骑五羊,衣服与五羊色。

observation of five immortals Refer to five immortals who rode on five sheep with the clothes similar to the color of the sheep.

W

五心【wǔ xīn】　指手、足心及心脏。

five hearts　Refer to the palms, the soles and the heart.

五心烦热【wǔ xīn fán rè】　气功学适应证,指手足心热,心胸烦热。

dysphoria in five centers　An indication of Qigong, referring to dysphoria of the hands, the feet and the heart.

五星【wǔ xīng】　指无方之星,即岁星、荧惑星、太白星、辰星、镇星。

five stars　Refer to Jupiter, Mars, Venus, Mercury and Saturn.

五行【wǔ xíng】　指木、火、土、金、水之生克乘侮。

five elements　Refers to the promotion, restriction, subjugation and counter-restriction among wood, fire, earth, metal and water in the five elements.

五行参差同根节【wǔ xíng cēn cī tóng gēn jié】　指木、火、土、金、水五行运动,其参差变化理性同一,根源相同。

irregularity of the five elements belonging to the same origin　Refers to the movement of the five elements (including wood, fire, earth, metal and water) with the same changes and ways of interactions.

五行颠倒术【wǔ xíng diān dǎo shù】　为静功。正坐,瞑目,调息,握固,心定,微息,则徐闭之,虽无所念,而卓然精明,毅然刚烈。

reversing techniques of the five elements　A static exercise, characterized by sitting, closing eyes, regulating respiration, holding hands, tranquilizing the heart and breathing slowly without any thought in order to naturally regulate the body and brilliantly to enrich the essence and the spirit.

五行归原论【wǔ xíng guī yuán lùn】

源自气功专论,主要阐述五行本于阴阳一气。

discussion about the five elements returning to the origin　Returning to the origin is collected from a monograph of Qigong, mainly describing that the promotion and restriction among the five elements depend on Qi from Yin and Yang.

五行还返【wǔ xíng huán fǎn】　源自气功专论,说明五行不顺行,才能降低生命速度,减少身体能源的消耗,保持身体的相对稳定状态。

reverse motion of the five elements　Collected from a monograph of Qigong, referring to the fact that only when the five elements fail to move naturally can it lower the speed of life, reduce exhaustion of energy in the body and stabilize the body.

五行配六字法【wǔ xíng pèi liù zì fǎ】　源自气功专论,主要阐述按五行相生,四时循序而行的六字排练功法。

technique of the five elements cooperating with six characters　Collected from a monograph of Qigong, mainly describing the dynamic exercise with six Chinese characters according to the promotion among the five elements and the circulation among the four seasons.

五行全【wǔ xíng quán】　指精气神三元合一,谓之五行全。

fulfillment of five elements　Refers to integration of essence, Qi and spirit that has fulfilled the movement of the five elements (including wood, fire, earth, metal and water).

五行全处虎龙蟠【wǔ xíng quán chù hǔ lóng pán】　指金、木、水、火运于中宫意土,精气神合而为一。

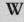

The five elements all move in the area occupied by the Loong and the tiger. This is a celebrated dictum, referring to movement of metal, wood, water and fire in the five elements (including wood, fire, earth, metal and water) in the central palace and ideal earth, indicating integration of the essence, Qi and the spirit.

五行生成【wǔ xíng shēng chéng】 指水之生成数为一、六；火之生成数为二、七；木之生成数为三、八；金之生成数为四、九；土之生成数为五、十。

generation of the five elements Refers to the fact that the generation numbers for water are one and six, for fire are two and seven, for wood are three and eight, for metal are four and nine and for earth are five and ten.

五行完坚【wǔ xíng wán jiān】 指头身、四肢、五脏坚固壮实。

strengthened five shapes Refers to strength of the head, the body, the four limbs and the five Zang-organs (including the heart, the liver, the spleen, the lung and the kidney).

五行相克【wǔ xíng xiāng kè】 指水克火、火克金、金克木、木克水。

restriction of the five elements Refers to the fact that water restricts fire, fire restricts metal, metal restricts wood and wood restricts water.

五行相生【wǔ xíng xiāng shēng】 指水生木、木生火、火生土、土生金、金生水。

interaction of the five elements Refers to the fact that water produces wood, wood produces fire, fire produces earth, earth produces metal and metal produces water.

五行相推反归一【wǔ xíng xiāng tuī fǎn guī yī】 指自然界五行，水、火、木、金、土相互作用，相互制约，维持五行间的协调统一。指逆五行而生，以达到合二而一。

integration of the five elements Refers to either harmony among the five elements of wood, fire, earth, metal and water that mutually promote and restrict each other; or integration achieved by reversing the five elements.

五行在人【wǔ xíng zài rén】 指肾为水、心为火、肝为木、肺为金、脾为土。

five elements in man Refers to the fact that the kidney belongs to water, the heart belongs to fire, the liver belongs to wood, the lung belongs to metal and the spleen belongs to earth.

五行之色【wǔ xíng zhī sè】 指青木、白金、黑水、赤火、黄土。

color of the five elements Refers to green wood, white metal, black water, red fire and yellow earth.

五行之时【wǔ xíng zhī shí】 指春木、夏火、秋金、冬水，四时各凡九十日，每时下十八日，黄土主之。

times of the five elements Refers to wood in the spring, fire in the summer, metal in the autumn and water in the winter. Each season contains ninety days, among which the yellow earth controls eighteen days in every season.

五行之位【wǔ xíng zhī wèi】 指东木、西金、北水、南火、中土。

positions of the five elements Refers to wood in the east, metal in the west, water in the north, fire in the south and earth in the center.

五行之象【wǔ xíng zhī xiàng】 指木

W

为青龙、火为朱雀、土为勾陈、金为白虎、水为玄武。

manifestations of the five elements Refers to the fact that wood represents Qinglong (green Loong), fire represents rosefinch, earth represents Gouchen (one of the six important gods), metal represents white tiger (one of the four benevolent animals) and water represents Xuanwu (one of the four benevolent animals).

五行总聚【wǔ xíng zǒng jù】 指五脏真气上聚于脑。

total accumulation of the five elements Refers to the fact that genuine Qi in the five Zang-organs (including the heart, the liver, the spleen, the lung and the kidney) concentrates on the brain.

五形【wǔ xíng】 指头与四肢。

five forms Refers to the head and the extremities.

五性【wǔ xìng】 ① 指五脏的特性,即肝性静,心性躁,脾性力,肺性坚,肾性智;② 指人的五种性情,即喜、怒、欲、惧、忧;③ 指道德规范,即仁、义、礼、智、信;④ 指五种紊乱精神的行为,即暴、淫、奢、酷、贼。

five features Refer to ① either the five qualities of the five Zang-organs (including the heart, the liver, the spleen, the lung and the kidney), such as quietness of the liver, restlessness of the heart, strength of the spleen, firmness of the lung and wisdom of the kidney; ② or five emotions, such as happiness, anger, desire, fear and anxiety; ③ or five moral standards, such as benevolence, righteousness, rite, wisdom and truth; ④ or five immoral

deeds, such as violence, obscene, luxury, cruel and thief.

五牙【wǔ yá】 ① 指五行之生气;② 指五脏之气。

five teeth Refer to ① either and Qi from the five elements; ② or Qi from the five Zang-organs (including the heart, liver, spleen, lung and kidney).

五眼【wǔ yǎn】 指肉眼、天眼、慧眼、法眼、佛眼。

five eyes Refer to the naked eyes, the unique eyes, the insight eyes, the wise eyes and the Buddhist eyes.

五阳【wǔ yáng】 指五脏的阳气。

five Yang Refers to Yang Qi in the the five Zang-organs (including the heart, liver, spleen, lung and kidney).

五养【wǔ yǎng】 指春养脾,夏养肺,秋养肝,冬养心,四季养肾。五脏得养,百病不生。

five kinds of nourishment Refer to nourishing the spleen in spring, nourishing the lung in summer, nourishing the liver in autumn, nourishing the heart in winter and nourishing the kidney in the four seasons. Only when the five Zang-organs (including the heart, the liver, the spleen, the lung and the kidney) are nourished can diseases be eliminated.

五液【wǔ yè】 指五脏所生的液体,即心为汗,肺为涕,肝为泪,脾为涎,肾为唾。

five humors Refers to the heart related to sweat, the lung related to snivel, the liver related to tears, the spleen related saliva and the kidney related to spittle.

五阴神祝法【wǔ yīn shén zhù fǎ】 为静功,指太极真人法,即以鸡鸣平旦之时,卧式或坐式均可,叩齿九通,然后行

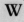

五法之神祝。

supernatural blessing of five kinds of Yin A static exercise, referring to supreme immortal exercise characterized by lying or sitting at dawn with nine times of clicking the teeth and taking steps of five elements.

五音【wǔ yīn】 指角、徵、宫、商、羽五种音调。古人把五音与五脏相配。

five sounds Refers to the five kinds of sound, i. e. Jiao, Zhi, Gong, Shang and Yu. In antiquity, the five sounds were connected with the five Zang-organs (including the heart, the liver, the spleen, the lung and the kidney).

五欲【wǔ yù】 ① 指耳、目、口、鼻、心的欲望；② 财、色、名、饮食、睡眠；③ 色、声、香、味、触五欲。

five desires Refers to ① either five desires from the ears, the eyes, the mouth, the nose and the heart; ② or five dreams, such as wealth, style, reputation, food and sleep; ③ or five desires like countenance, sound, fragrance, taste and contact.

五月节导引法【wǔ yuè jié dǎo yǐn fǎ】 为动功。其作法为，五月节每日寅卯时，正立，身后仰，两手朝上屈伸三十五次，引背上之气机流动，强腰肾，去积滞，身体轻快健康。

exercise of Daoyin in the feast days of May A dynamic exercise, marked by standing up in Yin (the period of a day from 3 a. m. to 5 a. m. in the morning) and Mao (the period of a day from 5 a. m. to 7 a. m. in the morning) in the feast days of May, turning the body backwards, bending and stretching the hands upwards for thirty-five times in order to promote the flow of Qi in the back. Such a way of dynamic exercise can strengthen the waist and kidney, eliminate stagnation and cultivate health.

五岳【wǔ yuè】 ① 指东岳、西岳、南岳、北岳、中岳；② 指人之头；③ 指五脏。

five mountains Refer to ① either five important mountains known as East Mountain, West Mountain, South Mountain, North Mountain and Central Mountain; ② or the head of human beings; ③ or the five Zang-organs (including the heart, the liver, the spleen, the lung and the kidney).

五岳之云【wǔ yuè zhī yún】 指五脏之气。

cloud in the five mountains Refers to Qi in the five Zang-organs (including the heart, the liver, the spleen, the lung and the kidney).

五运【wǔ yùn】 指五行之气流传。

five motions Refers to the movement and exchange of the five elements (including wood, fire, earth, metal and water).

五运相袭【wǔ yùn xiāng xí】 指木、火、土、金、水五行之气，随着时间的推移而依据五行的运转与时间的配合次序，相继承袭，用以说明某年或某一季节的气候特征。

patrimony among the five elements Refers to Qi in the five elements, i. e. wood, fire, earth, metal and water, which continue to inherit according to the process of time, the movement of the five elements and coordination of time, indicating the characteristics of Qi in any season or any year.

五蕴【wǔ yùn】 ① 指五种积集作用；

② 指五脏。

five accumulations　Refers to ① either five kinds of accumulation; ② or the five Zang-organs (including the heart, the liver, the spleen, the lung and the kidney).

五脏藏五神【wǔ zàng cáng wǔ shén**】** ① 指魂藏于肝,为肝之神;② 魄藏于肺,为肺之神;③ 精藏于肾,为肾之神;④ 志藏在脾,为脾之神;⑤ 神藏于心,为心之神。

the five Zang-organs storing the five spirits　Refers to ① the fact that the ethereal soul is stored in the liver and is the spirit of the liver; ② the corporeal soul is stored in the lung and is the spirit of the lung; ③ the essence is stored in the kidney and is the spirit of the kidney; ④ the will is stored in the spleen and is the spirit of the spleen; ⑤ the spirit is stored in the heart and is the spirit of the heart.

五脏横病【wǔ zàng héng bìng**】** 气功适应证,指本病非五脏按五行的乘克规律而自身致病,而多因生活起居变化,寒温失于节制,违背一般规律致血气虚弱所致的病证。

exogenous diseases of the five Zang-organs An indication of Qigong, referring to the fact that such diseases are not caused by the five Zang-organs according to the principles of subjugation and restriction in the five elements (including wood, fire, earth, metal and water), usually caused by changes of daily life, failure to control cold and warm conditions, and deficiency of blood and Qi due to violation of natural law.

五脏横病后导引法【wǔ zàng héng bìng hòu dǎo yǐn fǎ**】** 为静功。静心存想脐下有红光,内外相连,遮没全身。暖下元,治膝下有病。

exercise of Daoyin for diseases in the five Zang-organs A static exercise, marked by tranquilizing the heart and mind, imagining brightness below the navel, communicating the internal and external, covering the whole body, warming the lower and treating the disease located below the knee.

五脏化液【wǔ zàng huà yè**】** 指五脏的功能活动与五液有关,故五液分泌的异常即为五脏病变的表现。

five Zang-organs transforming into humor　Refers to the fact that the functional activities of the five Zang-organs (including the heart, the liver, the spleen, the lung and the kidney) are related to the five kinds of humor. Thus the abnormal secretion of five kinds of fluid represents pathological disorders of the five Zang-organs.

五脏六腑之海【wǔ zàng liù fǔ zhī hǎi**】** ① 指胃;② 指冲脉。

the sea in the five Zang-organs and six Fu-organs Refers to ① either the stomach; ② or the thoroughfare meridian.

五脏之长【wǔ zàng zhī zhǎng**】** 指肺,肺位胸腔,居脏腑中之最高位。

the highest one among the five Zang-organs Refers to the lung located in the chest, the location of which is highest among the five Zang-organs.

五脏之腧【wǔ zàng zhī shù**】** 指背部与五脏有密切联系的肺俞、心俞、肝俞、脾俞、肾俞五个脑穴。

acupoints of the five Zang-organs Refers to the five acupoints located on the back and closely related to the five

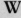

Zang-organs, i.e. lung acupoint, heart acupoint, liver acupoint, spleen acupoint and kidney acupoint.

五脏之专精【wǔ zàng zhī zhuān jīng】强调心在人体的重要作用。

special essence in the five Zang-organs Emphasizes the importance of the heart in the human body.

五贼【wǔ zéi】①指金、木、水、火、土;②又泛指损伤情志的非正常思维活动。

five thieves Refers to ① either the five elements, i.e. wood, fire, earth, metal and water; ② or abnormal thinking activity that damages the emotion.

五中【wǔ zhōng】指心、肝、脾、肺、肾五脏。

five centers Refers to the five Zang-organs, including the heart, the liver, the spleen, the lung and the kidney.

五中所主【wǔ zhōng suǒ zhǔ】指五脏所主时令:肝主春、心主夏、脾主长夏、肺主秋、肾主冬。

responsibility for five aspects Refers to the seasons controlled by the five Zang-organs (including the heart, the liver, the spleen, the lung and the kidney), indicating that the liver controls the spring, the heart controls the summer, the spleen controls the late summer, the lung controls the autumn and the kidney controls the winter.

五种散乱【wǔ zhǒng sǎn luàn】为佛家气功习用语,指自然散乱、外散乱、内散乱、粗重散乱、思维散乱。

five scattered disorders A common term of Qigong in Buddhism, referring to natural disorder, mental disorder, internal disorder, activity disorder and thinking disorder.

五种小衰【wǔ zhǒng xiǎo shuāi】为佛家气功习用语,指五种精神损伤。

five spiritual impairments A common term of Qigong in Buddhism, referring to five kinds of disorders that damage the spirit.

五主【wǔ zhǔ】指五脏所主的有关方面,即心主脉、肺主皮、肝主筋、脾主肉、肾主骨。

five dominations Refer to the five Zang-organs (including the heart, liver, spleen, lung and kidney), indicating that the heart controls the meridians, the lung controls the skin, the liver controls the sinews, the spleen controls the muscles and the kidney controls the bones.

五作业根【wǔ zuò yè gēn】佛家气功习用语,指语具(口或舌)、手、足、小便处、大便处。

five operational roots A common term of Qigong in Buddhism, referring to the mouth, the hands, the feet, the uterus and the anus.

午夜【wǔ yè】指午夜二十三时至次日凌晨一时。

midnight Refers to 11 p.m. to 1 a.m.

伍冲虚【wǔ chōng xū】明代著名的气功学家伍守阳的另外一个称谓,其撰有多部气功专著,对气功养生的发展做出了贡献。

Wu Chongxu Another name of Wu Shouyang, a great master of Qigong in the Ming Dynasty (1368 AD - 1644 AD) who wrote several monographs about Qigong, contributing a great deal to the development of Qigong and life cultivation.

伍守阳【wǔ shǒu yáng】明代著名的

W

气功学家,撰有多部气功专著,对气功养生的发展做出了贡献。

Wu Shouyang A great master of Qigong in the Ming Dynasty（1368 AD‑1644 AD）and wrote several monographs about Qigong，contributing a great deal to the development of Qigong and life cultivation.

伍真人丹道九篇【wǔ zhēn rén dān dào jiǔ piān】《伍真人丹道九篇》为气功专著,由明代气功学家伍守阳所著,阐述了道、儒、佛的气功理论。

Wuzhenren Dandao Jiupian（*Immortal Wu's Nine Chapters about Dandao*） A monograph of Qigong entitled I*mmortal Wu's Nine Chapters about Dandao*，written by Wu Shouyang in the Ming Dynasty（1368 AD‑1644 AD），mainly describing the theory of Daoism，Confucianism and Buddhism about Qigong.

武当山【wǔ dāng shān】 在湖北西北部,为武当派拳术发源地。

Wudang Mountian Located in the northwest in Hubei Province，which is the origin of Hudang school that developed free-hand boxing.

武火【wǔ huǒ】 ① 指大火、急火; ② 指呼吸匀、细、深、长,连绵不绝。

flaming fire Refers to ① either big fire and quick fire；② or incessantly even，thin，deep and long respiration.

舞蹈所以养血脉【wǔ dǎo suǒ yǐ yǎng xuè mài】 指经常进行舞蹈的训练,可以强壮筋骨、肌肉、舒通血脉,而达到健身抗病的作用。

Dancing can nourish the blood meridians and vessels. Indicates that constant dancing practice can strengthen the sinews，bones and muscles and promote the movement of the blood meridians and vessels for nourishing the body and preventing disease.

恶见【wù jiàn】 指违背事理的见解。

unreasonable idea Refers to the idea that violates the reasons and principles in doing anything.

勿忘勿助【wù wàng wù zhù】 指习练气功,养浩然正气,意识活动勿忘、勿助长,维持中和平衡的状态。

no forgetting and no fomenting Refers to cultivation of the great spirit，well remembering and promoting the activity of consciousness and keeping harmonization and balance in practicing Qigong.

勿药元诠【wù yào yuán quán】 《勿药元诠》为气功专著,为清代汪昂所著,主要论述气功养生的丰富内容。

Wuyao Yuanquan （*Discussion About Life Cultivation and Qigong Practice*） A monograph of Qigong entitled *Discussion About Life Cultivation and Qigong Practice*，written by Wang Ang in the Qing Dynasty（1636 AD‑1912 AD），mainly describing the abundant content of Qigong and life cultivation.

戊己【wù jǐ】 指脾的阴阳两个方面,故又称戊土和己土。

Wu and Ji Refers to Yin and Yang in the spleen，also known as Wu earth and Ji earth.

戊己合【wù jǐ hé】 即阴阳和合的意思。

combination of Wu and Ji Refers to harmonization of Yin and Yang.

戊土之腑【wù tǔ zhī fǔ】 指胃腑。

viscus of Wu earth Refers to the stomach in the six Fu-organs（including the gallbladder，the stomach，the small intestine，the large intestine，the bladder

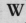

and the triple energizer).

物化【wù huà】　指事物之变化。

variation of things　Refers to changes of things.

物宜【wù yí】　指万物生成发育中，自然而然之貌。

natural development　Refers to natural style of anything that grows and develops.

悟性还易，了心甚难【wù xìng hái yì liǎo xīn shèn nán】　指认识觉悟自己本性容易，无念无欲，情识全无甚难。

It is easy to understand，but difficult to relieve desires.　Indicates that it is easy to understanding oneself nature，but difficult to keep no desires and dreams in the mind.

悟元子【wù yuán zǐ】　清代气功学家刘一明的另外一个称谓，其撰写了多部专著，介绍了气功的基本理论和方法。

Wu Yuanzi　Another name of Liu Yiming，a great master of Qigong in the Qing Dynasty（1636 AD－1912 AD）and wrote several monographs about Qigong to introduce the basic theory and practice of Qigong.

悟真篇【wù zhēn piān】　《悟真篇》为气功学专著，由宋代张伯瑞所著，说明阴阳及阴阳的相互作用是气功养生法的理论基础。

Wuzhen Pian（Book about Consciousness and Truth）　A monograph of Qigong entitled *Book about Consciousness and Truth*，written by Zhang Borui in the Song Dynasty（960 AD－1279 AD），describing that Yin and Yang and their mutual functions are the theoretical foundations of Qigong and life cultivation.

鹜行气【wù xíng qì】　为动功。其作法为，低头，身靠墙壁站立，闭气不息十二次，用意念推动，使痰饮和不消化的宿食，从下部排出。

Duck moving Qi　A dynamic exercise，marked by lowering the head，standing up against the wall，stopping respiration for twelve times，promoting it with consciousness for discharging phlegm，retained fluid and undigested food.

W

X

夕加夜甚【xī jiā yè shèn】 指患者在傍晚病情加重，夜间病势趋于严重。说明习练气功，应在疾病变重之先培养正气，才能获效。

worsening at dusk and night Refers to the fact that disease is worsened in midnight，indicating that Qigong should be practiced before disease worsened.

西川【xī chuān】 ① 即白虎，指二十八宿中西方的七宿；② 内丹书中指"心中元神谓之龙，肾中元精谓之虎"。

west plain The same as white tiger，referring to ① either the seven constellations in the west among the twenty-eight constellations；② or "the original spirit in the heart called Loong and the original essence in the kidney called tiger" mentioned in the books about internal Dan（pills of immortality）.

西方金母【xī fāng jīn mǔ】 指肺，肺在五行中属金，位西方。

west metal mother Refers to the lung which pertains to metal in the five elements（including wood，fire，earth，metal and water）and west when joining in the five directions.

西南乡【xī nán xiāng】 ① 为祖窍异名；② 为下丹田异名。

southwest village Refers to ① either a synonym of Zuqiao located right between the heart and navel；② or a synonym of the lower Dantian（the region below the navel）.

西山群仙会真记【xī shān qún xiān huì zhēn jì】 《西山群仙会真记》为气功学专著，由唐代施肩吾传，由李竦编。

Xishan Qunxian Huizhen Ji（*Pure Convergence and Record of Immortals in the West Mountain*） A monograph of Qigong entitled *Pure Convergence and Record of Immortals in the West Mountain*，described by Shi Jianwu and compiled by Li Song in the Tang Dynasty（618 AD‑907 AD）.

吸风以养神【xī fēng yǐ yǎng shén】 指调节呼吸，得自然太和之气，可以生神，荣养精神。

absorbing wind to nourish the spirit Refers to regulating respiration for the purpose of absorbing natural and harmonious Qi in order to produce and nourish spirit.

吸门【xī mén】 指人体的一个部位，及会厌。

absorbing gate Refers to a region in the body，known as epiglottis.

吸舐撮闭【xī shì cuō bì】 为动功，其作法为，呼吸时以鼻中吸气，借以接先天之气；吸取食物时，以舌上颚迎取甘露；紧摄谷道内中提，明月辉辉顶上飞；塞兑垂廉兼逆呷，久而神水落黄庭。

absorbing，lapping，pinching and closing A dynamic exercise，marked by receiving original celestial Qi when the nose is inhaling，receiving sweet dew when the tongue is taking food，pinching the grain trail（the anus）to enable the bright moon to raise，and concentrating the essence in order to transmit the spiritual water to flow into the yellow chamber（the region below the navel）.

吸引二景以集明【xī yǐn èr jǐng yǐ jí míng】　指交通心肾，水火既济，能够和调阴阳，明敏神识。

absorbing two images to accumulate brightness Refers to communicating the heart and the kidney，balancing water and fire，harmonizing Yin and Yang，clearing fancy and understanding the spirit.

希言【xī yán】　指少说话合乎自然之道，尤其是习练气功。

understatement Such a way of communication is natural，especial for practicing Qigong.

希夷府【xī yí fǔ】　为祖窍异名。

special mansion A synonym of Zuqiao which is an acupoint located in the area between the heart and navel.

希夷门【xī yí mén】　指神通达出入之门，即脑。

special gate Refers to the brain through which the spirit comes in and goes out.

郗俭【xī jiǎn】　汉末方士，通气功。

Xi Jian A necromancer in the late Han Dynasty（202 BC‑263 AD），who was quite familiar with Qigong.

息【xī】　① 指一呼一吸；② 指熄灭烦恼，安定精神、思维、意识，为佛家气功习用语。

respiration Refers to ① either the procedure of inhalation and exhalation；② or elimination of annoyance and stabilization of the spirit，consciousness and thinking，which is a common term of Qigong in Buddhism.

息道【xī dào】　指呼吸的通道。

respiratory way Refers to the way that leads and controls respiration.

息火沐浴说【xī huǒ mù yù shuō】　源自气功专论，主要阐述调节呼吸以行沐浴温养功夫。

idea about stalling fire for bathing Collected from a monograph of Qigong，mainly describing regulation of respiration for taking a bath and warmly nourishing the body.

息虑【xī lǜ】　即熄灭思虑、念虑。

eliminating contemplation Refers to elimination of any consideration，desires and hopes.

息念忘情【xī niàn wàng qíng】　指停止一切思维活动，保持情绪稳定。

purifying the mind and relieving emotion Refers to eliminating any activity of thought and stabilizing emotion.

息气【xī qì】　指肺主持下的呼吸之气。

Respiratory Qi Refers to Qi in respiration controlled by the lung.

息神气常在气海【xī shén qì cháng zài qì hǎi】　即神与气合于气海，为神气合而为一之意。

Spiritual Qi is usually absorbed from the sea of Qi. Indicates that the spirit and Qi are integrated in the sea of Qi.

息调心净【xī tiáo xīn jìng】　指呼吸调和，意识自然清净无杂。

regulating respiration to tranquilize the heart Indicates that tranquilization of respiration will clarify consciousness and eliminate any distracting thought.

息心和悦【xī xīn hé yuè】　指息灭妄念，和悦精神。

purifying the heart and enjoying pleasure Refers to eliminating avarice and harmonizing the spirit.

息心静虑【xī xīn jìng lǜ】　指保持身心安静，杜绝一切杂念。

purifying the heart and tranquilizing the mind　Refers to tranquilizing the heart and the body, eliminating all distracting thought.

息以踵【xī yǐ zhǒng】　指呼吸出入之气达于足跟。

inhaling to heel　Means that Qi in inhalation and exhalation should reach the heel.

翕聚【xī jù】　指阴阳交媾作用。

gathering　Refers to the effect of intercourse of Yin and Yang.

噏【xī】　指吸，即吸收之意。

absorbing　Refers to inhalation and breathing in.

噏日精法【xī rì jīng fǎ】　为动功。其作法为，调身、调气、调神。作行功前准备，自然站定，形神放松，正立向日。然后双臂徐徐向两侧伸开，手掌自然放松，指放平。伸平手臂后，手掌由阴掌变为阳掌，宽胸怀。鼻引自然清气，意念导引入丹田。少顷，引气从口出，连续九息之后，仰天向日。双臂缓缓抱日向口，意念有日精从口而入，随即吞而咽七噏或九噏，每日三次。

exercise for absorbing essence　A dynamic exercise for regulating the body, Qi and spirit, marked by naturally standing up for preparation of Qigong practice, relaxing the body and spirit, standing upright to see the sun; then stretching the arms mildly to the left and right sides, naturally relaxing the fists and smoothing the fists; then turning the fists from Yin fists into Yang fists after smoothing the arms, relaxing the chest; inhaling natural clear Qi through the nose and imagining to lead it to Dantian; exhaling Qi through the mouth after a while and looking up to see the sun after nine times of respiration; slowly holding the sun to the mouth with both arms, imagining to inhaling solar essence through the mouth, then swallowing seven or nine times. Dantian is divided into the upper Dantian (the region between the eyes), the middle Dantian (the region below the heart) and the lower Dantian (the region below the navel). Such a dynamic exercise is practiced three times every day.

膝【xī】　即大腿与小腿连接处。

knee　Refers to the region connected with the thighs and shanks.

膝风摩涌泉【xī fēng mó yǒng quán】　指对膝关节冷痛、风痛或精虚而气不通之病症。此穴位为气功习练之处。

knee wind rubbing Yongquan（KI 1）　Refers to the disease caused by coldness and pain of the knee joint as well as obstruction of Qi due to arthritic pain or deficient essence. This acupoint is a region usually used in practice of Qigong.

膝腘【xī huò】　即腘窝，位于膝关节后面。

knee and popliteal fossa　Refers to popliteal space located behind the knee joint.

习定【xí dìng】　指气功家居山养静入定。

exercise for tranquilization　Refers to the fact that the masters of Qigong lived in the mountains for nourishing the body and tranquilizing the mind.

习善【xí shàn】　佛家气功习用语，指习善灭恶，为转移精神活动之意。

exercise for perfection　A term of

X

Qigong in Buddhism, referring to elimination of wickedness with virtue for changing the activity of the spirit.

洗井灶【xǐ jǐng zào】 为动功,即用葱姜煎汤擦洗两鼻孔,通泄脏腑毒气,调和脏腑功能。

washing well and stove A dynamic exercise, marked by rinsing the nostrils with decoction of onion and ginger, eliminating toxic Qi in the five Zang-organs (including the heart, the liver, the spleen, the lung and the kidney) and six Fu-organs (including the gall-bladder, the stomach, the small intestine, the large intestine, the bladder and the triple energizer), regulating the functions of the five Zang-organs and six Fu-organs.

洗髓【xǐ suǐ】 指剔除一切欲念,清静虚无。

rinsing marrow A term of Qigong, referring to eliminating any desires and tranquilizing the mind with nothingness.

洗心【xǐ xīn】 ① 指内省思虑;② 排除杂念。

rinsing the heart Refers to ① either introspection and contemplation; ② or elimination of distracting thought.

洗心涤虑【xǐ xīn dí lǜ】 同洗心退藏,即通过调神、调身、调气以剔除烦躁和杂念。

rinsing the heart to cleanse consideration The same as rising the heart to retreat storage, referring to regulating the spirit, body and Qi for eliminating irritability and distracting thought.

洗心内听【xǐ xīn nèi tīng】 指排除杂念,内守精神,意念导引听觉向内。

rinsing the heart for internal listening Refers to eliminating distracting thought, internally concentrating the spirit, and leading listening to the internal with consciousness.

洗心退藏【xǐ xīn tuì cáng】 即通过调神、调身、调气以剔除烦躁和杂念。

rising the heart to retreat storage Refers to regulating the spirit, body and Qi for eliminating irritability and distracting thought.

喜怒不节【xǐ nù bù jié】 指人若不能调节情志,控制感情,稳定情绪,就会使气血逆乱,阴阳失去平衡而发生疾病。

intemperance of emotional changes Indicates that failure to regulate, control and stabilize emotion will cause diseases due to disorder of Qi and blood and imbalance of Yin and Yang.

喜怒伤气【xǐ nù shāng qì】 指喜怒等情志变化太过,损伤人体阴阳之气,影响健康。

happiness and anger damaging Qi Indicates that excessive changes of emotions like happiness and anger damages Qi from Yin and Yang in the human body and injures health.

喜则气缓【xǐ zé qì huǎn】 喜则使人心气和平,意志畅达。但过喜则伤心气,使心气涣散不收。

Happiness relaxes Qi. Indicates that happiness harmonizes heart Qi and pacifies the mind. But excessive happiness damages heart Qi and disperses heart Qi.

虾蟆行气法【xiā má xíng qì fǎ】 为动功,方法多样。如正坐自动摇臂,不息十二通,愈劳瘵水气;左右侧卧,不息十二通,治疾饮不消。

exercise of frog moving Qi A dynamic exercise with various methods, such as

X

sitting upright, naturally shaking the shoulders, reducing respiration in twelve ways in order to cure chronic disease; lying on the right side and left side, reducing respiration in twelve ways in order to solve indigestion.

侠以日月如连珠【xiá yǐ rì yuè rú lián zhū】 即精气沿着任督二脉运行,如连珠绵绵不已。

Follow the sun and the moon as holding the pearls. Refers to the essential Qi flowing incessantly along the conception meridian and governor meridian.

霞外杂俎【xiá wài zá zǔ】《霞外杂俎》为气功学养生学专著,主要论述摄生之要,注重精神修养,清心寡欲,养生炼气。作者不详。

Xiawai Zazu(*Miscellaneous Utensil Outside Sunlight*) A monograph of Qigong and life cultivation entitled *Miscellaneous Utensil Outside Sunlight*, mainly describing the importance of regimen, cultivation of the spirit, pure heart and few desires as well as nourishing life and refining Qi. The author was unknown.

下闭【xià bì】 指阴精闭藏而不外泄。

lower closure Refers to closure of Yin essence.

下晡【xià bū】 指一天之中未时,即下午一至三时。

afternoon Refers to the time from one to three hours p. m.

下不闭火不聚【xià bù bì huǒ bù jù】指练功时,当一阳来复之际,要提肛。

no lower closure and no fire convergence Refers to drawing up the anus when Yang has returned in practicing Qigong.

下部八景【xià bù bā jǐng】 指的是肾

神,大小肠神、胴神、胸神、膈神、两胁神、左阴左阳神、右阴右阳神。

eight lower spirits Refers to the spirit in the kidney, in the large intestine, in the small intestine, in the trunk, in the chest, in the midriff and double sides of hypochondrium.

下丹田【xià dān tián】 ① 指气海;② 指脐下。

lower Dantian(**the region below the navel**) Refers to ① either Qihai(CV 6) located below the navel; ② or the region below the navel.

下关【xià guān】 足少阴胆经的经穴名,位于下颌骨关节的前方。此穴位为气功习练之处。

Xiaguan(ST 7) An acupoint in the gallbladder meridian of foot Shaoyin, located anteriorly to the lower mandible. This acupoint is a region usually used in practice of Qigong.

下和六腑绍五宫【xià hé liù fǔ shào wǔ gōng】 指脑神调节五脏六腑的功能。

regulation of six Fu-organs and five Zang-organs Refers to the function of the brain spirit to regulate the five Zang-organs(including the heart, the liver, the spleen, the lung and the kidney) and the six Fu-organs(the gallbladder, stomach, small intestine, large intestine, bladder and triple energizer).

下焦如渎【xià jiāo rú dú】 形容下焦肾膀胱排泄水液和糟粕的功能,如同沟渠。

lower energizer like ditch Refers to the function of the kidney and the bladder in the lower energizer to excrete liquid and dregs.

下摩生门【xià mó shēng mén】 下摩

为静功。屏息闭气,用手摩脐腹部,能调理三焦之气,使无郁滞,助消化。

rubbing navel A dynamic exercise, referring to closure of the internal Qi in order to enrich lower abdomen, to regulate Qi in the triple energizer, to relieve stagnation and to improve transformation.

下脘【xià wǎn】　任脉中的一个穴位,位于前正中线,脐上 2 寸。此穴位为气功习练之处。

Xiawan（CV 10） An acupoint in the conception meridian, located 2 Cun above the navel. This acupoint is a region usually used in practice of Qigong.

夏令导引法【xià lìng dǎo yǐn fǎ】　为动功。其作法为,用呵字导引,可正坐,两手作拳用力,左右互相虚筑各五六度。又以两手交叉,以脚踏手中各五六,间气为之,行之良久,闭目三咽津,叩齿三通而止。

exercise of Daoyin in summer A dynamic exercise, marked by starting Daoyin with the Chinese character He（breathing out）, sitting upright, holding the fists strongly from the left to the right and vice versa for five to six degrees respectively, crossing the hands, stepping on the hands with the feet for five to six degrees respectively for a long time, closing the eyes, swallowing fluid for three times and clicking the teeth in three ways.

夏令治脾导引法【xià lìng zhì pí dǎo yǐn fǎ】　为动功。其作法为,用呼字导引,可大坐,伸一脚,屈一脚,以两手向后及掣三五度。又跪坐,以两手据地,回头用力作虎视各三五度。

exercise of Daoyin for curing the spleen in summer A dynamic exercise, marked by starting Daoyin with the Chinese character Hu（呼, exhaling）, sitting down, stretching one hand, bending the other hand, drawing the hands back for three to five degrees, then sitting on the knees, pressing the ground with both hands and turning the head to see tigers for three or five degrees.

夏云峰猛虎出洞法【xià yún fēng měng hǔ chū dòng fǎ】　为动功。其作法为,先自然站立,然后将身曲起伏地上,两膝跪下,手按地,行功运气左右各六口。

exercise of the fierce tiger running out of the mountain cave in summer A dynamic exercise, marked by standing naturally first, then bending the body to prostrate on the ground, sitting on the knees, pressing the ground with hands and moving Qi from the left to the right and vice versa for six times.

夏至五月中坐功【xià zhì wǔ yuè zhōng zuò gōng】　为动功。其作法为,每日寅卯时（三至七时）跪坐,伸手叉指,屈脚趾,换踏左右,各五七次,叩齿,纳清吐浊,咽液。

exercise of sitting in the middle of May A dynamic exercise, marked by sitting on the knees in（the period of the day from 3 a. m. to 5 a. m. in the early morning）and Mao（the period of a day from 5 a. m. to 7 a. m. in the morning）every day, stretching out the hands to fork the fingers, bending the toes and changing from the left to the right and vice versa for five to seven times, clicking the teeth, inhaling clear Qi, exhaling turbid Qi and swallowing humor.

仙道【xiān dào】　指气功养生之道。

immortal Dao Refers to the basic theory and methods of Qigong practice and life cultivation.

仙佛合宗语录【xiān fó hé zōng yǔ lù】《仙佛合宗语录》为气功学专著,为明代伍守阳所集,伍守虚校注。

Xianfo Hezong Yulu（*Combined Quotations of Immortals and Buddhism*） A monograph of Qigong entitled *Combined Quotations of Immortals and Buddhism*, compiled by Wu Shouyang and explained by Wu Shouxu in the Ming Dynasty（1368 AD - 1644 AD）.

仙赋【xiān fù】 气功专论,由汉代桓谭所作,主要论述气功的理法习要。

xian Fu（*Immoral Composition*） A monograph of Qigong entitled *Immoral Composition*, written by Huan Tan in the Han Dynasty（202 BC - 263 AD）, mainly describing the theory, practice and methods of Qigong practice.

仙经【xiān jīng】《仙经》为道家经典著作,部分内容阐述了养生的基本理论和实践方法。

Immortal Canon A canon of Daoism, describing the basic theory and practical methods about Qigong and life cultivation in some chapters.

仙人道士非有神,积精累气以成真【xiān rén dào shì fēi yǒu shén jī jīng lěi qì yǐ chéng zhēn】 意思是只有习练气功了才可能真正地有神气。

Immortals and Daoists may not really have the spirit and only when essence is enriched and Qi is fortified can spirit be really promoted. Refers to the fact that only practice of Qigong can enable people to have the spirit.

仙人之粮【xiān rén zhī liáng】 指吞咽口中唾液。

immortal grain Refers to swallowing saliva.

先觉【xiān jué】 指习练气功,导引入静,至静之中而觉悟,谓之先觉。

awakening Refers to tranquilization that increases consciousness in practicing Qigong.

先生【xiān shēng】 ① 指先醒,首先从人世中觉悟;② 指有德业之称。

early birth Refers to ① either awakening which means consciousness in the human world; ② or moral work.

先天【xiān tiān】 指无极,阴阳未分,一气处于混混沌沌之中。

innateness Refers to no extremity because Yin and Yang are not separated and Qi is in chaos.

先天金丹大道玄奥口诀【xiān tiān jīn dān dà dào xuán ào kǒu jué】《先天金丹大道玄奥口诀》为气功专著,为宋代霍济所述,论述习练气功重在药物和火候。

Xiantian Jindan Dadao Xuan'ao Koujue（*Supreme Rhyme of Primordial Golden Dan and Great Way*） A monograph of Qigong entitled *Supreme Rhyme of Primordial Golden Dan and Great Way*, written by Huo Ji in the Song Dynasty（960 AD - 1279 AD）, mainly describing the importance of medicinal and duration of heating in practicing Qigong.

先天景象【xiān tiān jǐng xiàng】 源自气功专论,主要阐述人与自然社会融为一体的征象。

primordial image Collected from a monograph, mainly describing the manifestation of man integrating with the natural world and social environment.

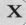

先天气【xiān tiān qì】 ① 指元始祖气；② 指静极一阳之气；③ 指子气；④ 指无极，天地混乱未分之前。

primordial Qi Refers to ① either the original Qi；② or Qi of Yang in extreme quietness；③ or Qi in the period of Zi（the period of the day from 11 p.m. to 1 a.m. in the afternoon）；④ or the condition before the sky and earth were separated.

先天一气【xiān tiān yī qì】 ① 指元始祖气；② 指静极一阳之气；③ 指子气；④ 指无极，天地混乱未分之前。

one primordial Qi Refers to ① either the original Qi；② or Qi of Yang in extreme quietness；③ or Qi in the period of Zi（the period of the day from 11 p.m. to 1 a.m.）；④ or the condition before the sky and earth were separated.

先天元神【xiān tiān yuán shén】 ① 指男女媾精候，形成生命之神；② 指静而生慧。

primordial and original spirit Refers to ① either coition of man and woman that has produced the spirit of life；② or tranquility that has increased wisdom.

先天主人【xiān tiān zhǔ rén】 "祖窍"之异名，位于心与脐之正中。

primordial master A term of Qigong, a synonym of Zuqiao which is an acupoint located in the region between the heart and the navel.

先知【xiān zhī】 指习练气功，导引入静，至寂至虚中而有知，谓之先知。

prophet Refers to tranquilization and silence that broaden the mind in practicing Qigong.

闲静【xián jìng】 指安静，无欲望。

leisure and quietness Refers to tranquilizing the mind and eliminating any desires.

闲居十德【xián jū shí dé】 佛家气功习用语，指佛家气功调节人与自然、社会而保持意识稳定的十种道德和行为。

ten moralities for leisure life A common term of Qigong in Buddhism, referring to ten moralities and activities in Buddhism for regulating the relationships between human beings and natural world and social environment in order to stabilize consciousness.

咸池【xián chí】 精气聚散常在此处，水火发端也在此处，阴阳变化也在此处，有无出入也在此处。

entire pond Refers to the region where the essential Qi concentrates and disperses there, water and fire appear there, Yin and Yang change there, exit and entrance exist there.

相入【xiāng rù】 佛家气功习用语，指你中有我，我中有你，彼此事物，相互融入。

blending A common term of Qigong in Buddhism, referring to combination of different things, just as the traditional Chinese idea that you can find yourself in myself and I can find myself in yourself.

相生相克【xiāng shēng xiāng kè】 即五行相生相克之理，亦为气功之理。

mutual promotion and restriction Explains the principles of mutual promotion and restriction among the five elements（including wood, fire, earth, metal and water）. These principles are also used in Qigong practice.

相似觉【xiāng sì jué】 佛家气功习用语，指习练佛家气功后，幡然大悟，增加认识能力。

ideal enlightenment A common term of Qigong in Buddhism, referring to sudden awareness and increased ability of knowledge after practicing Qigong in Buddhism.

相制【xiāng zhì**】** 指气功中阴阳之间相互制约。

mutual control Refers to mutual control of Yin and Yang in Qigong.

香山居士【xiāng shān jū shì**】** 指唐代诗人白居易,也是气功家。

Lay Buddhist in Xianshan Mountain Refers to Bai Juyi, a great poet and a master of Qigong in the Tang Dynasty (618 AD - 907 AD).

降伏【xiáng fú**】** ① 指纳气归丹田而不外散;② 指精神专一,排除杂念。

subduedness Refers to ① either inhalation of Qi entering Dantian without any dispersion; ② or concentration of the spirit without any distracting thought. Dantian is divided into the upper Dantian (the region between the eyes), the middle Dantian (the region below the heart) and the lower Dantian (the region below the navel).

降伏座【xiáng fú zuò**】** 佛家气功坐势,即盘腿而坐。

subdued sitting A sitting posture of Buddhism, referring to sitting with crossed legs.

降龙伏虎【xiáng lóng fú hǔ**】** 指精神内守,肾水上升而制火为降龙;精神内守,心火下降而济水,为伏虎。

subsiding Loong and bending tiger Refers to internal concentration of the spirit in order to raise kidney water and control fire, which means subsiding Loong; and internal concentration of the spirit in order to descend heart fire

and promote water, which means bending tiger.

降魔坐【xiáng mó zuò**】** 即以右趾押左股,后以左趾押右股。

sitting for expelling evil Means to press the left thigh with the right toes, and then to press the right thigh with the left toes.

享青龙之祉【xiǎng qīng lóng zhī sì**】** 为静功。其作法为,"以春三月朔旦,东面平坐,叩齿三通,闭气九息,吸震宫青气入口九吞之。以补嘘之损,享青龙之祉"。

enjoyment of sacrificing green Loong A static exercise, marked by "sitting to the east on the first day of every month in spring, clicking the teeth for three times, stopping respiration for nine times, inhaling green Qi from the east into the mouth for nine times in order to solve the problems caused by slow breath and to enjoy sacrificing green Loong".

想【xiǎng**】** 佛家气功习用语,指直接反映的影像,是精神活动的一种,相当于知觉、感觉。

thinking A term of Qigong, referring to direct reflection of shadow, which is an activity of the spirit, similar to consciousness and sensation.

项与手争【xiàng yǔ shǒu zhēng**】** 为动功。其作法为,先跳跃运动,平息后坐正,两手在项后相叉,仰视抬头,左右摇功,使项与手争。

struggle of neck and hand A dynamic exercise, marked by jumping first, sitting upright after quietness, crossing the hands behind the neck, raising the head to look up, shaking the head from the left to the right and vice versa for

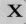

struggling the neck and hands.

项子食气法【xiàng zǐ shí qì fǎ】 为静功。其作法为，常以清旦鼻纳气咽之，经行勿休，口口吐之。

exercise for the neck to take Qi A static exercise, marked by inhaling through the nose, swallowing through the mouth in early morning, avoiding rest during practice and repeatedly vomiting turbid Qi.

逍遥游【xiāo yáo yóu】 《庄子》篇名，指人当破功、名、利、禄、权、势、尊位，处天时之和，可使精神意识思维活动自由自在，无牵无挂。

Happy Excursion A title of one chapter in *Zhuang Zi* writing by Zhuang Zhou, a great thinker, philosopher and litterateur in the Warring States Period (475 BC - 221 BC), refers to breaking exploit, reputation, benefit, emolument, power and high position in order to free the activities of the spirit, consciousness and thinking without any care and worry.

逍遥子搓涂法【xiāo yáo zǐ cuō tú fǎ】 为动静相兼功。其作法为，每晨静坐闭目，凝神存养，神运气自体内达外，停于面部，两手搓热，拂面七次。

free-unfettered man's exercise for rubbing and mudding An exercise combined with dynamic exercise and static exercise, marked by sitting quiet in the early morning, closing the eyes, gazing the spirit for nourishing the body, moving the spirit internally and externally to keep in the face, rubbing the hands warm and kneading the face for seven times.

逍遥子导引诀【xiāo yáo zǐ dǎo yǐn jué】 《逍遥子导引诀》为气功专著，阐述了各种各样的功法和静法，作者不详。

Xiaoyaozi Daoyin Jue（*Free-Unfettered Man's Formula of Daoyin*） Xiaoyaozi Daoyin Jue is a monograph of Qigong entitled *Free-Unfettered Man's Formula of Daoyin*, describing various dynamic exercises and static exercises. The author was unknown.

逍遥子兜礼法【xiāo yáo zǐ dōu lǐ fǎ】 动静相兼功。其作法为，自然、盘膝坐式均可。调气调神，静坐，安定身心。

free-unfettered man's exercise for praying An exercise combined with dynamic exercise and static exercise, marked by natural sitting with crossed legs, regulating Qi and spirit, sitting quietly, tranquilizing the body and heart.

逍遥子封金匮法【xiāo yáo zǐ fēng jīn kuì fǎ】 动静相兼功。其作法为，睡醒时调息思神，以左手搓脐一十四次，右手亦搓脐一十四次。再以两手搓胁腹，摇摆七次，咽气纳于丹田，握固良久乃止，屈足侧卧。

free-unfettered man's exercise for strengthening golden chamber An exercise combined with dynamic exercise and static exercise, marked by regulating respiration and thinking the spirit after waking up, rubbing the navel with the left hand and right hand for fourteen times respectively, rubbing the ribs and abdomen with both hands and shaking for seven times, swallowing Qi and inhaling it into Dantian, keeping it for a long period of time, bending the feet and lying on one side. Dantian is divided into the upper Dantian (the region between the eyes), the middle Dantian (the region below the heart) and the lower Dantian (the re-

X

gion below the navel).

逍遥子火起养生法【xiāo yáo zǐ huǒ qǐ yǎng shēng fǎ】 为静功。其作法为，子午二时，存想真火自涌泉穴起，先从左足行上玉枕，过泥丸，降入丹田三遍。次从右足亦行三遍，复从尾闾起，又行三遍。

free-unfettered man's exercise for increasing fire to cultivate life A static exercise, marked by imagining that genuine fire starts from Yongquan (KI 1) in Zi (the period of the day from 11 p.m. to 1 a.m.) and Wu (the period of a day from 3 a.m. to 5 a.m. in the early morning), moving it first from Yuzhen (BL 9) along the left foot and then along the right foot, through the mud bolus (the brain) and into Dantian for three times respectively.

逍遥子凝固法【xiāo yáo zǐ níng gù fǎ】 为静功。其作法为，平时静坐，存想元神入于丹田，随意呼吸，不可中途而废。

free-unfettered man's exercise for concentration A static exercise, marked by sitting quietly, imagining that the original spirit has entered Dantian, breathing naturally and preventing any ways of stopping the practice of Qigong. Dantian is divided into the upper Dantian (the region between the eyes), the middle Dantian (the region below the heart) and the lower Dantian (the region below the navel).

逍遥子升观法【xiāo yáo zǐ shēng guān fǎ】 为静功。其作法为，子午时握固端坐，凝神绝念，两眼含光，上视泥丸，存想追摄二气自尾闾上升，下降返还元海，每行九遍，日三次。

free-unfettered man's exercise for in-creasing vision A static exercise, marked by sitting upright in Zi (the period of the day from 11 p.m. to 1 a.m.), gazing the spirit, eliminating desires, keeping light in the eyes to see the mud bolus (the brain), imagining to rise two kinds of Qi from the coccyx and to return to the original sea for nine times a day in three days.

逍遥子守玉关法【xiāo yáo zǐ shǒu yù guān fǎ】 为静功。其作法为，行住坐卧，一意不散，固守丹田，默运神气，冲透三关。

free-unfettered man's exercise for keeping jade joint A static exercise, marked by either quietly walking or staying or sitting or lying, defending Dantian, silently moving the spirit and Qi thoroughly through three joints. Dantian is divided into the upper Dantian (the region between the eyes), the middle Dantian (the region below the heart) and the lower Dantian (the region below the navel).

逍遥子水潮除疾法【xiāo yáo zǐ shuǐ cháo chú jí fǎ】 为静功。其作法为，晨起睡醒时，起端坐，凝神息虑，舌舐上颚，闭口调息，津液自生，渐生满口，分作三次，以意送下。

free-unfettered man's exercise for eliminating disease through torrent A static exercise, marked by waking up in the early morning, gazing the spirit and stabilizing respiration, lapping the upper jaw with the tongue, closing the mouth and regulating respiration, sending downward fluid and humor full in the mouth for three times.

逍遥子胎息诀【xiāo yáo zǐ tāi xī jué】 静功口诀，重在平时养神爱气，加强修养。

free-unfettered man's formula for fetal respiration A static exercise, paying great attention to nourishing the spirit and loving Qi in order to increasing life cultivation.

逍遥子托踏法【xiāo yáo zǐ tuō tà fǎ】动静相兼功。其作法为,自然站立,平和呼吸。然后双手上托如举大石,两脚前踏,如履平地,存想神气,依按四时嘘呵二七次。

free-unfettered man's exercise for raising and treading An exercise combined with dynamic exercise and static exercise, marked by standing natural, peacefully breathing, raising the hands like holing a large stone, treading forward with both feet like walking on the flat ground, thinking of the spirit and breathing out for two or seven times according to the four seasons.

逍遥子消积聚法【xiāo yáo zǐ xiāo jī jù fǎ】为静功。其作法为,伸身闭息,鼓动胸腹,侍其气满,缓缓呵出。如此行三十五次,通快即止。

free-unfettered man's exercise for eliminating abdominal mass A static exercise, marked by stretching the body, stopping respiration, promoting the chest and abdomen, slowly breathing out when Qi is sufficient. Such a way of practice can be done for thirty-five times till all parts are unobstructed.

逍遥子掩耳法【xiāo yáo zǐ yǎn ěr fǎ】动静相兼功。其作法为,静坐伸身,闭息,以两手掩耳,缓慢折头五七次,存想元神逆上泥丸以逐其邪。

free-unfettered man's exercise for covering the ears An exercise combined with dynamic exercise and static exercise, marked by sitting quietly and stretching the body, stopping respiration, covering the ears with both hands, slowly turning the head for five to seven times, imagining that the original spirit reversely rising to the mud bolus (the brain) in order to expel pathogenic factors.

逍遥子意运法【xiāo yáo zǐ yì yùn fǎ】为静功。其作法为,行、住、坐、卧均可行功,取自然式,调气调神,安定精神,意识活动集中于丹田,待丹田精气盈满,意使精气流冲破三关(尾闾、夹脊、玉枕),上入泥丸,可反复行十数次。

free-unfettered man's exercise for consciousness activity A static exercise, marked by naturally walking, or staying, or sitting, or lying, regulating Qi and spirit, stabilizing the essence and spirit, concentrating the activity of consciousness in Dantian, enabling essential Qi to break through three joints and raise to the mud bolus (the brain) when essential Qi in Dantian is exuberant for dozens of time. The three joints include Weijian (an acupoint between the coccyx and anus), Jiaji (an acupoint located on both sides of the spine) and Yuzhen (BL 9). Dantian is divided into the upper Dantian (the region between the eyes), the middle Dantian (the region below the heart) and the lower Dantian (the region below the navel).

逍遥子远睛法【xiāo yáo zǐ yuǎn jīng fǎ】动静相兼功。其作法为,自然坐式或站式均可,姿势定后,闭目垂帘,正身,轮转双目,从左向右轮转七次,再从右向左轮转七次。

free-unfettered man's exercise for moving

the eyes An exercise combined with dynamic exercise and static exercise, marked by natural sitting or standing, closing the eyes, falling curtain, keeping the body upright, turning the eyes from the left to the right and vice versa for seven times respectively.

消除恶气出脐门【xiāo chú è qì chū qí mén】 指脑神将污秽、恶浊之气排出体外。

eliminating turbid Qi from navel gate Means that the brain spirit eliminates filth and turbid Qi.

消渴【xiāo kě】 气功适应证，泛指以多饮、多食、多尿症状为特点的病证。

consumptive thirst disease An indication of Qigong, referring to the disease with the symptoms of polydipsia, polyphagia and diuresis.

消渴候导引法【xiāo kě hòu dǎo yǐn fǎ】 为静功。其作法为，躺下，闭目、闭气不息，到极限时慢慢吐出十二次。理气消食，治饮食不消。

exercise for consumptive thirst A static exercise, marked by lying, closing the eyes, stopping respiration, slowly exhaling for twelve times when respiration is stopped to the maximum, regulating Qi and helping digestion. Such a static exercise can treat indigestion.

消息【xiāo xī】 指信息。

message Refers to information.

消阴魔法【xiāo yīn mó fǎ】 为静功。其作法为，静坐、端身竖脊，含胸勾腮，两手握固，凝神定息。

exercise for eliminating distraction A static exercise, marked by quietly sitting upright, stretching the spine, maintaining the chest and keeping the cheek, holding the hands, concentra-

ting the spirit and stabilizing respiration.

小便数候导引法【xiǎo biàn shù hòu dǎo yǐn fǎ】 为动功。其作法为，① 两足跟交替放膝上，利水，治小便频数；② 仰卧，两手放膝头，两足跟放臀下，口吸气，鼓腹，待气充满腹部时，用鼻呼出，利水通淋，治小便频数。

exercise of Daoyin for polyuria A dynamic exercise, marked by ① crossing the heels and pressing the knees, alleviating water and disposing frequent urination；② or lying on the back with both hands pressing on the knees, pressing the buttocks with both heels, inhaling with the mouth and exhaling with the nose for dealing with diuresis and stranguria.

小成【xiǎo chéng】 即小有成就。喻习练气功初获成功。

initial success Refers to success of initial practice of Qigong.

小寒十二月节坐功【xiǎo hán shí èr yuè jié zuò gōng】 为动功。其作法为，每日子丑时正坐，一手按足，一手上托，挽背互换，极力三五次，吐纳、叩齿、漱咽。

dhyana in the feast days of December A dynamic exercise, marked by sitting in Zi (the period of the day from 11 p.m. to 1 a.m.) and Chou (the period of a day from 1 a.m. to 3 a.m. in the morning) every day with one hand pressing the foot and the other hand popping up for three or five times respectively, breathing in and out, clicking the teeth, rinsing the throat and swallowing saliva. Such a dynamic exercise can treat various diseases.

小河车【xiǎo hé chē】 指的是羊车、

鹿车、牛车，或指小河车、大河车、紫
河车。

small river cart Refers to either sheep
cart, deer cart and cow cart, or small
river cart, large river cart and purple
cart, or attack cart, thunder cart and
broken cart.

小还丹【xiǎo huán dān】　即"自肾传
肝，自肝传心，自心传脾，传肺，周而复始
至丹田，曰小还丹"。

**returning to the small Dan（pills of im-
mortality）** Refers to the fact that "it
transmits to the liver from the kidney,
transmitting to the heart and spleen
from the liver, going round and round,
finally reaching Dantian called as returning to the small Dan（pills of im-
mortality）." Dantian is divided into the
upper Dantian（the region between the
eyes）, the middle Dantian（the region
below the heart）and the lower Dantian
（the region below the navel）.

小满四月中坐功【xiǎo mǎn sì yuè
zhōng zuò gōng】　为动功。其作法为，
每日寅卯时正坐，一手举托，一手拄按，
左右各三五次，叩齿、吐纳、咽液，可治
百病。

dhyana in the middle of April A dynamic exercise, marked y siting upright
in Yin（the period of a day from 3 a.m.
to 5 a.m. in the morning）and Mao
（the period of a day from 5 a.m. to
7 a.m. in the morning）every day with
one hand raising and the other hand
pressing three or five times, clicking
the teeth, breathing in and out and
swallowing fluid. Such a dynamic exercise can treat various diseases.

小年【xiǎo nián】　指朝菌大芝，天阴
生于粪上，见太阳即死，惠姑或各山蝉，

春生夏死，夏生秋死，故不知春秋。

short life Refers to the fact that bac-
teria appears from feces when it is
cloudy and disappears when it is bright;
cicada appears in spring and disappears
in summer or appears in summer and
disappears in autumn.

小暑六月节坐功【xiǎo shǔ liù yuè jié
zuò gōng】　为动功。其作法为，每日丑
寅时两手踞地，屈压一足，直伸一足，用
力掣三五次，叩齿、吐纳、咽液，可治
百病。

dhyana in the feast days of June A dynamic exercise, marked by pressing the
ground with both hands in Chou（the
period of a day from 1 a.m. to 3 a.m.
in the morning）and Yin（the period of
a day from 3 a.m. to 5 a.m. in the
morning）every day, bending and
pressing one foot, stretching the other
foot forcefully for three or five times,
clicking the teeth, breathing in and
out, and swallowing humor. Such a dynamic exercise can treat various diseases.

小雪十月中坐功【xiǎo xuě shí yuè
zhōng zuò gōng】　为动功。其作法为，
每日丑寅时正坐，一手按膝，一手挽肘，
左右争力，各三五次，吐纳、叩齿、咽液，
可治百病。

**dhyana in the middle of October with
small snow** A dynamic exercise,
marked by sitting upright in Chou（the
period of a day from 1 a.m. to 3 a.m.
in the morning）and Yin（the period of
a day from 3 a.m. to 5 a.m. in the
morning）every day, pressing the knee
with one hand, taking the elbow with
the other hand from the left to the
right and vice versa for three or five

times respectively, breathing in and out and clicking the teeth and swallowing fluid. Such a dynamic exercise can treat various diseases.

小玉液炼形法【xiǎo yù yè liàn xíng fǎ**】** 为静功。其作法为，气功锻炼中，练到一定时候，口中唾液增加，咽下此唾液有滋润脏六腑，健康形体的效果。

saliva exercise A static exercise, referring to saliva that has increased after practice of Qigong for a certain period of time and that swallowing saliva will enrich and moisten the five Zang-organs (including the heart, the liver, the spleen, the lung and the kidney) and the six Fu-organs (including the gallbladder, the stomach, the small intestine, the large intestine, the bladder and the triple energizer).

小指次指【xiǎo zhǐ cì zhǐ**】** 即第四指（趾）。

little finger Little finger refers to the fourth finger (toe).

小周天【xiǎo zhōu tiān**】** 为静功。其作法为，阴阳循环一小周天，闭目静坐，鼻吸清气，鼓腹使内气下降脐下丹田，运气过肛门，可强身却病。

small circulatory cycle A static exercise, referring to Yin and Yang circulating in a whole tiny sky. In practicing Qigong, the practitioner should close the eyes and sit quietly with the nose inhaling air, enabling internal Qi from the abdomen to descend to the lower Dantian below the navel and the anus in order to strengthen the body and cure disease. Dantian is divided into the upper Dantian (the region between the eyes), the middle Dantian (the region below the heart) and the lower Dantian (the region below the navel).

小周天鼎器【xiǎo zhōu tiān dǐng qì**】** 源自气功专论，主要阐述小周天功法中以坤腹为炉，乾首为鼎。

practice of small circulatory cycle Collected from a monograph of Qigong, referring to the chest taken as the stove while the head taken as the cauldron.

小周天神引说【xiǎo zhōu tiān shén yǐn shuō**】** 源自气功专论，阐述小周天功的含义及其神引息吹的具体做法。

miraculous explanation of small circulatory cycle Collected from a monograph of Qigong, referring to the meaning of the small circulatory cycle and the implication of the method in practicing Qigong under the guidance of the spirit.

小眦【xiǎo zì**】** 即目外眦。

small canthus Located in the region connected with the lower eyelid and temple.

哮喘导引法【xiào chuǎn dǎo yǐn fǎ**】** 为动功。其作法为，用手捏擦脊中穴数十次，然后用手摩擦乳下数次，擦背，擦双肩，定心咽津，调息降气。

exercise of Daoyin for asthma A dynamic exercise, marked by pinching and rubbing the acupoints located on the middle of the spine for dozens of times, then rubbing the region below the breasts for several times, rubbing the back and shoulders, tranquilizing the heart and swallowing fluid, regulating respiration and descending Qi.

哮证【xiào zhèng**】** 气功适应证，指发作性的痰鸣气喘疾患。

wheezing syndrome / pattern An indication of Qigong, referring to paroxysmal wheezing and panting.

笑一笑,少一少【xiào yī xiào shào yī shào】　指精神愉快、心情舒畅,气血流通,阴阳平衡,则显得年轻、有朝气。

Smile a while and lose a while.　Indicates that good mood，pleasant mind，unobstructed flow of Qi and blood and balance of Yin and Yang will make the practitioners young and vital.

啸父市上补履【xiào fù shì shàng bǔ lǚ】　为动功。其作法为,自然坐势,两足伸平放于席上。两手握住左足心(涌泉穴处),运气三口,然后两手换握右脚心,运气四口。主治强腰膝、固精。

Xiao Fu's exercise for mending shoes in city　A dynamic exercise，marked by naturally sitting，stretching the feet on the mat，holding the left sole with both hands，moving Qi for three times，then holding the right sole with both hands，and moving Qi for four times. Such a dynamic exercise can strengthen the waist，knees and essence.

消谷散气摄牙齿【xiāo gǔ sàn qì shè yá chǐ】　指脾的功能作用,磨谷,主运化,固摄牙齿。

exercise for promoting digestion，exhausting Qi and protecting teeth　Refers to the function of the spleen for digesting food，moving Qi and securing the teeth.

邪观【xié guān】　指练功时,眼神未能集中到"玄牝"处。玄牝①指身中一窍;②指二肾之间;③指天地;④指任督二脉;⑤指体内阴阳;⑥指中宫脾。

inattentive vision　Refers to failure to concentrate on Xuanpin in practicing Qigong. Xuanpin refers to ① either an orifice in the body；② or a region between the two kidneys；③ or the sky and the earth；④ or the conception

meridian and governor meridian；⑤ or Yin and Yang in the body；⑥ or the spleen.

邪火【xié huǒ】　① 指由身体内妄念所产生的火;② 指六淫之一的火邪。

evil fire　Refers to either fire produced by wild fancy；or fire evil，one of the six exogenous pathogenic factors.

邪魔腥【xié mó xīng】　指五谷之味,美味易引起欲念,影响入静。

evil stench　Refers to the tastes of five kinds of grain，the delicious taste of which causes desires that affects tranquility.

邪心【xié xīn】　指正常的意念活动。

evil heart　Refers to normal activity of consciousness.

胁【xié】　即腋下至第十肋下缘。

hypochondrium　Refers to the upper part of the side of the human body，the region from the oxter to the tenth rib.

胁痛【xié tòng】　气功适应证,指一侧或两侧胁肋疼痛为主要症状的病证。

hypochondriac pain　An indication of Qigong，marked by pain in the one side or two sides of the costal region.

胁痛候导引法【xié tòng hòu dǎo yǐn fǎ】　动静相兼功,作法多样。如静心存想,肝为青龙,左眼中有魂神,统帅五营兵,千乘万骑,从左胁下取病而去,治左胁痛。

exercise of Daoyin for hypochondriac pain　An exercise combined with dynamic exercise and static exercise with various methods，such as tranquilizing the heart and stabilizing the mind，in which the liver is known as green Loong，there is the ethereal soul and the spirit in the left eye，trying the best in imagining ways to expel disease from the left costal region in order to cure pain in the left costal region.

胁痛治法【xié tòng zhì fǎ】　动静相兼功，其作法多样，如突然左胁痛，用意念导气至左胁下取病。

treatment of hypochondriac pain An exercise combined with dynamic exercise and static exercise with various methods, such as leading Qi to the left costal region with consciousness if there is sudden pain in the left costal region.

泻肾经实火法【xiè shèn jīng shí huǒ fǎ】　为静功。其作法为，戌亥二时，仰卧，枕高四指，四肢宜伸。以鼻收气于右肾，火从口中嘻出，默数百次。以右肋着席，卧蹻两足，钩两腿，一手掩脐，一手掩外肾。

exercise for pouring fire from the kidney meridian A static exercise, marked by lying on the back in Xu period (the period of a day from 7 p. m. to 9 p. m. in the evening) and Hai period (the period of a day from 21 p. m. to 23 p. m. at night) with a pillow as high as four fingers, stretching the four limbs, inhaling Qi from the nose to the right kidney, spitting fire from the mouth silently for several hundred times, putting the right rib on the bed, curling up the feet, hooking the legs, pressing the navel with one hand and rubbing the external kidney with the other hand.

谢自然跌席泛海【xiè zì rán fū xí fàn hǎi】　为动功。其作法为，两手自然握拳按摩两胁，凝神运气，左右各廿四口。主治身体疲劳。

Xie Ziran's instep over the bed for floating sea A dynamic exercise, marked by naturally holding and rubbing the rib-sides with both hands, concentra-

ting the spirit for moving Qi from the left to the right and vice versa for twenty-four times. Such a dynamic exercise can cure fatigue.

懈怠【xiè dài】　佛家气功习用语，指断恶、修善之事不尽力，为烦恼之意，影响精神意识的稳定。

slack A common term of Qigong in Buddhism, indicating failure to break evil and to rehabilitate virtue, causing annoyance and affecting stability of the spirit and consciousness.

心【xīn】　① 指五脏之一的心脏；② 指精神；③ 指中心。

heart Refers to ① either one of the five Zang-organs (including the heart, the liver, the spleen, the lung and the kidney); ② or the spirit; ③ or the center.

心痹【xīn bì】　气功适应证，指冠心病及其他心脏病。

Heart impediment An indication of Qigong, refers to coronary disease and other heart diseases.

心病【xīn bìng】　① 指精神损伤；② 指心及心经所生病。

Heart disease Refers to ① either spirit damage；② or disease located in the heart and the heart meridian.

心病导引【xīn bìng dǎo yǐn】　指正面坐好，两手握拳，双手暗自用力各六次。

Exercise of Daoyin for heart disease Refers to sitting frontally with both hands clenching each other forcefully for six times.

心荡【xīn dàng】　指精神震悸不宁。

Heart restlessness Refers to palpitation and inquietude.

心灯【xīn dēng】　指气功景象，即静坐时神思明亮，如灯照光明。

cardiac lamp Refers to scene of Qigong practice，indicating brightness of thought in quiet sitting.

心地【xīn dì】　指存养心性，佛家认为心为万法之本。

heart status Refers to keeping cardiac disposition. According to Buddhism，the heart is the origin of all things in the world.

心典【xīn diǎn】　同心意，指精神意识活动。

heart canon Refers to intention，indicating activities of the spirit and consciousness.

心定【xīn dìng】　指精神意识合乎自然、社会变化的道理，而趋于稳定。

heart harmony Refers to the fact that the spirit and consciousness conform to the principles of natural and social changes，and tend to be stabilized.

心顿于息【xīn dùn yú xī】　指意念与呼吸相合，即神息相依。

heart focusing on respiration Refers to combination of consciousness and respiration，indicating that the spirit and respiration depend on each other.

心法【xīn fǎ】　① 指修身养性的方法；② 指以心相传授的佛法；③ 指气功养生法。

heart method Refers to ① either the method for cultivating the body；② or passing on knowledge or skills through the heart，which is an exercise in Buddhism；③ or exercise for practicing Qigong and cultivating life.

心风【xīn fēng】　指心系病及其临床特征。

heart wind Refers to heart disease and clinical features.

心府【xīn fǔ】　指神，即记忆、思维等。

heart palace Refers to the spirit，indicating memory and thought.

心腹痛【xīn fù tòng】　气功适应证，多有寒邪客于脏腑之间，与血气相互搏结所致。

cardiac and abdominal pain An indication of Qigong，refers to invasion of pathogenic cold into the five Zang-organs（including the heart，the liver，the spleen，the lung and the kidney）and the six Fu-organs（including the gallbladder，the stomach，the small intestine，the large intestine，the bladder and the triple energizer），related to confrontation of the blood and Qi.

心腹痛候导引法【xīn fù tòng hòu dǎo yǐn fǎ】　为静功，经常静心存想日月星辰，凌晨鸡鸣时，安卧于床，以唾液漱口，待津液满口时，分三次咽下。

exercise of Daoyin for cardiac and abdominal pain A static exercise，marked by tranquilizing the heart and mind every time，lying quietly on bed before dawn when chickens begin to crow，rinsing the mouth with saliva，and swallowing three times when fluid and humor are full in the mouth.

心腹痛治法【xīn fù tòng zhì fǎ】　动静相兼功，习练方法多样，如指仰卧，展两腿手，跷足趾，用鼻吸气，尽力行气七息。

treatment of cardiac and abdominal pain An exercise combined with dynamic exercise and static exercise，such as lying on the back，stretching the legs and hands，raising the toes，inhaling through the nose and promoting circulation of Qi for seven times.

心腹胀【xīn fù zhàng】　气功适应证，多因脏气内虚，邪气乘袭心脾二经所致。

cardiac and abdominal distension An indication of Qigong, is caused by internal deficiency of visceral Qi and invasion of pathogenic Qi into the heart meridian and the spleen meridian.

心腹胀候导引法【xīn fù zhàng hòu dǎo yǐn fǎ】 为静功,指伸右腿,左膝弯曲压在右腿上,入静,呼吸五次。

exercise of Daoyin for cardiac and abdominal flatulence A static exercise, marked by stretching the right leg, bending the left knee to press the right leg, promoting tranquility, inhaling and exhaling for five times.

心肝【xīn gān】 ① 指精神现象;② 指肝脏、心脏。

heart and liver Refers to ① spiritual manifestation;② two important organs in the five Zang-organs (including the heart, the liver, the spleen, the lung and the kidney).

心功【xīn gōng】 为静功,此功法可调心,固神气,治七情所致之病。

heart exercise A static exercise, indicating that it can regulate the heart, keeping the spiritual Qi and treating diseases caused by seven emotions.

心花【xīn huā】 指精神宁静,喻行功中,静而生慧。

cardiac flower Refers to quietness of the spirit, indicating great wisdom in tranquil practice of Qigong.

心灰【xīn huī】 ① 指意识消沉;② 指心中杂念。

distracted heart Refers to depression of will and distracting thought.

心火【xīn huǒ】 ① 指心,五行中心属于火;② 指心和心经实火;③ 指心的生理功能作用。

heart fire Refers to ① either heart

that pertains to fire in the five elements (including wood, fire, earth, metal and water);② or fire in the heart and the heart meridian;③ or the physiological function of the heart.

心稽【xīn jī】 指心计,为意识思维活动。

heart investigation Refers to heart management, indicating activities of consciousness and thought.

心疾【xīn jí】 ① 指意识活动;② 指神形疾病。

heart gale Refers to ① either the activity of consciousness;② or physical and spiritual diseases.

心悸【xīn jì】 气功适应证,指患者自觉心中悸动,惊惕不安。

palpitation An indication of Qigong, refers to patient's feeling of throb or fearful intranquility.

心经【xīn jīng】 指通过气功习练,达到"常乐我净"的精神境界。

Heart sutra Refers to the state of happiness and quietness in practicing Qigong.

心经导引法【xīn jīng dǎo yǐn fǎ】 为静功,闲居静坐,两目垂帘,安定神志,调节呼吸,精神内守,降心火于丹田。

exercise of Daoyin for the heart meridian A static exercise, marked by sitting quietly, closing the eyes, tranquilizing the mind, regulating respiration, keeping the spirit inside and descending heart fire to the Dantian. Dantian is divided into the upper Dantian (the region between the eyes), the middle Dantian (the region below the heart) and the lower Dantian (the region below the navel).

心静【xīn jìng】 指思维活动减少到静

止的状态。

heart quietness Refers to thinking activity tending to tranquil state.

心静可通神明【xīn jìng kě tōng shén míng】 指心静无杂念,阴阳平衡,可康健无病。

heart tranquility ensuring mental activity Refers to no distracting thought and balance of Yin and Yang, effective for cultivating health and relieving any disorders.

心境【xīn jìng】 指精神意识,认为静默作功,可以调节意识活动。

heart state Refers to spirit and consciousness, indicating that quietness in practicing Qigong can regulate consciousness activity.

心镜【xīn jìng】 ① 指习练气功,精神明净如镜,能提高智慧,认识事物;② 泛指精神活动。

heart mirror Refers to ① either quietness of the spirit like a mirror in practicing Qigong which can improve wisdom and knowledge; ② or the spirit activity.

心镜通【xīn jìng tōng】 指习练气功出现的潜能。

heart enlightenment Indicates the potency of Qigong practice.

心君【xīn jūn】 意识、念头。

heart monarch Refers to consciousness and thought.

心空【xīn kōng】 指情性广远,可容万物。

Heart vacuum Refers to broad mentalism that can contain anything.

心灵【xīn líng】 ① 指意识、精神、思维;② 指心;③ 指思想情感。

heart soul Refers to ① consciousness, spirit and thought; ② or the heart;

③ or emotional thought.

心马【xīn mǎ】 指精神躁动不安,喻气功中不能入静。

cardiac horse Refers to restlessness of the spirit, indicating failure to tranquilize the mind in practicing Qigong.

心目【xīn mù】 心指意识,目指眼识,泛指精神活动。

heart and eyes Refers to consciousness and ocular observation, indicating the spiritual activities.

心念【xīn niàn】 指意念,意念专一而静,才能排除杂念,灭除烦恼。

heart idea Refers to thought. Only when thought is tranquilized can distracting thought be removed and annoyance be eliminated.

心念病处【xīn niàn bìng chù】 指意识活动集中于疾病所患之部位,然后运气以攻之。

heart activity focusing diseases Refers to concentration of consciousness activity on the location of diseases which is attacked by movement of Qi.

心平德和【xīn píng dé hé】 指精神意识平和稳定。

cardiac peace and moral harmony Refers to mildness and stability of the spirit and consciousness.

心气【xīn qì】 ① 指心的功能作用;② 指心系神形疾病。

heart Qi Refers to ① either the function of the heart; ② or the physical and spiritual disorders.

心若驰散,即便摄来【xīn ruò chí sàn jí biàn shè lái】 指习练气功时,一有杂念,即便排除,守神于内。

taking measures to relieve dispersion from the heart Refers to elimination of distracting thought in practicing Qigong in order to keep the spirit inside the body.

心神【xīn shén】 ① 指心含藏精神；② 指心之神；③ 指意念活动。

heart spirit Refers to ① either the essence and the spirit contained in the heart；② or the spirit in the heart；③ or activity of consciousness.

心神去【xīn shén qù】 指心神损伤于神散失唇见青白。

loss of the heart spirit Refers to the fact that the spirit in the heart is damaged by loss of the spirit and change of the lips.

心术【xīn shù】 ① 指调节精神的方法；② 指心的功能。

heart technique Refers to ① either the method to regulate the spirit；② or the function of the heart.

心死【xīn sǐ】 ① 指意志消沉到极点；② 指排除杂念。

cardiac death Refers to ① either extreme depression of will；② or elimination of distracting thought.

心死性废【xīn sǐ xìng fèi】 指习练气功，意识思维活动相对静止，形体放松。

quiet heart and stable property Refers to the tranquil activities of consciousness and thought as well as relaxation of the body.

心随转法【xīn suí zhuǎn fǎ】 为静功，指盘膝坐式行功，呼吸自然平顺。

formula for regulating the heart A static exercise，marked by sitting and crossing the knees with natural respiration.

心所【xīn suǒ】 指心王而起的精神意识思维活动。

heart holder Refers to activities of the spirit，consciousness and thought controlled by the heart king.

心体寂静【xīn tǐ jì jìng】 指神形放松，协调合一。

quietness and harmony of the heart and body heart and body refers to relaxation and integration of the spirit and the body.

心体圆融【xīn tǐ yuán róng】 心指的是神，体指的是形，指神形和合为一，融为一体。

integration of the heart and body Refers to integration of the spirit and the body. In this term，the heart refers to the spirit.

心田【xīn tián】 指意识活动。

cardiac field Refers to the activity of consciousness.

心痛【xīn tòng】 ① 指心病出现的症状；② 泛指胸部、上腹部胆、胃疾病出现的症状；③ 指病名，如真心痛。

heart pain Refers to ① either symptoms of heart disease；② or symptoms of gallbladder and stomach diseases；③ or true heart pain.

心王【xīn wáng】 ① 指精神作用的元首；② 指心。

cardiac king Refers to ① either the ruler of the spirit；② or the heart.

心忘【xīn wàng】 指意识思维活动的相对静止。

heart forgetting Refers to relative and static activities of consciousness and thinking.

心无所住法【xīn wú suǒ zhù fǎ】 为静功，指自然坐势或盘膝坐势，呼吸自然而然。

free formula for the heart A static exercise，marked by sitting naturally or sitting with crossed knees with natural respiration.

心息相依【xīn xī xiāng yī】 指意识与

呼吸结合,以意领气,用气摄神,交相作用。

interdependence of the heart and respiration Refers to combination of consciousness and respiration characterized by consciousness taking Qi and Qi controlling the spirit.

心系【xīn xì】 ① 指心与各脏相连的组织;② 指与肺相连的组织。

heart system Refers to ① either the system of the heart with other Zang-organs (including the heart, the liver, the spleen, the lung and the kidney); ② or the system of the heart with the lung.

心想欲事,恶邪大起【xīn xiǎng yù shì è xié dà qǐ】 指人的欲念无穷会极大地耗损元气精血,造成严重病变。

excessive desires triggering evils Refers to the fact that excessive desires may damage original Qi and essential blood, causing serious diseases.

心晓根基养华采【xīn xiǎo gēn jī yǎng huá cǎi】 指补脑安神,和调意识思维,神形合一。

foundation of the heart promoting life cultivation Refers to tonifying the brain, stabilizing the spirit, harmonizing consciousness and thought, and integrating the spirit and the body.

心邪【xīn xié】 指不正常的精神活动。

heart evil Refers to abnormal activity of the spirit.

心心【xīn xīn】 指形神合一,喻行功中,阴平阳秘,协调平衡。

heart and heart Refer to integration of the body and spirit, indicating that Yin is stable while yang is compact in practicing Qigong.

心性【xīn xìng】 ① 指思维意识活动;

② 指不变的心体;③ 指静寂、和平。

heart disposition Refers to ① the activities of thought and consciousness; ② or natural property without any changes; ③ or quietness and peace.

心虚【xīn xū】 ① 指精神静谧、安泰;② 指理亏。

heart deficiency Refers to ① either tranquility and quietness; ② or wrongness.

心虚而神一【xīn xū ér shén yī】 指脑神虚静,则意识活动专一而不杂。

quietness of the heart and tranquility of the spirit Refers to tranquility of the spirit in the brain with quiet activity of consciousness.

心学【xīn xué】 指宋明理学的一个流派,以人心宇宙为本体,常应用气功知识,论述哲学问题。

heart philosophy Refers to a school of neo-confucianism of the Song Dynasty (960 AD‐1279 AD) and Ming Dynasty (1368 AD‐1644 AD) that took the human heart and the universe as noumenon and analyzed philosophy according to the knowledge of Qigong.

心眼【xīn yǎn】 指认识、思维活动。

heart eye Refers to knowledge and activity of thought.

心一境性【xīn yī jìng xìng】 指精神意识活动集中于一点、一片、一个景物,或身体的某一部位。

heart concentration Refers to concentration of the spirit and consciousness activity on one point, one field, one state, or one part of the body.

心意【xīn yì】 指精神活动平和安适,神形协调自然。

heart consciousness Refers to peaceful and quiet activity of the spirit with nat-

X

ural coordination.

心印【xīn yìn**】** 指用心体验。

heart feeling Refers to experience with the heart.

心俞【xīn yú**】** 足太阳膀胱经的一个穴位,位第五胸椎棘突下旁开1.5寸处。这一穴位为气功运行的一个常见部位。

Xinshu（BL 15） An acupoint in the gallbladder meridian of foot Taiyang, located in 1.5 Cun below the thoracic vertebral furcella. This acupoint is a region usually used for keeping the essential Qi in practice of Qigong.

心猿【xīn yuán**】** 指人的精神意识活动躁动浮游,如猿动而不止。

heart ape Refers to restlessness of the spirit and consciousness activities, like an ape that is running all the way.

心源【xīn yuán**】** 指心及心神,亦指脑神。

heart origin Refers to either the heart and the heart spirit, or the brain spirit.

心在灵关身有主,气归元海寿无穷
【xīn zài líng guān shēn yǒu zhǔ qì guī yuán hǎi shòu wú qióng**】** 指神不外驰,元气不耗散,是健康长寿的关键。

When the heart is in the spiritual custom, there is a king in the body; when Qi enters the original sea, life is prolonged. Refers to the fact the only when the spirit is not dispersed can the original Qi not be dissipated, which is the key for cultivating health and prolonging life.

心脏导引法【xīn zàng dǎo yǐn fǎ**】** 为动功,以两手作拳用力,左右互相筑;又可正坐,以一手按膝上,一手向上托空如重石。

exercise of Daoyin for the heart A dynamic exercise, marked by boxing both hands forcefully to stretch the left and the right; or sitting upright with one hand pressing the knee and the other hand holding up like a heavy stone.

心斋法【xīn zhāi fǎ**】** 指精神集中,返听内视,功效在于稳定精神,调节神形。

heart dhyana Refers to concentration of the spirit, self-listening and internal observation in order to stabilize the spirit and regulate the spirit and the body.

心症治法【xīn zhèng zhì fǎ**】** 动静相兼功,指凡心虚疼痛,静坐,擦两手安膝,用意在中,右视左提、左视右提,各十二次。

treatment of heart disease An exercise combined with dynamic exercise and static exercise, marked by sitting quietly when the heart is weak and painful, characterized by rubbing hands, pressing the knees, concentrating consciousness on the center, viewing the right and enhancing the left as well as viewing the left and enhancing the right for twelve times.

心枝【xīn zhī**】** 指精神意识之外,又派生出意念。

heart branch Refers to derivate idea beyond the spirit and consciousness.

心止于符【xīn zhǐ yú fú**】** 指神气合一的境界。

concentration of the heart on the spirit Refers to the state characterized by integration of the spirit and Qi.

心咒【xīn zhòu**】** 指说念口诀。如默念"紫气东来"或"我一定能恢复健康"。专一定志,以稳定情绪。

heart reading Refers to reading rhymes, such as "The purple air comes from the east" and "I will certainly recuperate health". Reading rhymes can stabilize the will and emotion.

心珠【xīn zhū**】** 指人的精神气质明洁如珠。

heart pearl Refers to the quality of the spirit as pure as the pearl.

心主【xīn zhǔ**】** 指手厥阴心包经。

heart master Refers to the pericardium meridian of hand Jueyin.

心主神明【xīn zhǔ shén míng**】** 指脑主意识思维活动,故有头为身之元首。

heart governing mental activities Refers to the activities of consciousness and thought governed by the brain. That is why the head is known as the king of the body.

心专不横【xīn zhuān bù hèng**】** 指习练气功,意识专注于一境,但又不能僵硬、放纵。

heart concentration without confrontation Refers to concentration of consciousness on one state without any stiffness and indulgence in practicing Qigong.

心传述证录【xīn zhuàn shù zhèng lù**】** 《心传述证录》为气功专著,清代蒋日纶著,主要辑养生炼气之功图二十余幅。

Xin Zhuanshu Zhenglu(*Collection of Demonstratoin and Discussion about Heart Inheritance*) A monograph of Qigong entitled *Collection of Demonstratoin and Discussion about Heart Inheritance*, written by Jiang Yuelun in the Qing Dynasty(1636 AD – 1912 AD), mainly compiling twenty pictures about practice of Qigong for nourishing the body.

心作主【xīn zuò zhǔ**】** 指脑的精神意识作主。

heart domination Refers to decision made by the spirit and consciousness in the brain.

辛金之脏【xīn jīn zhī zāng**】** 指肺脏。

metal viscus Refers to the lung.

刑德【xíng dé**】** 为独立的两个方面。刑为降,德为升;刑为罚,德为育。

Xing and De Refers to two independent sides, in which Xing means descent and punishment, De means ascent and education.

刑德并会【xíng dé bìng huì**】** 指阴阳相会,交合作用,而处于相对稳定状态。

combination of Xing and De Refers to combination and integration of Yin and Yang for stabilizing all parts of the body. In this term, Xing means descent and punishment, De means ascent and education.

行【xíng**】** 佛家气功习用语,① 指神形活动;② 指精神思维活动;③ 指进行气功实践。

motion A term of Qigong, referring to ① either the activities of the spirit and the body; ② or the activities of the spirit and consciousness; ③ or the practice of Qigong.

行痹【xíng bì**】** 即风痹,为气功适应证,指肌肉、筋骨、关节酸痛,痛处游走不定,关节屈伸不利。

wind impediment An indication of Qigong, referring to aching pain of muscles, sinews, bones and joints that causes wandering pain and inflexibility of joints.

行不欲离于世,举不欲观于俗【xíng bù yù lí yú shì jǔ bù yù guān yú sú**】** 指举止言行符合道德规范,不离开社会的一般准则。

Any activity should not be aloof from the world and any behavior should not pay attention to mortal life. Refers to the fact that any words, deeds and manners must fit in with ethics and must follow the general principles of this world.

行禅法【xíng chán fǎ**】** 为动功,行时气和心定,或往或来,时行时止,行时眼注视于丹田。

dhyana exercise A dynamic exercise, marked by balancing Qi and stabilizing the heart, or acting to and fro, or sometimes doing and sometimes stopping in practicing Qigong. In practicing, the eyes can focus on Dantian. Dantian is divided into the upper Dantian (the region between the eyes), the middle Dantian (the region below the heart) and the lower Dantian (the region below the navel).

行大道,常度日月星辰【xíng dà dào cháng dù rì yuè xīng chén**】** 即做重要的导引,上乘功法,要常存想日月星辰。

To walk along the great way must follow the sun, the moon and the stars. Refers to practicing Daoyin with the methods of Buddhism and contemplation of the sun, the moon and the stars.

行动【xíng dòng**】** 源自气功专论,阐述了习练气功的一些方法及感受。

action Collected from a monograph of Qigong, mainly describing the methods and experiences of Qigong practice.

行端直【xíng duān zhí**】** 指道德端方,行为正直。

behaving properly Refers to moral and correct aspects. That means to be honest in doing anything, especially in practicing Qigong.

行禁戒【xíng jìn jiè**】** 指行功期间,不符合气功规则的言行,就不说不做。

following disciplines Refers to the fact

that the words and deeds unconfirmed to the principles of Qigong should not be said or done during the procedure of Qigong practice.

行利【xíng lì**】** 即处理痢疾,习练气功之前习练者可能有大便稀溏的问题,故称为行利。

dealing with dysentery Refers to relieving dysentery in practicing Qigong. Before practicing Qigong, some practitioners may suffer from sloppy stool.

行气【xíng qì**】** 指呼吸吐纳,调息均匀细微。

respiration Refers to respiration with exhalation of the old and inhalation of the new as well as well-distributed and fine regulation of breath.

行气法【xíng qì fǎ**】** 为静功。其作法为,常以鸡鸣生气时,正值卧,握固,两足间相去五寸,两臂去体,相去亦各五寸。

method for circulating Qi A static exercise, usually marked by lying on bed when cocks begin to crow, holding the fists, during which two feet separate from each other in about 5 Cun, and two shoulders keep aloof from the body in about 5 Cun.

行气绝谷景象【xíng qì jué gǔ jǐng xiàng**】** 源自气功专论,阐述行气绝谷术后的人体变化情况。

scene of Qi circulation without any grain Collected from a monograph about Qigong, mainly describing the changes of human body after circulating Qi without taking any food.

行气须知【xíng qì xū zhī**】** 源自气功专论,主要阐述行气时的注意事宜。

attention to circulation of Qi Collected from a monograph about Qigong, mainly describing matters needing attention in circulating Qi.

行气宜思精【xíng qì yí sī jīng**】** 源自气功专论,主要阐述行气法的宜忌。

necessity to think essence in circulating Qi Collected from a monograph about Qigong, mainly describing suitability and avoidance in practicing Qigong.

行气玉佩铭【xíng qì yù pèi míng**】**《行气玉佩铭》为气功专论,问世于战国时期,主要阐述小周天功的作法和行功时的注意事项。作者不详。

Xingqi Yupei Ming(*Inscription of Qi Circulation with Jade Pendant*) A monograph of Qigong entitled *Inscription of Qi Circulation with Jade Pendant*, written in the Warring States Period, mainly describing matters needing attention in practice related to the small celestial circle. The author was unknown.

行气主【xíng qì zhǔ**】** 指目。

host of Qi circulation Refers to the eyes.

行如盲无杖【xíng rú máng wú zhàng**】** 即行走时要如盲人无杖而行,抬脚低,速度慢,步步踏实。

walking like blind person without cane Indicates practitioners of Qigong walking like blind persons without any cane, lowly lifting the feet and slowly taking a step forward in order to make every step steady.

行庭法【xíng tíng fǎ**】** 为静功,取自然坐式,或盘膝坐式。然后鼻引清气入,意念导引下入丹田,然后再引气到背,意念活动集中于背,然后沿督脉,意引气行背十数回,随即引气入丹田。

courtyard sitting exercise Courtyard sitting exercise is a static exercise, marked by natural sitting or sitting with crossed legs. During this practice, clear Qi can be inhaled through the nose inside Dantian with consciousness. Then the clear Qi can be transmitted to the back. At the same time the activity of consciousness is concentrated on the back. Under such a condition, the clear Qi is again transmitted to the back from the governor meridian for about ten times and finally transmitted to Dantian. Dantian is divided into the upper Dantian (the region between the eyes), the middle Dantian (the region below the heart) and the lower Dantian (the region below the navel).

行位三道【xíng wèi sān dào**】** 佛家气功习用语,指习练见道、修道、无学道。见道指应用"空观",稳定情绪,消除烦恼。修道指理解认识道理,并行之实践。无学道指学习佛家气功戒、定、慧三法,断自然与社会的烦恼,以实现精神世界的理想境界。

three ways to know Daoism A common term of Qigong in Buddhism, referring to refining perspective of Dao, practicing Dao and avoidance of studying Dao. Perspective of Dao refers to stabilizing the mind and eliminating annoyance in order to cultivate health. Practicing Dao refers to understanding the knowledge and the principles in order to well practice. Avoidance of studying Dao refers to relieving social and natural annoyance when studying the methods of Qigong in Buddhism.

行五行气法【xíng wǔ xíng qì fǎ**】** 为静功,春季巳时,食气一百二十次,致气于心,令心胜肺,无令肺伤肝;夏季未时,食气一百二十次,以助脾令胜肾,使肾不伤心;季夏申时,食气一百二十次,以助肺令胜肝，使肝不伤脾；秋季亥时，食气一百二十次，以助肾令胜心，使心不伤肺；冬季寅时，食气一百二十次，以助肝令胜脾，使脾不伤肾。

exercise of for circulating Qi from the five elements（including wood，fire，earth，metal and water） A static exercise，marked by inhaling Qi for one hundred and twenty times in Shi（the period of a day from 9 a. m. to 11 a. m. in the morning）in the days of spring，transmitting Qi to the heart in order to enable the heart superior to the lung and prevent the lung to injure the liver；inhaling Qi for one hundred and twenty times in Wei（the period of a day from 1 p. m. to 3 p. m. in the afternoon）in the days of summer，helping the spleen to be superior to the kidney and preventing the kidney to injure the heart；inhaling Qi for one hundred and twenty times in Shen（the period of a day from 3 p. m. to 5 p. m. in the afternoon）in the days of late summer，helping the lung to be superior to the liver and preventing the liver to injure the spleen；inhaling Qi for one hundred and twenty times in Hai（the period of a day from 9 p. m. to 11 p. m. in the evening）in the days of autumn，helping the kidney to be superior to the heart and preventing the heart to injure the lung；inhaling Qi for one hundred and twenty times in Yin（the period of a day from 3 a. m. to 5 a. m. in the early morning）in the days of winter，helping the liver to be superior to the spleen and preventing the spleen to injure the kidney.

行与神俱【xíng yǔ shén jù】 指形体与精神和谐，整个生命力旺盛。

harmonized body and spirit Refers to harmony of the body and the spirit as well as vigorous vitality.

行圆【xíng yuán】 指行"一心三观"。

active cycle Refers to one mind with three visions.

形骸【xíng hái】 指人的形体。

physical skeleton Actually refers to the human body.

形气【xíng qì】 即人之身体及功能活动。

physical Qi Refers to functional activity of the human body.

形神【xíng shén】 ① 指神为生命的主宰；② 指神由气生；③ 指神形不相离，相互为用；④ 指神形相离则死；⑤ 指气功养生以养神为主；⑥ 指气功的作用是使神形表里既济；⑦ 指习练气功即是调节神形，神形合一是气功的理想境界。

body and spirit Refers to ① either the fact that the spirit controls life；② or that the spirit is produced by Qi；③ or that the body and the spirit cannot seperate from either other；④ or that the spirit and body will be destroyed if they are separated from either other；⑤ or that practice of Qigong mainly nourishes the spirit；⑥ or that the effect of Qigong enables the spirit and body to depend on each other；⑦ or that practice of Qigong is to regulate the spirit and the body and the ideal effect of Qigong is to integrate the spirit and body.

形神俱妙【xíng shén jù miào】 指形神合一而具的妙趣。

miraculous integration of the body and the spirit Refers to the interest of the harmonization and integration of the body and the spirit.

形神乃全【xíng shén nǎi quán】　指神形协调,功用齐全。

coordination of the body and spirit　Refers to regulation of the body and spirit with complete functions.

形神相亲【xíng shén xiāng qīn】　指形神相互作用而合一。

blind date of the body and spirit　Refers to interactional function and integration of the body and the spirit.

性【xìng】　佛家气功习用语,指精神意识思维,亦指精神活动的稳定。

nature　A common term of Qigong in Buddhism, referring to either the spirit, consciousness and thought; or stability of the spirit activity.

性根命蒂【xìng gēn mìng dì】　性即神,性根即神根,神根即脑;命即气,命蒂即气蒂,气蒂即脐。亦指丹田。

root of nature and pedicle of life　In this term, nature refers to the spirit, the root of nature refers to the root of the spirit and the root of the spirit refers to the brain; life refers to Qi, pedicle of life refers to pedicle of Qi and pedicle of Qi refers to the navel. Root of nature and pedicle of life also refers to Dantian. Dantian is divided into the upper Dantian (the region between the eyes), the middle Dantian (the region below the heart) and the lower Dantian (the region below the navel).

性功【xìng gōng】　指调节精神意识活动为主的功法。

mental exercise　Refers to the exercise of Qigong for regulating the activities of the spirit and consciousness.

性汞命铅【xìng gǒng mìng qiān】　喻阴阳两神气方面,为炼金丹大药的基本

物质。在这个术语中,性为神,汞即阳;命为气,铅即阴。

nature with lead and life with mercury　Refers to the fields of the spirit and Qi in Yin and Yang, which is the basic foundation for refining golden Dan (pills of immortality) and great medicinal. In this term, nature refers to the spirit and mercury refers to Yang while life refers to Qi and lead refers to Yin.

性海【xìng hǎi】　① 指心及心神;② 亦指脑神。

nature and sea　Refers to ① either the heart and the heart spirit; ② or the brain spirit.

性空子胎息诀【xìng kōng zǐ tāi xī jué】　静功口诀,指人体本性。

formula of vacuum respiration　Formula of vacuum respiration is a static exercise, referring to the natural root of human body.

性命【xìng mìng】　① 指意识活动,其中性为神,命为气;② 指性为先天,命为后天;③ 指生命;④ 指气功,性为性功,命为命功。

nature and life　Refers to ① either consciousness activity, in which nature refers to the spirit and life refers to Qi; ② or another exercise of Qigong practice, in which nature refers to the innate and life refers to the postnatal; ③ or life; ④ or Qigong practice, in which nature refers to nature exercise and life refers to life exercise.

性命圭旨全书【xìng mìng guī zhǐ quán shū】　《性命圭旨全书》为气功专著,明代以来较有影响的理论与实践相结合的气功学著作,作者不详。

Xingming Guizhi Quanshu（*A Pandect

about Imperial Edict of Nature and Life) A monograph of Qigong entitled *A Pandect about Imperial Edict of Nature and Life*, which is an impressive monograph about the theory and practice of Qigong since the Ming Dynasty (1368 AD－1644 AD). The author was unknown.

性命合一【xìng mìng hé yī】 指意识思维活动与呼吸之气合而为一,亦谓神气合一。

integration of nature and life Refers to either combination of the consciousness and thought with Qi in respiration; or combination of the spirit and Qi.

性命混融【xìng mìng hùn róng】 指习练气功进入理想境界时,神气合而为一,融为一体。

integration of nature and life Refers to reaching the ideal state in practicing Qigong. In this ideal state, the spirit and Qi are integrated fused into one.

性命双修【xìng mìng shuāng xiū】 性指性功,即以炼神为主的功法;命指命功,即以炼精气为主的功法。

double cultivation of nature and life In this term, nature refers to nature exercise for refining the spirit, life refers to life exercise for refining the essence.

性命双修之道【xìng mìng shuāng xiū zhī dào】 源自气功专论,主要阐述修炼精、气、神并使之合三为一之理。

the way for double cultivation of nature and life Collected from a monograph of Qigong, mainly describing cultivation and integration of the essence, Qi and the spirit.

性命说【xìng mìng shuō】 源自气功专论,阐述性命的含义及其相互关系。

idea about life Collected from a monograph of Qigong, mainly describing the meaning of life and interrelation.

性命圆通【xìng mìng yuán tōng】 指神气和合为一。其中性为神,命为气。

accommodation of nature and life Refers to integration of the spirit and Qi. In this term, nature refers to the spirit and life refers to Qi.

性命之本【xìng mìng zhī běn】 指神。

origin of life Refers to the spirit.

性潜于顶,命归于脐【xìng qián yú dǐng mìng guī yú qí】 顶为脑,指精神意识思维活动藏于脑;脐即腹,指呼吸自然太和之下沉坤腹。

Nature hides in the top and life returns to the navel. The top refers to the brain, indicating the storage of the activities of the spirit, consciousness and thought in the brain; the navel refers to the abdomen, indicating respiration naturally deepening into the abdomen.

性情【xìng qíng】 ① 指人的本性及其向外的反应;② 指人的禀赋及气质。

human characteristics Refers to either the nature and external response of human beings; or the gift and temperament.

性情合【xìng qíng hé】 即金木并而魂魄协调之意。其中金为性,木为情。

combination of nature and feeling Refers to combination of metal and wood as well as regulation of the ethereal soul and corporeal soul. In this term, nature refers to metal and feeling refers to wood according to the five elements (including wood, fire, earth, metal and water).

性天【xìng tiān】 ① 指人的自然本性;② 指性由天赋,得之自然。

celestial nature Refers to either the

natural humanity; or innate nature.

性天风月通玄记【xìng tiān fēng yuè tōng xuán jì】《性天风月通玄记》为气功专著,由明代兰茂所著,专论气功的基本理论及具体功法。

Xingtian Fengyue Tongxuan Ji (*Thoroughfare and Supreme Record of Scenery of Celestial Nature*) A monograph of Qigong entitled *Thoroughfare and Supreme Record of Scenery of Celestial Nature*, written by Lan Mao in the Ming Dynasty (1368 AD - 1644 AD), mainly describing the basic theory and actual practice of Qigong.

性在泥丸命在脐 【xìng zài ní wán mìng zài qí】 即调节意识思维活动。

Nature is in the brain and life is in the navel. Refers to regulating the activities of consciousness and thought.

性真纯静【xìng zhēn chún jìng】 指习练气功,耳逐声而不闻,目逐色而不见,意识稳定而不思,神形协调安适,不受外界之干扰。

genuine nature with pure tranquility Refers to practice of Qigong marked by listening nothing with the ears, seeing nothing with the eyes, stabilizing the consciousness without any contemplation, coordinating the spirit and body, and avoiding disturbance of the external world.

性之根【xìng zhī gēn】 指头顶。

root of nature Refers to the top of the head.

性质【xìng zhì】 指个性禀之于先天,即先天因素。

individuality Refers to innate humanity.

性宗【xìng zōng】 指以炼神为主的气功流派。

nature school Refers to the school for refining the spirit in practicing Qigong.

胸痹【xiōng bì】 气功适应证,指胸部闷痛,甚则胸痛彻背,短气,喘息不得卧为主要症状的疾病。

chest impediment An indication of Qigong, referring to stuffy pain or the disease with the symptoms of chest and back pain, shortness of breath and inability to sleep due to panting.

胸膈气症治法【xiōng gé qì zhèng zhì fǎ】 为动功。其作法为,凡胸膈痞闷,八字立定,将手向内相叉,由胸前往下擦十二次,闭气一口,再擦十二次,共三五遍。然后用左右手上下伸十二次,双拳相交,轻捶臂肩各十数次,调咽一口,轻呵一口,叩齿一遍止。

treatment of disorder in chest and diaphragm A dynamic exercise, marked by standing up with silent reading eight Chinese characters when there is fullness and oppression in the chest and diaphragm; crossing the hands internally to rub from the chest and the abdomen for twelve times; stopping breath for a while, and rubbing again for twelve times, altogether for three or five times; then stretching the hands from the left to the right and from the upper to the lower and vice versa for twelve times respectively; crossing the fists to mildly thump the shoulders for dozens of times; regulating swallow for a while, mildly breathing out for a while and clicking the teeth for a while.

胸堂穴【xiōng táng xué】 膻中的另外一个称谓,是人体的穴位,在前正中线上,两乳头连线的中点。此穴位为气功习练之处。

Xiongtangxue A synonym of Danzhong

X

(CV 17)，an acupoint located in the front midline between the breasts. This acupoint is a region usually used in practice of Qigong.

雄金【xióng jīn】　指阳火，为阴中之阳。

grand metal　Refers to Yang fire, indicating Yang within Yin.

雄里藏雌【xióng lǐ cáng cí】　指阴阳两个方面，亦谓阳中有阴。

woman within man　Refers to either Yin and Yang; or Yin within Yang.

雄阳玄施【xióng yáng xuán shī】　为阳极阴生出现的微妙变化。

grand Yang and tiny change　Refers to tiny changes of extreme Yang and growing Yin.

熊经【xióng jīng】　为动功。其作法为，临睡时，将两手拘定两足，直伸其腰，头回顾后视，左右各七次，自无痰症。

bear imitating　A dynamic exercise, marked by holding the feet with both hands before sleeping, stretching the waist, turning the head to view backward from the left to the right and vice versa for seven times respectively. Such a dynamic exercise will cure phlegm syndrome.

熊经鸟申【xióng jīng niǎo shēn】　指熊攀援树木，鸟嚬呻阴气。

bear climbing and bird groaning　Indicates that the bear climbs up the tree and the bird groans Yin Qi.

熊戏【xióng xì】　为动功。其作法为，正仰，以两手抱膝下，举头，左僻地七，右亦七。蹲地，以手左右而托地。

bear playing　A dynamic exercise, marked by looking up, holding the regions below the knees with both hands, raising the hands, secluding the ground

from the left side and right side for seven times respectively, squatting on the ground, and pressing the ground with both hands from the left to the right and vice versa.

休粮【xiū liáng】　辟谷，即不食饮食。练功到一定程度出现不感饥饿，不进饮食而精神不减，身体轻快而无不适。

stopping diet　Refers to the marvel in practicing Qigong, characterized by no hunger in practicing Qigong to a certain level. Although food is not taken in practicing Qigong, the spirit is still energetic and the body is still brisk.

修【xiū】　泛指学习研究气功养生法。

cultivation　Refers to studying and researching the exercise of Qigong and life cultivation.

修存补脑法【xiū cún bǔ nǎo fǎ】　为静功。其作法为，凡胎息气者，先叩齿三十六通，集诸神然后转颈一次。其胎息已，咽之，如此三通。其功效为补脑，润五脏，通经活络，滋助正气，预防疾病。

exercise for cultivating existence and tonifying the brain　A static exercise, marked by clicking the teeth for thirty-six times during fetal respiration, concentrating various spirits and turning to the neck, and swallowing for three times if fetal respiration is finished. Such a static exercise can tonify the brain, moisten the five Zang-organs (including the heart, the liver, the spleen, the lung and the kidney), unblock the meridians and activate the collaterals, enrich healthy Qi and prevent diseases.

修存休粮法【xiū cún xiū liáng fǎ】　为静功。其作法为，每至食时，漱口，存想上元两条白气从脑中出，沿流项至背脊过，入于脐下气海中。

exercise for cultivating existence and ceasing meal A static exercise, marked by rinsing the mouth when taking food, imagining two kinds of white Qi from the brain flowing along the neck to the spine and entering the sea of Qi below the navel.

修存咽气法【xiū cún yàn qì fǎ**】** 为静功。其作法为，每日夜半之后，五更睡觉之初，先以舌漱掠唇齿之间，咽下津液，吐出浊气三口，鼻收清凉气入于胸膈之中，淘隔宿来秽滞之气，呵出三口。

exercise for cultivating existence and swallowing Qi A static exercise, marked by rinsing the tongue between the lips and teeth after midnight and before dawn, swallowing fluid and humor, vomiting turbid Qi for three times, inhaling clear Qi through the nose into the chest and diaphragm and vomiting filthy Qi for three times.

修道【xiū dào**】** ① 指学习道家学问，或躬身实践道法；② 为佛家气功学习用语，指理解认识真理，并行之实践；③ 指教育；④ 指习练气功。

cultivation according to Dao Refers to either ① studying the theory of Dao or practicing the exercise of Daoism; ② or the common term of Qigong in Buddhism, referring to understanding the truth and putting into practice; ③ or education; ④ or practice of Qigong.

修短寿夭，皆自人为【xiū duǎn shòu yāo jiē zì rén wéi**】** 指人的健康、疾病、寿命、夭亡，都是由人的本身所决定的。

Longevity or ephemerality after short time of cultivation depend self-behavior. Indicates that health, disease, longevi-ty and ephemerality are all related to oneself body.

修昆仑【xiū kūn lún**】** 即补脑。

cultivating the Kunlun (the brain) Re-fers to nourishing the brain. In this term, Kunlun refers to the brain.

修昆仑法【xiū kūn lún fǎ**】** 为动功，"发宜多梳，齿宜多叩，液宜常咽，气宜清炼，手宜在面，此为修昆仑之法"。

exercise for cultivating Kunlun (brain) A dynamic exercise, marked by repeat-edly combing hair, clicking the teeth, swallowing humor, refining Qi and rubbing the face with hands. This is the way to cultivate the brain.

修昆仑真诀【xiū kūn lún zhēn jué**】** 源自气功专论，主要阐述修昆仑真诀是常养元神。

genuine formula for cultivating Kunlun (the brain) Collected from a mono-graph of Qigong, mainly describing the fact that to cultivate the brain is actual-ly to nourish the original spirit.

修炼待时说【xiū liàn dài shí shuō**】** 源自气功专论，讨论了炼丹的择时问题。

idea about how to cultivate and prac-tice Collected from a monograph of Qigong, discussing the issues of alche-my.

修炼须知【xiū liàn xū zhī**】** 《修炼须知》为气功学专著，内容介绍了练功中需要知道的七个方面。作者不详。

***Xiulian Xuzhi**(**Announcement of Culti-vation and Practice**)* A monograph of Qigong entitled *Announcement of Cul-tivation and Practice*, mainly introdu-cing seven aspects of Qigong practice. The author was unknown.

修龄要旨【xiū líng yào zhǐ**】** 《修龄要旨》为气功养生专著，由明代冷谦所著，论述起居调摄、四季却病、延年长生等导引法。

Xiuling Yaozhi（*Essentials for Cultivating Age*） A monograph of Qigong and life cultivation entitled *Essentials for Cultivating Age*, written by Leng Qian in the Ming Dynasty（1368 AD - 1644 AD）, describing the exercises for regulation of daily life, elimination of diseases in the four seasons and prolonging life.

修身【xiū shēn】 ① 指端正形神,提高智慧,富足知识;② 指修养精神,习练气功。

cultivating body Refers to ① either regularizing the body and the spirit, increasing wisdom and enriching knowledge; ② or cultivating the spirit and practicing Qigong.

修身法【xiū shēn fǎ】 为静功,即调身、调气、调神。其作法为,自然站立或正坐,调和呼吸,正心,安定精神,自然微合双目,排除杂念,意识活动独立于身体之中。

exercise for cultivating the body A static exercise for regulating the body, Qi and spirit, marked by natural standing up or sitting upright, regulating respiration, tranquilizing the heart, naturally and mildly closing the eyes, eliminating distracting thought and independently keeping the activity of consciousness in the body.

修身之道贵乎中和【xiū shēn zhī dào guì hū zhōng hé】 阐明气功养生保健最根本的道理在于调整人体阴阳及保存精神活动的平衡。

The important way for cultivating the body is concentration and harmony. Expounds that the basic way for practicing Qigong and cultivating life is to regulate Yin and Yang in the body and to balance the activity of the spirit.

修神【xiū shén】 即调节精神思维意识活动,为气功中习练的重要一环。

cultivating the spirit A term of Qigong, referring to regulating the activities of the spirit, thinking and consciousness, which is an important way to practice Qigong.

修天庭法【xiū tiān tíng fǎ】 为动功,其作法为,将两手掌擦热后,频频按摩额部。天庭指额部。

exercise for cultivating celestial hall A dynamic exercise, marked by repeatedly rubbing the forehead with both hands after rubbing the hands hot. In this term, the so-called celestial hall refers to the forehead.

修无为【xiū wú wéi】 指习练气功,调节意识思维活动,使之保持平和。

achieving harmony Refers to practice of Qigong in order to regulate the activities of consciousness and thinking and to keep balance.

修习止观坐禅法要【xiū xí zhǐ guān zuò chán fǎ yào】 《修习止观坐禅法要》为气功专论,由隋代智𫖮所撰,深刻地论述了气功的理论、方法、功效和要求。

Xiuxi Zhiguan Zuotan Fayao（*Essentials of Dhyana for Perfect Cultivation and Practice*） A monograph of Qigong entitled *Essentials of Dhyana for Perfect Cultivation and Practice*, written by Zhi Kai in the Sui Dynasty（581 AD - 618 AD）, discussing the theory, methods, effects and requirements of Qigong practice.

修心【xiū xīn】 指炼己,持心。

cultivating the heart　Refers to refining the body and concentrating the heart.

修心炼性【xiū xīn liàn xìng】　指习练气功,调节精神意识活动,涵养本性。

cultivating the heart to refine nature Refers to regulating the activities of the spirit and consciousness in order to well cultivate nature in practicing Qigong.

修心正行【xiū xīn zhèng xíng】　指调节精神活动,可以端正形体。

cultivating the heart to strengthen the body Means to regularize the body through regulating the activity of the spirit

修行【xiū xíng】　指按理修习作行,泛指习练气功。

improving practice Refers to improve activities according to the principles and rules, usually referring to practice of Qigong.

修行径路【xiū xíng jìng lù】　指气功功法。

cultivating pathway Refers to an exercise in practicing Qigong.

修性说【xiū xìng shuō】　源自气功专论,主要阐述修性的道理与方法。

idea about cultivating nature Collected from a monograph of Qigong, mainly describing the theory and methods for cultivating nature.

修性直指天元章【xiū xìng zhí zhǐ tiān yuán zhāng】　源自气功专论,主要阐述养神在练功中的重要性。

cultivating nature directly according to celestial original section Collected from a monograph of Qigong, mainly describing the importance of nourishing the spirit in practicing Qigong.

修羊公卧石榻【xiū yáng gōng wò shí tà】　为静功。其作法为,侧卧、屈膝、以两手擦热,一手握住生殖器及阴囊,另一手置于耳部,运气二十四口。主治四时外感、伤寒。

exercise of Yang Gong's sleeping on stone bed A static exercise, marked by lying on one side, bending the knees, rubbing the hands hot, holding the genital organ and scrotum with one hand, covering the aural region with the other hand and moving Qi for twenty-four times in order to treat external contraction and cold damage in the four seasons.

修养【xiū yǎng】　指内守精神,外养形体,延年益寿。

life cultivation Refers to internal concentration of the spirit, external cultivation of the body and prolonging life.

修养须知【xiū yǎng xū zhī】　《修养须知》为养生学专著,兼论气功,由清代朱本中所著,介绍了气功习练的具体方法。

Xiuyang Xuzhi(*Announcement of Cultivation and Nourishment*)　A monograph of life cultivation and Qigong entitled *Announcement of Cultivation and Nourishment*, written by Zhu Benzhong in the Qing Dynasty (1636 AD - 1912 AD), introducing the methods for practicing Qigong.

修养杂诀【xiū yǎng zá jué】　源自气功专论,阐述调神、炼气、导引、咽液的具体做法和功用。

formula for cultivating life Collected from a monograph of Qigong, mainly describing the methods and effects of regulating the spirit, refining Qi and Daoyin and swallowing humor.

修一却邪法【xiū yī què xié fǎ】　为静功。其作法为,端身正坐,意识思维活动稳定于顶,或目目,或脐,或气(呼吸),或心，或手足心，或脊，或肠胃，不使其分散。其功效为和调神形，调节脏腑功能，轻身延年。

exercise for cultivating core to eliminate distraction A static exercise, marked by sitting upright, concentrating the activities of consciousness and thinking on the top, or the eyes, or the navel, or Qi (respiration), or heart, or soles and palms, or spine, or intestines and stomach, avoiding dispersion of anything. Such a static exercise can harmonize the spirit and the body, regulate the functions of the five Zang-organs (including the heart, the liver, the spleen, the lung and the kidney) and the six Fu-organs (including the gallbladder, the stomach, the small intestine, the large intestine, the bladder and the triple energizer), relax the body and prolong life.

修真【xiū zhēn】① 指调养真性；② 指保养神气，使神气不散。

cultivating essence Refers to ① either regulating and cultivating genuine nature; ② or protecting and cultivating the spirit and Qi in order to avoid dispersion.

修真秘录【xiū zhēn mì lù】《修真秘录》为气功专著，由宋代符度仁编，介绍调食养气之术。

Xiuzhen Milu(*Secret Record of Cultivating Genuineness*) A monograph of Qigong entitled *Secret Record of Cultivating Genuineness*, compiled by Fu Duren in the Song Dynasty (960 AD - 1279 AD), introducing the techniques for regulating food and cultivating Qi.

修真秘要【xiū zhēn mì yào】《修真秘要》为养生气功专著，由明代王蔡所著，

论述了起居饮食等调养，深入研究了吐纳导引。

Xiuzhen Miyao(*Secret Record of Cultivating Genuineness*) A monograph of life cultivation and Qigong entitled *Secret Record of Cultivating Genuineness*, written by Wang Cai in the Ming Dynasty (1368 AD - 1644 AD), describing life cultivation with daily life and diet, and researching inhalation, exhalation and Daoyin.

修真十书【xiū zhēn shí shū】《修真十书》为气功学丛书，收集了隋唐两宋时期重要的气功学著作数十种。作者不详。

Xiuzhen Shishu(*Ten Books of Cultivating Genuineness*) A series of Qigong entitled *Ten Books of Cultivating Genuineness*, collected over ten books about Qigong from the Sui Dynasty (581 AD - 618 AD), Tang Dynasty (618 AD - 907 AD), North Song Dynasty (960 AD - 1127 AD) and South Song Dynasty (1127 AD - 1279 AD). The author was unknown.

修真太极混元图【xiū zhēn tài jí hùn yuán tú】《修真太极混元图》为气功专著，由宋代萧道存撰，以文解图，论述气功功法。

Xiuzhen Taiji Hunyuan Tu(*Repairing the Primeval Pictures of Genuine Supreme Pole*) A monograph of Qigong entitled *Repairing the Primeval Pictures of Genuine Supreme Pole*, written by Xiao Daocun in the Song Dynasty (960 AD - 1279 AD), explaining the pictures with characters and analyzing the exercises for Qigong practice.

修真太极混元指玄图【xiū zhēn tài jí hún yuán zhǐ xuán tú】《修真太极混元指玄图》为气功专著，以图为主，附有口

诀，论述气功的理论、方法、功效和要求。作者不详。

Xiuzhen Taiji Hunyuan Zhixuan Tu（*Supreme and Primeval Pictures for Repairing Genuine Supreme Pole*） A monograph of Qigong entitled *Supreme and Primeval Pictures for Repairing Genuine Supreme Pole*, discussing the theory, methods, effects and requirements of Qigong practice mainly according to pictures with certain pithy mnemonic formulae. The author was unknown.

修真旨要【xiū zhēn zhǐ yào】 《修真旨要》为气功养生专著，重点论述调神，认为精气神为人体三宝。作者与年代不详。

Xiuzhen Zhiyao（*Essentials of Cultivating Genuineness*） A monograph of Qigong and life cultivation entitled *Essentials of Cultivating Genuineness*, mainly describing regulation of the spirit and the three important elements（essence，Qi and spirit）in the human body. The author and the related dynasty were unknown.

修治城廓法【xiū zhì chéng kuò fǎ】 为动功。其作法为，端身正坐，用两于摩揉两耳郭，不拘遍数，摩时不用力，意念集中在耳廓上。

exercise for repairing enceinte A dynamic exercise，marked by sitting upright，rubbing the auricles with both hands for without any limit and strength，and concentrating consciousness in the auricle.

虚静【xū jìng】 指习练气功时，无思无念，意识思维活动处于相对静止的状态。

tranquil and peaceful activity Refers to no any thoughts and no any ideas，and comparatively tranquilized the activity of consciousness and thought in practicing Qigong.

虚静无为【xū jìng wú wéi】 指意识思维活动安静、不妄为，是习练气功获得成功的根本。

tranquility and inaction Refers to tranquilized activities of consciousness and thinking without any absurd action，which is the root for successful practice of Qigong.

虚空【xū kōng】 佛家气功习用语，指虚是无形质，空为无障碍。

deficiency and vacuum A term of Qigong. In this term，deficiency means no form of quality and vacuum means no obstacle.

虚空藏【xū kōng cáng】 祖窍的异名，指位于心与脐之正中。

deficiency and vacuum storage Another way to describe ancestral orifice，referring to the central region between the heart and the navel.

虚空界【xū kōng jiè】 佛家气功习用语，指宇宙无际。

deficiency and vacuum boundary A common term of Qigong in Buddhism，referring to universal vacuum.

虚空无为【xū kōng wú wéi】 佛家气功习用语，① 指宇宙自然，无边无际，永不变易；② 指真如即神形和谐的理想境界。

emptiness and inaction A common term of Qigong in Buddhism，indicating that ① the universe is natural without any limit and change；② or that integration of the spirit and body is the ideal state.

虚劳寒冷【xū láo hán lěng】 气功适应证，指因虚劳病致气血虚弱，阴阳不能维持正常状态(不平衡)，阳气偏衰，则内生寒冷之证。

consumptive disease with coldness An indication of Qigong, referring to deficiency of Qi and blood due to consumptive disease that causes imbalance of Yin and Yang, decline of Yang Qi and internal cold syndrome.

虚劳寒冷候导引法【xū láo hán lěng hòu dǎo yǐn fǎ**】** 为动功。其作法为,正坐,交叉两脚,手从脚弯中入,低头,两手交叉放在项上。温经通阳,增进听力。主治肢体久寒不温,耳聋。

exercise of Daoyin for consumptive disease with coldness A dynamic exercise, marked by sitting upright, crossing the feet, putting the hands from the soles, lowering the head, overlapping the hands and putting them on the neck for warming the meridians, dredging Yang and increasing listening ability. Such a dynamic exercise can cure chronic coldness and deafness.

虚劳候导引法【xū láo hòu dǎo yǐn fǎ**】** 为动静相兼功,方法多样。如早晨鸡叫时叩齿三十六遍,搅舌漱口,令津液满口时咽下,作三次。杀虫补虚,令人强壮。

exercise of Daoyin for consumptive disease An exercise combined with dynamic exercise and static exercise with various methods, such as clicking the teeth for thirty-six times in the early morning when the cock crows, agitating the tongue and rinsing the mouth, swallowing when the fluid and humor are enriched in the mouth for three times. Such an exercise combined with dynamic exercise and static exercise can kill worms to tonify deficiency and strengthen the body.

虚劳口干燥【xū láo kǒu gān zào**】** 气功适应证,由劳损血气,阴阳断隔,冷热不通,上焦生热令口干燥。

consumptive disease with dryness of the mouth An indication of Qigong, caused by overstrain and injury of the blood and Qi, separation of Yin and Yang due to coldness and heat, and heat increasing in the upper energizer that makes the mouth dry.

虚劳口干燥候导引法【xū láo kǒu gān zào hòu dǎo yǐn fǎ**】** 为静功。其作法为,向东而坐,仰头,闭气不息,至极限时慢慢吐出五遍,以舌在口中搅动,漱口满十四次,咽下。生津止渴,治口干口苦。

exercise of Daoyin for consumptive disease with dryness of the mouth A static exercise, marked by sitting to the east, raising the head, stopping respiration, slowly exhaling for five times when respiration is stopped to the extreme, gargling the mouth for fourteen times and swallowing saliva. Such a static exercise can produce fluid and stop cough as well as cure oral dryness and pain.

虚劳羸瘦【xū láo léi shòu**】** 气功适应证,指精髓萎竭,血气虚弱,不能充盈肌肤,故而造成羸瘦。

consumptive disease with emaciation An indication of Qigong, usually caused by exhaustion of essence and marrow, deficiency of the blood and Qi that fails to exuberate the skin.

虚劳羸瘦候养生方【xū láo léi shòu hòu yǎng shēng fāng**】** 为静功。其作法为,每日早晨,未起床时,用舌在口腔内搅动,作漱口状,待津液满口时咽下,叩齿十四次,如此三遍,名叫炼精。补虚损,使人强壮。

exercise of nourishing life for consumptive disease with emaciation A static exercise, marked by stirring the mouth like gargling with the tongue in the morning before getting up, swallowing it when fluid and humor are enriched, clicking the teeth for fourteen times. To practice in such a way for three times is called refining the essence. Such a static exercise can tonify deficiency and strengthen the body.

虚劳里急【xū láo lǐ jí】 气功适应证,指肾气内损,冲脉失于濡养,致腹部拘挛紧缩不舒。

consumptive disease with contraction of genitals An indication of Qigong, referring to internal injury of kidney Qi and failure of the thoroughfare meridian to nourish the body, which causes the abdomen contracted and bent.

虚劳里急候导引法【xū láo lǐ jí hòu dǎo yǐn fǎ】 动静相兼功,其作法为,仰卧,用口慢慢吸气,用鼻呼出。疏肝理气,缓挛急,治腹痛拘急。饱食后,小咽气九十次。温中散寒,治里寒证。用口吸气七十次,令气充满腹部,再小咽气几十次,然后,两手掌摩擦,到极热时,以手掌按摩腹部,使气下行。温中理气,治干呕腹痛。

exercise of Daoyin for consumptive disease with contraction of genitals An exercise combined with dynamic exercise and static exercise, marked by lying on the back, slowly inhaling Qi through the mouth, exhaling Qi through the nose, soothing the liver and regulating Qi, relieving spasm, mildly swallowing Qi for ninety times after taking food for warming the center, dispersing cold and curing cold syndrome; then inha-

ling Qi for seventy times through the mouth, enriching Qi in the abdomen, and slowly swallowing Qi for dozens of times; then rubbing the palms to become very hot, pressing and rubbing the abdomen with the palms to promote Qi flow downwards. Such an exercise combined with dynamic exercise and static exercise can warm the center, regulate Qi and cure retching and abdominal pain.

虚劳少气【xū láo shǎo qì】 气功适应证,指虚劳患者因肺气损伤,致呼吸微弱而不足之证。其病多为阳气不足所致。

consumptive disease with less Qi An indication of Qigong, referring to the syndrome pattern caused by damage of lung Qi that makes respiration feeble. Such a disease is usually caused by insufficiency of Yang Qi.

虚劳少气候导引法【xū láo shǎo qì hòu dǎo yǐn fǎ】 为静功。其作法为,整天不吐唾液,常含枣核,待津液满口时咽下,益气生津。

exercise of Daoyin for asthenic short breath A static exercise, marked by no vomiting saliva every day, keeping date stone in the mouth and swallowing when fluid and humor are enriched for fortifying Qi and producing fluid.

虚劳体痛【xū láo tǐ tòng】 气功适应证,指虚劳患者因阴阳皆虚,经络血脉凝涩,血气运行不畅所致。

consumptive disease with body pain An indication of Qigong, caused by deficiency of both Yin and Yang, stagnation of the blood in the meridians and collaterals and inhibited circulation of the blood and Qi.

虚劳体痛候导引法【xū láo tǐ tòng

X

hòu dǎo yǐn fǎ】 为动功,方法多样。如正坐,伸直腰,右手上举,手掌向上,左手掌压右手掌上,用鼻呼吸七次,同时左手稍振动。舒筋活络,治臂背疼痛。

exercise of Daoyin for asthenic body pain A dynamic exercise with various methods, such as sitting upright, stretching the waist, raising the right hand with the palm rising up, pressing the right palm with the left palm, breathing through the nose for seven times, and slowly vibrating the left hand. Such a dynamic exercise can soothe the sinews and activate the collaterals as well as treat shoulder pain and back pain.

虚劳膝冷【xū láo xī lěng】 气功适应证,因肾虚弱髓虚,为寒冷所搏。

consumptive disease with coldness of the knees An indication of Qigong, caused by weakness of the kidney and deficiency of marrow that cause coldness in the body.

虚劳膝冷候导引法【xū láo xī lěng hòu dǎo yǐn fǎ】 为动功,方法多样。如仰卧,伸展两足,两足趾向左,两手伸直放身旁,鼻吸气七次。活血散寒,治肌肉麻痹,胫寒。

exercise of Daoyin for consumptive disease with knee coldness A dynamic exercise with various methods, such as lying on the back, stretching the feet, turning the toes of both feet to the left side, unwinding the hands and putting on the sides of the body, inhaling Qi through the nose for seven times for activating the blood and expelling cold. Such a method in this dynamic exercise can cure muscle paralysis and shank coldness.

虚劳阴痛【xū láo yīn tòng】 气功适应证,指肾虚复受风冷之邪侵袭,邪入于肾经,邪正交争,致前阴疼痛之症。

consumptive disease with Yin pain An indication of Qigong, referring to kidney deficiency with invasion of pathogenic cold and struggle between pathogenic factors and healthy Qi, which causes pain in the external genitalia.

虚劳阴痛候导引法【xū láo yīn tòng hòu dǎo yǐn fǎ】 为动功。其作法为,两足趾向下撑地,两足跟相靠,坐足跟上,两膝向外,两手从身体前面向下,尽量作七遍。补益脏腑,温阳散寒。

exercise of Daoyin for consumptive disease with genital pain A dynamic exercise, marked by pushing the ground with toes from both feet with connection of the heels, sitting on the heels, turning the knees externally, lowering the hands from the front of the body for seven times. Such a dynamic exercise can tonify and replenish the five Zang-organs (including the heart, the liver, the spleen, the lung and the kidney) and the the six Fu-organs including the gallbladder, the stomach, the small intestine, the large intestine, the bladder and the triple energizer as well as warm Yang and relieve cold.

虚劳阴下痒湿【xū láo yīn xià yǎng shī】 气功适应证,指虚劳患者前阴部瘙痒之证。

consumptive disease with itching and wetting in Yin An indication of Qigong, referring to syndrome /pattern of pudendum itching in patients with consumptive disease.

虚劳阴下痒湿候导引法【xū láo yīn xià yǎng shī hòu dǎo yǐn fǎ】 为静功。

其作法为,仰卧,两手放膝头,两足跟放臀下,用口服气,待气充满腹部时,用鼻慢慢呼出。通阳利温,治阴下湿,少腹痛,膝冷活动不便。

exercise of Daoyin for consumptive disease with genital itching and dampness A static exercise, marked by lying on the back, putting the hands on the knees, putting the heels behind the buttocks, inhaling Qi through the mouth, and exhaling Qi through the nose when Qi is enriched in the abdomen. Such a static exercise can dredge Yang, increase warmth and cure dampness below the scrotum, lower abdominal pain and knee coldness.

虚室生白【xū shì shēng bái】 指空明的意境能生出光明。泛指气功状态下,虚静而出智慧。

vacuum chamber producing whiteness Indicates that quiet and effulgent state can produce brightness. In Qigong, tranquility can increase wisdom.

虚妄【xū wàng】 佛家气功习用语,指虚为无实,妄为反真。虚妄的行为影响入静。

whim A common term of Qigong in Buddhism, referring to deficiency without any excess and absurdity without any truth, making it difficult to be tranquil.

虚危穴【xū wēi xué】 即九灵铁鼓,精气聚散常在此处,水火发端也在此处,阴阳变化也在此处,有无出入也在此处。

deficient and anxious point The same as nine genius-fire drums, refers to the region where the essential Qi concentrates and disperses there, water and fire appear there, Yin and Yang

change there, exit and entrance exist there.

虚无【xū wú】 意识活动相对静止之意,即眼不视物,耳不闻声,鼻不辨气,舌不知味,神守于内。

tranquil and free from any avarice Means that the activity of consciousness is comparatively quiet, indicating that the eyes will not see anything, the ears will not listening any sounds, the nose will not differentiate any Qi, the tongue will not know any tastes and the spirit will concentrate in the internal.

虚无论【xū wú lùn】 源自气功专论,阐述虚无的含义,说明切断外界的干扰,才能合于气功之道。

discussion about tranquility and freedom from any avarice Collected from a monograph of Qigong, mainly describing the meaning of tranquility and freedom, indicating that only when disturbance of the external world is prevented can one really follow the law of Qigong.

虚无身【xū wú shēn】 佛家气功习用语,指进行气功养生之后,身体与自然、社会相适应,逍遥自在,神形合适。

tranquilized body A term of Qigong, indicating adaption of the body to the natural environment and society that makes it carefree and suitable after practice of Qigong.

虚无为体【xū wú wéi tǐ】 指气功以无念,意识思维活动相对静止为本体。

vacuum as foundation Indicates that there is no contemplation in Qigong practice which is the foundation for tranquilizing the activity of consciousness and thinking.

虚无之谷【xū wú zhī gǔ】 祖窍的异

名,指位于心与脐之正中。

vacuum valley Another way to describe ancestral orifice, referring to the central region between the heart and the navel.

虚无自然【xū wú zì rán】 指意识活动如太空,广漠无垠空空如也,无有牵挂,谓之虚无自然。

natural vacuum Refers to the activity of consciousness just as the sky without any limit and care.

虚心【xū xīn】 指脑内无纤尘邪念。

Purifying the heart Means that there is no fine dust and evil idea in the brain.

虚心合掌【xū xīn hé zhǎng】 佛家气功习用语,指两手相合而中稍空。为佛家调身时姿势之一。

tranquilizing the heart and closing the palms A common term of Qigong in Buddhism, referring to combination of both hands with slight vacuum in the palms, which is one of the ways for regulating the body in Buddhism.

虚心实腹【xū xīn shí fù】 指圣人调节神形,稳定意识,吐故纳新,纳气归于丹田。

tranquilizing the heart and solidifying the abdomen Refers to the ways of sages to regulate the spirit and body, to stabilize mentality, to get rid of the stale and to take in the fresh, and to inhale Qi and to enter it in Dantian. Dantian is divided into the upper Dantian (the region between the eyes), the middle Dantian (the region below the heart) and the lower Dantian (the region below the navel).

虚心实腹论【xū xīn shí fù lùn】 源自气功专论,主要阐述练功要使神清净(虚心)一身精气充实(实腹)。

idea about tranquilizing the heart and enriching the abdomen Collected from a monograph of Qigong, mainly describing tranquilization of the spirit and enriching essence and Qi in the body. In this term, tranquilizing the heart refers to tranquilizing the spirit while enriching the abdomen refers to enriching the essence and Qi.

虚壹而静【xū yī ér jìng】 指意识思维活动专一宁静,镇定而不乱。

tranquilized concentration Refers to tranquilized activities of consciousness and thinking without any disorder.

虚证【xū zhèng】 气功适应证,精气神损伤出现的一系列病证,即面色苍白、精神萎靡、疲倦无力、心悸气短、自汗盗汗、手足厥逆、头昏眩晕、脉沉细无力,或虚弱。

deficiency symptom An indication of Qigong, referring to a series of diseases caused by damage of the essence, Qi and spirit, such as pale face, dispiritedness, fatigue, palpitation with shortness of breath, spontaneous perspiration and night sweating, reversal cold of hands and feet, dizziness and vertigo, deepness, thinness and weakness of the meridians.

虚中恬惔自致神【xū zhōng tián tán zì zhì shén】 指意守虚无,神形和调,智慧由生。

tranquility can purify the mind and stabilize the spirit Refers to purification of the mind and coordination of the spirit and body that have increased wisdom.

虚筑【xū zhù】 出拳作打的动作,并非真打。

false construction Means false activity of hitting with the fists is false.

徐春圃【xú chūn pǔ】　明代医学家,通气功,其学术专著中载有气功养生导引按摩法。

Xu Chunpu　A doctor of traditional Chinese medicine in the Ming Dynasty (1368 AD‐1644 AD) who was also familiar with Qigong and always studied and practiced Qigong. In his monographs of traditional Chinese medicine, the exercises of Qigong, life cultivation and kneading were all introduced and analyzed.

徐春圃吞日精法【xú chūn pǔ tūn rì jīng fǎ】　为静功。其作法为,日出卯时,坐西面向东,意想日如车轮形象,吞七十二口。

Xu Chunpu's exercise for absorbing solar essence　A static exercise, marked by sitting at the west and facing the east in Mao (the period of the day from 5 a.m. to 7 a.m. in the morning) at sunrise, imagining the sun as the wheel and absorbing for seventy-two times.

徐春圃吞月华法【xú chūn pǔ tūn yuè huá fǎ】　为静功。其作法为,每逢每月阴历初八日,晚饭后背向月坐,月华入于口,八十一咽。至二十三日下弦即停止,到下月初八日再依前法吞之。

Xu Chunpu's exercise for absorbing lunar essence　A static exercise, marked by sitting with the back to the moon at night after taking dinner on 8th in every month, absorbing lunar essence into the mouth and swallowing for eighty-one times. Such a static exercise should be stopped at the last quarter (23th) and starts to absorb lunar essence again from 8th at the next month.

徐大椿【xú dà chūn】　清代医学家徐灵胎的另外一个称谓,其对气功养生有

一定的研究。

Xu Dachun　Another name of Xu Lingtai, a doctor of traditional Chinese medicine in the Qing Dynasty (1636 AD‐1912 AD), who also studied Qigong and life cultivation.

徐大业【xú dà yè】　清代医学家徐灵胎的另外一个称谓,其对气功养生有一定的研究。

Xu Daye　Another name of Xu Lingtai, a doctor of traditional Chinese medicine in the Qing Dynasty (1636 AD‐1912 AD), who also studied Qigong and life cultivation.

徐灵胎【xú líng tāi】　清代医学家,对气功养生有一定的研究。

Xu Lingtai　A doctor of traditional Chinese medicine in the Qing Dynasty (1636 AD‐1912 AD), who also studied Qigong and life cultivation.

徐神公胎息诀【xú shén gōng tāi xī jué】　静功口诀,意在守神,保持精神意识活动相对静止。

Xu Shengong's formula for fetal respiration　A static exercise, emphasizing the importance to concentrate the spirit as well as to tranquilize and to stabilize the activities of the spirit and consciousness.

徐文弼【xú wén bì】　清代气功养生学家,有专著传世,书中推崇气功养生。

Xu Wenbi　A master of Qigong and life cultivation in the Qing Dynasty (1636 AD‐1912 AD), who wrote a monograph about how to practice Qigong and cultivate life.

许旌阳【xǔ jīng yáng】　晋代著名的气功养生家许逊的另外一个称谓,曾撰写了多部专著。

Xu Jingyang　Another name of Xu

Xun，a great master of Qigong and life cultivation in the Jin Dynasty（266 AD - 420 AD）. He wrote several monographs of Qigong.

许旌阳飞剑斩妖【xǔ jīng yáng fēi jiàn zhǎn yāo】 为动功。其作法为，丁字步站立，右手扬起，扭身左视，左手置于后，运气九口。治一切心痛。

Xu Jingyang's exercise for killing devil A dynamic exercise，marked by standing straight，raising the right hand，turning the body for looking the left side，turning the left hand to the back and circulating Qi for nine times in order to relieve heart pain.

许敬之【xǔ jìng zhī】 晋代著名的气功养生家许逊的另外一个称谓，曾撰写了多部专著。

Xu Jingzhi Another name of Xu Xun，a great master of Qigong and life cultivation in the Jin Dynasty（266 AD - 420 AD）. He wrote several monographs of Qigong.

许迈【xǔ mài】 东晋气功养生学家，曾写十二首诗，论及神仙之事。

Xu Mai A great master of Qigong and life cultivation in the East Jin Dynasty （317 AD - 420 AD）. He wrote twelve poems to analyze the important activities in the immortals.

许栖岩胎息法【xǔ qī yán tāi xī fǎ】 为静功。其作法为，"纳气于丹田，定心于觉海。心定而神宁，神宁则气住，气住则胎长矣"。

Xu Qiyan's exercise for fetal respiration A static exercise，referring to "transmitting Qi to Dantian and stabilizing the heart in the conscious sea；only when the heart is stabilized can the spirit be tranquilized；only when the

spirit is tranquilized can Qi be concentrated；only when Qi is concentrated can fetus be improved". Dantian is divided into the upper Dantian（the region between the eyes），the middle Dantian（the region below the heart）and the lower Dantian（the region below the navel）.

许碏插花满头【xǔ què chā huā mǎn tóu】 为动功。其作法为，身体自然站立，两手托天，两脚着地，不离地面，坐提肛动作，运气九口。主治腹胀、身痛。

flowers arranged over the head of Xu Que A dynamic exercise，marked by standing up naturally，raising the hands upwards，keeping the feet on the ground，lifting the anus and circulating Qi for nine times in order to treat abdominal distension and body pain.

许叔玄【xǔ shū xuán】 东晋气功养生家许迈的另外一个称谓。

Xu Shuxuan Another name of Xu Mai，a great master of Qigong and life cultivation in the East Jin Dynasty（317 AD - 420 AD）.

许仙观【xǔ xiān guān】 位于湖北荆州，为晋代著名气功家许逊修练之处。

Immortal Xu's Temple Located in Jingzhou City in Hunan Province，where Xu Xun，a great master of Qigong and life cultivation in the Jin Dynasty（266 AD - 420 AD），studied，practiced and developed Qigong.

许逊【xǔ xùn】 晋代著名的气功养生家，曾撰写了多部专著。

Xu Xun A great master of Qigong and life cultivation in the Jin Dynasty（266 AD - 420 AD）. He wrote several monographs of Qigong.

许逊服气法【xǔ xùn fú qì fǎ】 为静

功,指调身、调气、调神,以补脑髓、益精血、安神明、调形神。

Xu Xun's exercise for regulating respiration　A static exercise, referring to regulating the body, Qi and the spirit in order to tonify the brain, to nourish essence and blood, to stabilize the spirit and intelligence as well as to regulate the body and the spirit.

许逊五脏导引法【xǔ xùn wǔ zàng dǎo yǐn fǎ】　为动功。其作法为,春季补肝三势,季春补脾一势,夏季补心三势,季夏补脾一势,秋季补肺三势,季秋补脾一势,冬季补肾三势,季冬补脾一势。

Xu Xun's exercise of Daoyin for the five Zang-organs　A dynamic exercise, referring to tonifying the liver in spring in three ways; tonifying the spleen in late spring in one way; tonifying the heart in summer in three ways; tonifying the spleen in late summer in one way; tonifying the lung in autumn in three ways; tonifying the spleen in late autumn in one way; tonifying the kidney in winter in three ways; tonifying the spleen in late winter in one way.

许远游【xǔ yuǎn yóu】　东晋气功养生家许迈的另外一个称谓。

Xu Yuanyou　Another name of Xu Mai, a great master of Qigong and life cultivation in the East Jin Dynasty (317 AD－420 AD).

呴吹【xǔ chuī】　① 指习练气功,调节呼吸;② 指功法,呴暖吹冷。

mild respiration　Refers to ① either regulation of respiration in practicing Qigong; ② or the method of Qigong practice, marked by mildly warming the body and slowly blowing cold Qi.

序古名论【xù gǔ míng lùn】　源自其中专论,主要阐述养生却病大法在保精、行气。

expression of antiquity and reputation for development　Collected from a monograph of Qigong, mainly describing that protection of essence and movement of Qi are the major methods for nourishing life.

续骊山老母胎息诀【xù lí shān lǎo mǔ tāi xī jué】　为静功,说明习练时保持形体"不动不静""似有似无"的重要性,稳定形神的方法。

great grandmother's formula for continued fetal respiration in Lishan Mountain　A static exercise, indicating the importance of quietness, silence and seeming to have and not to have as well as the methods for stabilizing the body and spirit.

宣导【xuān dǎo】　指宣通经络,导引气血流畅。

flowing and leading　Refers to promoting the flow of the meridians and collaterals as well as leading Qi and the blood to circulate smoothly.

玄【xuán】　① 指太极,为创造天地万物之母;② 指精神活动;③ 指道,为变化之义。

mystery　Refers to ① either the Supreme Ultimate, the mother of all things in the sky and the earth; ② or the activity of spirit; ③ or the way of changes.

玄禅二门【xuán chán èr mén】　指道家气功和佛家气功。玄指的是道,禅指的是佛。

two gates of supreme dhyana　Refers to Qigong in Daoism and Qigong in Buddhism. In this term, Xuan refers to

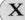

Daoism and Chan refers to Buddhism.

玄丹【xuán dān】 ① 指心神；② 指脑内九宫之一；③ 同内丹。

Supreme Dan（pills of immoratility） Refers to ① either heart spirit； ② or one of the nine chambers in the brain； ③ or internal Dan（pills of immoratility）.

玄道【xuán dào】 气功专论，为晋代葛洪所著，主要阐述气功养生的道理。

Xuan Dao（*Supreme Dao*） A monograph of Qigong entitled *Supreme Dao*, written by Ge Hong, a great scholar and master of Qigong in the Jin Dynasty（226 AD - 420 AD），mainly describing the principles and rules for practicing Qigong.

玄都道藏【xuán dū dào cáng】 指金元两代所修道藏的总称。

Daoist supreme sutra Refers to the general designation of Daoist sutra in the Jin Dynasty（1115 AD - 1234 AD）and Yuan Dynasty（1271 AD - 1368）.

玄根【xuán gēn】 ① 指身体；② 指口中津液。

supreme root Refers to ① either the body； ② or the fluid in the mouth.

玄功【xuán gōng】 指气功。

supreme merit Refers to Qigong, a very important art for cultivating health and prolonging life.

玄宫黑气【xuán gōng hēi qì】 指北方自然之气。

Black Qi in supreme chamber Refers to the natural Qi（air）in the north.

玄谷【xuán gǔ】 指肾。

Supreme grain Refers to the kidney, one of the five Zang-organs, including the heart, liver, spleen, lung and kidney.

玄关【xuán guān】 ① 指入道之门，泛指气功基础；② 指丹田。

supreme pass Refers to ① either the gate of Daoism, indicating the function of Qigong； ② or Dantian which is divided into the upper Dantian（the region between the eyes），the middle Dantian（the region below the heart）and the lower Dantian（the region below the navel）.

玄关露象【xuán guān lù xiàng】 指气功现象，为静极一阳生之象。

supreme phenomena Refers to phenomena of Qigong practice, indicating appearance of Yang after extreme quietness.

玄含黄芽【xuán hán huáng yá】 指行气功时阴中阳生之象。

supreme convergence Refers to the manifestation of Yang produced in Yin in practicing Qigong.

玄和子十二月卦金诀【xuán hé zǐ shí èr yuè guà jīn jué】《玄和子十二月卦金诀》为气功专论，主要阐述习练气功，调节阴阳，应随十二月气候变化而变化、以顺应自然。

practicing Qigong in the twelve months with Trigrams Collected from a monograph of Qigong, mainly describing the importance of regulating Yin and Yang as well as transformation according to the changes of weather in the twelve months in practicing Qigong.

玄葫真人胎息诀【xuán hú zhēn rén tāi xī jué】 静功口诀，本法以炼神为主，通过宁神协调脏腑功能，保持全身的稳定。

Immortal's exercise for fetal respiration A formula of static exercise, marked by mainly practicing the spirit and regulating the functions of the viscera through stabilizing the spirit in order to balance the whole body.

玄华【xuán huá】 指发之神。

supreme magnificence Refers to the spirit in the hair.

玄黄醇精【xuán huáng chún jīng】 指天地太和之精气。

supreme pure essence Refers to the essence and Qi based on the harmonization of the sky and the earth.

玄际【xuán jì】 指气功中阴阳二气进入和合状态的时机。

supreme abstruseness Refers to the chance for entering and harmonizing Yin and Yang in practicing Qigong.

玄鉴导引法【xuán jiàn dǎo yǐn fǎ】 为动功,方法多样。如左手按右手指,五息,右手按左手指亦如之。治大肠中恶气。

exercise of Doayin for supreme reflection A dynamic exercise with various methods, such as pressing the right fingers with the left hand for five times of respiration and pressing the left fingers with the right hand for relieving pathogenic Qi in the large intestine.

玄教宗主论【xuán jiào zōng zhǔ lùn】 源自气功专论,阐述气功养生法的历史沿革。

supreme discussion about the importance of Qigong Collected from a monograph about Qigong, describing the historical development of Qigong for nourishing life.

玄精【xuán jīng】 指人体的元精。

supreme essence Refers to the original essence in the human body.

玄静先生【xuán jìng xiān shēng】 唐代医药家和道界气功家李含光的另外一个称谓。

Mr. Xuan Jing Another name of Li Hanguang, a great doctor and a great master of Qigong in Daoism in the Tang Dynasty (618 AD - 907 AD).

玄览【xuán lǎn】 指气功中,静而生慧,提高智力。

supreme cognition Refers to the fact that quietness improve wisdom in practicing Qigong.

玄理【xuán lǐ】 ① 指气功基本理论; ② 指道家微妙的道理。

supreme theory Refers to ① either the basic theory of Qigong; ② or the subtle principles in Daoism.

玄灵宫真人【xuán líng gōng zhēn rén】 小肠所主神名。

immortal in supreme spiritual chamber Refers to the name of the spirit controlled by the small intestine.

玄门【xuán mén】 ① 指道; ② 指气功。

supreme gate Refers to ① either Daoism; ② or Qigong.

玄门以止念为本【xuán mén yǐ zhǐ niàn wéi běn】 指道家气功,以止除杂念为根本。

Elimination of reading is foundation of supreme gate. Refers to the fact that elimination of distracting thought is the root for Qigong in Daoism.

玄妙之业【xuán miào zhī yè】 指气功养生法。

supreme course Refers to the methods of Qigong practice for nourishing life.

玄冥【xuán míng】 指肾之神。

supreme obscurity Refers to the spirit in the kidney.

玄牝【xuán pìn】 ① 指身中一窍;

②指二肾之间；③指天地；④指任督二脉；⑤指体内阴阳；⑥指中宫脾。

xuanpin Refers to ① either an orifice in the body; ② or a region between the two kidneys; ③ or the sky and the earth; ④ or the conception meridian and the governor meridian; ⑤ or Yin and Yang in the body; ⑥ or the spleen.

玄牝之门【xuán pìn zhī mén】 ①指天地；②指口鼻；③指人体正中。

gate of Xuanpin A term of Qigong, referring to ① either the sky and the earth; ② or the mouth and the nose; ③ or the middle of the body. In this term, Xuanpin refers to the sky and the earth, the nose and the mouth, the upper and the lower etc.

玄气【xuán qì】 指元气，即自然之气。

supreme Qi Refers to the original Qi which is the natural Qi.

玄窍【xuán qiào】 ①指身中一窍；②指二肾之间；③指天地；④指任督二脉；⑤指体内阴阳；⑥指中宫脾。

supreme orifice A term of Qigong, referring to ① either a orifice in the body; ② or a region between the two kidneys; ③ or the sky and the earth; ④ or the conception meridian and the governor meridian; ⑤ or Yin and Yang in the body; ⑥ or the spleen.

玄穹主【xuán qióng zhǔ】 指脑。

supreme master Refers to the brain.

玄泉【xuán quán】 ①指元海；②指口中唾液，气功状态下口中练就的津液；③指肾液。

supreme spring A term of Qigong, referring to ① either the original sea; ② or saliva in the mouth, a fluid produced in practicing Qigong; ③ or hu-

mor in the kidney.

玄阙圆【xuán què yuán】 指肾的外形。

supreme shape Refers to the external form of the kidney.

玄师【xuán shī】 ①指有较高修养的道士；②泛指气功医师。

supreme master A term of Qigong, referring to ① either Daoists with great life cultivation; ② or important doctors in the Qigong field.

玄书【xuán shū】 ①指《老子》；②指道家气功著述。

supreme book Refers to ① either *Lao Zi*, a great book about Dao written by Lao Zi who was the founder of the most important Chinese thought known as Dao; ② or the books about Qigong in Daoism.

玄术【xuán shù】 指方术，泛指气功养生法。

supreme techniques Refers to the arts of necromancy, astrology, medicine, etc. Usually it refers to the exercise of Qigong for nourishing life.

玄俗形无影【xuán sú xíng wú yǐng】 为动功。其作法为，身体盘膝端坐，两手擦左脚心，同时运气二十四口，再擦右脚心，亦运气二十四口。

supreme secular invisibility A dynamic exercise, marked by sitting with crossed legs, pressing the left sole with both hands, and directing Qi for twenty-four times; then pressing the right sole with both hands and directing Qi for twenty-four times.

玄胎【xuán tāi】 指人体阴阳二气相合而生。

supreme embryo Refers to the embryo formed through combination of Qi in

Yin and Yang.

玄天【xuán tiān】　① 指北方之天；② 指天色玄，"黑而有赤色"。

supreme sky　Refers to ① either the sky in the north；② or mysterious color of the sky，such as "black and red".

玄武【xuán wǔ】　① 指北方太阳之神；② 指肾。

supreme martial　Refers to ① either the spirit of the sun in the north；② or the kidney，one of the five Zang-organs（including the gallbladder，the stomach，the small intestine，the large intestine，the bladder and the triple energizer）.

玄息【xuán xī】　指习练气功，降低身体能源的消耗，调节身体各部的功能，延年益寿。

supreme respiration　Refers to the function of Qigong practice that can reduce consumption of energy source in the body，regulate the functions of all parts in the body and prolong life.

玄心【xuán xīn】　指深入认识事物奥秘的精神活动。

supreme heart　Refers to the activity of the spirit for recognizing anything and any mystery.

玄虚【xuán xū】　① 指气功；② 指气功高深的义理；③ 指性情平和，神志清明。

supreme deficiency　Refers to ① either Qigong；② or the view of righteousness in Qigong；③ or harmonious property or clear and bright spirit and will.

玄玄子【xuán xuán zǐ】　明代气功学家张三丰的另一称谓。张三丰为明代的气功学家，深入系统地研究和发展了气功的理论和方法。

Xuan Xuanzi　Another name of Zhang Sanfeng，a great master of Qigong in the Ming Dynasty（1368 AD - 1644 AD），thoroughly and systematically studied and developed the theory and practice of Qigong.

玄学【xuán xué】　① 指魏晋时期的哲学流派；② 指古代学习道家学说的学校，为南朝宋文帝所创建。

supreme study　Refers to either a school of philosophy in the Wei and Jin Dynasties（220 AD - 420 AD）；or a university of Daoism created by Emperor Wendi in the South Song Dynasty（1127 AD - 1276 AD）.

玄一【xuán yī】　既指深奥、神妙，也指本源、根本。气功学文献中泛指气功养生法的基础理论及重要功法。

supreme source　Refers to either abstruseness and supreme；or origin and root. In the literature of Qigong，it refers to the theory and exercise for practicing Qigong and cultivating life.

玄膺【xuán yīng】　指气管，亦指重楼。

supreme chest　Refers to air tube；or important building.

玄元【xuán yuán】　① 指道，泛指气功养生法；② 指丹田；③ 或指玄牝。

supreme origin　Refers to ① either Daoism，indicating the function of Qigong in nourishing life；② or Dantian，which is divided into the upper Dantian（the region between the eyes），the middle Dantian（the region below the heart）and the lower Dantian（the region below the navel）；③ or Xuanpin which refers to the sky and earth，nose and mouth，upper and lower etc.

玄奘【xuán zàng】　唐代高僧，俗家姓名"陈祎（yī）"，促进了气功养生法的传播，与鸠摩罗什、真谛并称为中国佛教三大翻译家。

X

Xuan Zang A dignitary in the Tang Dynasty（618 AD - 907 AD）whose original name was Chen Yi. In transmitting Buddhism in China, he not only developed Qigong, but also developed translation. He was one of the three important translators in ancient China, the other two were kumarajiva and Parama˘rtha.

玄真【xuán zhēn】 指气功养生法。

supreme truth Refers to the exercise of Qigong for nourishing life.

玄真法【xuán zhēn fǎ】 为静功。其作法为,清斋休粮,存日月在口中,昼存日,夜存月。

supreme true exercise A static exercise, marked by fasting in sacrifice, keeping the sun and the moon in the mouth, keeping the sun in the daytime and keeping the moon in the nighttime.

玄真子【xuán zhēn zǐ】 《玄真子》为气功养生书,由唐代张志和所撰,阐述气功养生知识及具体方法。也是唐代气功学家张志和的另外一个称谓。

Xuan Zhenzi（Supreme Truth） Refers to either a monograph about Qigong entitled *Supreme Truth* written by Zhang Zhihe, a great master of Qigong in the Tang Dynasty（618 AD - 907 AD）; or another name of Zhang Zhihe.

玄真子啸咏坐席浮水【xuán zhēn zǐ xiào yǒng zuò xí fú shuǐ】 为动功,身体盘膝端坐,两手上举托天运气九口,手放下亦运气九口,可治肚腹虚肿。

Xuan Zhenzi floating exercise A dynamic exercise, marked by sitting with crossed legs, raising both hands to direct Qi for nine times and descending the hands to direct Qi for nine times in order to treat deficiency and dropsy of the abdomen.

玄中颠倒【xuán zhōng diān dǎo】 指五行颠倒,三归二,二合一,一归虚或无,即神形合一。

Supreme overthrow Refers to the five elements（including wood, fire, earth, metal and water）overthrow, marked by three returning to two, two integrating into one and one returning to deficiency or nothingness, indicating integration of the spirit and the body.

玄中之玄【xuán zhōng zhī xuán】 指脑。

supreme in supreme Refers to the brain.

玄珠【xuán zhū】 指内丹,即阴精阳气在神的作用下形成的特殊物质。

supreme pearl Refers to the internal Dan（pills of immortality）which is a special substance formed by Yin essence and Yang Qi under the control of the spirit.

玄珠成象【xuán zhū chéng xiàng】 指气功中,入静后进入高深境界时,内气运行,阴平阳秘,身体处于稳定状态。

supreme pearl image Refers to reaching the highest state after tranquilization in practicing Qigong, marked by movement of internal Qi, stable Yin and compact Yang as well as stabilization of the body.

玄珠歌【xuán zhū gē】 气功歌诀。

supreme pearl song Refers to the songs usually sung in practicing Qigong.

玄作【xuán zuò】 指习练气功的道理。

supreme action Refers to the rule for practicing Qigong.

悬衡【xuán héng】 即精神意识思维活动处于安静和平的状态。

outstanding balance Refers to tranquil-

X

ized and pacified activities of the spirit, consciousness and thinking.

悬解【xuán jiě**】**　指面对纷乱的社会环境而不受束缚,情绪稳定,意识平和。

outstanding comprehension Refers to emotional stability and mild consciousness without any fettering from the disordered society.

悬阳【xuán yáng**】**　① 指心;② 指目。

outstanding Yang Refers to ① the heart; ② or the eyes.

旋台骨【xuán tái gǔ**】**　即第四、五、六颈椎骨。

rotary platform bone Refers to the fourth, fifth and sixth cervical vertebrae.

璇玑【xuán jī**】**　① 指北斗七星;② 为任脉中的一个穴位,位于胸骨中线上。

armillary sphere　① Refers to seven stars in the Big Dipper. ② It also refers to Xuanji (CV21), an acupoint in the conception meridian, located above the middle line of the sternum.

璇玑停轮【xuán jī tíng lún**】**　指胎息法呼吸之深功夫。

armillary sphere stopping wheel Refers to fetal respiration exercise for deep skill of breath.

璇玑悬珠环无穷【xuán jī xuán zhū huán wú qióng**】**　指小周天功法,精气运行的状态。

armillary sphere with suspension beads and infinite link Refers to exercise of small celestial cycles and the condition of essential Qi movement.

眩晕【xuàn yūn**】**　指头脑晕转、眼目昏花,临床上分为虚实两型。

dizziness Refers to dizziness with blurred vision which is divided into deficiency syndrome/pattern and excess

syndrome/pattern in clinical practice.

薛道光【xuē dào guāng**】**　宋代气功学家,著有气功专著,介绍和分析气功的理论与方法。

Xue Daoguang A master of Qigong in the Song Dynasty (960 AD - 1279 AD), who wrote monographs of Qigong to introduce and to analyze the theory and exercises of Qigong.

薛道光摩踵法【xuē dào guāng mó zhǒng fǎ**】**　动静相兼功。其作法为,用手擦左脚心至热,运气二十四口,再以手擦右脚心至热,行功如左。功效为养元护精、治元气虚弱。

Xue Daoguang's exercise for rubbing foot An exercise combined with dynamic exercise and static exercise, marked by rubbing the left sole hot with the hands, moving Qi for twenty-four times, rubbing the right sole hot with the hands. Such an exercise combined with dynamic exercise and static exercise can nourish the original spirit, protect the essence and cure deficiency of the original Qi.

薛道原【xuē dào yuán**】**　宋代气功学家薛道光的另外一个称谓,其著有气功专著,介绍和分析气功的理论与方法。

Xue Daoyuan Another name of Xue Daoguang, a master of Qigong in the Song Dynasty (960 AD - 1279 AD), who wrote monographs of Qigong to introduce and to analyze the theory and exercises of Qigong.

薛式【xuē shì**】**　宋代气功学家薛道光的另外一个称谓,其著有气功专著,介绍和分析气功的理论与方法。

Xue Shi Another name of Xue Daoguang, a master of Qigong in the Song Dynasty (960 AD - 1279 AD), who wrote monographs of Qigong to introduce and to analyze the theory and exercises of Qigong.

薛太源【xuē tài yuán】　宋代气功学家薛道光的另外一个称谓，其著有气功专著，介绍和分析气功的理论与方法。

Xue Taiyuan Another name of Xue Daoguang, a master of Qigong in the Song Dynasty（960 AD – 1279 AD），who wrote monographs of Qigong to introduce and to analyze the theory and exercises of Qigong.

薛子养寿法【xuē zǐ yǎng shòu fǎ】为静功。其作法为，端身正坐，常沉静含蓄。厚重、静定、宽缓，乃进德之基，义理深而应事有力。为老人养寿之要。

Mr. Xue's exercise for cultivating life A static exercise, marked by sitting upright, tranquilizing and veiling the spirit, relaxing the body and purifying the mind. Such a static exercise is a good way for old people to prolong their life.

学道【xué dào】　指学习气功养生法。

Studying Dao Refers to studying the methods of Qigong and life cultivation.

雪里花开【xuě lǐ huā kāi】　同水中火发。水为阴，水中为阴之极，火为阳，火发为阳生。火发于水中，即阴极一阳生。

Flowers blooming in snow The same as fire appearing in water. Water pertains to Yin and the central part of water reflects the extreme stage of Yin; fire pertains to Yang and hyperactivity of fire indicates the production of Yang. That is why fire occurs in water, indicating that extreme Yin produces Yang.

雪山一味好醍醐，倾入东阳造化炉【xuě shān yí wèi hǎo tí hú qīng rù dōng yáng zào huà lú】　指肺津还入丹田。雪山色白喻肺色白，东阳造化炉即丹田。

The taste of snow in the mountain is just like finest cream which flows to the east Yang and makes furnace. Indicates that fluid in the lung enters Dantian. In this celebrated dictum, snow in the mountain refers to the whiteness of the lung and the east Yang making furnace refers to Dantian. Dantian is divided into the upper Dantian（the region between the eyes），the middle Dantian（the region below the heart）and the lower Dantian（the region below the navel）.

血海【xuè hǎi】　足太阴脾经的一个穴位，位髌骨内上缘2寸，也是四海之一的冲脉。这一穴位为气功运行的一个常见部位。

Xuehai（SP 10）　An acupoint in the spleen meridian of foot Taiyin, located 2 Cun above the kneecap. It also refers to the thoroughfare meridian, one of the four seas. This acupoint is a region usually used for keeping the essential Qi in practice of Qigong.

血淋【xuè lín】　气功适应证，多因湿热下注膀胱，热盛伤络，迫血妄行所致。

bloody stranguria An indication of Qigong, usually caused by downward pouring of damp heat into the bladder, making intense heat that damages the collaterals and frenetically forces the blood.

血轮【xuè lún】　眼科五轮之一，指眼睛中的内眦和外眦。

blood wheel One of the five wheels in the eyes, referring to the inner canthus and outer canthus in the eyes.

血脉【xuè mài】　血液运行的通道。在气功文献中,血脉为精气运行的通道。

blood vessel　Refers to thoroughfare of blood in the body. In the literature of Qigong, the blood vessel is described as the thoroughfare of the spirit and Qi.

血盟【xuè méng】　指古代师傅对学徒讲授气功养生术,需歃血誓盟。

blood oath　Refers to swearing an oath made by the teacher in teaching the students to practice Qigong for nourishing life.

血气朝囟门【xuè qì cháo xìng mén】指血气涌向头顶,是气功中出现的一种自身感应,也称气功现象。

blood and Qi in fontanelles　Refers to blood and Qi surging up to the top of the head, indicating self-response in practicing Qigong.

血气精神【xuè qì jīng shén】　指人体生命活动的物质基础。

essence and spirit of the blood and Qi　Refers to the material basis of life activity.

血之府【xuè zhī fǔ】　指脉。

blood mansion　Refers to meridians and vessels.

熏心【xūn xīn】　即守真,指内守精神,调和形神,使之达到神形高度稳定的状态。

fumigating the heart　The same as defending genuineness, refers to internal concentration of the essence and the spirit as well as combination of the body and the spirit in order to enable the spirit and boy to reach the stable state.

熏蒸诸宫【xūn zhēng zhū gōng】　指精气上至泥丸,熏蒸脑中诸宫。

fumigating and steaming all chambers　Refers to essential Qi ascending to the mud bolus (the brain) to fumigate and steam all the chambers in the brain.

荀况【xún kuàng】　战国时杰出的思想家、教育家荀子的另外一个称谓,其对气功学的发展有较大的贡献。

Xun Kuang　Another name of Xun Zi, a great thinker and educator in the Warring States Period (475 BC – 221 BC), contributing a great deal to the development of Qigong.

荀卿【xún qīng】　战国时杰出的思想家、教育家荀子的另外一个称谓,其对气功学的发展有较大的贡献。

Xun Qing　Another name of Xun Zi, a great thinker and educator in the Warring States Period (475 BC – 221 BC), contributing a great deal to the development of Qigong.

荀子【xún zǐ】　战国时杰出的思想家、教育家,对气功学的发展有较大的贡献。

Xun Zi　A great thinker and educator in the Warring States Period (475 BC – 221 BC), contributing a great deal to the development of Qigong.

循身观【xún shēn guān】　为静功。其作法为,结跏趺坐,意想身体头颈、胸腹、背腰、四肢,从上到下,从后向前,反复循观意想九次。功效防治贪欲,稳定情绪。

following physiological view　A static exercise, marked by sitting in lotus position, imagining the head, the neck, the chest, the abdomen, the back, the waist and the four limbs from the upper to the lower and from the back to the front for nine times. Such a static exercise can prevent greediness and stabilize emotion.

循数勿失【xún shù wù shī】　指遵循四时阴阳的变化规律,使人体的气机不得与之相失。

following number and avoiding loss Refers to following the principles for changes of Yin and Yang in the four seasons in order to prevent loss of the activities of Qi in the body.

巽【xùn】 ① 指卦名，为风；② 指取象比类；③ 指行为符合事理；④ 指长女。

xun Refers to ① either Xun Trigram, indicating wind；② or analogy；③ or behavior fitting in with the reason；④ eldest girl. Xun Trigram is one of the Eight Trigrams from Yijing (*Canon of Simplification*, *Change and No Change*).

巽风【xùn fēng】 指肺呼吸之气。

xun wind Refers to Qi related to pulmonary respiration.

Y

牙龋【yá qǔ】 气功适应证，多因口腔不洁，或风痰湿热熏蒸手、足阳明二经所致。

dental caries An indication of Qigong, usually caused by impurity of the mouth, or evaporation of the stomach meridian of foot Yangming at both sides with wind phlegm and damp heat.

牙痛治法【yá tòng zhì fǎ】 动静相兼功，具体做法是，凡牙痛，双手托住下巴骨，闭气，口麻方止。

toothache treatment exercise An exercise combined with dynamic exercise and static exercise, marked by holding the jaw with both hands and stopping respiration till the mouth is numb when there is suffering from toothache.

哑门【yǎ mén】 督脉中的一个穴位，位于后正中线。这一穴位为气功运行的一个常见部位。

Yamen（GV 15） An acupoint in the governor meridian, located in the back middle line. This acupoint is a region usually used for keeping the essential Qi in practice of Qigong.

咽喉【yān hóu】 ① 指咽；② 指咽喉的总称。

throat Refers to ① either pharynx; ② or the general term of pharynx and larynx.

咽门【yān mén】 即咽。由于咽是进入食管和气管的门户，故将咽称咽门。

throat gate Refers to throat. The throat is the way to enter the esophagus and trachea. That is why is called the throat gate.

咽日【yān rì】 即对日咽气，亦称咽日气。

inhaling the sun Indicates that practitioners face the sun for inhaling Qi. That is why it is also called inhaling solar Qi.

咽唾【yān tuò】 指咽下自己的唾液。气功学家认为咽唾可强身延年。

swallowing saliva Refers to saliva. Masters of Qigong believe that swallowing saliva can strengthen the body and prolong life.

烟火【yān huǒ】 ① 指人烟；② 指熟食。

smoke and fire Refers to ① either signs of human habitation; ② or cooked food.

烟萝子【yān luó zǐ】 为晋代气功学家，精于内丹，撰写多部专著，影响巨大。

Yan Luozi Yan Luozi was a master of Qigong and life cultivation in the Jin Dynasty（266 AD - 420 AD）, proficient in internal Dan（pills of immortality）. He wrote several important monographs of Qigong and life cultivation.

烟萝子胎息诀【yān luó zǐ tāi xī jué】 为静功，本法以动静交相养立论，安神定息为法，意在"气住神定"。

Yan Luozi's formula for fetal respiration Yan Luozi's formula for fetal respiration is a static exercise, marked by combination of dynamic exercise and static exercise for cultivating health as the principles, and pacification of the spirit and stabilization of respiration as the methods in order to keep Qi and to stabilize the spirit.

烟霞志【yān xiá zhì】　指习练气功,自然经脉通达,五藏之神灵明,能清能净,三丹田之气升腾有如烟霞。

will of smoke and cloud　Indicates that in practicing Qigong, the meridians are unobstructed; the spirit in the five Zang-organs (including the heart, the liver, the spleen, the lung and the kidney) is bright, clear and clean; Qi from the three kinds of Dantian rises like smoke and cloud. The three kinds of Dantian refer to the upper Dantian (the region between the eyes), the middle Dantian (the region below the heart) and the lower Dantian (the region below the navel).

延陵先生集新旧服气经【yán líng xiān shēng jí xīn jiù fú qì jīng】　《延陵先生集新旧服气经》为气功专著,作者不详,阐述了气功养生的理论与方法。

Yanling Xiansheng Jixinjiu Fuqijing（*Mr. Yanling's Compilation of the New and Old Ways for Respiration*）　A monograph of Qigong entitled *Mr. Yanling's Compilation of the New and Old Ways for Respiration*, mainly describing the theory and methods for practicing Qigong. The author was unknown.

延龄纂要【yán líng zuǎn yào】　《延龄纂要》为气功养生学专著,为清代罗福至所撰,主张习练气功当动静结合。

Yanling Zuanyao（*Essential Compilation of Longevity*, *written by Luo Fuzhi*）A monograph of Qigong entitled *Essential Compilation of Longevity*, *written by Luo Fuzhi*, a great master of Qigong in the Qing Dynasty（1636 AD–1912 AD）, suggesting to combine dynamics and statics in practicing Qigong.

延年九转法【yán nián jiǔ zhuǎn fǎ】《延年九转法》为气功学专著,由清代方开编辑,主要强调摩腹及捏拿。

Yannian Jiuzhuan Fa（*Exercise of Nine Exchanges for Prolonging Life*）　A monograph of Qigong entitled *Exercise of Nine Exchanges for Prolonging Life*, compiled by Fang Kai, a master of Qigong in the Qing Dynasty（1636 AD–1912 AD）, emphasizing the importance of kneading, pinching and holding the abdomen.

延年九转功【yán nián jiǔ zhuǎn gōng】　为动功,作法多样。如以两手中三指按心窝,由左顺摩圆转二十一次。

exercise of nine turns for longevity　A dynamic exercise with various methods, such as pressing the precordium with three fingers in both hands and kneading round from the left for twenty-one times, etc.

延养之理【yán yǎng zhī lǐ】　源自气功专论,阐述延养之理在于习练气功时,和调神形,减少身体能源的消耗。

principle for prolonged cultivation　Collected from a monograph of Qigong, mainly describing the way to harmonize and to regulate the spirit and body in practicing Qigong in order to reduce consumption of the energy in the body.

颜【yán】　① 指额部;② 指面容、脸色;③ 指眉目之间。

countenance　Refers to ① either frontal part; ② or facial feature and complexion；③ or the part between the eyes.

颜回【yán huí】 孔子的门生，提倡"静坐"，主张"坐忘"的练功方法。

Yan Hui A student of Confucius，advocating to sit quietly and silently for practicing Qigong.

颜渊【yán yuān】 孔子的门生颜回的另外一个称谓，提倡"静坐"，主张"坐忘"的练功方法。

Yan Yuan Another name of Yan Hui who was a student of Confucius，advocating to sit quietly and silently for practicing Qigong.

掩蔽【yǎn bì】 指习练气功，阴阳之间的气化作用，细微而不显著。

shelter Refers to the function of Qi transformation in Yin and Yang without obvious scene in practicing Qigong.

掩耳屈头【yǎn ěr qū tóu】 为动功，指两手掌掩住两耳，屈颈数次。能治眩晕、头痛、散风邪。

exercise for covering the ears and bending the head A dynamic exercise，marked by covering the ears with the palms and bending the neck for several times. Such a dynamic exercise can cure vertigo and headache as well as expel pathogenic wind.

掩耳去头旋法【yǎn ěr qù tóu xuán fǎ】 为动静功。其作法为，静坐、闭息，以两手掩耳，折头五七次，存想元神，逆上泥丸。

exercise for covering the ears and moving the head An exercise combined with dynamic exercise and static exercise，marked by sitting quietly，stopping respiration，covering the ears with both hands，breaking the head for five to seven times，imagining the original

spirit and raising to the mud bolus（the brain）.

眼不见【yǎn bú jiàn】 指守神于内，精神集中，眼不视外物。

seeing nothing Refers to keeping the spirit inside，concentrating the essence and spirit，and avoiding seeing anything in the external world.

眼观心动，耳听神移，口谈气散【yǎn guān xīn dòng ěr tīng shén yí kǒu tán qì sàn】 极简明地谈练功中闭塞眼、耳、口外三关，才不耗散神气。

Seeing anything agitates the heart，listening any sound transfers the spirit and talking anything disperses Qi. Indicates that only when the eyes，the ears and the mouth are closed in practicing Qigong can the spirit and Qi not be dispersed.

眼目症治法【yǎn mù zhèng zhì fǎ】 动静相兼功。其作法为，凡三焦血热眼睛昏花，正坐，将两手掌擦热后摩脐及两膝，待气定后做第二遍，日行三五次。

exercise for treating ocular disease An exercise combined with dynamic exercise and static exercise，marked by sitting upright when the blood in the triple energizer is hot and the eyes are dim-sighted，scraping the palms hot and then rubbing the navel and knees with the palms. After Qi is stabilized，such a way of practice can be done for twice，and three or five times a day.

眼目治法【yǎn mù zhì fǎ】 动静相兼功，方法多样。如踞坐，伸右脚，两手抱左膝，伸腰，用鼻吸气，尽力行七息。

exercise for treating the eyes An exercise combined with dynamic exercise and static exercise with various methods，such as squatting and sitting，

Y

stretching the right foot, holding the left knee with both hands, stretching the waist, inhaling Qi through the nose and trying to move for seven times.

眼前【yǎn qián】　指面前,用以说明气功并不难寻。

in sight　Refers to in front of the face, indicating that Qigong is not difficult to find.

偃伏【yǎn fú】　即双膝跪地,前额着地,披发在地。

laying down and bending over　Refers to kneeling on the knees, putting the forehead on the ground and stretching hair on the ground.

偃卧行气法【yǎn wò xíng qì fǎ】　为静功。其作法为,先去鼻中之毛,偃卧,两足相去五寸,两臂去身亦五寸,瞑目握固。精念玉房,内视丹田,内气致之于丹田,令气充形和,亦可却病。

exercise of bending and lying for moving Qi　A static exercise, marked by eliminating hair in the nose, lying on bed with the feet separating from each other for 5 Cun and the shoulders separating from the body for 5 Cun, closing the eyes to hold the hands, imagining jade house, internally observing Dantian, promoting internal Qi to enter Dantian, enriching Qi and balancing the body. Dantian is divided into the upper Dantian (the region between the eyes), the middle Dantian (the region below the heart) and the lower Dantian (the region below the navel). Such a static exercise can cure disease.

偃仰之方【yǎn yǎng zhī fāng】　指导引,即动功。

formula for bending and lifting　Refers to Daoyin, indicating exercise of

Qigong.

偃月炉【yǎn yuè lú】　即偃月炉中玉蕊生,指腹中偃月炉为阴炉,阴中一阳生而曰玉蕊。

half month furnace　Refers to the celebrated sentence that barringtonia racemosa grows in furnace in half month, indicating that half month furnace in the abdomen is Yin furnace and barringtonia racemosa furnace is Yang within Yin.

偃月炉中玉蕊生【yǎn yuè lú zhōng yù ruǐ shēng】　指腹中偃月炉为阴炉,阴中一阳生而曰玉蕊。

Barringtonia racemosa grows in furnace in half month.　Indicates that half month furnace in the abdomen is Yin furnace and barringtonia racemosa furnace is Yang within Yin.

咽气【yàn qì】　指咽下自然太和之气,使气归本返元,便可神守根固,延年益寿。

inhalation　Refers to natural and peaceful Qi that leads to Qi into the root and the origin in order to protect the root with the spirit, to prolong life and to cultivate health.

咽气诀【yàn qì jué】　静功口诀,即每次咽气吐纳,则内外气相应,气自海中随吐而上,直至喉中,使内气相固。

exercise for inhalation　A static formula, marked by correspondence of the external Qi and internal Qi after swallowing Qi, exhaling Qi and inhaling Qi, enabling Qi from the sea to flow upwards into the throat and finally stabilizing the internal Qi.

晏晡【yàn bū】　指戌时。

late time　Refers to Xu (the period of a day from 7 p. m. to 9 p. m. in the evening）.

晏食【yàn shí】　指习练气功者，黄昏戌时饮食。

dusk diet　Refers to taking food in Xu（the period of a day from 7 p. m. to 9 p. m. in the evening）for practitioners of Qigong.

晏坐【yàn zuò】　佛家气功功法。其作法为，结跏趺坐，安住根本净禅，乃至灭定，息外劳尘，安置心中，形神高度协调统一。

tranquilized sitting　The exercise of Qigong practice in Buddhism, marked by sitting with crossed feet, tranquilizing the mind to eliminate any desires, breathing out according to the condition of the external world, stabilizing the heart, and highly coordinating and unifying the spirit and body.

雁行气法【yàn xíng qì fǎ】　为动功。其作法为，低头倚臂，不息十二通。以意排留饮、宿食，从下部出饮邪即愈。

exercise of wild goose moving Qi　A dynamic exercise, marked by lowering the head to the shoulders and stopping respiration in twelve ways. Such a dynamic exercise can eliminate retention of fluid and dyspepsia and disperse pathogenic fluid from the lower region.

羊车【yáng chē】　指尾闾关到夹脊关，其行缓慢。

sheep cart　Refers to slow movement from the coccyx to the point located in the vertebra.

羊车小乘【yáng chē xiǎo chéng】　动静相兼功。其作法为，抽缩外肾，使膀胱下昧民火，下合外肾左文右武之地，火从下上达，直透三关，行之四十九日内，自有甘露降于玉池。

slowly riding sheep cart　Exercise combined with dynamic exercise and static exercise, marked by shrinking the external kidney, enabling the bladder to conceal human fire in order to fit in with the position of the external kidney marked by mild fire in the left and great fire in the right, transmitting fire from the upper to the lower through the three passes directly. Such a way of practice should be done for forty-nine days in order to descend best water to the immortal pool.

阳白【yáng bái】　足少阳胆经的一个穴位，位于前额眉中直上 1 寸，正视时与瞳孔垂直处。这一穴位为气功运行的一个常见部位。

Yangbai（GB 14）　An acupoint in the gallbladder meridian of foot Shaoyang, located 1 Cun directly above the forehead at the middle of the eyebrow, looking squarely at the vertical region with the pupil. This acupoint is a region usually used for keeping the essential Qi in practice of Qigong.

阳返负阴【yáng fǎn fù yīn】　阳指肾阳，阴指心阴，气功状态下肾阳含心阴上归心中，此种现象称"阳返负阴气"。

yang returning to Yin　A special term, in which Yang refers to kidney Yang and Yin refers to heart Yin. In practicing Qigong, kidney Yang contains heart Yin and therefore returns to the heart. That is why it is called Yang returning to Yin.

阳风【yáng fēng】　指热风。

yang wind　Refers to hot wind.

阳宫【yáng gōng】　指离宫心。

yang chamber　Refers to the heart away from the chamber.

阳光三现【yáng guāng sān xiàn】　指

在炼精化气阶段中,眼前三次出现闪光,这是炼精化气止火之机。

three flashes of light Indicates that flash lightens for three times in the eyes during the time of refining and transforming Qi. This is the time to refine the essence and transform Q, making it possible to cause fire.

阳化气【yáng huà qì】 指阳主生化,气功中阳动而生,故化气养精,温养形体。

yang transforming Qi Refers to the fact that Yang is responsible for growth and transformation. In Qigong practice, Yang acts and produces the necessary elements. That is why transformation of Qi nourishes the essence and warmly cultivates the body.

阳还阴丹【yáng huán yīn dān】 阳极生阴,阴中有正阳之气,其气随阴下降,所以叫"阳还阴丹"。

yang producing Yin Dan (pills of immortality) Refers to the fact that extremity of Yang produces Yin and that in Yin there is Qi of righteous Yang which descends together with Yin. That is why it is called Yang producing Yin Dan (pills of immortality).

阳既索阴【yáng jì suǒ yīn】 指阴阳交合。

intercourse of Yang and Yin Refers to combination and integration of Yin and Yang.

阳交【yáng jiāo】 足少阳胆经,位于外髁尖上 7 寸,腓骨后缘处。

Yangjiao (GB 35) An acupoint in the gallbladder of foot Shaoyang, located 7 Cun above the top of the lateral malleoli and at the back of the fibula. This acupoint is a region usually used in practice of Qigong.

阳精【yáng jīng】 指真精。

yang essence Refers to genuine essence.

阳陵泉【yáng líng quán】 足少阳胆经中的一个穴位,位于小腿外侧。这一穴位为气功运行的一个常用部位。

Yanglingquan (GV 34) An acupoint in the gallbladder of foot Shaoyang, located in the lateral side of the calf. This acupoint is a region usually used for keeping the essential Qi in practice of Qigong.

阳龙【yáng lóng】 心属火,心为液源,液中有正阳之气,称为"阳龙"。

yang Loong In the human body, the heart pertains to fire and is the origination of humor in which there is positive Yang. That is why it is called Yang Loong.

阳陇【yáng lǒng】 指阳气隆盛。

vigorous Yang Refers to exuberance of Yang Qi.

阳脉之海【yáng mài zhī hǎi】 阳脉即督脉,督脉为诸阳之会,故称阳脉之海。

sea of Yang meridian Yang meridian refers to the governor meridian which is the association of all kinds of Yang. That is why it is called sea of Yang meridian.

阳门【yáng mén】 指七窍之门,亦指玄牝之门。所谓"玄牝"指的是有天与地、鼻与口、上与下、父精与母血和肾、元神、中丹田、心之左右二窍等诸说。

Yang gate Refers to the gate of the seven orifices or the gate of the Xuanpin. The so-called Xuanpin refers to the sky and the earth, or the nose and the mouth, or the upper and the lower, or the paternal semen and the maternal blood, or the kidney, the original spirit, the middle Dantian (the region below the heart) and the left and the right orifices of the heart.

阳明阴灵【yáng míng yīn líng】 目视向外,为阳;耳听在内,为阴。指目、耳的生理功能作用。

Yang bright and Yin flexible Refers to the function and effect of the eyes and ears. In this term, Yang refers to the eyes that see externally and Yin refers to the ears that listen internally.

阳气【yáng qì】 与阴气相对,指人体内生理功能。

Yang Qi Refers to the internal physiological function of the body, opposite to that of Yin Qi.

阳气者,精则养神,柔则养筋【yáng qì zhě jīng zé yǎng shén róu zé yǎng jīn】 精指的是精微,柔指的是津液。阳气可生化,运输精微以养神气,又可输布津液以养筋脉。

Nourished by Yangqi, the spirit becomes refreshed; tonified by Yangqi, the sinew appears soft. The spirit refers to refined nutrient while softness refers to fluid and humor. Yang Qi can grow and transform in order to transmit refined nutrient to nourish the spirit and Qi as well as transport fluid and humor to nourish sinews and meridians.

阳蹻脉【yáng qiāo mài】 人体奇经八脉之一,起于足跟外侧。这一经脉为气功运行的一个常见部位。

Yang heel meridian One of the eight extraordinary meridians, starting from the lateral side of the heel. This meridian is a region usually used for practicing Qigong.

阳窍【yáng qiào】 指眼睛。

Yang orifice Refers to the eyes.

阳伸阴屈【yáng shēn yīn qū】 为气功的呼吸方法,呼伸吸屈以进行气体交换,吐故纳新。

Yang extending while Yin bending Refers to the method of respiration which exchanges Qi and the body through extending exhalation and bending inhalation, known as exhaling the old and inhaling the new.

阳神【yáng shén】 指习练气功,获得遥视、遥感之力为阴神。阴神再进一步坚固,出由人间,飞腾变化,任意所为,称之为阳神。

Yang spirit Refers to great change of Yin spirit which reflects the power of remote vision and sense in practicing Qigong. When Yin spirit is greatly strengthened and flies swiftly upwards with complete change, it will turns into Yang spirit.

阳神出现【yáng shén chū xiàn】 指习练气功,不受外魔内障的干扰,意识思维活动稳定而出现的良性现象。

appearance of Yang spirit Refers to practice of Qigong with stable activities of consciousness and thinking, during which it is not disturbed by external evil and internal cataract.

阳神主宰【yáng shén zhǔ zǎi】 指阳神变化,主使于性,即意念导引。

dictator of Yang spirit Means that Yang spirit changes and controls the activities of every aspects, known as consciousness Daoyin.

阳生阴长,阳杀阴藏【yáng shēng yīn cháng yáng shā yīn cáng】 指阴阳双方互相依存,阳气生化正常,能使阴气不断滋长。

Yang manages germination while Yin gov-

erns growth，Yang manages killing while Yin controls storage. Indicates that Yin and Yang depend on each other and Yang Qi naturally grows and transforms，enabling Yin Qi to constantly increase.

阳生阴长【yáng shēng yīn zhǎng】指阴阳相互为根。

Yang growing and Yin developing Indicates that Yin and Yang depend on each other.

阳盛则热，阴盛则寒【yáng shèng zé rè yīn shèng zé hán】 指阴阳失去平衡而有所偏胜，就会出现热象或寒象。阳气偏胜就会出现热象，阴气偏胜就会出现寒象。

Exuberant Yang causes heat while exuberant Yin causes cold. This is a celebrated dictum，indicating that imbalance of Yin and Yang will cause heat or cold phenomena. Usually unilateral dominance of Yang Qi causes heat while unilateral dominance of Yin Qi causes cold.

阳燧【yáng suì】 利用聚光原理，于日取火的器物称阳燧。

Yang apparatus Traditionally the principle of spotlight that takes fire from the sun is called Yang apparatus.

阳台宫【yáng tái gōng】 位于王屋山下，为晋代气功学家烟萝子修炼处。

Yangtai Mansion Located in the Wangwu Mountain where Yan Luozi, a great master of Qigong in the Jin Dynasty (266 AD - 420 AD)，studied and practiced Qigong.

阳维脉【yáng wéi mài】 人体奇经八脉之一，起于足跟外侧。这一经脉为气功运行的一个常见部位。

Yang link meridian One of the eight extraordinary meridians，starting from the lateral side of the heel. This meridian is a region usually used for practicing Qigong.

阳虚【yáng xū】 指身体阳气不足，功能衰退。临床治疗以练动功为主。

Yang deficiency Refers to insufficiency of Yang Qi in the body and decline of physiological functions. Clinical treatment of this disease depends on dynamic practice of Qigong.

阳虚则外寒，阴虚则内热 【yáng xū zé wài hán yīn xū zé nèi rè】 "阳虚"指命门火衰，"阴虚"指阴液不足。命门火衰，卫阳不足，不能温煦体表，就会出现怕冷之寒象。阴液不足，水不济火，阴不胜阳而发生内热（一种虚热）。

Yang deficiency leads to external cold while Yin deficiency results in external heat. Indicates that Yin deficiency refers to decline of fire in the life gate while Yin deficiency refers to insufficiency of Yin humor. When fire in the life gate is declined，defense Yang will be insufficient and cannot warm the body，causing coldness in the body. When Yin humor is insufficient，water cannot support fire. If Yin fails to surpass Yang，it will cause internal heat （deficiency heat）.

阳溢阴损【yáng yì yīn sǔn】 指阳气不固，阴精耗伤，多为情志喜哀太过所致。

Yang spilling and Yin wasting Refers to the fact that Yang Qi is weakened and Yin essence is injured，usually caused by excessive emotions of pleasure and anger.

阳中之阳【yáng zhōng zhī yáng】 指阳中有阳。

Yang within Yang　Yang within Yang indicates that there is Yang in Yang.

阳中之阴【yáng zhōng zhī yīn】　指阳中有阴。

Yin within Yang　Indicates that there is Yin in Yang.

杨继洲【yáng jì zhōu】　明代著名的针灸学家,重视气功研究,其学术著作中注重用引导法调理五脏。

Yang Jizhou　A great scholar of acupuncture and moxibustion in the Ming Dynasty (1368 AD–1644 AD) who also emphasized the study of Qigong. The monographs written by him paid great attention to the application of Qigong for regulating the five Zang-organs (including the heart, the liver, the spleen, the lung and the kidney).

杨氏周天功【yáng shì zhōu tiān gōng】　为静功,先扫除妄念,收视返听,以静定为基本,然后缓慢调息,精神内守,含光默默,注意丹田。

Yang's celestial exercise　A static exercise, marked by eliminating distracting thought first, contracting vision and returning listening, tranquilizing the mind as the foundation, then slowly regulating respiration, internally stabilizing the essence and spirit, silently containing brightness and paying attention to Dantian. Dantian is divided into upper Dantian (the region between the eyes), the middle Dantian (the region below the heart) and the lower Dantian (the region below the navel).

杨西山接气法【yáng xī shān jiē qì fǎ】　为静功。其作法为,虚心一志,内忘一己,外忘人物。朝则迎向东光,夕则广步月下。

Yang Xishang's exercise for obtaining

Qi　A static exercise, marked by stabilizing the heart with less desires, internally forgetting selfishness, externally forgetting any people and anything, turning to the east at sunrise and walking under the moon at sunset.

杨西山论宁神【yáng xī shān lùn níng shén】　源自气功学专论,主要论述宁神之道贵在"静"字,而静并非不动,宜动静结合。

Yang Xishan's discussion about tranquilizing the spirit　Collected from a monograph of Qigong, mainly discussing the importance of quietness for tranquilizing the spirit. Tranquility means to combine dynamic exercise with static exercise, not meaning without any action.

杨西山调气法【yáng xī shān tiáo qì fǎ】　为静功。其作法为,静坐,平心委气,呼吸勿令太急,勿令太缓,勿令有声,不急行,不久立,不多睡。

Yang Xishan's exercise for regulating Qi　A static exercise, marked by sitting quietly, stabilizing the heart, enriching Qi and preventing rapid breath with any voice as well as avoiding walking quickly, standing for a long time and sleeping for a long time.

杨羲【yáng xī】　晋代著名的气功学家,对道家气功的传播有积极作用。

Yang Xi　A great master of Qigong in the Jin Dynasty (226 AD–420 AD) who made great contribution to the dissemination of Qigong in Daoism.

仰和天真【yǎng hé tiān zhēn】　为动功,与对修常居同。常以两手按眉后小穴中十八次,坚持锻炼一年,能夜间看书、写字。

looking　and　harmonizing　celestial

truth A dynamic exercise, the same as normal residence for life cultivation, marked by pressing the small acupoints behind the eyes for eighteen times, persevering practice for a year, reading and writing at night.

养病庸言【yǎng bìng yōng yán】《养病庸言》为气功学专著，由清代沈子复所著，主要论述了气功养生疗病的方法。

Yangbing Yongyan（*General Discussion about Curing Diseases*） A monograph of Qigong entitled *General Discussion about Curing Diseases*, written by Shen Zifu in the Qing Dynasty（1636 AD – 1912 AD）, mainly describing the methods for curing diseases in practicing Qigong and life cultivation.

养齿法【yǎng chǐ fǎ】 为动功。其作法为，浓茶漱口，坚齿去蠹；夜漱齿，垢污尽除。

exercise for nourishing the teeth A dynamic exercise, marked by drinking strong tea rinsing the mouth and strengthening the teeth to eliminate turbidity; or rinsing the teeth in the evening to eliminate dirt.

养丹【yǎng dān】 源自气功专论，阐述习练气功的基本要领及功用。

nourishing Dan（**pills of immortality**） Collected from a monograph of Qigong, describing the requirements and function of Qigong practice.

养德【yǎng dé】 养德即养阴，德为阴。

nourishing virtue Refers to nourishing Yin. In Qigong, virtue refers to Yin.

养肺坐功法【yǎng fèi zuò gōng fǎ】为动功。其作法为，正坐，用两手着地缩身曲脊向上三举，两手反拳捶脊左右各三五次，闭目调息，咽液、叩齿为止。能养肺去胸间风毒邪气。

sitting exercise for nourishing the lung A dynamic exercise, marked by sitting upright, pressing the ground with both hands, shrinking the body and bending the spine upwards for three times, turning the fists to press the spine from the left to the right and vice versa for three to five times, closing the eyes, regulating respiration and stopping swallowing humor and clicking the teeth in three ways. To practice Qigong in such a way can nourish the lung and expel accumulation of toxic wind and pathogenic Qi in the chest.

养肝坐功法【yǎng gān zuò gōng fǎ】为动功。其作法为，正坐，两手相重，按股部，缓慢左右扭转身体。又用两手相交，翻复向胸，调息、咽津、叩齿止。可养肝，去肝经风邪积聚。

sitting exercise for nourishing the liver A dynamic exercise, marked by sitting upright, crossing the hands, pressing the thighs with both hands, turning round the body from the left to the right and vice versa, intersecting the hands to reach the chest for regulating respiration and stopping swallowing fluid and clicking the teeth. To practice Qigong in such a way can nourish the liver and expel accumulation of pathogenic wind in the liver meridian.

养老奉亲书【yǎng lǎo fèng qīn shū】《养老奉亲书》为医学专著，兼述气功养生，由宋代陈直所著。系统地论述了老年病的病机、病理及其防治。

Yanglao Fengqin Shu（*A Fragrant Book about Nourishing the Aged*） A monograph of traditional Chinese medicine with the discussion of Qigong and life cultivation entitled *A Fragrant Book*

about Nourishing the Aged, written by Chen Zhi yin the Song Dynasty（960 AD－1279 AD）, systematically discussing the pathogenesis, pathology, prevention and treatment of senile diseases.

养脑【yǎng nǎo】 指养肾才能养唾, 养唾才能养血,养血才能养精,养精才能养脑。

nourishing the brain Refers to the fact that only when the kidney is nourished can salvia be nourished, only when the saliva is nourished can the blood is nourished, only when the blood is nourished can the essence be nourished, and only when the essence is nourished can the brain be nourished.

养内【yǎng nèi】 指宁心定志,调养内在的形体。

nourishing the internal Refers to stabilizing the heart and deciding the will in order to regulate and to nourish the body.

养脾坐功法【yǎng pí zuò gōng fǎ】 为动功。其作法为,坐稳,伸一脚屈一脚,两手向后反擊。或跪坐,两手撑地,用力回头虎视,调息、咽津、叩齿止。能养脾,去脾脏积聚、风邪。

sitting exercise for nourishing the spleen A dynamic exercise, marked by sitting stably, stretching one foot and bending the other foot, turning the hands backwards; or sitting with kneeling, forcibly turning the head to observe, and stopping regulating respiration, swallowing fluid and clicking the teeth. To practice Qigong in such a way can nourish the spleen and expel accumulation of pathogenic wind in the spleen.

养气【yǎng qì】 指习练气功,纳自然清气入丹田。

Nourishing Qi Refers to entering the natural clear Qi into Dantian in practicing Qigong. Dantian is divided into the upper Dantian（the region between the eyes）, the middle Dantian（the region below the heart）and the lower Dantian（the region below the navel）.

养气以保神气清则神爽【yǎng qì yǐ bǎo shén qì qīng zé shén shuǎng】 阐明了气与神之间的关系。

Nourishing Qi can protect the spirit and clearing Qi can refresh the spirit. Expound the relation between Qi and the spirit.

养神【yǎng shén】 指习练气功,调节意识思维活动,不使神外散。

nourishing the spirit Refers to regulating the activities of consciousness and thinking in order to prevent dispersion of the spirit in practicing Qigong.

养神气法【yǎng shén qì fǎ】 为静功。其作法为,静坐、端身、屏尽万缘,使之表里清静,绵绵固守不动。

exercise for nourishing the spirit and Qi A static exercise, marked by sitting quietly and upright, eliminating any disturbance in order to tranquilize the external and internal sides and to concentrate the spirit and Qi in the body.

养神之道【yǎng shén zhī dào】 指养神的方法,即形体欲得劳动而不能疲极,精用而不能耗竭,意识纯和而没有杂念,神形合一而又保持稳态,恬淡而不妄为。

the way for nourishing the spirit Refers the methods for nourishing the spirit, including work without any tiredness, application of the essence without any exhaustion，purifying the mind without any distracting thought，integrating the spirit and body with stability and sincerity without any absurdity.

养肾坐功法【yǎng shèn zuò gōng fǎ】 为动功。其作法为，正坐，两手揉摩两耳至两胁肋，左右挽臂向空抛射，放松身体，两足向前后迈十余步，调息、咽津、叩齿止。能养肾，去腰间、肾、膀胱风邪、积聚。

sitting exercise for nourishing the kidney A dynamic exercise，marked by sitting upright，rubbing the ears and ribs with both hands，raising the shoulders to the space from the left to the right and vice versa，relaxing the body，walking forwards and backwards with both feet for dozens of steps，regulating respiration and stopping swallowing fluid and clicking the teeth. To practice Qigong in such a way can nourish the kidney and expel accumulation of pathogenic wind in the waist，the kidney and the bladder.

养生【yǎng shēng】 即调养身体，延续生命。养生内容广泛，方法众多，计有气功、食养、药养等。

nourishing life Regulating and nourishing the body in order to prolong life. The content of nourishing life is extensive with various methods，including Qigong and cultivation with food and medicinal.

养生辨疑诀【yǎng shēng biàn yí jué】 《养生辨疑诀》为气功专著，由唐代施肩吾所著，论述了气功养生的基本理论和方法。

Yangsheng Bianyi Jue（*Formula for Differentiating the Ways to Cultivate Life*） A monograph of Qigong enti-tled *Formula for Differentiating the Ways to Cultivate Life*，written By Shi Jianwu in the Tang Dynasty（618 AD - 907 AD），mainly describing the basic theory and practice of Qigong.

养生尽理【yǎng shēng jìn lǐ】 指通晓养生的道理。

awareness of life cultivation Refers to the ways to understand the principles for cultivating life.

养生揽要【yǎng shēng lǎn yào】 《养生揽要》为气功养生专著，收录了清代以前历代养生家的修身养性、延年益寿之术。作者不详。

Yangsheng Lanyao（*Key Points of Life Cultivation*） A monograph of Qigong entitled *Key Points of Life Cultivation*，collecting the techniques for cultivating health and prolonging life used by the masters of life cultivation before the Qing Dynasty（1636 AD - 1912 AD）. The author was unknown.

养生秘录【yǎng shēng mì lù】 《养生秘录》为气功学专著，记载了各种各样的气功养生专论，作者不详。

Yangsheng Milu（*Important Collection of Life Cultivation*） A monograph of Qigong entitled *Important Collection of Life Cultivation*，collecting various discussions and analyses of Qigong and life cultivation. The author was unknown.

养生秘旨【yǎng shēng mì zhǐ】 《养生秘旨》为气功养生专著，论述气功养生之道，介绍各种功法及作用。作者及成书年代不详。

Yangsheng Mizhi（*Important Principles for Cultivating Life*） A monograph of Qigong entitled *Important Principles for Cultivating Life*，describing the principles for practicing Qigong and cultivating life, and introducing th[...] ercises and effects of Qigong pract[...] The author and the related dyna[...] were unknown.

养生十三则【yǎng shēng shí sān zé】动静相兼功。其作法为,两手握固,闭目冥心;舌舐上腭,一意调心;神游水府,双擦两肾;心注(意想)尾闾,颇耸两肩;目视顶门,叩齿搅口;静运两目,频频咽气;澄神摩肤,手攀两足,俯身鸣鼓,数息凝神;摆腰洒腿,两手托天;左右开弓,平心静气;无人无我,心如止水;血遍体常暖,昼夜冲和;动静不二,和光同尘。久行之,补脑安神,调节脏腑功能,轻身耐老延年。

thirteen courses of life cultivation An exercise combined with dynamic exercise and static exercise, marked by firmly holding the hands, closing the eyes and tranquilizing the heart; licking the upper jaw with the tongue and regulating the heart with consciousness; promoting the spirit to move in water chamber and rubbing the kidneys with both hands; imagining the coccyx and raising the shoulders; observing the top, clicking the teeth and stirring the mouth; quietly moving the eyes and frequently swallowing Qi; clarifying the spirit, rubbing the skin and holding the feet with both hands; bending the body, clicking teeth and concentrating the spirit with several ways of respiration; shaking the waist, relaxing the legs and raising the hands to the sky; stretching the hands from the left to the right and vice versa in order to stabilize the heart and tranquilize Qi; quieting the heart like water without any sense of oneself and others; warming

[...]he blood in the whole body and har[...] [...]onizing the blood day and night; [...]eeping dynamic and static exercise for [...]rmony and balance. A long period of [...]acticing Qigong in such a way can [...]ify the brain, stabilize the spirit, [...]ulate the visceral functions, relax [...] body and prolong life.

养生息命诗【yǎng shēng xī mìng shī】[...]气功专论,主要阐述勤学气功可以[...]生长寿。

poems about nourishing life and protecting life Collected from a monograph of Qigong, mainly describing that diligently studying Qigong can nourish life and prolong life.

养生咏元集【yǎng shēng yǒng yuán jí】《养生咏元集》为气功专著,论述了气功的基本理论和方法。作者不详。

Yangsheng Yongyuan Ji (*Collection of Cultivating Life and Chanting the Origin*) A monograph of Qigong entitled *Collection of Cultivating Life and Chanting the Origin*, describing the theory and methods of Qigong practice. The author was unknown.

养生之道【yǎng shēng zhī dào】 指气功养生法。

the way for cultivating life Refers to the method for cultivating life in practicing Qigong.

养生至论【yǎng shēng zhì lùn】 清代《养生至论》为气功养生专著,汇集气功论述,介绍气功养生诸法。作者不详。

Yangsheng Zhilun (*Sincere Discussion about Life Cultivation*) A monograph of Qigong in the Qing Dynasty (1636 AD - 1912 AD) entitled *Sincere Discussion about Life Cultivation*, collecting all the discussions about Qigong and in-

Y

troducing all the exercises for prac
cing Qigong and cultivating life. The
author was unknown.

养生主【yǎng shēng zhǔ】 指养生
主要方面是养神。

nourishing the essential Refers to nourishing the spirit which is the most important stage for nourishing life.

养五脏五行【yǎng wǔ zàng wǔ xíng】
指培养五脏真气以协调各脏之间关系。

nourishing the five Zang-organs and activities Refers to nourishing the genuine Qi in the five Zang-organs (including the heart, the liver, the spleen, the lung and the kidney) in order to coordinate the relations among the five Zang-organs.

养五脏五行气法【yǎng wǔ zàng wǔ xíng qì fǎ】 为静功,利用五脏五行关系调气以养五脏,周而复始,精心为之,令五脏功能协调,可健身益寿。

exercise of Qi for nourishing the five Zang-organs and five activities A static exercise, referring to continuously and elaborately nourishing the five Zang-organs (including the heart, the liver, the spleen, the lung and the kidney) with the relation between the five Zang-organs and five activities in order to regulate the five Zang-organs, to fortify the body and to prolong life.

养心【yǎng xīn】 指爱养神明,安神,莫过于减少杂念,排除情欲。

nourishing the heart Refers to nourishing the mental activities, stabilizing the spirit, reducing distracting thought and eliminating lust.

养心坐功法【yǎng xīn zuò gōng fǎ】
为动功。其作法为,正坐,两手握拳用力

以一手按腕上,一手向下拓空如重
又以两手相叉,以脚踏手中。闭目
,三咽三叩齿而止。能养心去心胸间
,邪诸疾。

sitting exercise for nourishing the heart A dynamic exercise, marked by sitting upright, holding the fists with both hands in the same way, pressing the wrist with one hand, expanding the lower region with the other hand like a heavy stone, crossing the hands, treading the palms with the feet, closing the eyes to regulate respiration till swallowing saliva and clicking the teeth for three times respectively in order to nourish the heart, to eliminate pathogenic wind and to cure various diseases in the heart and chest.

养形不如养神【yǎng xíng bù rú yǎng shén】 指肾是形体生命活动中的表现,神去则行死。

Nourishing the body is no better than nourishing the spirit. Indicates that the spirit is more important than the body and that loss of the spirit will lose life.

养性【yǎng xìng】 指涵养本性,喻气功养生法入静,淡泊无为,意在涵养人的自然本性。

nourishing nature Refers to moistening and nourishing human nature, comparing to tranquility in indifference to fame and wealth in order to nourish the original and spiritual nature.

养性延命录【yǎng xìng yán mìng lù】
《养性延命录》为气功专著,由梁代陶弘景所著,为现存最早介绍五禽戏动作的文献。

Yangxing Yanming Lu (*Records of Cultivating Life and Prolonging Life*) A monograph of Qigong entitled *Records of Cultivating Life and Prolonging Life*, written by Tao Hongjing in the Liang Dynasty（502 AD－557 AD），which is the earliest literature to introduce the activities of Five Animals Exercises.

养性延命录运气治病法【yǎng xìng yán mìng lù yùn qì zhì bìng fǎ】　为静功。其作法为，"凡行气欲除百病，随所在念之，头痛念头，足痛念足，和气往攻之，从时至时，便自消矣"。

exercise for moving Qi and curing disease recorded by nourishing the body and prolonging life　A static exercise，marked by "moving Qi to cure various diseases，silently thinking the related region to relieve headache and foot pain，harmonizing Qi for a long time to disperse it naturally".

养正【yǎng zhèng】　指习练气功养生法，蒙昧静默，意识平和内存以养正气。

nourishing healthy Qi　Refers to the life cultivation exercise for practicing Qigong，marked by tranquilization of the mind and harmonization of consciousness in order to nourish the healthy Qi.

养志【yǎng zhì】　指涵养其志，喻气功养生法旨在调节意识活动，使之平和。

increasing will　Refers to moistening and nourishing the mind in order to decide the will，comparing to regulating and balancing the activity of consciousness in practicing Qigong and cultivation of life.

养中【yǎng zhōng】　指意识稳定以养身体中之精气。

nourishing the center　Refers to stabilizing the consciousness in order to nourish the essence and Qi in the body.

夭折【yāo zhé】　即寿命短，未及天年。

short life　Refers to failure to prolong life.

腰【yāo】　① 指人体部位名，躯干两侧，肋以下，髂嵴以上部分；② 指肾之府。

waist　Refers to ① either the name of the lateral sides of the trunk below the ribs and above the crista iliaca；② or the chamber of the kidney.

腰背疼痛症治法【yāo bèi téng tòng zhèng zhì fǎ】　动静相兼功。其作法为，立定，低头弯腰如下拜，闭气，手与脚尖齐，然后起身。息定再行，连行五七次止，日行三次。

exercise for curing lumbago and backache　An exercise combined with dynamic exercise and static exercise，marked by standing up，lowering the head，bending the waist，stopping respiration，corresponding the hands to the tiptoe，then standing up，practicing again when respiration is stabilized，continuing to practice for five to seven times，and practicing three times everyday.

腰功【yāo gōng】　为动功。其作法为，两手握固柱两胁肋，摆摇两肩二十四次。两手擦热，以鼻吸清气，徐徐从鼻放出，用两热手擦精门。

waist exercise　A dynamic exercise，marked by holding the rib-sides with both hands，shaking the shoulders for twenty-four times；then rubbing the hands hot，inhaling clear Qi through the nose，slowly exhaling through the nose and rubbing the essence gate with hot hands.

腰痛【yāo tòng】　气功适应证，主要由少阴虚、肾虚、风痹、坠堕伤腰、寝卧湿地

Y

所致。

lumbago An indication of Qigong, usually caused by deficiency of Shaoyin, deficiency of the kidney, wind impediment, damage of the waist and sleep in damp place.

腰痛不得俯仰候导引法【yāo tòng bù dé fǔ yǎng hòu dǎo yǐn fǎ】 为动功。其作法为,伸展两足而坐,两手放足趾上,活血通络,治腰痛如折,不能弯曲,瘀血唾血,久痛入络。伸展两足而坐,用两手握足趾七遍。

exercise of Daoyin for unmovable lumbago A dynamic exercise, marked by sitting, stretching the feet, putting the hands on the toes, activating the blood and dredging the collaterals for curing severe lumbago with inability to bend, blood stasis, spitting blood and chronic pain in the collaterals; then stretching the feet to sit and hold the toes with both hands for seven times.

腰痛候导引法【yāo tòng hòu dǎo yǐn fǎ】 为动功,方法多样。如一手向上尽量伸展,手掌向四方回转,一手向下用力按,两手掌相合,手指对撑,然后侧身,使身向一侧倾斜,旋转身体,似乎在看手掌向上。

exercise of Daoyin for lumbago A dynamic exercise with various methods, such as stretching one hand upward, turning the palm toward the four sides, pressing the lower region forcefully with the other hand, crossing both palms, corresponding the fists with the fingers, then leaning the body to one side, rotating the body, and seeming to see the palms raised up.

腰阳关【yāo yáng guān】 督脉中的一个穴位,位于后正中线,第四腰椎棘突下凹陷中,为气功中常用的意守部位。

Yaoyangguan（GB 34） An acupoint in the governor meridian, located in the back midline and below the spinous process of the fourth lumbar vertebra, which is the region for concentrating consciousness in practicing Qigong.

瑶池【yáo chí】 出于丹阙之前。

abode of immortals Refers to the abode before the red palace.

杳冥恍惚【yǎo míng huǎng hū】 指意识思维活动若有若无的状态。

distant obscure trance Refers to trance state of consciousness and thinking activities.

杳冥之事【yǎo míng zhī shì】 指气功状态下静寂则神守于内,目不外视,耳不外闻。

extreme tranquilization Refers to that only when Qigong practice is tranquilized can the spirit maintain inside the body, the eyes avoid to see anything outside and the ears refuse to listen any news outward.

咬实【yǎo shí】 为动功,即咬牙,每日行之可固齿。

clenching teeth Means to click the teeth in order to strengthen the teeth.

窅冥府【yǎo míng fǔ】 指真人呼吸处,为身体中空窍。

vacuum chamber Indicates that the breathing region of the immortal is the orifice in the body that communicates with the external world.

药火论【yào huǒ lùn】 源自气功专论,主要阐述气功中神是火,气是药,炼丹就是以神御气。

discussion about medicinal and fire Collected from a monograph of Qigong, mainly describing that in Qigong the spirit refers to fire and Qi refers to medicinal, and that refining Dan (pills of immortality) means to resist Qi with the spirit.

药取先天气【yào qǔ xiān tiān qì】 源自气功专论,主要阐述气功中药火的关系。

taking innate Qi from medicinal Collected from a monograph of Qigong, mainly describing the relationship between medicinal and fire in Qigong.

药物【yào wù】 ① 指结成内丹的阴阳两个方面的物质;② 指内丹;③ 指元阳。

medicinal Refers to ① either Yin and Yang in constituting internal Dan (pills of immortality); ② or internal Dan (pills of immortality); ③ or original Yang.

药物火候论【yào wù huǒ hòu lùn】 源自气功专论,阐述药物、火候、性命、真息的含义。

discussion about medicinal and heating Collected from a monograph of Qigong, describing the meaning of medicinal, heating, life and respiration.

药物阳内阴,火候阴内阳【yào wù yáng nèi yīn huǒ hòu yīn nèi yáng】 药物中精气属阴,神属阳。火候中武火为阳,文火为阴,进火为阳,退火为阴。

There is Yin within Yang in medicinal and there is Yang within Yin in heating. The essential Qi in medicinal pertains to Yin and the spirit pertains to Yang. In heating, strong fire is Yang, mild fire is Yin, flaming fire is Yang and annealing fire is Yin.

药祖丹基【yào zǔ dān jī】 指产丹之所,即丹田。

foundation of medicinal and Dan (pills of immortality) Refers to the place where Dan (pills of immortality) is produced, indicating Dantian. Dantian is divided into the upper Dantian (the region between the eyes), the middle Dantian (the region below the heart) and the lower Dantian (the region below the navel).

要道【yào dào】 即捷迳、关键。指习练气功的关键在于循序渐进,由浅入深,意诚志坚,定信不疑。

access Refers to crosscut and key, indicating that the importance of Qigong practice is to proceed step by step from the shallower to the deeper with firmness and confidence.

要知金液还丹法,自向家园下种栽【yào zhī jīn yè huán dān fǎ zì xiàng jiā yuán xià zhǒng zāi】 指习练金液还丹法,只在自己身内修炼,不必向外寻觅。

To know the exercise for turning golden humor to Dan (pills of immortality), one must plant in the homeland. Refers to only cultivating and refining inside the body without looking for externally in practicing Qigong for turning golden humor into Dan (pills of immortality).

野战【yě zhàn】 指龙(元神)虎(元精)交合的意思。

field operations Refer to combination of Loong (the original spirit) and tiger (the original essence).

业【yè】 佛家气功习用语,泛指一切神形活动。

action A common term of Qigong in Buddhism, usually referring to the activities of the spirit and the body.

业报【yè bào】 佛家气功习用语。佛学认为相应于善、恶业而得到的苦、乐果报,称为业报。

Y

occupational result　A common term of Qigong in Buddhism, referring to unhappy result and happy result due to moral action and immoral action.

业障【yè zhàng】　佛家气功习用语,指影响习练气功入静的精神活动和行为。

obstacle　A common term of Qigong in Buddhism, referring to failure to tranquilize in practicing Qigong due to the spiritual activity and action.

夜半【yè bàn】　指夜间二十三时至次日凌晨一时,也称"子时"。

midnight　Refers to Zi (the period of the day from 11 p.m. to 1 a.m.) at night.

夜半灵根灌清水,丹田浊气切须呵【yè bàn líng gēn guàn qīng shuǐ dān tián zhuó qì qiē xū hē】　为功法,即夜半练功,舌舐上腭,津液满口,慢慢咽下,以灌溉五脏。

At midnight spiritual root can irrigate clear water and turbid Qi in Dantian should breathe out.　This is a method for practicing Qigong, marked by practice at midnight, licking the upper palate with the tongue, enriching the mouth with fluid and humor, slowly swallowing saliva to irrigate the five Zang-organs (including the heart, the liver, the spleen, the lung and the kidney). Dantian is divided into the upper Dantian (the region between the eyes), the middle Dantian (the region below the heart) and the lower Dantian (the region below the navel).

液行夫妇【yè xíng fū fù】　五行相克,克者为夫,受克者为妇。如火克金,心液传肺液,即所谓液行夫妇。

movement of humor like parents　In the five elements (including wood, fire, earth, metal and water), restraint refers to father and being restrained refers to mother according to the theory and practice of Qigong. The so-called movement of humor like parents refers entrance of heart humor into lung humor, just like fire restraining metal among the five elements.

腋【yè】　肩下胁上之陷窝。

armpit　Refers to the depression below the shoulder and above the rib.

一【yī】　指根本,即生命之本,① 道家修心养性,守中抱一;② 儒家为存心养性,执中贯一;③ 佛家为明心见性,万法规一;④ 医家为虚心定性,抱元守一。指规律,即万事万物运动的法则。

one　Refers to the root, which means the origin of life. ① In Daoism, the root means to cultivate the mind for improving the disposition and to keep concentration for maintaining the integrity; ② in Confucianism, the root means to purify the heart for improving the disposition and to execute concentration for implementing the integrity; ③ in Buddhism, the root means to clear the heart for clarifying the disposition and to integrate all the principles; ④ in traditional Chinese medicine, the root means to tranquilize the heart for purifying the disposition and to protect the origin for keeping the integrity. One also refers to the principle for the movement and development of all the things.

一尘【yī chén】　指一世。儒谓之世,释谓之劫,道谓之尘。

a dirt　Refers to one century which was called century by Confucianism, calamity by Buddhism and dirt by Daoism.

一诚【yī chéng】 指专心专意。

a concentration Refers to concentrated contemplation and consciousness.

一乘【yī chéng】 佛家气功习用语,泛指最佳气功功法,能使人通向理想境界。

a passageway A common term of Qigong in Buddhism, referring to the best method in practicing Qigong, enabling people to reach the ideal state.

一秤金诀【yī chèng jīn jué】 这一术语与"十六字诀法"意思相同,为静功。一吸便提,气气归脐;一提便咽,水火相见。

a scale of golden formula Similar to the formula of sixteen-characters, is a static exercise, referring to sixteen important ways for strengthening health and treating any disease which are described with sixteen special Chinese characters. In practice, after inhalation, it must be enhanced. When any Qi is inhaled, it should be returned to the navel. When it is enhanced, it must be swallowed in order to coordinate water and fire.

一得永得【yī dé yǒng dé】 指习练气功,获得成效,终身有益。

constant benefit Refers to achievement of success and benefit in all life after practice of Qigong.

一鼎【yī dǐng】 指脑。

a cauldron Refers to the brain, which is the most important organ in the human body.

一动一静【yī dòng yī jìng】 指神形俱静,意识思维无一毫杂念。

activity and tranquility Refers to tranquility of both the spirit and body, indicating that there is no distracting thoughts in the mind.

一二三【yī èr sān】 气功文献中,一指一气,二指阴阳,三指阴阳交媾所生之物之丹。

one-two-three In the literature of Qigong, one refers to Qi, two refers to Yin and Yang, and three refers to Dan (pills of immortality) which is an object formed by integration of Yin and Yang.

一分为二【yī fēn wéi èr】 指世间一切事物,都可以分而为二。这是个普遍现象,这就是辩证法。从无限大到无限小的事物,均有阴阳对立的双方,一分为二,乃至于无穷。人体也不例外,含阴含阳,阴阳双方对立而存在于一体。一体中的任何一个部分,都可分而为二。

division of one into two Means that all the things in this world can be divided into two, which is an ordinary phenomenon and dialectics. From the infinitely largest things to the infinitely smallest things, all things contain two different sides like Yin and Yang, and thus dividing into two in infinity. The human body is the same, containing Yin and Yang in the whole body. Thus any part in the human body all can be divided into two aspects like Yin and Yang.

一符【yī fú】 指时间概念,一个时辰分三符,炼丹采药只在一符之间。

a mark Refers to an idea about time. In traditional Chinese calendar, one day is divided into twelve periods and one period is divided into three marks. To refine Dan (pills of immortality) and to collect medicinal are all just done in one mark.

一故神【yī gù shén】 指以脑神为主的

Y

全身各部神,集中统一于一。

spiritual concentration　Refers to unification of the spirit, mainly the mental spirit, in all parts of the body.

一好【yī hǎo】　①指纯一其好,思虑不杂;②又指唯一不二。

a goodness　Refers to ① either concentrated mind without any distracting thought; ② or only one without two, which means integration or combination.

一候【yī hòu】　指五日为一候。

a Hou　A Hou refers to a period of five days.

一壶天地【yī hú tiān dì】　指身体。气功家把人体喻为宇宙,人体即一小天地。

a small sky and earth　Refers to the human body which is compared to the universe in Qigong. It means that the human body is a small sky and earth.

一即一切,一切即一【yī jí yī qiè yī qiè jí yī】　佛家气功习用语,指一分为二,合二而一,事物对立而又统一。

One is all and all is one.　This is a common term of Qigong in Buddhism, indicating that one divides into two and two forms into one, which means that all the things are not only opposite to each other, but also unified to each other.

一纪【yī jì】　①指十二年为一纪;②《黄帝内经》指四年为一纪。

a period　Refers to ① either a period of twelve years; ② or a period of four years mentioned in Huangdi Neijing (entitled *Yellow Emperor's Internal Canon of Medicine*).

一节【yī jié】　指十五天为一气,三气为一节。

one Jie (a section of time)　Traditionally in China a period of fifteen days is called one Qi and a period of three Qi (45 days) is called one Jie (a section of time).

一竞【yī jìng】　指七日,即今之一周。

a Jing　Refers to a period of seven days, similar to one week.

一开一阖【yī kāi yī hé】　指呼吸,连续不绝。亦指一阴一阳。

constant respiration　Refers to constant breath. It also refers to Yin and Yang.

一灵【yī líng】　指人身之元神,即生命活动的主宰。

a destiny　Refers to the primordial spirit in the human body, which refers to the dominator of the life activities.

一门【yī mén】　指的是一类、一派也。门指道之门。《淮南子》说:"百事之根,皆出一门。"

one gate　Refers to one genre or one school or one style. In *Huai Nan Zi*, a great canon of traditional Chinese culture compiled in the West Han Dynasty (202 BC – 8 AD), it says that "The root of all things originates from one gate".

一面之神宗泥丸【yī miàn zhī shén zōng ní wán】　指头部眼、耳、鼻、舌、齿、发等神,均宗于泥凡,故有"脑中丹田,百神之主"。

Mud bolus (the brain) in spiritual temple　Indicates that the spirit in the eyes, ears, nose, tongue, teeth and hair all belongs to muddy pill. That is why it is traditionally believed that "Dantian in the brain is the controller of all the spirits in the body". Dantian refers to the upper Dantian (the region between the eyes), the middle Dantian (the region below the heart) and the lower Dantian (the region below the navel).

一念【yī niàn】 ① 指单一的精神活动;② 佛家气功习用语,指极短促之时刻;③ 指一心;④ 指念一次;⑤ 指意识活动。

a thought Refers to ① either a single activity of the spirit; ② or a short period of time, which is a common term of Qigong in Buddhism; ③ or the heart, which means concentrated contemplation; ④ or a thought; ⑤ or the activity of consciousness.

一念不生【yī niàn bù shēng】 佛家气功习用语,指行功中,思想意识活动相对静止。

no mental activity A common term of Qigong in Buddhism, indicating to relatively tranquilize the activities of thinking and consciousness in practicing Qigong.

一念动时皆是火,万缘寂处即生春
【yī niàn dòng shí jiē shì huǒ wàn yuán jì chù jí shēng chūn】 心头产生杂念,会导致人身产生烦恼,烦恼就会成为损坏健康的邪火。清除杂念,就能生机盎然。

Distracting thought causes fire while elimination of distracting thought protects life. Indicates that distracting thought makes people distraught and harms people's health. Only when distracting thought is eliminated can people live a healthy life.

一念相应【yī niàn xiāng yìng】 佛家气功习用语,指精神活动的相对静止,得到神形的稳定状态。

correspondence of tranquilization A common term of Qigong in Buddhism, indicating relatively tranquilizing the activity of the spirit and stability of the spirit and the body.

一气【yī qì】 ① 指构成万物的基本物质;② 指一气含阴阳两方面;③ 指三候为一气。

one Qi Refers to ① the basic materials that have formed various things; ② or Qi containing the two sides of Yin and Yang; ③ or the period of fifteen days.

一气化三清【yī qì huà sān qīng】 指一生二,二生三,三生万物。即万物从一气中来。三清即太清、玉清、上清。

one Qi transforming triple purity Indicates that one produces two, two produces three and three produces all things. It means that all the things come from Qi. In this term, the triple purity refers to great purity, beautiful purity and high purity.

一气生两仪【yī qì shēng liǎng yí】 指一气含阴、含阳两个方面。一气又指太极。

one Qi producing two forces Means that one Qi contains Yin and Yang, which means two different sides. In this term, the so-called one Qi also refers to Taiji which is the supreme pole of the universe.

一气盛而一气弱【yī qì shèng ér yī qì ruò】 指五脏之气一年四时之中相互制约,如春季木旺,肝属木,脾属土,木克土,故肝旺而脾弱。此五行相克的现象称为"一气盛而一气弱"。

exuberance of one Qi and deficiency of another Qi Indicates that Qi in the five Zang-organs (including the heart, the liver, the spleen, the lung and the kidney) controls each other in a year. For instance, in spring wood is exuberant. The liver pertains to wood, the spleen pertains to earth. Since wood restricts earth, the liver also restricts

Y

the spleen. Thus when the liver is exuberant, the spleen is weak. That is why the mutual restriction among the five elements (including wood, fire, earth, metal and water) is called "exuberance of one Qi and deficiency of another Qi".

一窍【yī qiào】　专指人身体中玄关一窍。指七窍之一，如眼、耳、鼻等。

an orifice　Refers to an abstruse orifice in the human body or one of the seven important orifices in the human body.

一切禅【yī qiē chán】　佛家气功功法。行功时，排除杂念，精神内守，形体放松；行功时，凝神入静，专注一境，静而生慧；行功时，常存善念，稳定精神，利己利他（众生）。

all meditation　A common term of Qigong in Buddhism, which means to avoid distracting thought, to keep the spirit inside the body, to relax the body, to tranquilize the mind, to concentrate on a special state, to calm down in order to increase wisdom, to keep good will, to stabilize the spirit and to benefit all the people.

一切法【yī qiē fǎ】　指诸法而言：一者有为法，二者无为法，三者无尽法。

all rules　Refer to the rules in all the fields, in which the first indicates existence of all rules, the second indicates no existence of rules and the third indicates existence of part of the rules.

一切门禅【yī qiē mén chán】　佛家气功习用语，指有觉有观禅，与喜俱禅，与乐俱禅，与舍具之禅。四种禅即一法的四个阶段。从静虚而入寂定，协调全身各部，清净形神（身心）。

all meditation　A common term of Qigong in Buddhism, referring to con-sciousness of dhyana, enjoying of dhyana, happiness of dhyana and contribution of dhyana. The four ways of dhyana refer to the four stages of Qigong practice, which can enter into tranquilization from quietness, regulate all regions in the body and tranquilize the body and spirit.

一切时【yī qiē shí】　佛家气功习用语，指一天中任何时间，均可练功。

all time　A term of Qigong, indicating that Qigong can be practiced at any time in a day.

一切智【yī qiē zhì】　佛家气功习用语。① 指无所不知；② 指三智之一；③ 指对现象共性的认识。

all wisdom　A common term of Qigong in Buddhism, referring to ① either omniscience; ② or one of three wisdoms; ③ or consensus.

一切法通【yī qiè fǎ tōng】　佛家气功习用语。指习练气功，认识各种功法的基础理论，应用技能，具有分析研究的能力。

perforation of all practice　A common term of Qigong in Buddhism, referring to practice of Qigong with special function based on the theoretical foundation of various Qigong exercise, practical techniques and analytic ability.

一切行禅【yī qiè xíng chán】　佛家气功功法。为行禅的汇集，初禅摄心止念，正念思维，逐步排除邪念，而入寂静。久行之，通达心性，圆明无碍，清净而无染着，自利利他。并能作种种变现，以慧相应，洞察明了世间事物。

Constant practice of dhyana　The way of practicing Qigong in Buddhism, indicating the collection of dhyana practice. To practice dhyana, one must tranquilize the mind, purify the ideas and eliminate demon. A long period of constant dhyana practice will enable one to understand mental temperament, to eliminate any obstacle, to avoid any confusion and to benefit oneself and others, enabling one to reform anything, to correspond anything and to understand the whole world.

一切种智【yī qiè zhǒng zhì】　佛家气功习用语。① 指三智之一智；② 指对一切现象的认识；③ 指用作个性和共性的综合认识。

all kinds of wisdom　A common term of Qigong in Buddhism, ① one of the three wisdoms；② knowledge of all phenomena；③ comprehensive knowledge of individuality and generality.

一如【yī rú】　佛家气功习用语，指不二不异，为真如之理也。

a steadfastness　A common term of Qigong in Buddhism, referring to reality without any change.

一三昧【yī sān mèi】　佛家气功习用语，指的是专心一事。

one-three concentration　A common term of Qigong in Buddhism, which means concentrated attention.

一三五【yī sān wǔ】　指阳数为一、三、五，始于一，终于九，中为五。

one-three-five　One, three and five all refer to the numbers of Yang. In terms of numbers, Yang ends at nine and five is the middle number of Yang.

一赏【yī shǎng】　意识活动集中之意，指习练儒家气功，意识集中，神形合一。

an appreciation　Refers to concentrated contemplation and consciousness in order to integrate the body and the spirit.

一生二【yī shēng èr】　指一分为二，一种事物可分为阴阳对立的两个方面。

two from one　Means that one can be divided into two, indicating that one thing can be divided into two different aspects like Yin and Yang.

一生两尔【yī shēng liǎng ěr】　指世间一切事物，都可以分而为二。这是个普遍现象，这就是辩证法。从无限大到无限小的事物，均有阴阳对立的双方。一分为二，乃至于无穷。人体也不例外，含阴含阳，阴阳双方对立而存在于一体。一体中的任何一个部分，都可分而为二。

two sides in life　Means that all the things in this world can be divided into two, which is an ordinary phenomenon and dialectics. From the infinitely largest things to the infinitely smallest things, all things contain two different sides like Yin and Yang, and thus dividing into two in infinity. The human body is the same, containing Yin and Yang in the whole body. Thus any part in the human body all can be divided into two aspects like Yin and Yang.

一时【yī shí】　指的是四季之一季及一个时期。

a time　Refers to either one season in a year, or a certain period of time.

一体【yī tǐ】　指神形和一。

an integration　Refers to the integration of the body and spirit.

一妄【yī wàng】　佛家气功习用语，指迷妄之心，为意识散乱。

a confusion　A common term of Qigong in Buddhism, referring to perplexed mind or mental confusion.

一物【yī wù】　指一类事物。

a matter　Refers to a category of objects in the world.

一息【yī xī】　时间单位，一呼一吸为一

Y

息。指念头，为意识活动。

a breath Refers to breathing in and breathing out, indicating idea and consciousness activity.

一息尚存皆可复命【yī xī shàng cún jiē kě fù mìng**】** 指生命一息尚存，均可习练气功，救护命宝。

Embodiment of vitality preserves life. Indicates that when a person is alive he must practice Qigong in order to protect his life.

一息神气注于气海而长生 【yī xī shén qì zhù yú qì hǎi ér cháng shēng**】** 源自气功专论。主要阐述神与气相守则能健康长寿。

Entrance of spiritual Qi into the Qi sea can prolong life. This sentence is collected from a monograph of Qigong and is a special description about Qigong, describing that combination of the spirit and Qi protects health and longevity.

一向【yī xiàng**】** 佛家气功习用语，指意向于一处而无余念，意识活动不分散。

a direction A common term of Qigong in Buddhism, referring to a concentrated contemplation without any different ideas.

一心【yī xīn**】** ① 指专心一志；② 指一个念头，更无余念；③ 指脑及其精神活动。

concentrated heart Refers to ① either concentrated emotion; ② or a concentrated idea without any other ideas; ③ or concentrated mental and spiritual activities.

一心不乱【yī xīn bù luàn**】** 佛家气功习用语，指习练气功，精神专注无散乱。

the heart without any chaos A common term of Qigong in Buddhism, referring

to practice of Qigong with concentrated meditation and without any confusion.

一心三观法【yī xīn sān guān fǎ**】** 为静功。其作法为，结跏趺坐，先修空观，破见思之惑，得一切智，而证真谛之理；次修假观，破尘沙之惑，得道种智，而知假谛恒沙之法门；后修中观，破无明之惑，得一切种智，而证中道法身。

one heart and triple observation A static exercise, marked by sitting in lotus position, revising empty concept first, eliminating confusion, cultivating the mind to increase wisdom, testifying truth; then revising false sense, eliminating foul confusion, increasing wisdom and understanding any ways of mendacity; and finally revising medium perception, clearing any confusion, obtaining any wisdom in order to reach the perfect stage.

一心三智【yī xīn sān zhì**】** 佛家气功习用语，认为修习般若，集中精神，专注于一（一个念头、一个景物），即所谓"一念心"，可顿得三智之果，从而丰富智慧，用不着分阶段进行。三智指一切智，一切种智，道种智。得三智后即能断除烦恼，稳定情绪，获得安乐。

one mind and three wisdoms A common term of Qigong in Buddhism, referring to earnestly practice of Qigong with highest wisdom in order to concentrate the spirit and to focus on one idea. Traditionally it is known as "one mental idea", expressing the result of the three kinds of wisdom that has constantly enriched the wisdom without separating any stages. The so-called three kinds of wisdom refer to all wisdom, all kinds of wisdom and all difference of wisdom. If the three kinds of wisdom have been obtained, one can eliminate annoyance, stabilize emotion and obtain peace and happiness.

一阳来复【yī yáng lái fù】 古人认为，天地之间有阴阳二气，每年到了冬至日，阴气尽，阳气开始复生，叫阳来复。意义非凡。

reflex of Yang Believed in ancient times that there were Yin Qi and Yang Qi between the sky and earth and that Yin Qi began to dispel and Yang Qi began to resuscitate each year in winter solstice. That is why it is called reflex of Yang.

一阳生【yī yáng shēng】 指冬至后白天见长，古人认为阳气初生，故称冬至为一阳生。以一天而言，子时阳气初生，故称子时为一阳生。

growth of all Yang After winter solstice, daytime gradually becomes longer, and, according to the idea of people from ancient times, Yang Qi begins to grow. That is why winter solstice is called growth of all Yang. In every day, Yang Qi begins to grow from Zi (the period of a day from 11 p. m. to 1 a. m.). That is why the period from Zi (the period of a day from 11 p. m. to 1 a. m.) is called growth of all Yang.

一叶蔽目【yī yè bì mù】 指小能蔽大，切断目耳听视之觉，可以存神于内而不散。

shading the eyes with a leaf Means that the small can shelter the large, indicating to cut off the hearing and seeing of the ears and eyes in order to keep the spirit inside the body without any dispersion.

一异法【yī yì fǎ】 佛家气功功法。其作法为，结跏趺坐，调节精神，稳定意识活动，保持形神松静自适。其功效为治理偏执、妄念、烦恼、惊怖。

a special method An exercise of Qigong in Buddhism, marked by sitting in lotus position, regulating the essence and the spirit, stabilizing the activity of consciousness, ensuring tranquilization the body and the spirit. Such an exercise of Qigong practice in Buddhism can relieve bigotry, delusion, annoyance and terror.

一意【yī yì】 ① 指意识集中为一；② 指一个意念活动，为专心一意。

a thought Refers to ① either integration of consciousness in the mind; ② or concentrated thinking, which means greatest attention.

一意归中【yī yì guī zhōng】 这一概念中的中为气穴，意为神，即神驭气，凝神入气穴。

entrance of mentality in the middle Refers to Qi acupoint and mentality refers to the spirit, indicating that the spirit controls Qi and enters the Qi acupoint.

一阴生【yī yīn shēng】 指夏至后白天渐短，古人认为阴气初生，故称夏至为一阴生。以一日而言，午为阴气初生，故称午时为一阴生。

growth of all Yin After summer solstice, daytime gradually becomes shorter, and, according to the idea of people from ancient times, Yin Qi begins to grow. That is why summer solstice is called growth of all Yin. In every day, Yin Qi begins to grow from Wu (the period of a day from 11 a. m. to 1 p. m.). That is why the period from Wu (the period of a day from 11 a. m.

to 1 p.m.) is called growth of all Yin.

一阴一阳【yī yīn yī yáng】 指事物的阴、阳两个方面。

one Yin and one Yang Refers to the two sides of anything like Yin and Yang.

一阴一阳之谓道论【yì yīn yì yáng zhī wèi dào lùn】 源自论气功专论。主要说明气功动静、有无、龙虎、水火、日月等为阴阳两个方面。练功的作用在于调节身体阴阳，使之阴平阳秘。

discussion of Yin and Yang pertaining to Dao Collected from a monograph of Qigong, indicating that movement and quietness, existence and nothingness, Loong and tiger, water and fire as well as the sun and the moon all belong to the performance of Yin and Yang. The function of Qigong practice depends on regulating and balancing Yin and Yang in the body.

一元【yī yuán】 ① 指的是事物的开始；② 指阴阳未分的混沌状态；③ 指合二而一，即阴阳和合之意。

primary origin Refers to ① either the beginning of anything; ② or chaotic condition of Yin and Yang; ③ or two combined into one, indicating the integration of Yin and Yang.

一真【yī zhēn】 指精气神合而为一，或阴阳相互育。

a truth Refers to either integration of the essence, Qi and spirit; or combination of Yin and Yang.

一指头禅【yī zhǐ tou chán】 为静功，即思想活动集中于指头而不分散。

one finger zen Refers to a static exercise, indicating that the activity of thinking focuses on the finger without any dispersion.

一致不久【yī zhì bù jiǔ】 指神形合调，神守于内，须臾即能使意识活动保持稳定状态。

constant stability Indicates that the body and the spirit are harmonized, the spirit is kept inside the body, and the activity of consciousness is stabilized.

医衡【yī héng】 《医衡》为中医学专著，由明末清初沈时誉所著，论述了中医的理法方药，也论述了气功养生。

Yi Heng A monograph of traditional Chinese medicine, written by Shen Shiyu in the late Ming Dynasty (1368 AD‑1644 AD) and early Qing Dynasty (1636 AD‑1912 AD). This monograph not only discussed the theory and practice of traditional Chinese medicine, but also discussed the exercises of Qigong for nourishing life.

医家功【yī jiā gōng】 指以医学理论为指导创制的功法，原于医家。

medical achievement Refers to the achievement method created according to the theory of traditional Chinese medicine.

医说【yī shuō】 《医说》为中医学专著，由宋代张杲所著，书中除论述医学外，也论述了气功的理论和方法。

Yi Shuo(*Theory of Traditional Chinese Medicine*) A monograph of traditional Chinese medicine entitled *Theory of Traditional Chinese Medicine*, written by Zhang Gao in the Song Dynasty (960 AD‑1279 AD). This monograph not only discussed the theory and clinical practice of traditional Chinese medicine, but also discussed the theory and exercises of Qigong.

医统调法【yī tǒng tiáo fǎ】 为静功。其作法为，通过调身、调气、调神以补脑安神,调和五脏,通经活络之功。

exercise of medical regulation A static exercise, referring to regulation of the body, Qi and spirit for tonifying the brain, stabilizing the spirit, regulating the five Zang-organs (including the heart, the liver, the spleen, the lung and the kidney), unblocking the meridians and activating the collaterals.

壹气孔神兮,于中夜存 【yī qì kǒng shén xī yú zhōng yè cún】 指气合于神,神合于气,于夜中交融,不相悖离。

concentrating Qi in the spirit and coordinating at night Indicates that Qi is combined with the spirit and the spirit is combined with Qi at night without any deviation.

壹于道【yī yú dào】 即精神意识活动专一。

concentrating in Dao Refers to concentrating the activities of the spirit and consciousness.

移精变气【yí jīng biàn qì】 ① 指移易和改变病人的精气,使之精神内守,则病自愈;② 指转移患者的精神,改变患者脏气紊乱的状况。

moving essence and changing Qi Refers to ① either moving and changing the essence and Qi in patients for internally concentrating the essence and spirit for curing disease; ② or transferring the essence and the spirit of patients for improving the disorder of visceral Qi.

遗精导引法【yí jīng dǎo yǐn fǎ】 为动动。其作法为,半夜子时,阳正兴时仰卧,瞑目闭口,舌舐上腭,将腰拱起,左手中指顶住尾闾穴,右手大指顶住无名指根,将两腿伸直,两足十趾上翘,提起一口气,心中存想着脊背脑后,上贯至顶门,慢慢直下至丹田,方将腰腿脾手从容

放下,再照前行,阳则衰矣。

exercise of Daoyin for curing spermatorrhea A dynamic exercise, marked by lying on the back at midnight with exciting Yang, closing the eyes and mouth, licking the upper jaw with the tongue, and hunching up the waist; pushing the acupoint in the coccyx with the middle finger in the left hand, pushing the root of the fourth finger with the thumb in the right hand, stretching the feet, raising the ten toes, and lifting Qi in the mouth; imagining to observe from the spine, body back and brain back to the top of the head and finally to the lower Dantian (the region below the navel); then laying down the waist, legs, spleen and hands, then walking forward along the light to decline Yang.

遗精治法【yí jīng zhì fǎ】 为动静相兼功。其作法为,侧坐,用双手扳两脚心,先搬左脚心,擦热,运气行功九口。次搬右脚心,同前行之。

exercise for curing spermatorrhea An exercise combined with dynamic exercise and static exercise, marked by sitting at one side, pulling the soles with both hands, pulling the left sole first to rub hot, moving Qi for nine times; then pulling the right sole with the previous way.

遗尿【yí niào】 气功适应证,指膀胱失于制约,小便不禁。多因肾气不足,膀胱之气不固所致。

enuresis An indication of Qigong, referring to incontinence of urine due to failure of the bladder to control caused by insufficiency of kidney Qi and weakness of bladder Qi.

Y

遗尿候导引法【yí niào hòu dǎo yǐn
fǎ】 为动功。其作法为,蹲下,臀部离
地约一尺,用两手从膝外侧弯曲处深入
至足背上,以手握住足五趾,尽力握一
次,使五趾内弯,通利腰髋。

exercise of Daoyin for enuresis A dynamic exercise, marked by squatting
with one Chi from the buttocks to the
ground, reaching the hands deeply to
the acrotarsium from along the lateral
side of the knees, holding the five toes
with one hand for one time to bend the
five toes for normalizing the waist and
hip.

遗泄治法【yí xiè zhì fǎ】 为动静相兼
功。其作法为,晚七至十一时,一手兜阴
囊,一手搓擦脐下丹田处八十一次,然后
换手,每手各行九次。九日可见效,八十
一日功成。

exercise for curing emission An exercise combined with dynamic exercise
and static exercise, marked by practicing from 7 - 11 hours at night; holding
the scrotum with one hand and rubbing
the lower Dantian (the region below
the navel) with the other hand and vice
versa for eighty-one times respectively,
during which each hand moves for nine
times. After nine days of practice, the
treatment is effective; after eighty-one
days of practice, the treatment is succeeded.

颐【yí】 ① 指人体部位,即颊、腮;
② 指修养、保养。

cheek Refers to ① either a part of the
body; ② or cultivating life and nourishing health.

颐养诠要【yí yǎng quán yào】 《颐养
诠要》为气功养生学专著,由清代冯曦所
著,主要阐述养生而调神,其推崇太乙真

人养生七法。

Yiyang Quanyao(*Nourishing the cheek
and explaining the importance*) A
monograph of Qigong and life cultivation entitled *Nourishing the cheek and
explaining the importance*, written by
Feng Xi in the Qing Dynasty (1636
AD - 1912 AD), mainly describing the
ways to cultivate life and to regulate the
spirit, highly praising Taiyi Immortal's
seven ways for cultivating life.

颐真【yí zhēn】 为养真之意,即习练
气功养生法。

genuine cheek Refers genuine cultivation, indicating the exercise for practicing Qigong and cultivating life.

乙木之脏【yǐ mù zhī zàng】 指肝脏,
肝在五行属木,配天干为乙,故为乙木
之脏。

Yimu viscus Refers to the liver which
pertains to wood in the five elements
(including wood, fire, earth, metal
and water). In the ten Heavenly
Stems, the liver pertains to Yi, that is
why the liver is also called Yimu.

已漏【yǐ lòu】 指已婚,精漏泄者。

excretion Refers to seminal emission
after marriage.

以黑见红【yǐ hēi jiàn hóng】 指运北
方水中之金(即黑),以制南方火中之木
(即红)。

seeing red from black A term of
Qigong, refers to the metal in the water in the north and the wood in the
fire in the south. In this term, the so-
called metal refers to black and the so-
called wood refers to red.

以红投黑【yǐ hóng tóu hēi】 即"运南
方离宫之火(即红),以炼北方水中之金
(即黑),是为以红投黑,则凝神入坤脐而

生药"。

Red promoting black Refers to using detached palace (red) in the south to practice metal (black) in water, indicating red promoting black, finally entering the spirit into the navel as a medicinal to relieve any disorders.

以火炼药【yǐ huǒ liàn yào】 指神为火,气为药。即神御气之谓也。

refining spiritual medicine with fire Refers to the fact that the spirit is fire and Qi is medicinal, indicating that the spirit controls Qi.

以空为本【yǐ kōng wéi běn】 指习练气功时,调节精神意识活动,以精神意识活动相对静止为入静安神的根本。

taking vacuum as root Refers to regulating the activities of the spirit and consciousness in practicing Qigong. Only when the activities of the spirit and consciousness are static can the mind be tranquilized and the spirit be stabilized.

以乐和阴阳法【yǐ lè he yīn yáng fǎ】 为静功。其作法为,正身安坐,凝神息虑良久,意想乐从慎重处,然后默念。久行之,脑通神明,形养精气,阴变于阳,阳变于阴,阴阳相得,乃能成治。

exercise for harmonizing Yin and Yang A static exercise, marked by sitting quietly, concentrating the spirit for a long time, thinking prudently and reading silently. Such a way of practicing Qigong for a long time will clarify the brain, nourish the essential Qi and coordinate Yin and Yang marked by Yin changing into Yang and Yang changing into Yin.

以神归气穴,丹道自然成 【yǐ shén guī qì xué dān dào zì rán chéng】 指极精炼地,凝神入气穴,就是内丹之道。

Transmiting the spirit into Qi point, the way of Dan will be perfect. Refers to the fact that extreme practice of Qigong in the quiet place will transmit the spirit into the Qi point, which is the right way of internal Dan (pills of immortality).

以恬愉为务【yǐ tián yú wéi wù】 指排除一切干扰,以心情安静、愉快为目的。

tranquil and calm as task Refers to eliminating any disturbance in order to tranquilize the mind.

以意气攻病法【yǐ yì qì gōng bìng fǎ】 为静功。其有宿患,但用意并气,注之患处。不过三五日必愈。

curing disease with consciousness and Qi A static exercise, marked by transmitting consciousness and Qi into the location of disease. After three to five days of practicing Qigong in such a day, the disease will be cured.

以意想注【yǐ yì xiǎng zhù】 即用意念运气攻逐病所,以祛除病邪。

elimination of disease without consciousness Refers to movement of Qi with consciousness in order to expel diseases and to eliminate pathogenic factors.

以自得为功【yǐ zì dé wéi gōng】 指气功养生要随遇而安。

self-satisfaction as contribution Refers to reconciliation oneself to one's situation in practicing Qigong for cultivating health.

忆【yì】 ① 指回忆,意念;② 指想念;③ 指佛家气功专心一处而不忘。

memory Refers to ① either recalling and consciousness; ② or missing; ③ or concentration without any obliviousness

Y

in Buddhism.

忆持【yì chí】　佛家气功用语,指记忆力强而不忘。

strong memory　A common term of Qigong in Buddhism, referring to good memory without any obliviousness.

异人【yì rén】　即不同一般,异于常人。常指习练气功后,出现的一种奇特现象。

unusual person　Refers to a person different from ordinary people, indicating a special phenomenon after practice of Qigong.

抑喜以养阳气【yì xǐ yǐ yǎng yáng qì】　喜则伤心,心阳受损,故欲养阳气务使过喜,以调节精神,益养阳气。

restraining excitement to nourish Yang Qi　A celebrated dictum, indicating that excitement injures the heart and damages Yang in the heart, and that only when excitement is restrained and the spirit is regulated can Yang Qi be nourished.

役神之舍【yì shén zhī shè】　泛指两眼,眼为神之窍。

special orifice of the spirit　Refers to the eyes that act as the orifices of the spirit.

易【yì】　①指《易经》;②指日月的相互运动;③指阴阳;④指刚柔。

Yi　Refers to ① either Yijing (*Simplification, Change and No Change*), the first canon in China, which is the origin of traditional Chinese civilization; ② or mutual movement of the sun and the moon; ③ or Yin and Yang; ④ or hardness and softness.

易伏猛兽,难降寸心【yì fú měng shòu nán jiàng cùn xīn】　指猛兽容易降伏,但人的意念却不容易控制。说明初学气功者在练功过程中思想入静的不

易,需要在入静、意守上狠下功夫,才能进入气功状态。

It is easy to tame wild animals, but it is difficult to control human heart.　Refers to the fact that those who first practice Qigong are not easy to tranquilize the mind. Only when the mind is tranquilized and the consciousness is well controlled can those who practice Qigong really reach the state of Qigong.

易简【yì jiǎn】　指学习气功在于明白天地阴阳,又指气功基本理论易简不繁杂。

easiness and simplification　Refers to either understanding the sky and the earth as well as Yin and Yang in studying Qigong; or the basic theory of Qigong that is simple, not complicated.

易筋【yì jīn】　易即变化之意,易筋是改变体质之意。

physique change　Refers to changing the physique through the practice of Qigong.

易筋经图势功法【yì jīn jīng tú shì gōng fǎ】　动静相兼功,方法多样。如站立,两足并拢,身体正直,两手如拱放于胸前,定心息气,心存静极。

exercise for activating sinews and postures　An exercise combined with dynamic exercise and static exercise with various methods. One of the methods is to stand up with both feet put together, straightening the body, putting the hands over the chest, stabilizing the heart with respiration and tranquilizing the mind.

易筋图说功法【yì jīn tú shuō gōng fǎ】　为动功,方法多样。如面向东而站,头微上仰,目微上视,两足与肩宽窄

相齐，脚站平，不可前后参差。两臂下垂，肘微弯曲，掌心向下，十指尖朝前点，数四十九。

exercise for vividly activating sinews　A dynamic exercise with various methods. One of the methods is to stand up in the east side，mildly raising the head，mildly raising the eyes，aligning the extent of the two feet and the two shoulders，keeping the feet stable without any irregularity，drooping the arms，slowly bending the elbows with the palms turning downwards and the ten fingers stretching forwards for forty-nine times.

易经【yì jīng】　《易经》为哲学名著，约成书于殷周之际，战国时即列为经典，被誉为众经之首，是中国文明的源头。其内容主要反映上古自然、社会的复杂关系，是研究人与自然、社会的珍贵历史文献。

Yijing（*Simplification，Change and No Change*）　The most important canon of philosophy in ancient China，was compiled in the Shang Dynasty（1600 BD - 1046 BD）and Zhou Dynasty（1046 BD - 256 BD），the first canon in China and the origin of Chinese civilization. This first Chinese canon and first Chinese philosophy mainly reflects the complicated relationship between the natural world and the social world，and is the most important historic literature about human beings，natural world and social world.

易外别传【yì wài bié zhuàn】　《易外别传》为气功专著，由元代俞琰所述，解说气功的基本理论和功法。

Yiwai Beichuan（*Special Inheritance of Yijing*）　A monograph of Qigong enti-

tled *Special Inheritance of Yijing*，compiled by Chao Yuyan in the Yuan Dynasty（1271 AD - 1368 AD），explaining the basic theory and practice of Qigong.

易益之道【yì yì zhī dào】　指气功养生法荣养精神，变易形体，并使之轻健、延年。

exercise for improvement and change　Refers to nourishing the essence and spirit and simply changing the body in order to cultivate health and to prolong life.

益龄单【yì líng dān】　《益龄单》为气功养生学专著，由明代周履靖所著，主要收集前任养生学经验，注重气功调摄。

Yiling Dan（*Collection of Beneficial Experiences*）　A monograph of Qigong and life cultivation entitled *Collection of Beneficial Experiences*，written by Zhou Lǚjing in the Ming Dynasty（1368 AD - 1644 AD），collecting previous experiences in practicing life cultivation and paying great attention to Qigong for nourishing the body.

益龄养生法【yì líng yǎng shēng fǎ】　源自气功专论，主要阐述气功及饮食，睡眠养生的基本道理及具体作法。

beneficial exercise for life cultivation　Collected from a monograph of Qigong，mainly describing Qigong and diet as well as the basic theory and methods for cultivating life by sleeping.

益易【yì yì】　指有益于精的生成，形体的变易。即通过习练气功，强壮体质，改变身体不健康的面貌。

beneficial change　Refers to benefit for producing essence and changing the body. That means practice of Qigong

Y

can strengthen the body and change unhealthy body into healthy body.

意【yì】 ① 指思量、思虑；② 指末那识为意；③ 指一切精神活动；④ 指意根，为六根之一，即意产生的精神活动。

contemplation Refers to ① either consideration；② or manas consciousness；③ or all activities of the spirit；④ or the root of consciousness，which is one of the six roots，referring to the activity of the spirit produced by consciousness.

意地【yì dì】 佛家气功习用语，指精神意识活动产生的根源。

contemplation source A common term of Qigong in Buddhism，referring to the original source produced by the activities of the spirit and consciousness.

意马心猿【yì mǎ xīn yuán】 指意识活动如马奔驰在外，如猿活动不止。

horse mind and monkey heart（restless and whimsical） Indicates that the activity of consciousness is just like a horse running outside and like a monkey acting incessantly.

意气常饱【yì qì cháng bǎo】 以意念导引气入腹中，如食物后之饱满。

constant fullness of conscious Qi Indicates that consciousness leads Qi into the abdomen，just like eating enough food.

意生身【yì shēng shēn】 指习练气，意识稳定，神形和调，形体精神，通达无碍。

consciousness promoting the body Refers to stabilizing consciousness，regulating the spirit and body，clearing the body and the spirit in practicing Qigong.

意识【yì shí】 ① 指精神活动，为意念、意想、记忆、识别、认识之意；② 指佛

家气功习用语，指意根引起的识。

consciousness Refers to ① activity of the spirit related to idea，imagination，memory，recognition and cognition；② or insight formed by the root of consciousness，which is a common term of Qigong in Buddhism.

意为媒【yì wéi méi】 源自气功专论，说明意念是调节形神，使之稳定的关键。

consciousness for intermediary Collected from a monograph of Qigong，indicating that consciousness regulates the body and the spirit and is the key to stability.

溢饮【yì yǐn】 气功适应证，指饮溢于四肢体表肌肤，多因外感风寒，脾肺输布水液失致致水饮溢于四肢肌肤而成。

fluid detention An indication of Qigong，referring to fluid detention into the skin in the four limbs，usually caused by invasion of external pathogenic wind and coldness as well as accumulation of water into the skin in the four limbs due to failure of the spleen and the lung to circulate body fluid.

翳风【yì fēng】 手少阳三焦经中的一个穴位，位于耳垂后方。此穴位为气功习练之处。

Yifeng（TE 17） An acupoint in the triple energizer meridian of hand Shaoyang，located at the rear area of earlobe. This acupoint is a region usually used in practice of Qigong.

因【yīn】 佛家气功习用语，指能引起结果的原因。

cause A common term of Qigong in Buddhism，referring to the cause of result.

因果【yīn guǒ】 佛家气功习用语，指任何精神活动、行为必须产生相应的

结果。

cause and result A common term of Qigong in Buddhism, referring to the fact that any spiritual activity and action must produce the corresponding result.

因内【yīn nèi】 指引起疾病的内在原因,一般指情志损伤。

internal cause Refers to the cause of diseases, usually indicating emotional damage.

因形而生病【yīn xíng ér shēng bìng】 指不同类型的人在不同时间里,由于五行生克、反侮关系而导致生病。

diseases caused by different types Refers to diseases caused by promoting, restricting, reverse restriction and reverse restraint activities among the five elements (including wood, fire, earth, metal and water) related to different types of people at different times.

因阴取阴【yīn yīn qǔ yīn】 指接近或靠近阴位而取阴气协调之。

taking Yin when facing Yin Refers to taking Yin Qi to regulate anything when near the Yin position.

因圆【yīn yuán】 佛家气功术语,指的是能调节精神意识活动,和谐行为的八法之一。

successful generation A common term of Qigong in Buddhism, referring to one of the eight ways in Buddhism for regulating mental activities and harmonizing the spirit and body.

因缘【yīn yuán】 佛家气功习用语,指原因,或直接作用的条件为因。

reason A common term of Qigong in Buddhism, referring to the cause or the direct condition.

因缘观【yīn yuán guān】 佛家气功

法,具体作法是:观十二因缘、三世相续之理,而停止愚痴之法。

reason inspection An exercise of Qigong in Buddhism, marked by inspecting twelve reasons and the principles in three generations and stopping use of feebleminded exercise.

阴藏【yīn cáng】 佛家气功习用语,指阴为佛之阴茎,藏于腹中而不显现,犹马阴不可见也。

Yin hiding A common term of Qigong in Buddhism, in which Yin refers to penis in Buddhism and hiding refers to invisibility of the abdomen like concealed penis.

阴成形【yīn chéng xíng】 指阴形成了形体。

Yin forming shape Means that Yin constitutes the human body.

阴丹【yīn dān】 指津液,即口中唾液。

Yin Dan (pills of immortality) Refers to saliva in the mouth.

阴都【yīn dū】 足少阴肾经的一个穴位,位于脐上 4 寸。这一穴位为气功运行的一个常见部位。

Yindu (KI 19) An acupoint in the kidney meridian of foot Shaoyin, located 4 Cun above the navel. This acupoint is a region usually used for keeping the essential Qi in practice of Qigong.

阴端【yīn duān】 ① 指会阴;② 指龟头。

Yin aspect Refer to ① either pudendal region; ② or balanus.

阴返抱阳【yīn fǎn bào yáng】 指气功状态下肾阴含心阳纳入肾中,其中阴指肾阴,阳指心阳。

Returning Yin and holding Yang Refers to the fact that there is heart Yang in kidney Yin and is transmitted into the kidney in practicing Qigong. In this term, Yin refers to kidney Yin and Yang refers to heart Yang.

阴符经【yīn fú jīng】 《阴符经》即《黄帝阴符经注》,为气功专著,由宋代唐淳所注。

Yinfu Jing(*Yellow Emperor's Yin Conception Canon*) A monograph of Qiong entitled *Yellow Emperor's Yin Conception Canon*, analyzed by Tang Chun, a great scholar and master of Qigong in the Song Dynasty (960 AD - 1279 AD).

阴宫【yīn gōng】 指肾,为五脏之一。

Yin chamber Refers to the kidney in the five Zang-organs (including the heart, the liver, the spleen, the lung and the kidney).

阴关【yīn guān】 大赫的一个别称,是足少阴肾经的穴位,位于横骨上 1 寸,为气功常用意守部位。

Yinguan A synonym of Dahe (KI 12), which is an acupoint in the kidney meridian of foot Shaoyin, located 1 Cun above the transversum. This acupoint is a region usually used in practice of Qigong.

阴核【yīn hé】 睾丸的别称。

Yin nucleus A synonym of scrotum.

阴虎【yīn hǔ】 指肾中真一之水。

Yin tiger Refers to the genuine water in the kidney.

阴还阳丹【yīn huán yáng dān】 指肾水上济心火,水火既济。

Yin returning to Yang Dan Refers to kidney water connecting with heart fire and coordination between water and fire.

阴精【yīn jīng】 ①指体内不受制约的气;②指阴液。

Yin essence Refers to ① either Qi in the body that cannot not be restricted; ② or Yin humor.

阴陵泉【yīn líng quán】 足太阳脾经中的一个穴位,位于胫骨内侧下缘。这一穴位为气功运行的一个常见部位。

Yinlingquan(SP 9) An acupoint in the spleen meridian of foot Taiyin, located in the lower side of the internal edge on the tibia. This acupoint is a region usually used for keeping the essential Qi in practice of Qigong.

阴陇【yīn lǒng】 指阴气隆盛。

Yin vigorousness Refers to exuberance of Yin Qi.

阴卵【yīn luǎn】 指睾丸,又称阴核、肾子、卵势。

Yin ovum Refers to scrotum, also called Yin nucleus, kidney seed and scrotum style.

阴脉之海【yīn mài zhī hǎi】 阴脉即为任脉,任脉为诸阴之会,故称阴脉之海。

sea of Yin meridians In the term of sea of Yin meridians, Yin meridian refers to the conception meridian which is the region for all kinds of Yin to communicate. That is why it is called the sea of Yin meridians.

阴魔【yīn mó】 指邪念。

Yin demon Yin demon refers to wicked idea.

阴平阳秘【yīn píng yáng mì】 ① 指阴阳互根;② 指阴阳相合;③ 指形神统一。

Yin stable and Yang compact Refers to ① either the interdependence of Yin and Yang; ② or combination of Yin and Yang; ③ or unification of the body and spirit.

阴气【yīn qì】 与阳气相对,指人体内有形物质,如五脏之气。习练气功,调阴气固秘,荣养全身。

Yin Qi Opposite to Yang Qi. It refers to physical objects in the body, such as Qi in the five Zang-organs (including the heart, the liver, the spleen, the lung and the kidney). Practice of Qigong can regulate Yin Qi for nourishing the body.

阴器【yīn qì】　指外生殖器。

Yin joint Refers to external genitals.

阴跷【yīn qiāo】　即虚危穴和九灵铁鼓,精气聚散常在此处,水火发端也在此处,阴阳变化也在此处,有无出入也在此处。

Yin Qiao The same as Xuwei point and nine genius-fire drums, referring to the region where the essential Qi concentrates and disperses there, water and fire appear there, Yin and Yang change there, exit and entrance exist there.

阴跷脉【yīn qiāo mài】　奇经八脉之一,起于足舟骨后方,经内踝,沿下肢内侧向下,进入阴部。此经脉为气功习练之处。

Yin heel meridian One of the eight extraordinary meridians, starting from the backside of the central navicular bone and entering the Yin region through the medial malleolus and along the internal side of the legs downwards. This meridian is a region usually used in practice of Qigong.

阴胜则阳病阳胜则阴病【yīn shèng zé yáng bìng yáng shèng zé yīn bìng】指阴阳失去平衡就会出现阴阳偏胜偏衰的现象,发生疾病。

Predominance of Yin results in the disease of Yang while predominance of Yang leads to the disease of Yin. Refers to imbalance of Yin and Yang that causes unilateral predominance or unilateral of decline, eventually causing various diseases.

阴维【yīn wéi】　大赫的一个别称,是足少阴肾经的穴位,位于横骨上 1 寸,为气功常用意守部位。

Yinwei A synonym of Dahe (KI 12), which is an acupoint in the kidney meridian of foot Shaoyin, located 1 Cun above the transversum. This acupoint is a region usually used in practice of Qigong.

阴维脉【yīn wéi mài】　奇经八脉之一。起于小腿内侧,沿大腿内侧上行到腹部,与足太阴经相合,过胸部,与任脉会于颈部。此经脉为气功习练之处。

Yin link meridian One of the eight extraordinary meridians, starting from the internal side of the shank, moving to the abdomen from the internal side of the thigh, connected with the spleen meridian of foot-Taiyin and joining with the conception meridian in the neck through the chest. This meridian is a region usually used in practice of Qigong.

阴虚【yīn xū】　指身体阴虚发热,阴液损耗,水不制火而为病。

Yin deficiency Refers to fire in the body caused by Yin deficiency. Exhaustion of Yin humor and failure of water to control fire will cause certain diseases.

阴阳【yīn yáng】　古代哲学名词,阴指暗,阳指明。日称太阳,月称太阴。

Yin and Yang A term of ancient Chinese philosophy, in which Yin refers to darkness while Yang refers to bright-

Y

ness. Traditionally the sun is called Great Yang and the moon is called Great Yin.

阴阳变化之乡【yīn yáng biàn huà zhī xiāng】 指任脉、督脉交会之处，即会阴，一说尾闾，亦指虚危。虚危穴为精气聚散常在此处，水火发端也在此处，阴阳变化也在此处，有无出入也在此处。

changing place of Yin and Yang Refers to place where the conception meridian and governor meridian interact with each other. It is also called perinaeum, coccyx or Xuwei acupoint which is the region where the essential Qi concentrates and disperses there, water and fire appear there, Yin and Yang change there, exit and entrance exist there.

阴阳不交【yīn yáng bù jiāo】 不交之禁欲。

no association of Yin and Yang Refers to asceticism.

阴阳出入门户【yīn yáng chū rù mén hù】 指阴阳之转枢，子午卯酉四个时辰为阴阳转枢的时间。

Yin and Yang leaving and entering gateway Refers to Yin and Yang turning pivot in the periods of Zi (the period of a day from 11 p.m. to 1 a.m.), Wu (the period of a day from 11 a.m. to 1 p.m. in the noon), Mao (the period of a day from 5 a.m. to 7 a.m. in the morning) and You (a period of a day from 5 p.m. to 7 p.m. in the dusk).

阴阳处中【yīn yáng chù zhōng】 即阴中有阳，阳中有阴，阴阳尽在其中。

Yin and Yang staying in the center Indicates that there is Yang in Yin and there is Yin in Yang. That is why Yin and Yang all stay in the center.

阴阳得类【yīn yáng dé lèi】 源自气功专论，主要阐述炼内丹靠自身之阴阳协调，非自然界之朱砂、水银。

category of Yin and Yang Collected from a monograph of Qigong, mainly describing that practice of Qigong depends on coordination of Yin and Yang, not cinnabar and mercury in the natural world.

阴阳递迁【yīn yáng dì qiān】 指一日之中阴阳是不断消长变化的。

transmission and transference of Yin and Yang Refers to constant growth, decline and transformation of Yin and Yang in everyday.

阴阳颠倒【yīn yáng diān dǎo】 源自气功专论，阐述阴阳互根在气功中的应用情况。

overthrow of Yin and Yang Collected from a monograph of Qigong, mainly describing the application of interdependence between Yin and Yang in practicing Qigong.

阴阳老少【yīn yáng lǎo shào】 源自气功专论，阐述气功中阴阳之间的气化作用。

old and young in Yin and Yang Collected from a monograph of Qigong, mainly describing the effect of the transformation of Qi in Yin and Yang in practicing Qigong.

阴阳离决精气乃绝【yīn yáng lí jué jīng qì nǎi jué】 指阴阳分离，内体的精气就会随之衰竭。

If Yin and Yang separate from each other, essence and Qi will be completely exhausted. Refers to exhaustion of essence and Qi in the body when Yin and Yang separate from each other.

阴阳气化说【yīn yáng qì huà shuō】

源自气功专论,说明形体在气功状态下,阴阳相互为根,互相转化,以维持相对稳定。

discussion about transformation of Qi from Yin and Yang Collected from a monograph of Qigong, referring to mutual dependence and transformation of Yin and Yang in order to maintain comparative balance in practicing Qigong.

阴阳升降【yīn yáng shēng jiàng】 指人体内阳主胜,阴主降,阴阳升降指阴阳相互作用,协调共济之意。

ascent and descent of Yin and Yang Refers to Yang controlling ascent while Yin controlling descent. The ascent of Yang and descent of Yin indicates mutual influence and coordination of Yin and Yang.

阴阳始末【yīn yáng shǐ mò】 指阳气之生始于子时,午后减而至无;阴气之生始于午时,子后减而至无。

beginning and ending of Yin and Yang Refers to the fact that Yang Qi starts from Zi (the period of the day from 11 p.m. to 1 a.m.) and diminishes to exhaustion after Wu (the period of the day from 11 a.m. to 1 p.m.); and that Yin Qi starts from Wu (the period of the day from 11 a.m. to 1 p.m.) and diminishes to exhaustion after Zi (the period of the day from 11 p.m. to 1 a.m.).

阴阳相失【yīn yáng xiāng shī】 即气血散乱不调,其中阴指血,阳指内气。

mutual decline of Yin and Yang Refers to disorder and imbalance of Yin and Yang. In this term, Yin refers to blood and Yang refers to internal Qi.

阴阳消息【yīn yáng xiāo xī】 指一年

中自然阴阳的变化规律。

information of Yin and Yang Refers to natural principles of Yin and Yang change in every year.

阴阳耀光赫真内景法【yīn yáng yào guāng hè zhēn nèi jǐng fǎ】 为静功。其作法为,于夏历每月初一日清净室内静坐,排除杂念。

exercise of Yin and Yang for shining the grand genuine internal state A static exercise, marked by cleaning the room and sitting quietly in the room to eliminate distracting thought on the first day of every month according to traditional Chinese calendar.

阴阳应象【yīn yáng yìng xiàng】 指应阴阳是自然界的基本规律。

intercourse of Yin and Yang Refers to the basic principle of combination between Yin and Yang in the natural world.

阴阳应象大论【yīn yáng yìng xiàng dà lùn】 用阴阳学说的理论,阐发事物的阴阳属性及其对立、互根、转化的运动,并用取类比象的方法,论述阴阳五行的属性特点,及在人体生理、病理、诊断、治疗等方面的运用,强调阴阳是自然界的根本规律。

major discussion on the theory and principles of Yin and Yang Describes the nature, opposition, interdependence and transformation of Yin and Yang in anything according to the theory of Yin and Yang. According to analogy, it discusses the property and characteristics of Yin, Yang and five elements (including wood, fire, earth, metal and water) as well as physiology, pathology, diagnosis and treatment of human body, emphasizing that Yin and

Y

Yang are the fundamental principles of the natural world.

阴阳者万物之能始也【yīn yáng zhě wàn wù zhī néng shǐ yě】 指阴阳是一切事物发生、发展、变化、消亡的根本原因。气功与养生均着眼于调和阴阳。

Yin and Yang are the source of everything. Refers to the fact that Yin and Yang are the primary causes of occurrence, development, change and exhaustion of all things. Qigong and life cultivation all depend on regulation of Yin and Yang.

阴阳之变【yīn yáng zhī biàn】 指阴阳互相消长变化。

changes of Yin and Yang Refers to mutual wane and wax of Yin and Yang.

阴阳之根【yīn yáng zhī gēn】 指天地之元,即神。

root of Yin and Yang Means the origin of the sky and the earth, referring to the spirit.

阴真君还丹歌注【yīn zhēn jūn hái dān gē zhù】 《阴真君还丹歌注》为气功专著,由陈抟注,成书于宋代。书中根据天地方位,五行所属,阴阳交感,四时运转的道理,说明人体脏腑部位,练功的时机、方法和功效。

Yinzhenjun Huandan Gezhu(*Explanation of Yin Genuine Monarch's Song for Returning Dan*) A monograph of Qigong entitled *Explanation of Yin Genuine Monarch's Song for Returning Dan* (*Pills of Immortality*), compiled in the Song Dynasty (960 AD - 1279 AD) and explained by Chen Tuan. This book describes the location of the five Zang-organs (including the heart, the liver, the spleen, the lung and the kidney) and the six Fu-organs (including the gallbladder, the stomach, the small intestine, the large intestine, the bladder and the triple energizer) as well as the time, method and effect of Qigong practice according to the position of the sky and earth, the existence of the five elements (including wood, fire, earth, metal and water), the interaction of Yin and Yang and the revolution of the four seasons.

阴中【yīn zhōng】 指外生殖器。

Yin center Refers to the external genitals.

阴中之阳【yīn zhōng zhī yáng】 指阴中有阳,与肝有关。

Yang within Yin Means that there is Yang in Yin related to the liver.

阴中之阴【yīn zhōng zhī yīn】 指阴中有阴,与肾有关。

Yin within Yin Means that there is Yin in Yin related to the kidney.

音声相和【yīn shēng xiāng hé】 指音声谐和。气功中喻阴阳和合,安宁平静。

harmony of sound and voice Refers to balance of Yin and Yang with stability and quietness in Qigong.

氤氲【yīn yūn】 亦称缊缊,原意指气或光色混合,气功文献中指阴阳交媾。

suffusing The same as enshrouding, originally refers to the blend of Qi and light color. In the literature of Qigong, it refers to intercourse of Yin and Yang.

缊缊【yīn yùn】 亦称氤氲,原意指气或光色混合,气功文献中指阴阳交媾。

enshrouding Originally refers to the blend of Qi and light color. In the literature of Qigong, it refers to intercourse of Yin and Yang.

鄞鄂成【yín è chéng】 指习练气功,

持续不断所取得的成功。

continuity without stop　Refers to success in continuously practicing Qigong without any stop.

尹清和安寝法【yǐn qīng hé ān qǐn fǎ】 为动功。其作法为，平身仰卧，右脚架左脚上，直舒两手搬肩，治脾胃虚弱，五谷不消。

Yin Qinghe's method for lying quietly　A dynamic exercise, marked by lying on the back quietly, raising the right foot above the left foot, and holding the shoulders with both hands. Such a dynamic exercise can treat spleen and stomach deficiency and indigestion of five cereals.

尹志平【yǐn zhì píng】 元代气功家，著有两部气功专著，传承和发展了气功学。

Yin Zhiping　A great master of Qigong in the Yuan Dynasty (1169 – 1251) who wrote two monographs of Qigong for inheriting and developing Qigong.

引火逼金【yǐn huǒ bī jīn】 顺为金生水，逆为火逼金行，引金生之水上行济火，水火既济。

promoting fire to force metal　Refers to metal producing water, fire forcing metal to move, and promoting water produced by metal to flow up in order to coordinate fire and water.

引颈咽气法【yǐn jǐng yàn qì fǎ】 为动静相兼法。在寅时（清晨三至五点钟）面向南方，精神集中，消除杂念，闭住气息，吸而不呼，连作七次，伸直颈项，用力咽气，像咽很硬的东西一样，连作七遍，然后吞咽舌下的津液。

method for stretching the neck to inhale air　An exercise combined with dynamic exercise and static exercise,

marked by turning to the south in Yin (3 a.m. to 5 a.m. in the morning), concentrating the spirit, eliminating distracting thought, suspending respiration, inhaling without exhaling for seven times, stretching the neck, breathing like taking a very hard substance for seven times, and finally swallowing fluid and humor behind the tongue.

引肾【yǐn shèn】 即用意念行气导引，使津液上达咽喉及人体上部，以治疗消渴及津液干枯的疾病。

promoting kidney　Refers to promoting the movement of Qi with consciousness, enabling fluid and humor to flow into the throat and the upper part of the body in order to treat consumptive thirst disease and loss of fluid.

饮刀圭【yǐn dāo guī】 刀指水中金，圭指戊己真土。练功时，先采水中金，借戊己土化火，逼金行，上升至泥丸。

drinking with knife and jade　In this term, knife refers to gold in water and jade refers to genuine earth in Wu (the fifth Heavenly Stem) and Ji (the sixth Heavenly Stem). In practicing Qigong, measures should be taken to take gold from the water first and transform fire according to Wu (the fifth Heavenly Stem) and Ji (the sixth Heavenly Stem), promoting the gold to move upwards to the mud bolus (the brain).

饮酒中毒候导引法【yǐn jiǔ zhòng dú hòu dǎo yǐn fǎ】 为动静相兼功。其作法为，正坐，安定精神，调节呼吸，抬头向天，呼出酒食醉饱之气，气出后酒醒，有饥饿感。

exercise of Daoyin for disinfecting toxin from alcohol　A method combined with dynamic exercise and static exercise,

Y

marked by sitting upright, stabilizing the essence and spirit, regulating respiration, raising the head towards the sky and exhaling Qi from alcohol. Such a way of practicing Qigong will make the practitioners sober up and feel hungry.

饮食自然【yǐn shí zì rán】 指咽唾液。
naturally taking diet Refers to swallowing saliva.

隐白【yǐn bái】 足太阴脾经中的一个穴位，位于蹞趾内侧，为气功中常用的意守部位。
Yinbai（SP 1） An acupoint in the spleen meridian of foot Taiyin, located in the medial side of the first toe, which is the region for concentrating consciousness in practicing Qigong.

隐藏气穴【yǐn cáng qì xué】 指意守气穴，目内视气穴，勿忘勿助，自然息调神静，为气功中常用的意守部位。
hiding Qixue（KI 13） Refers to concentrating Qixue（KI 13）（an acupoint in the kidney meridian of foot Shaoyin）with the mind, internally observing Qixue（KI 13）with the eyes, and naturally regulating respiration and tranquilizing the spirit without any neglecting and supporting, which is the region for concentrating consciousness in practicing Qigong.

隐地回八术【yǐn dì huí bā shù】 指隐遁变化之法。
hiding and escaping eight techniques Refers to the ways for reclusion and changes.

隐芝翳郁【yǐn zhī yì yù】 ① 指阴阳；② 指内丹成就。
hiding ganoderma and nebula Refers to ① either Yin and Yang；② or achievement of internal Dan（pills of immor-

tality）.

英玄【yīng xuán】 与明上同，指眼神，即目光精彩。
outstanding supremeness The same as supreme brightness, refers to the spirit in the eye, indicating brilliant vision.

婴儿姹女【yīng ér chà nǚ】 ① 指肾精、心穴；② 指药物，为阴阳两个方面。
baby and beauty Refers to ① either the kidney essence and the heart acupoint；② or medicinal which refers to two sides of Yin and Yang.

撄宁【yīng níng】 指精神意识思维活动在面对万物生死成毁的纷争中保持宁静。
stabilizing contact Refers to keeping quietness of the activities of consciousness and thinking in contacting with various situations of life and death as well as success and failure.

膺【yīng】 指胸前上部的肌性隆起处，即胸大肌部。
breast Refers to ectopectoralis or the breast muscle.

迎风冷泪【yíng fēng lěng lèi】 气功适应证，由肝肾两虚，精血耗散所致。
cold tearing with wind An indication of Qigong practice, usually caused by deficiency of the liver and kidney and dissipation of acupoints in the meridians.

迎风热泪【yíng fēng rè lèi】 气功适应证，由风热外袭，肝肺火炽或肝肾阴虚，虚火上炎所致。
pyretic tearing with wind An indication of Qigong, usually caused by external invasion of wind heat, intense fire in the liver and lung, or deficiency of the liver and kidney and flaming up of deficiency fire.

迎气法【yíng qì fǎ】 为静功。其作法

为,早晨起床,面向南,两手伸展放于膝上,静心存想,内观其气上入于头顶,下达涌泉。此法交通心肾,治上热下寒诸症。

exercise for receiving Qi A static exercise, marked by getting up in the morning, facing the south, putting the hands on the knees, tranquilizing the heart and contemplating inwards, internally observing Qi ascending to the head and descending to Yongquan (KI 1). Such a way of practicing Qigong can coordinate the heart and the kidney and cure any disease with fever in the upper and cold in the lower.

迎香【yíng xiāng】 为手阳明大肠经中的一个穴位,位于鼻唇沟中。这一穴位为气功运行的一个常见部位。

Yingxiang (LI 20) An acupoint in the large intestine meridian of hand Yangming, located in between the nose and lip. This acupoint is a region usually used for keeping the essential Qi in practice of Qigong.

莹蟾子【yíng chán zǐ】 元代气功学家李道纯的另外一个称谓,其著有多部气功学专著,对后世影响很大。

Ying Chanzi Another name of Li Daochun, a great master of Qigong in the Yuan Dynasty (1271 AD - 1368 AD), whose monographs of Qigong greatly influenced the later generations.

影人【yǐng rén】 即意念中人的影像,非真人也。

imagined figure Refers to the image of a person in contemplation, not a real person.

影人法【yǐng rén fǎ】 为静功。其作法为,分身作影人,长三四寸许,立影人鼻上,令影人取天边太空太和之气,从天

而下,穿屋及头,直入四肢百脉,无处不彻。其功效为治一切疾病。

exercise for imagined figure A static exercise, marked by separating the body as an imaged figure for three or four Cun, putting the imaged figure on the nose, leading the imaged figure to take celestial Qi from the sky into the room and the head, and directly entering the celestial Qi in the four limbs and all the meridians in the whole body. Such a static exercise can cure all diseases.

瘿【yǐng】 气功适应证,指颈部结喉两旁,结块肿大的疾病。多与情志内伤及水土因素有密切关系。

goiter An indication of Qigong, referring to swollen mass at both sides of the neck, usually caused by internal damage due to emotional changes and water changes.

应节顺时【yìng jié shùn shí】 指一年、一月、一日中,练功要顺应自然阴阳变化的时节。

seasonal compliance Refers to following the natural changes of Yin and Yang in a year, a month and a day in practicing Qigong.

涌泉【yǒng quán】 足少阴肾经中的一个穴位,位于足心前三分之一的凹陷中,为气功中常用的意守部位。

yongquan (KI 1) An acupoint in the kidney meridian of foot Shaoyin, located in the depression one-third to the sole, which is the region for concentrating consciousness in practicing Qigong.

涌泉观【yǒng quán guān】 位于庐山西南七十里,为晋代气功家葛玄炼丹处。

Yongquan Temple Located in the southwest about seventy Li towards the

Y

Lushan Mountain, where Ge Xuan, a great master of Qigong in the Jin Dynasty (266 AD – 420 AD), refined Dan (pills of immortality).

用和安神【yòng hé ān shén】 指调节精神意识思维活动,使之协调稳定,能于安神补脑。

tranquilizing the spirit through harmonization Refers to regulating the activities of the spirit, consciousness and thinking in order to stabilize the body, to tranquilize the spirit and to tonify the brain.

用神静【yòng shén jìng】 指圣人用神少而协调,即爱惜精神之意。

exercise for tranquilizing the spirit Refers to the fact that sage seldom used the spirit in order to regulate anything, indicating treasure of the spirit.

用神躁【yòng shén zào】 指用神多可耗散精气。

spiritual exhaustion Refers to consumption and dissipation of essential Qi due to excessive use of the spirit.

用意与不忘【yòng yì yǔ bù wàng】 源自气功专论,指习练气功既要用意,又不能太过与不及。

Intention without forgetting Collected from a monograph of Qigong, referring to the importance of intention and crisis of hyperactivity and hypoactivity in practicing Qigong.

优游【yōu yóu】 指习练气功,意守景物。

leisurely travel Refers to concentrating mind on photographic field in practicing Qigong.

忧【yōu】 ① 指病;② 指思;③ 指病因。

anxiety Refers to ① either disease; ② or consideration; ③ or cause of disease.

忧悲【yōu bēi】 指情志的不愉和伤感,为人体致病之因,是气功之戒。

depression Refers to unpleasantness and sentiment, which are the causes of diseases and are admonishments of Qigong.

忧陀那【yōu tuó nà】 指丹田。

youtuona Refers to Dantian which is divided into the upper Dantian (the region between the eyes), the middle Dantian (the region below the heart) and the lower Dantian (the region below the navel).

幽谷【yōu gǔ】 指耳。

deep valley Refers to the ears.

幽关【yōu guān】 指肾,位于人体的深部。

deep joint Refers to the kidney located in the deep region of the body.

幽门【yōu mén】 足少阴肾经中的一个穴位,位于脐下6寸。这一穴位为气功运行的一个常见部位。

Youmen(KI 21) An acupoint in the kidney meridian of foot Shaoyin, located 6 Cun below the navel. This acupoint is a region usually used for keeping the essential Qi in practice of Qigong.

幽阙【yōu què】 ① 指两肾之间的幽深之处;② 指肾之后。

deep palace Refers to ① either the deep region between the kidneys; ② or the region behind the kidneys.

幽室【yōu shì】 指肾。

deep chamber Refers to the kidney.

幽室内明【yōu shì nèi míng】 指守神于内,身体内极幽隐之室,明朗如日月。

brightness in the deep chamber Refers

to the spirit in the deep and latent region in the body, as bright as the sun and the moon.

游神【yóu shén**】** 指游走不定的意念活动。

migrating spirit Refers to indeterminate activity of consciousness.

游心于虚【yóu xīn yú xū**】** 指意识思维活动的无欲状态。

tranquilized heart Refers to tranquil activity of consciousness and thinking.

游行天地之间,视听八达之外【yóu xíng tiān dì zhī jiān shì tīng bā dá zhī wài**】**《黄帝内经》中的名言,指气功中自我控制精神的练功方法。

Roaming around on the earth and in the sky, seeing and hearing beyond the eight directions. A celebrated dictum in Huangdi Neijing (entitled *Yellow Emperor's Internal Canon of Medicine*), referring to the exercise for controlling the spirit in practicing Qigong.

有【yǒu**】** 佛家气功习用语,指存在,亦指意识存在引起的行为。

possession A common term of Qigong in Buddhism, referring to ① either existence; ② or action due to existence of consciousness.

有胎中息【yǒu tāi zhōng xī**】** 指练功调息时,控制呼吸的枢机在丹田。

existence of fetal respiration Refers to regulation of respiration in practicing Qigong, in which the helm that controls respiration and is located in Dantian. Dantian is divided into the upper Dantian (the region between the eyes), the middle Dantian (the region below the heart) and the lower Dantian (the region below the navel).

有头疽【yǒu tóu jū**】** 气功适应证,多因外感风温湿热之毒,内有脏腑蕴毒,凝聚肌表,营卫不和,气血凝滞,经络阻塞所致。

gangrene An indication of Qigong, usually caused by toxin from external contraction of wind warmth and damp heat, and internal accumulation of toxin in the viscera, the muscles and superficies, disharmony of nutrient and defense aspects, stagnation of Qi and blood as well as obstruction of the meridians and collaterals.

有为【yǒu wéi**】** 即意识的作为,气功中指用意念导引杂念外出,使神有专向。

promise Refers to deed made by consciousness. In Qigong practice, consciousness can eliminate distracting thought and direct the function of the spirit.

有无相生【yǒu wú xiāng shēng**】** 指自然、社会之中,有与无相对立而存在。气功文献中,说明有生于无,无生于有,相互滋生。

mutual promotion of being and non-being A celebrated dictum, referring to opposite existence of being and non-being in natural and social environments. In the literature of Qigong, it says that the things of this world come from being and being comes from non-being.

有象【yǒu xiàng**】** 即太极生二仪之象,分阴分阳。

image Refers to the image of Taiji (Supreme Pole) that has produced two appearances which pertain to Yin and Yang.

有作【yǒu zuò**】** 练功之始,炼己持心,降龙伏虎,采药结丹之类称为有作。

action Refers to concentrating the

Y

heart, descending Loong and controlling at the beginning of practicing Qigong. The so-called action refers to collecting medicinal in order to form Dan (pills of immortality) in practicing Qigong.

于真人胎息法【yú zhēn rén tāi xī fǎ】静功口诀。其作法为，"凡所修行，先定心气，心气定则神疑，神凝则心安，心安则气升，气升则境空，境空则清静，清静则无物，无物则命全，命全则道生"。本口诀法主要是定心神，兼有佛家功法于内，其法即金液还丹之法。

immortal's exercise for fetal respiration A static exercise. According to this static exercise, heart Qi must be stabilized in practicing Qigong; only when heart Qi is stabilized can the spirit be concentrated; only when the spirit is concentrated can the heart be stabilized; only when the heart is stabilized can Qi be increased; only when Qi is increased can the state be vacuumed; only when the state is vacuumed can the mind be tranquilized; only when the mind is tranquilized can nothingness be produced; only when nothingness is produced can the life be perfected; only when the life be perfected can Dao be formed. Such a dynamic exercise mainly can stabilize the heart spirit with the application of the exercise of Qigong practice in Buddhism, which means to lead golden humor to Dan (pills of immortality).

鱼【yú】　指手足大指（趾）。

fish Refers to the thumbs and big toes.

鱼际【yú jì】　指手足大指（趾）后，鱼之外侧赤白肉分界处。

thenar eminence Refers to the region between the back of the thumbs and big toes as well as the dorsoventral boundary of hand or foot.

鱼尾【yú wěi】　足少阳胆经中的一个穴位瞳子髎的另外一个称谓，位于目外眦外侧 0.5 寸。

Yuwei A synonym of Tongziliao (GB 1) which is an acupoint in the gallbladder meridian of foot Shaoyang, located 0.5 Cun lateral to the outer canthus.

俞曲园【yú qǔ yuán】　清代著名学者、文学家和精气功俞樾的另外一个称谓，气论著中论述了三种习练气功的方法。

Yu Quyuan Another name of Yu Yue, a great scholar, litterateur and master of essential Qi in the Qing Dynasty (1636 AD – 1912 AD). He wrote a monograph of Qigong, describing three important exercises for practicing Qigong.

俞琰【yú yǎn】　宋末元初的气功理论家，著有多部气功学专著，精详阐述了气功的理论和方法，对后世颇有影响。

Yu Yan A theorist of Qigong in the late Song Dynasty (960 AD – 1279 AD) and early Yuan Dynasty (1271 AD – 1368 AD). He wrote several monographs about Qigong, particularly describing the theory and practice of Qigong, greatly influenced the later generations.

俞荫甫【yú yīn fǔ】　清代著名学者、文学家和精气功俞樾的另外一个称谓，气论著中论述了三种习练气功的方法。

Yu Yinfu Another name of Yu Yue, a great scholar, litterateur and master of essential Qi in the Qing Dynasty (1636 AD – 1912 AD). He wrote a monograph of Qigong, describing three important exercises for practicing Qigong.

俞玉吾【yú yù wú】　宋末元初的气功理论家俞琰的另外一个称谓,著有多部气功学专著,精详阐述了气功的理论和方法,对后世颇有影响。

Yu Yuwu　Another name of Yu Yan, a theorist of Qigong in the late Song Dynasty (960 AD – 1279 AD) and early Yuan Dynasty (1271 AD – 1368 AD). He wrote several monographs about Qigong, particularly describing the theory and practice of Qigong, greatly influenced the later generations.

俞樾【yú yuè】　清代著名学者、文学家和精气功,气论著中论述了三种习练气功的方法。

Yu Yue　A great scholar, litterateur and master of essential Qi in the Qing Dynasty (1636 AD – 1912 AD). He wrote a monograph of Qigong, describing three important exercises for practicing Qigong.

渔父词【yú fù cí】　《渔父词》为气功专论,作者为唐末五代时期的道士吕岩,概要介绍了凝神、一阳来复、火候、沐浴等内容。

Yufu Ci（*Cold Fisherman's Poetry*）　A monograph of Qigong entitled *Cold Fisherman's Poetry*, written by Daoist Lǔ Yan in the late Tang Dynasty (618 AD – 907 AD) and early Five Dynasties (907 AD – 979 AD), mainly introducing the contents of concentrating the spirit, returning of one Yang, duration-degree of heating, and bath.

瑜伽【yú jiā】　佛家气功习用语,泛指佛家气功。

yoga　A common term of Qigong in Buddhism, usually referring to Qigong in Buddhism.

髃骨【yú gǔ】　即肩前骨,为肩胛骨的肩峰与锁骨的外侧端。

scapular bone　Refers to the anterior bone in the shoulder at the top of the scapula and at the lateral side of the clavicle.

与天地为一【yǔ tiān dì wèi yī】　指出人若能明白恬淡虚无,去除杂念、欲望,保持心的宁静,则能健康长寿。

integration with the sky and earth　A celebrated dictum, referring to the idea that man should integrate with the sky and the earth in order to eliminate distracting thought and desire for the purpose of tranquilizing the heart, cultivating health and prolonging life.

与天为一【yǔ tiān wéi yī】　指形体健全,精力充沛,即是与自然合二为一。

integration with the sky　Refers to full health of the body and abundance of the spirit, indicating integration of the mind and nature.

宇泰定【yǔ tài dìng】　指脑神安定。

celestial stability　Refers to tranquilization of the spirit in the brain.

羽【yǔ】　① 指鸟类的毛;② 指古代五音之一,即角、徵、宫、商、羽。

yu　Refers to ① either feathers of birds; ② or one of the five notes, including Jiao, Zheng, Gong, Shang and Yu.

羽翼戊己【yǔ yì wù jǐ】　指阴阳相互为用。其中的羽翼为阴阳之意。戊和己指一阴一阳之土。

consciousness with Wu and Ji　Refers to interaction of Yin and Yang. In this term, consciousness refers to the meaning of Yin and Yang, Wu and Ji refers to the position of one Yin and one Yang.

雨水正月中坐功【yǔ shuǐ zhēng yuè zhōng zuò gōng】 为动功。其作法为，每日子丑时，叠手按腥，拗颈转身，左右偏引，各三五次，叩齿，吐纳，漱咽。

rain and water sitting exercise in the middle of January A dynamic exercise, marked by holding the hands to press the body every day in Zi (the period of the day from 11 p. m. to 1 a. m.) and Chou (the period of a day from 1 a. m. to 3 a. m. in the morning), immobilizing the neck and turning the body from the left to the right and vice versa for three to five times, clicking the teeth, inhalation and exhalation as well as rinsing the mouth and swallowing saliva.

玉蟾【yù chán】 玉兔的别称，传说在月中，气功文献中指代月。

jade toad A synonym of jade rabbit, is in the moon according to legendary story. In the traditional literature of Qiong, jade rabbit refers to the moon.

玉晨君【yù chén jūn】 指脑神居上清，主宰一身意识思维活动，有感觉、知觉、协调全身各部，作用至上。

jade monarch Refers to the brain spirit that is in the upper and controls the activities of consciousness thinking in order to regulate sensation and consciousness in the whole body.

玉池【yù chí】 ① 指唇齿之内；② 指口。

jade pool Refers to ① the region between the lips and teeth; ② or the mouth.

玉珰【yù dāng】 指两眉间直入一寸。

jade ornament Refers to 1 Cun directly into the region between the eyes.

玉珰紫阙【yù dāng zǐ què】 指眉额部。

jade ornament and violet palace Refers to the eyes and the forehead.

玉帝【yù dì】 ① 指玉液；② 指津液润泽通达一身。

jade emperor Refers to ① either saliva; ② or fluid that flows along all parts of the body.

玉鼎汤液【yù dǐng tāng yè】 指元精经河车搬运入泥丸时的景象。

jade cauldron decoction Refers to the image of the original essence flowing into the mud bolus (the brain) along the river cart.

玉都【yù dū】 指身体，亦指脑。

jade capital Refers to either the body; or the brain.

玉房【yù fáng】 为气功中心的别称。

jade house Refers to a synonym of the heart in Qigong.

玉房宫真人【yù fáng gōng zhēn rén】 指膀胱所主神名。

genuine man in jade ornament palace Refers to the name of the spirit in the bladder.

玉关【yù guān】 ① 指脑中神室，或神门；② 指丹田。

jade col Refers to ① spirit chamber or spirit gate in the brain; ② or Dantian. Dantian is divided into the upper Dantian (the region between the eyes), the middle Dantian (the region below the heart) and the lower Dantian (the region below the navel).

玉光澄辉高明内景【yù guāng chéng huī gāo míng nèi jǐng】 为静功。其作法为，于夏历每月十三日夜间，清净的室内坐定，入静后，意想自己飞升坐在昆仑山顶,仰望天上皎洁的月光,叩齿,咽津各三十六次,调息良久收功。

internal image of brightness at night A static exercise, marked by sitting quietly in the room at the night of 13th in every month in summer, imagining to fly to the top of the Kunlun Mountain after being tranquilized, looking at the moonshine in the sky, clicking the teeth and swallowing fluid for thirty-six times respectively. After regulating respiration for a long period of time, this a static exercise can be finished.

玉环【yù huán】　指练气功时的意守部位。

jade ring Refers to the position of mind concentration in practicing Qigong.

玉醴金浆【yù lǐ jīn jiāng】　指服炼口中津液。

jade wine and golden syrup Refers to fluid and humor swallowed in the mouth.

玉炼颜【yù liàn yán】　指习练气功养生法,肤肌如霜雪,绰约如处子。

jade practice image Refers to the technique for practicing Qigong and cultivating life, characterized by the skins and the muscles like frost and snow, as graceful as a virgin.

玉灵宫真人【yù líng gōng zhēn rén】指胆腑所主神名。

genuine man in jade spiritual palace Refers to the name of the spirit in the gallbladder.

玉垄【yù lǒng】　指鼻神。

jade ridge Refers to the nose spirit.

玉庐【yù lú】　指鼻。

Jade cottage Refers to the nose.

玉门【yù mén】　①指印堂穴;②又指妇女阴道外口。

jade gate Refers to ① either the region between the eyes; ② or the external aperture of vagina.

玉清金笥青华秘文金宝内炼丹诀【yù qīng jīn sì qīng huá mì wén jīn bǎo nèi liàn dān jué】《玉清金笥青华秘文金宝内炼丹诀》为气功学专著,为紫阳真人张平叔撰。

Yuqing Jinsi Qinghua Miwen Jinbao Neilian Danjue (*Jade Cleanness, Golden Basket, Green Magnificience, Secret Literature and Golden Treasure About Internal Dan Practice Formula*) A monograph of Qigong entitled *Jade Cleanness, Golden Basket, Green Magnificience, Secret Literature and Golden Treasure About Internal Dan Practice Formula*, written by Zhang Pingshu, a great Daoist and master of Qigong in the Song Dynasty (960 AD - 1279 AD).

玉泉【yù quán】　①指口中唾液;②为中极穴别名,位于体前正中线,脐下4寸。

jade spring Refers to ① saliva in the mouth; ② or a synonym of Zhongji (CV 3) located in the front midline and about 4 Cun below the navel.

玉树【yù shù】　①指身体;②亦专指脑。

jade tree Refers to ① either the body; ② or the brain.

玉堂【yù táng】　①指上颚;②指经穴名,属任脉;③指右肾。

jade hall Refers to ① either the upper jaw; ② or an acupoint called Yutang (CV 18) in the conception meridian; ③ or the right kidney.

玉堂宫【yù táng gōng】　指五脏中的肺脏。

jade palace Refers to the lung in the five Zang-organs (including the heart, the liver, the spleen, the lung and the kidney).

玉兔【yù tù】 玉兔传说在月中,气功文献中指代月。

jade rabbit Jade rabbit is in the moon according to legendary story. In the traditional literature of Qiong, jade rabbit refers to the moon.

玉兔与金乌相抱【yù tù yǔ jīn wū xiāng bào】 玉兔为阴,金乌为阳,喻身体阴阳两方,指阴阳相互作用,维持平衡,即阴平阳秘之意。

embrace of jade rabbit and golden crow Jade rabbit refers to Yin and golden crow refers to Yang, comparing to the interaction and balance between Yin and Yang, indicating the mutual effects of Yin and Yang that keep balance and harmony. This term actually refers to the fact that Yin is stable while yang is compact.

玉溪子【yù xī zǐ】 南宋气功家李简易的另外一个称谓,其编写的气功专著对后世有一定的影响。

Yu Xizi Another name of Li Jianyi, a great master of Qigong in the South Song Dynasty (1127 AD - 1279 AD), whose monographs of Qigong influenced the later generations.

玉溪子丹经指要【yù xī zǐ dān jīng zhǐ yào】 《玉溪子丹经指要》为气功学专著,为宋代李简易所著,对后世有一定的影响。

Yu Xizi's Danjing Zhiyao (Yu Xizi's Discussion About Dan Canon) A monograph of Qigong entitled *Yu Xizi's Discussion About Dan Canon*, written by Li Jianyi, a great master of Qigong in the Song Dynasty (960 AD - 1279 AD), whose monographs of Qigong influenced the later generations.

玉阳真人【yù yáng zhēn rén】 金代气功学家王处一的另外一个称谓,为全真道嵛山派的创始人。

Yuyang Zhenren Another name of Wang Chuyi, a great master of Qigong in the Jin Dynasty (1142 - 1217), who was the founder of Yushan school in Acme Genuine Dao.

玉液【yù yè】 ① 指用矿物经炼制变成可服用的丹药;② 指唾液;③ 指经外奇穴;④ 指肾液。

jade humor Refers to ① either a medicinal made by mineral; ② or saliva; ③ or Yuye (EX - HN 13), an extraordinary acupoint; ④ or kidney humor.

玉液还丹【yù yè huán dān】 玉液是指肾液,肾液随元气上升而朝于心,自心经中丹田而复还下丹田。

jade humor entering Dan (pills of immortality) In this term, jade humor refers to kidney humor that flows up along the original Qi into the heart and descends to the lower Dantian (the region below the navel) from the middle Dantian (the region below the heart) in the heart meridian.

玉液炼形法【yù yè liàn xíng fǎ】 为静功。其作法为,意守玄膺(气管),不久则津液满口,慢慢将此津液以意引下,渐达膻中、鸠尾、中脘、神阙,至气海而止。

exercise for practicing jade humor A static exercise in practicing Qigong, marked by keeping the mind in the trachea that eventually enriches fluid and humor in the mouth. The fluid and humor are gradually introduced through the mind to Danzhong (CV 17), Jiuwei

(CV 15), Zhongwan (CV 12), Shenque (CV 8) and Qihai (CV 6).

玉饴【yù yí】　指舌上之津液。

jade maltose　Refers to fluid above the tongue.

玉云张果老胎息诀【yù yún zhāng guǒ lǎo tāi xī jué】　为静功口诀,本法重在意守丹田,存神气精于丹田。

Zhang Guolao's jade cloud formula about fetal respiration　A static exercise of table, referring to concentration of mind in Dantian and keeping the spirit, Qi and essence in Dantian. Dantian is divided into upper Dantian (the region between the eyes), the middle Dantian (the region below the heart) and the lower Dantian (the region below the navel).

玉枕【yù zhěn】　为足太阴膀胱经中的一个穴位,位于头正中入后发际 2.5 寸,旁开 1.3 寸处。这一穴位为气功运行的一个常见部位。

Yuzhen (BL 9)　Refers to an acupoint in the bladder meridian of foot Taiyin, located 2.5 Cun to and 1.3 Cun beside the hair line from the middle center of the head. This acupoint is a region usually used for keeping the essential Qi in practice of Qigong.

郁冒【yù mào】　气功适应证,多见于血虚、亡津液或肝气郁结所致,也指血厥。

depression and dizziness　An indication of Qigong, referring to either the disease caused by blood deficiency, loss of fluid and humor or stagnation of liver Qi; or blood syncope.

郁仪结璘善相保【yù yí jié lín shàn xiāng bǎo】　郁仪为阳,结璘为阴,即阴阳相互作用,以维持相对平衡以稳定。

Luxuriance connected with luster is excellent for protection.　Luxuriance refers to Yang while luster refers to Yin, indicating that combination of Yin and yang can maintain balance and stability.

郁证【yù zhèng】　气功适应证,泛指气机郁滞不得发越所致的病证。

Stagnation syndrome　An indication of Qigong, usually referring to the disease caused by stagnation of Qi activity that cannot be active.

欲【yù】　① 指情欲、欲念等精神活动;② 指希望、想要、欲望、希求等思维活动;③ 佛家气功指欲念之后而养性。

desire　Refers to ① either spirit activity with passions and desires; ② or thinking activity with hope, desire, requirement and expectation; ③ or exercise of Qigong for nourishing life after desire in Buddhism.

欲安神,炼元气【yù ān shén liàn yuán qì】　源自气功专论,主要阐述神气相依,气海盈则心安。

refining the original Qi for stabilizing the spirit　Collected from a monograph of Qigong, mainly describing interdependence of the spirit and Qi and exuberance of Qihai (CV 6) stabilizing the heart.

欲得长生,先须久视【yù dé cháng shēng xiān xū jiǔ shì】　源自气功专论,主要阐述意守三丹田的作用。

Watching for a long time can prolong life.　This sentence is collected from a monograph of Qigong, mainly describing the effects of protecting the three kinds of Dantian. Dantian is divided into the upper Dantian (the region between the eyes), the middle Dantian

Y

（the region below the heart）and the lower Dantian（the region below the navel）.

欲海【yù hǎi】 指个人的欲望无边。

ideal sea Refers to oneself boundless desires.

欲界定【yù jiè dìng】 指练禅功达到定的境界时，感觉自己的身体非常明朗，心理"爽爽清凉"，没有一丝牵挂。

ideal relief Indicates that the body is quite clear and the heart is quite fresh without any worry when reaching a certain state after refining dhyana exercise.

欲神【yù shén】 有为之动为欲神。

ideal spirit Refers to ideal action.

元【yuán】 ① 指头；② 同玄。

origin Refers to ① either the head; ② or secret.

元儿穴【yuán ér xué】 膻中的另外一个称谓，是人体的穴位，在前正中线上，两乳头连线的中点。

Yuan'erxue A synonym of Danzhong（CV 17），an acupoint located in the front midline between the breasts.

元火【yuán huǒ】 指肾中真阳。

original fire Refers to true Yang in the kidney.

元见穴【yuán jiàn xué】 膻中的另外一个称谓，是人体的穴位，在前正中线上，两乳头连线的中点。此穴位为气功习练之处。

Yuanjianxue A synonym of Danzhong（CV 17），an acupoint located in the front midline between the breasts. This acupoint is a region usually used in practice of Qigong.

元精【yuán jīng】 指的是生命之本、元气之精华、气功作用下的内控力。

original essence Refers to either the

origin of life; or the essence of the original Qi; or intrinsic control under the function of Qigong.

元明【yuán míng】 佛家气功习用语，指本来就有的自性清净的精神活动。

original brightness A common term of Qigong Buddhism, referring to natural tranquilized activity of the spirit.

元冥【yuán míng】 指的是肾神。

original abstruseness Refers to the kidney spirit.

元气【yuán qì】 指自然之气、生之本、天地之精气、元气。

original Qi Refers to either the natural air; or the base of life; or the natural essence; or the original Qi.

元气实,不思食【yuán qì shí bù sī shí】 指习练气功，内气形成，使元气充实，则不感饥饿。

enrichment of the original Qi and no hunger in practice of Qigong Refers to no feeling of hunger in practicing Qigong because the internal Qi is formed and original Qi is concentrated.

元气所合【yuán qì suǒ hé】 指神气相合。

integration of original Qi Refers to integration of the spirit and Qi.

元气有限,人欲无限【yuán qì yǒu xiàn rén yù wú xiàn】 指人要善于调节情志，节制欲望，使元气充足，阴阳平衡，延年益寿。

Original Qi is limited, but human desires are unlimited. Refers to the fact that human beings should be good at regulating emotion, controlling desires, enriching the original Qi, and balancing Yin and Yang in order to prolong life and to replenish health.

元神【yuán shén】 指脑神、意识思维活动、性命之根、精神、呼吸之主。

original spirit　Refers to either the celebral spirit; or the activities of consciousness and thinking; or the root of life; or the spirit; or the foundation of respiration.

元神宫【yuán shén gōng**】**　指脑。

original spiritual mansion　Refers to the brain.

元神会，不思睡【yuán shén huì bù sī shuì**】**　指习练气功，意念集中，使元神聚汇，则精力充沛，不感疲乏。

concentration of the original spirit and no fatigue in practice of Qigong　Refers to no feeling of fatigue in practicing Qigong because consciousness is concentrated and the original Qi is accumulated, effectively enriching the spirit and expelling fatigue.

元神之府【yuán shén zhī fǔ**】**　指脑。

mansion of original spirit　Refers to the brain.

元神足，不思欲【yuán shén zú bù sī yù**】**　指习练气功，增强生命之根本，使元气之精华充足，保持阴阳平衡，则无欲望。

Enrichment of the original spirit and no desire in practice of Qigong　Refers to no feeling of desire in practicing Qigong because the root of life is increased, the essence of original Qi is enriched, Yin and Yang are balanced. That is why there is no desire.

元潭【yuán tán**】**　指小肠。

original pool　Refers to the lower part of the small intestine.

元宪真人胎息诀【yuán xiàn zhēn rén tāi xī jué**】**　静功口诀，指保持形体和精神稳定，机体动静平衡。

immoral Yuanxian's fetal respiration for-mula　A static exercise, referring to stabilization and balance of the body and the spirit in practicing Qigong.

元心【yuán xīn**】**　佛家气功习用语，指产生一切精神意识思维活动的根本。

original heart　A common term of Qigong in Buddhism, referring to origin of spiritual, emotional and mental activity.

元阳【yuán yáng**】**　指命门火、肾阳。

original Yang　Refers to fire in the life gate and Yang in the kidney.

元一【yuán yī**】**　指元气。

original one　Refers to the original Qi.

元因【yuán yīn**】**　佛家气功学习用语，指气功习练中的重要因由。

original cause　A term of Qigong in Buddhism, referring to the important cause for normalizing all activities in practicing Qigong.

元阴【yuán yīn**】**　指肾阴。

original Yin　Refers to kidney Yin.

元阴元阳【yuán yīn yuán yáng**】**　指的是真阴真阳，即肾之阳，心之阴。

original Yin and original Yang　Refers to genuine Yin and genuine Yang, i.e. Yang in the kidney and Yin in the heart.

元元子【yuán yuán zǐ**】**　明代气功学家张三丰的另一称谓。张三丰指为明代的气功学家，深入系统地研究和发展了气功的理论和方法。

Yuan Yuan Zi　Another name of Zhang Sanfeng, a great master of Qigong in the Ming Dynasty (1368 AD - 1644 AD), thoroughly and systematically studied and developed the theory and practice of Qigong.

元脏【yuán zàng**】**　指肾。

original viscus　Refers to the kidney.

元中颠倒颠 【yuán zhōng diān dǎo diān】 源自气功专论《悟真篇》，阐述坎离颠倒、神息天人为炼丹关键。

avoidance of coition in practice of Qigong Collected from Wuzhen Pian which the monograph of Qigong entitled *Canon of Perception and Truth*, referring to discussion about how to normalize spiritual activities and respiration in practicing Qigong.

袁坤仪 【yuán kūn yí】 明代气功养生家，著有气功养生专著，研究气功养生的理论与方法。

Yuan Kunyi A master of Qigong and life cultivation in the Ming Dynasty (1368 AD - 1644 AD), who wrote a monograph of Qigong to study the theory and practice of Qigong.

袁天纲胎息诀 【yuán tiān gāng tāi xī jué】 为静功。以阴阳变化为理，说明子午卯酉四时习练气功，取自然之气以助机体阴阳变化，保持身体"四定"。

Yuan Tiangang's formula for fetal respiration A static exercise, referring to taking the changes of Yin and Yang as the principles to practice Qigong in Zi (the period of the day from 11 p.m. to 1 a.m.), Wu (the period of the day from 11 a.m. to 1 p.m. in the noon), Mao (the period of the day from 5 a.m. to 7 a.m. in the early morning) and Yin (the period of the day from 3 a.m. to 5 a.m. in the early morning), and take natural Qi to assist the changes of Yin and Yang in the human body in order to protect four stabilities in the body.

圆成实性 【yuán chéng shí xìng】 佛家气功习用语，指习练气功获得的神形稳定状态。

seeking the truth A common term of Qigong in Buddhism, referring to stabilization of the body and the spirit in practicing Qigong.

圆顿止观 【yuán dùn zhǐ guān】 佛家气功习用语，指静止妄念，真智通达。

perfect harmony A common term of Qigong in Buddhism, referring to tranquilizing the mind, eliminating distracting thought and increasing the genuine wisdom.

圆光灵明洞照内景 【yuán guāng líng míng dòng zhào nèi jǐng】 为静功。其作法为，於夏历每月十五日在清净的室内坐定，入静后，意想自己立于昆仑山顶，见月圆光满，月光上降下云彩形成一座桥，月亮发出银白色的光芒。默念道家符咒三十六遍，叩齿咽津亦各三十六，静坐良久收功。

perfect observation of the internal light scene A static exercise, marked by sitting quietly in a clear and quiet room on 15th in every month in summer, imagining to have reached the top of Kunlun Mountain after tranquilization, observing the round moon with bright light that descends to form a bridge with silvery white light, silently reading charms in Daoism for thirty-six times, clicking the teeth and swallowing fluid for thirty-six times respectively, and sitting quietly for a long period of time till the practice is succeeded.

圆合 【yuán hé】 佛家气功习用语，即协调统一，使身体各部协调稳定。

concord A common term of Qigong in Buddhism, referring to coordination and unification of all parts in the body.

圆寂 【yuán jì】 佛家气功习用语，①指消除烦恼；②指精神活动相对静止；③ 指达到健康安乐境界；④ 指坐忘。

nirvana A common term of Qigong in Buddhism，referring to ① either eliminating annoyance；② or tranquilizing spirit activity；③ or reaching the state of health，peace and happiness；④ or sitting without memorizing anything.

圆觉【yuán jué】　佛家气功习用语，指圆满的灵觉，昭昭不昧，了了常知，常住清净。

perfect consciousness A common term of Qigong in Buddhism，referring to perfect mentality，bright memory，full knowledge，peaceful and quiet life.

圆觉海【yuán jué hǎi】　指脑。

perfect understanding the sea Refers to the brain.

圆觉三关【yuán jué sān guān】　佛家气功功法，① 指奢靡他观；② 指三摩钵底观；③ 指禅那观。

three states of perfect consciousness An exercise of Qigong in Buddhism，referring to ① either tranquilized activity of the spirit；② or imagined vision with or without any scene；③ or concentrating on the center without any other changes.

圆元【yuán yuán】　佛家气功学习用语，指调节人的精神活动，与众人和平相处。

circular origin A common term of Qigong in Buddhism，referring to regulating spirit activity and peacefully getting along with other people.

援生四书【yuán shēng sì shū】　《援生四书》为养生学专著，兼论气功，由清代田绵淮所著。

Yuansheng Sishu（*Four Books for Supporting Life*）　A monograph of life cultivation with discussion of Qigong entitled *Four Books for Supporting Life*，written by Tian Jinhuai in the Qing Dynasty（1636 AD‑1912 AD）.

缘【yuán】　佛家气功习用语，① 指意识活动攀缘一切之境界；② 事物间彼此的联系和影响。

edge A common term of Qigong in Buddhism，referring to ① either the activity of consciousness that has reached various states；② or relation and influence of various things.

缘督【yuán dū】　为静功。其作法为，精神意识活动集中于督脉，维持精神意识与督脉之间的稳定状态即可。

governing edge A static exercise，marked by concentrating the activities of the spirit and consciousness in the governor meridian for maintaining stability between the spirit and consciousness with the governor meridian.

缘境【yuán jìng】　即人之思维与外界事物相攀缘，指气功中没有脱离尘事，没有入静的状态。

edge state Indicates that human thinking climbs up to the things in the external world. In Qigong，it refers to failure to separate from social affairs and failure to be tranquilized.

缘务【yuán wù】　为杂念之意。

edge affairs Refers to distracting thought.

缘中【yuán zhōng】　佛家气功习用语。指行功时，意守的事物。

central edge A common term of Qigong in Buddhism，referring to things concentrated by consciousness in practicing Qigong.

猿臂【yuán bì】　为动功。其作法为，"将左手伸直，以右手探左手心，头却尽力右顾,右手亦然,此法当于食后行之一二次,能消食"。

monkey arm A dynamic exercise，marked by "stretching the left hand，touching the left palm with the right hand，turning the head forcefully to the right and stretching the right hand. Such a dynamic exercise can be done for one or twice after eating for digesting food".

猿臂导引法【yuán bì dǎo yǐn fǎ】 为动功。其作法为,"左手伸直,以右手探左掌心,头向右顾,右手亦然。此法宜食后炼一、二次。消食、助分娩"。

exercise of Daoyin for monkey arm A dynamic exercise，marked by "stretching the left hand，touching the left palm with the right hand，turning the head to the right side，and stretching the right hand. Such a dynamic exercise can be done for one or twice after eating for digesting food and assisting childbirth".

猿经鸱顾【yuán jīng chī gù】 是一种模仿猿猴及鸟的导引术。

monkey movement and owl management Refers to a technique of Daoyin imitating the style of monkey and bird.

猿戏【yuán xì】 为动功。其作法为,"猿戏者,攀物自悬,伸缩身体,上下一七,以脚拘物自悬、左右七,手钩起立,按头各七"。

monkey game A dynamic exercise，marked by "climbing naturally, stretching and shrinking the body upward and downward for seven times, restraining things with the feet from the left to the right and vice versa for seven times, hooking with the hands for standing up, and pressing the head for seven times".

远罢河车君再睡【yuǎn bà hé chē jūn zài shuì】 即练罢河车搬运法再睡。

Only when river cart is stopped can the sovereign sleep again. It is a celebrated dictum, indicating that only when the movement of the river cart is stopped can the practitioner sleep again.

远尘【yuǎn chén】 指避免尘世的干扰以安定情绪。

far away from this world Means to avoid interference and disturbance of this world in order to stabilize the emotion.

月窟【yuè kū】 指阴之根,为阳极阴生之处。

root of Yin Refers to the place where Yang is terrific and Yin is growing.

月与日两半【yuè yǔ rì liǎng bàn】 指月为液,日为神气。神气与液合而为一。

Half is the moon and half is the sun. Refers to integration of humor and the spiritual Qi, among which the moon refers to humor while the sun refers to the spiritual Qi.

云光集【yún guāng jí】 《云光集》为气功学专著,共四卷,介绍和分析气功的理论、方法和功效。作者不详。

Yun Guang Ji（*Cloud and Brightness Monograph*） A monograph of four volumes entitled *Cloud and Brightness Monograph*，describing the theory, practice and effects of Qigong. The author was unknown.

云笈七签【yún jí qī qiān】 《云笈七签》为道教类书,兼述气功。

Yunji Qiqian（*Integration of Seven Essences*） Book in Daoism containing Qigong, entitled *Integration of Seven Essences*.

Y

云鸾法师服气法【yún luán fǎ shī fú qì fǎ】 为静功。其作法为,功前准备,解带宽衣,放松形体。起坐时两手置膝,闭目举舌,渐渐长吐气。

master Yun Luan's respiration exercise A static exercise, marked by softening the belt and clothes and relaxing the body for preparing practice of Qigong, then sitting upright, pressing the knees with both hands, closing the eyes, raising the tongue and gradually breathing out.

云气罗【yún qì luó】 即黄庭之外象。

manifestation of cloud and Qi Refers to the external manifestation of the yellow chamber which refers to the lower Dantian (the region below the navel).

云卧天行【yún wò tiān xíng】 指调息静极时的意境。

cloudy lying and celestial movement Refers to the state of tranquilization in respiration and practice of Qigong.

云牙子【yún yá zǐ】 即东汉时期杰出的气功学家魏伯阳的另外一个称谓。

Yun Yazi Another name of Wei Boyang who was a great master of Qigong in the East Han Dynasty (25 AD – 220 AD).

云仪玉华【yún yí yù huá】 指的是发、鬓。

cloudy style and magnificent jade Refers to hair and temples.

允执厥中【yǔn zhí jué zhōng】 指不偏不倚,两在其中。

neutrality Refers to balance and center.

运动水土【yùn dòng shuǐ tǔ】 动静相兼功,饮食后散步,两手按摩腹胁上下,又再将两手转到背后摩擦肾堂使之发热。

moving water and earth An exercise combined with dynamic exercise and static exercise, marked by walking after taking food, rubbing the upper and the lower sides of the abdomen with both hands and turning the hands to the back to rub the kidney position in order to generate heat.

运符行火【yùn fú xíng huǒ】 动静相兼功。其作法为,子后午前,存神端坐,闭息,蓄两外肾,缩谷道,定息七十二数。子后行功半个时辰,午前行功半个时辰。

moving symbol to act fire An exercise combined with dynamic exercise and static exercise, marked sitting quietly after Zi (the period of the day from 11 p.m. to 1 a.m.) and Wu (the period of the day from 11 a.m. to 1 p.m. in the noon), holding breath, storing up the two external kidneys, shrinking the grain trail (anus) and stabilizing respiration for seventy-two times. The practice is continued for half a period of time (one hour) after Zi (the period of the day from 11 p.m. to 1 a.m.) and before Wu (the period of the day from 11 a.m. to 1 p.m. in the noon).

运膏肓【yùn gāo máng】 为动功。其作法为,肘曲摇转肩关节,带动肩胛骨,以作用于背部的膏肓俞。

moving Gaohuang (BL 43) A dynamic exercise, marked by rotating the shoulders with the elbows which drives the scapula in order to act Gaohuang (BL 43) located in the back.

运火【yùn huǒ】 指习练小周天,待丹田精气盈满时,用意收腹提肛,促精气流过尾闾间关上行。

moving fire Refers to practice the

Y

small celestial circle as well as concentrating the abdomen and lifting the anus with consciousness when the essence and Qi in Dantian are exuberant in order to promote the essence and Qi to flow upwards from the coccyx. Dantian is divided into the upper Dantian (the region between the eyes), the middle Dantian (the region below the heart) and the lower Dantian (the region below the navel).

运火于脐【yùn huǒ yú qí】 为动功。其作法为,左右掌连心,心火暗自达,手心与心脉相通,右手掌擦左手心,左手掌擦右手心,双手互擦,意念集中于左右手心。

moving fire to the navel A dynamic exercise, marked by connecting the left and the right hands with the heart with secret arrival of heart fire, connecting the palms with the heart meridian, kneading the left palm with the right fist, kneading the right palm with the left fist, and concentrating consciousness in the right palm and the left palm.

运睛【yùn jīng】 为动功,即眼睛经常上下左右旋转运动,治目暗不明。

moving eyes A dynamic exercise, referring to always moving the eyes upwards and downwards as well as to the left and to the right in order to cure blurred vision.

运睛除睛翳法【yùn jīng chú jīng yì fǎ】 为静功。其作法为,紧闭目,左右转睛各七次。转眼珠时,口鼻闭气,睁眼时尽力呵出浊气,吸入清,各七次。

moving eyes to eliminate negula A static exercise, marked by closing the eyes and turning the eyes from the left to the right for seven times, turning the eyeball, closing Qi in the mouth and nose, breathing out turbid Qi when opening the eyes and breathing in pure air for seven times.

运精气要诀【yùn jīng qì yào jué】 为动功。其作法为,以两手上交,左右努力,各三遍;以两手下交,左右努力,各七遍;以两手屈跃,左右手七遍;以两手叉腰,左右努力,各七遍;以两手抱颈,以两肩左右努力,各七遍。能使气和则神和。

formula for transporting essence and Qi A dynamic exercise, marked by crossing hard the both hands upwards for three times, crossing forcefully the both hands downwards for seven times, bending forcefully the both hands upwards for seven times, pressing hard the waist with both hands for seven times, holding the neck with both hands and the shoulders for seven times. Such a way of practice will harmonize Qi and the spirit.

运气按摩【yùn qì àn mó】 为动功,气功医师运用体内之气,通过手指或手掌等部位发功,作用于患者经络穴位或病变部位而治疗疾病。

circulating Qi for kneading A dynamic exercise. Usually doctors take Qi from the body with the fingers or fists to pump the acupoints in the meridians of patients or location of disease in order to treat disease.

运气还精补脑法【yùn qì huán jīng bǔ nǎo fǎ】 为静功,一撞三关,常使气冲关节透,自然精满谷神存。

exercise of moving Qi and returning essence to tonify the brain A static exercise, marked by bumping three passes and making Qi rush joints in order to enrich essence in Gushen (mental faculties).

运气却病法【yùn qì què bìng fǎ】　为静功,运气如屋漏注连相续,送至病处,一便除病。

Emitting Qi to cure disease　An exercise combined with dynamic exercise and static exercise, marked emitting Qi like leakage in the room and transmitting it to the location of disease in order to cure the disease.

运手法【yùn shǒu fǎ】　为动功,每朝自然站立,放松形体,将左右手放前绞纽,不计遍数。

exercise for moving hands　A dynamic exercise, marked by sitting naturally every morning, relaxing the body and putting the hands in front to cross and turn for many times.

运天经【yùn tiān jīng】　指五脏六腑各有所司,皆有法象,运行径路依经脉而行。

moving celestial meridian　Refers to the fact that the five Zang-organs (including the heart, the liver, the spleen, the lung and the kidney) and six Fu-organs (including the gallbladder, the stomach, the small intestine, the large intestine, the bladder and the triple energizer) all have their own advantages and manifestations, which move all along the meridians.

运足法【yùn zú fǎ】　为动功。其作法为,行步时,将脚朝前踢,如踢球状,如此常行数百步。

exercise for moving feet　A dynamic exercise, marked by kicking the feet forwards in walking like kicking a ball for hundreds of steps.

熨目【yùn mù】　为动功。指经常按摩腹部,能健脾胃,帮助消化,防治水谷积滞不化。为内伤调中之法。

rubbing the eyes　A dynamic exercise, marked by often rubbing the abdomen for fortifying the spleen and stomach, digesting food, preventing and curing indigestion. Such a dynamic exercise is for curing internal damage and regulating the middle.

Y

Z

杂念【zá niàn】 指气功锻炼中，初学调神时，各种念头纷乱杂至的情况。排除这些杂念是调神之第一步。

distracting thought Refers to various chaotic distracting thoughts in primary study of spirit regulation. To eliminate such distracting thoughts is the first step in regulating the spirit.

载营魄抱一【zǎi yíng pò bào yī】 指行动中，形体与精神意识协调统一。

integration of the body and spirit in action Means to coordinate and to integrate the body with the spirit and consciousness.

攒簇五行【zǎn cù wǔ xíng】 指气功习练时，在脑神的作用下，五脏神及全身各部神聚会和谐，而使全身处于稳定协调的状态。

accumulating and gathering the five elements Refers to combination and harmonization of the spirit in the five Zang-organs (including the heart, the liver, the spleen, the lung and the kidney) and all parts in the body under the influence of the brain spirit in practicing Qigong for stabilizing and coordinating the whole body.

攒竹【zǎn zhú】 足太阳膀胱经中的一个穴位，位于眉毛内侧端。此穴位为气功习练之处。

Cuanzhu（BL 2） An acupoint in the bladder meridian of foot Taiyang, located in the interior of the eyebrow. This acupoint is a region usually used in practice of Qigong.

脏腑配八卦【zàng fǔ pèi bā guà】 震为肝，坎为肾，艮为膀胱，巽为胆，离为心，兑为肺。

combination of the viscera with the Eight Trigrams Zhen Trigram refers to the liver, Kan Trigram refers to the kidney, Gen Trigram refers to the bladder, Xun Trigram refers to the gallbladder, Li Trigram refers to the heart and Dui Trigram refers to the lung.

脏象【zàng xiàng】 包括五脏六腑，气功文献称为"内景"（或内境），为内视、内观的对象。

visceral manifestations Include the five Zang-organs (including the heart, the liver, the spleen, the lung and the kidney) and the six Fu-organs (the gallbladder, stomach, small intestine, large intestine, bladder and triple energizer). In the literature of Qigong, it refers to internal scene, including internal vision and internal observation.

早服【zǎo fú】 指爱惜精神，预防疾病。

early prevention Refers to cherishing the spirit and preventing disease.

造化【zào huà】 指创造化育。

creation Refers to creation and fostering.

造化真功【zào huà zhēn gōng】 指使身体神形相对稳定的方法，即是造化真功。

genuine exercise for creation Refers to

the way to stabilize the spirit and the body.

造化真机【zào huà zhēn jī**】** 指一阳来复之时机。

genuine opportunity of creation Refers to the advantage for Yang to return.

造化之源【zào huà zhī yuán**】** 为"祖窍"的异名,指位于心与脐之正中。

source of creation A synonym of ancestral orifice, referring to the central region between the heart and the navel.

躁静之决在于气【zào jìng zhī jué zài yú qì**】** 指烦躁和安静决定于气。气盛则躁,气平则静。

Annoyance and tranquility all depend on Qi. Indicates that dysphoria and tranquility decides the condition of Qi. When Qi is exuberant, dysphoria will be caused; when Qi is stable, tranquility will be formed.

曾伯瑞【zēng bó ruì**】** 宋代诗人兼气功学家曾慥的另外一个称谓,撰写了重要的气功专著。

Zeng Borui Another name of Zeng Zao, a poet and master of Qigong in the Song Dynasty (960 AD － 1279 AD), who wrote a very important monograph of Qigong.

曾慥【zēng zào**】** 宋代诗人兼气功学家,撰写了重要的气功专著。

Zeng Zao A poet and master of Qigong in the Song Dynasty (960 AD － 1279 AD), who wrote a very important monograph of Qigong.

斋戒【zhāi jiè**】** ① 指调节饮食,按摩身体;② 指调节精神意识活动的方法;③ 指古人祭祀时,沐浴更衣,不饮酒吃荤,止伏妄念。

fasting Refers to ① either regulating food and kneading the body; ② or re-

gulating the activities of the spirit and consciousness; ③ or bathing and changing clothes in sacrifice in ancient China without drinking alcohol, eating meat and keeping distracting thought.

宅中有真【zhái zhōng yǒu zhēn**】** 宅指脑。真指赤诚童子,即赤城童子居脑中。

sincerity in residence Refers to the brain. In this term, sincerity refers to boy, which means the sincere boy in the brain.

斩赤龙【zhǎn chì lóng**】** 指女性练功后身体生理的变化。

chopping red Loong Refers to physiological changes of women after practicing Qigong.

斩魔【zhǎn mó**】** 指去除杂念,调节意识思维活动。

chopping devil Means to eliminate distracting thought and to regulate the activities of consciousness and thinking.

湛然安静【zhàn rán ān jìng**】** 指治身,应当意识思维活动安静。

transparent stability and tranquility Means that the activities of consciousness and thinking should be stabilized and tranquilized for curing the body.

张安道养生诀【zhāng ān dào yǎng shēng jué**】** 为动静相兼功。其作法为,每日子时后,面向东或南,披衣盘足而坐,叩齿三十六次,握固,闭息,内视五脏,肺白肝青脾黄心赤肾黑,次想心为炎火,光明洞彻,入下丹田中,待腹满气极,则徐徐出气,候出息匀调,即以舌搅唇齿内外,漱炼津液,不得咽下。

Zhang Aandao's life cultivation formula An exercise combined with dynamic exercise and static exercise, marked by sitting with face toward the east or south after Zi (the period of the day from 11 p. m. to 1 a. m.) every day, clicking the teeth for thirty-six times; holding respiration, internally observing the five Zang-organs (including the heart, the liver, the spleen, the lung and the kidney) in which the lung is white, the liver is green, the spleen is yellow, the heart is red and the kidney is black, imagining that the heart is hot and transmitting brightness into the lower Dantian (the region below the navel), mildly breathing when Qi in the abdomen is rich, equally regulating respiration with the tongue stirring the internal and external of the lips and teeth, rinsing and refining fluid and humor without swallow.

张白【zhāng bái】 唐代著名学者和气功学家,深入系统地研究和发展了气功的理论和方法。

Zhang Bai A great scholar and master of Qigong in the Tang Dynasty (618 AD－907 AD), thoroughly and systematically studied and developed the theory and practice of Qigong.

张伯端【zhāng bó duān】 北宋气功学家,著有气功专著,分析研究了气功的基本理论和方法。

Zhang Boduan A great master of Qigong in the North Song Dynasty (960 AD－1127 AD), who wrote a monograph of Qigong, analyzing and studying the basic theory and practice of Qigong.

张谌【zhāng chén】 古代著名的学者和气功学家,他博学习儒,晚年通气功,能服气辟谷。

Zhang Chen A great scholar and mas-

ter of Qigong in ancient China. He studied and inherited Confucianism. In his old age, he well studied Qigong and could naturally move Qi and practice inedia (stopping diet).

张从正【zhāng cóng zhèng】 金代著名医学家和气功学家,所撰写的医学专著里积累了丰富的气功资料。

Zhang Congzheng A great scientist of traditional Chinese medicine and master of Qigong in the Jin Dynasty (1115 AD－1234 AD). The monographs of traditional Chinese medicine written by him collected rich literature of Qigong.

张果【zhāng guǒ】 唐代著名气功学家,八仙之一张果老的另外一个称谓。

Zhang Guo Another name of Zhang Guolao, a great master of Qigong and one of the eight immortals in the Tang Dynasty (618 AD－907 AD).

张果老【zhāng guǒ lǎo】 唐代著名气功学家,八仙之一。

Zhang Guolao A great master of Qigong and one of the eight immortals in the Tang Dynasty (618 AD－907 AD).

张果老抽添火候法【zhāng guǒ lǎo chōu tiān huǒ hòu fǎ】 为动静相兼功。其作法为,正坐,用两手摩热脐轮。然后按两膝,闭口静坐,候气定,运气九口。

Zhang Guolao's exercise for taking and increasing duration of heating Zhang Guolao's exercise for taking and increasing duration of heating is an exercise combined with dynamic way and static way, marked by sitting upright, rubbing the navel warm with both hands, pressing the knees with both hands, closing the mouth and sitting quietly in order to concentrate Qi and moving Qi for nine times.

张果老先生服气法【zhāng guǒ lǎo xiān shēng fú qì fǎ】　为静功。其作法为，每日常平卧，摄心绝想，闭气握固。鼻引口吐，无令耳闻，唯是细微，满即闭之。

Mr. Zhang Guolao's exercise for taking Qi　Mr. Zhang Guolao's exercise for taking Qi is a static exercise, marked by lying on the back every day, controlling the heart and thought, concentrating Qi, breathing through the nose and vomiting through the mouth, purify listening and micronizing any activities.

张金【zhāng jīn】　张三丰的另外一个称谓。张三丰为明代的气功学家，深入系统地研究和发展了气功的理论和方法。

Zhang Jin　Another name of Zhang Sanfeng, a great master of Qigong in the Ming Dynasty（1368 AD – 1644 AD）, thoroughly and systematically studied and developed the theory and practice of Qigong.

张景和胎息诀【zhāng jǐng hé tāi xī jué】　张景和胎息诀为静功。其作法为，真玄真牝，自呼自吸，似春沼鱼，如百虫蛰，灏气融融，灵风习习。

Zhang Jinghe's fetal respiration exercise　A static exercise, marked by purifying the nature, natural inhaling and exhaling like ponding fish in spring and stinging of all insects, making Qi rich and warm as well as wind pure and gentle.

张君宝【zhāng jūn bǎo】　张三丰的另外一个称谓。张三丰为明代的气功学家，深入系统地研究和发展了气功的理论和方法。

Zhang Junbao　Another name of Zhang Sanfeng, a great master of Qigong in the Ming Dynasty（1368 AD – 1644 AD）, thoroughly and systematically studied and developed the theory and practice of Qigong.

张君房【zhāng jūn fáng】　中国古代的道学家和气功学家，撰写了气功学专著，为保留宋以前的气功著述做出了较大的贡献。

Zhang Junfang　A great Daoist and master of Qigong in ancient China who wrote a monograph of Qigong, contributing a great deal to the inheritance of Qigong monographs compiled before the Song Dynasty（960 AD – 1279 AD）.

张君实【zhāng jūn shí】　张三丰的另外一个称谓。张三丰为明代的气功学家，深入系统地研究和发展了气功的理论和方法。

Zhang Junshi　Another name of Zhang Sanfeng, a great master of Qigong in the Ming Dynasty（1368 AD – 1644 AD）, thoroughly and systematically studied and developed the theory and practice of Qigong.

张邋遢【zhāng lā tā】　张三丰的另外一个称谓。张三丰为明代的气功学家，深入系统地研究和发展了气功的理论和方法。

Zhang Lata　Another name of Zhang Sanfeng, a great master of Qigong in the Ming Dynasty（1368 AD – 1644 AD）, thoroughly and systematically studied and developed the theory and practice of Qigong.

张留侯辟谷处【zhāng liú hóu bì gǔ chù】　又名汉张留侯祠、张良庙，位于陕西留坝紫柏山，为古人习练气功之处。

Zhang Liuhou's inedia place Also called Zhang Liuhou's temple and Zhang Liang's temple, located in Zibo Mountain in Shaanxi Province. In ancient China, the practitioners in Shaanxi Province studied and practiced Qigong in this temple.

张平叔【zhāng píng shū】 北宋气功学家张伯端的另外一个称谓,著有气功专著,分析研究了气功的基本理论和方法。

Zhang Pingshu Another name of Zhang Boduan, a great master of Qigong in the North Song Dynasty (960 - 1127), who wrote a monograph of Qigong, analyzing and studying the basic theory and practice of Qigong.

张全一【zhāng quán yī】 张三丰的另外一个称谓。张三丰为明代的气功学家,深入系统地研究和发展了气功的理论和方法。

Zhang Quanyi Another name of Zhang Sanfeng, a great master of Qigong in the Ming Dynasty (1368 AD - 1644 AD), thoroughly and systematically studied and developed the theory and practice of Qigong.

张三丰【zhāng sān fēng】 为明代气功学家,深入系统地研究和发展了气功的理论和方法。

Zhang Sanfeng A great master of Qigong in the Ming Dynasty (1368 AD - 1644 AD), thoroughly and systematically studied and developed the theory and practice of Qigong.

张三丰大周天【zhāng sān fēng dà zhōu tiān】 为静功。其作法为,作河车真动,中间若有一点灵光,觉在丹田,尔时一阳来复,恍惚如红日初升,照于沧海之内。

Zhang Sanfeng's great celestial exercise A static exercise, marked by activating the river cart (lead). If there is a feeling of miraculous brightness, it is in Dantian. If Yang returns like sunrise, it shines in the great sea. Dantian is divided into the upper Dantian (the region between the eyes), the middle Dantian (the region below the heart) and the lower Dantian (the region below the navel).

张三丰九转大还【zhāng sān fēng jiǔ zhuǎn dà huán】 即张三丰周天法,为静功。其作法为,打坐,将神气抱住,意系住息,在丹田中宛转悠扬,聚而不散。

Zhang Sanfeng's exercise of circulatory cycle The same as Zhang Sanfeng's celestial exercise, is a static exercise, marked by sitting, holding the spirit and Qi, concentrating respiration with consciousness, melodiously turning Dantian and accumulation it without any dispersion. Dantian is divided into the upper Dantian (the region between the eyes), the middle Dantian (the region below the heart) and the lower Dantian (the region below the navel).

张三丰炼精化气法【zhāng sān fēng liàn jīng huà qì fǎ】 为静功。其作法为,坐下闭目存神,使心静息调,即能炼精化气。

Zhang Sanfeng's exercise for refining essence and generating Qi A static exercise, marked by sitting with closed eyes and concentrated spirit, tranquilizing the heart and regulating respiration in order to refine the essence and to generate Qi.

张三丰炼气化神法【zhāng sān fēng liàn qì huà shén fǎ】 为静功。其作法

为，回光返照，凝神丹穴，使真息往来，内中静极而动，动极而静，无限生机，即能炼气化神。

Zhang Sanfeng's exercise for refining Qi and generating spirit　A static exercise, marked by observing rightness at sunset, accumulating the spirit in Danxue (alchemic cave), continuing real inhalation and exhalation, activating after extreme tranquilization, tranquilizing after extreme activation. Such a way of practicing Qigong will cultivate health and prolong life.

张三丰论修心炼性【zhāng sān fēng lùn xiū xīn liàn xìng】　源自气功专论，主要阐述何谓修心、炼性，认为修心炼性是气功内丹法的最基本要求。

Zhang Sanfeng's cultivating the heart and refining the nature　Collected from a monograph of Qigong, mainly describing the ways to cultivate the heart and refine the nature which are the basic exercises for practicing Qigong with internal Dan (pills of immortality).

张三丰先生全集【zhāng sān fēng xiān shēng quán jí】　《张三丰先生全集》为清代李四月所辑，收录了与气功学家张三丰有关的所有气功文献资料。

Zhangsanfeng Xiansheng Quanji（Complete Collection of Mr. Zhang Sanfeng）　Quanji was a collected edition compiled by Li Siyue in the Qing Dynasty (1636 AD - 1912 AD), entitled *Complete Collection of Mr. Zhang Sanfeng*, collecting all the literature of Qigong related to Zhang Sanfeng, a great master of Qigong in the Ming Dynassty.

张三丰周天法【zhāng sān fēng zhōu tiān fǎ】　为静功。其作法为，打坐，将神气抱住，意系住息，在丹田中宛转悠扬，聚而不散。

Zhang Sanfeng's celestial exercise　A static exercise, marked by sitting, holding the spirit and Qi, concentrating respiration with consciousness, melodiously turning Dantian and accumulation it without any dispersion. Dantian is divided into the upper Dantian (the region between the eyes), the middle Dantian (the region below the heart) and the lower Dantian (the region below the navel).

张三峰【zhāng sān fēng】　张三丰的另外一个称谓。张三丰为明代的气功学家，深入系统地研究和发展了气功的理论和方法。

Zhang Sanfeng　Another name of Zhang Sanfeng, a great master of Qigong in the Ming Dynasty (1368 AD - 1644 AD), thoroughly and systematically studied and developed the theory and practice of Qigong.

张善【zhāng shàn】　古代著名的气功学家，深有内养之功，年八十七岁离世。

Zhang Shan　A great master of Qigong in ancient China who deeply and thoroughly practiced Qigong, grasped the exercises of Qigong and lived eight-seven years.

张思廉【zhāng sī lián】　张三丰的另外一个称谓。张三丰为明代的气功学家，深入系统地研究和发展了气功的理论和方法。

Zhang Silian　Another name of Zhang Sanfeng, a great master of Qigong in the Ming Dynasty (1368 AD - 1644 AD), thoroughly and systematically studied and developed the theory and practice of Qigong.

张天师胎息诀【zhāng tiān shī tāi xī jué】 静功口诀,旨在心定、气定、神定,保持精神意识活动相对静止,并无成法。
Master Zhang's fetal respiration formula A static exercise, referring to stabilizing the heart, Qi and spirit in order to tranquilize the activities of the essence, spirit and consciousness without any requirements.

张通【zhāng tōng】 张三丰的另外一个称谓。张三丰为明代的气功学家,深入系统地研究和发展了气功的理论和方法。
Zhang Tong Another name of Zhang Sanfeng, a great master of Qigong in the Ming Dynasty (1368 AD – 1644 AD), thoroughly and systematically studied and developed the theory and practice of Qigong.

张虚白【zhāng xū bái】 唐代著名学者和气功学家张白的另外一个称谓,深入系统地研究和发展了气功的理论和方法。
Zhang Xubai Another name of Zhang Bai, a great scholar and master of Qigong in the Tang Dynasty (618 AD – 907 AD), thoroughly and systematically studied and developed the theory and practice of Qigong.

张玄化【zhāng xuán huà】 张三丰的另外一个称谓。张三丰为明代的气功学家,深入系统地研究和发展了气功的理论和方法。
Zhang Xuanhua Another name of Zhang Sanfeng, a great master of Qigong in the Ming Dynasty (1368 AD – 1644 AD), thoroughly and systematically studied and developed the theory and practice of Qigong.

张玄素【zhāng xuán sù】 张三丰的另外一个称谓。张三丰为明代的气功学家,深入系统地研究和发展了气功的理论和方法。
Zhang Xuansu Another name of Zhang Sanfeng, a great master of Qigong in the Ming Dynasty (1368 AD – 1644 AD), thoroughly and systematically studied and developed the theory and practice of Qigong.

张玄玄【zhāng xuán xuán】 张三丰的另外一个称谓。张三丰为明代的气功学家,深入系统地研究和发展了气功的理论和方法。
Zhang Xuanxuan Another name of Zhang Sanfeng, a great master of Qigong in the Ming Dynasty (1368 AD – 1644 AD), thoroughly and systematically studied and developed the theory and practice of Qigong.

张玄玄牢栓猿马【zhāng xuán xuán láo shuān yuán mǎ】 为静功。其作法为,侧卧,沐浴,练功中重点在排除杂念。
Zhang Xuanxuan strictly controlling thiller A static exercise, marked by lying on one side and eliminating distracting thought which is the most important act in practicing Qigong.

张铉一【zhāng xuàn yī】 张三丰的另外一个称谓。张三丰为明代的气功学家,深入系统地研究和发展了气功的理论和方法。
Zhang Xuanyi Another name of Zhang Sanfeng, a great master of Qigong in the Ming Dynasty (1368 AD – 1644 AD), thoroughly and systematically studied and developed the theory and practice of Qigong.

张怡堂炼成灵宝【zhāng yí táng liàn chéng líng bǎo】 为静功。其作法为,右侧卧,精神内守,意念专一。可治失

Z

眠、多梦、梦游等。

Zhang Yitang's success and treasure in practice Qigong A static exercise, marked by lying on the right side, internally concentrating the essence and spirit, and purifying consciousness in order to cure insomnia, dreaminess and sleepwalking.

张映汉【zhāng yìng hàn】 清代气功养生家，著有气功养生专著，介绍了较多气功导引按摩方法。

Zhang Yinghan A master of Qigong and life cultivation in the Qing Dynasty (1636 AD – 1912 AD) who wrote a monograph, introducing the theory and methods of Qigong and tuina.

张用成【zhāng yòng chéng】 北宋气功学家张伯端的另外一个称谓，著有气功专著，分析研究了气功的基本理论和方法。

Zhang Yongcheng Another name of Zhang Boduan, a great master of Qigong in the North Song Dynasty (960 AD – 1127 AD), who wrote a monograph of Qigong, analyzing and studying the basic theory and practice of Qigong.

张云衢【zhāng yún qú】 清代气功学家张映汉的另外一个称谓，著有气功专著，介绍了较多气功导引按摩方法。

Zhang Yunqu Another name of Zhang Yinghan, a great master of Qigong in the Qing Dynasty (1636 AD – 1912 AD), who wrote a monograph of Qigong, introducing the basic theory and methods of Qigong and tuina.

张真奴神注法【zhāng zhēn nú shén zhù fǎ】 为动功。其作法为，盘膝端坐，两手按膝，用意在中，右视左提，左视右提，左右运气各二十二口。

Zhang Zhennu's exercise for spiritual motion A dynamic exercise, marked by sitting upright with crossed legs, pressing the knees with both hands, concentrating consciousness on the center, seeing the right and lifting the left, seeing the left and lifting the right, moving Qi from the left to the right and vice versa for twenty-two times respectively.

张志和【zhāng zhì hé】 唐代气功学家，著有气功养生书《玄真子》。

Zhang Zhihe A great master of Qigong in the Tang Dynasty who wrote a monograph about Qigong entitled *Supreme Truth*.

张子和【zhāng zǐ hé】 金代著名医学家和气功学家张从正的另外一个称谓，所撰写的医学专著里积累了丰富的气功资料。

Zhang Zihe Another name of Zhang Congzheng, a great scientist of traditional Chinese medicine and master of Qigong in the Jin Dynasty (1115 AD – 1234 AD). The monographs of traditional Chinese medicine written by him collected rich literature of Qigong.

张子坚【zhāng zǐ jiān】 为古代著名的学者和气功学家张谌的另外一个称谓，他博学习儒，晚年通气功，能服气辟谷。

Zhang Zijian Another name of Zhang Chen, a great scholar and master of Qigong in ancient China. He studied and inherited Confucianism. In his old age, he well studied Qigong and could naturally move Qi and practice inedia.

张子同【zhāng zǐ tóng】 唐代气功学家张志和的另外一个称谓。

Zhang Zitong Another name of Zhang

Z

Zhihe.

章门【zhāng mén】 足厥阴肝经中的一个穴位,位于腹部两侧,为气功中常用的意守部位。

Zhangmen（LR 13） An acupoint in the liver meridian of foot Jueyin, located on the lateral sides of the abdomen, which is the region for concentrating consciousness in practicing Qigong.

长谷玄乡绕郊邑【zhǎng gǔ xuán xiāng rào jiāo yì】 指体象。长谷为鼻,玄乡为肾,郊邑为五脏、肢节。

long distance between the head and the five viscera A celebrated dictum, referring to the manifestations of the body, such as the nose, kidney, five Zang-organs（including the heart, the liver, the spleen, the lung and the kidney）and the limbs.

长强【zhǎng qiáng】 督脉的一个穴位,位于尾骨尖与肛门连线之中点。这一穴位为气功运行的一个常见部位。

Changqiang（GV 1） An acupoint in the governor meridian, located in the region between the coccyx and anus. This acupoint is a region usually used for keeping essential Qi in practice of Qigong.

胀满治法【zhàng mǎn zhì fǎ】 动静相兼功,其作法多样。如蹲坐,宁心,卷曲两手以心向下,左右摇动两臂,交替侧斜身体,两肩尽量用力,低头向肚,两手沿冲脉按到脐下,上下反复二十二次。

treatment of distension and fullness An exercise combined with dynamic exercise and static exercise with various methods. One of the practice method is marked by sitting, stabilizing the heart, bending the hands to raise with heart, shaking the shoulders from the left to the right and vice versa, slanting the body alternatively, straightening the shoulders, lowering the head to the abdomen, pressing the region below the navel with the hands along the thoroughfare meridian upwards and downwards for twenty-two times respectively.

障道【zhàng dào】 指习练气功,引起精神失调,杂念丛生的各种原因。

distraction Refers to the imbalanced spirit and weedy distracting thought in practicing Qigong.

朝暮子午【zhāo mù zǐ wǔ】 指一天中十二个时辰的四个时辰,朝指卯时(早晨五至七时),暮指酉时(晚上五至七时),子为夜半(夜间十一至一时),午为正午(中午十一至一时)。

Zi and Wu in the morning and evening Refers to the four periods in the twelve periods in every day, i. e. Mao（the period of a day from 5 a.m. to 7 a.m. in the morning）, You（the period of a day from 5 p.m. to 7 p.m. in the dusk）, Zi（the period of the day from 11 p.m. to 1 a.m.）and Wu（the period of the day from 11 a.m. to 1 p.m. in the noon）.

朝霞【zhāo xiá】 ① 指春天日欲出时东方的赤黄气;② 指早晨天空的云霞。

spectacular sunrise Refers to ① either red and yellow Qi in the east when the sun is going to rise in spring; ② or rosy clouds in the morning.

照海【zhào hǎi】 足少阴肾经中的一个穴位,位于内踝尖直下 1 寸处,为气功中常用的意守部位。

Zhaohai（KI 6） An acupoint in the kidney meridian of foot Shaoyin, located 1 Cun directly below the medial malleolus, which is the region for concentrating consciousness in practicing Qigong.

贞白先生【zhēn bái xiān shēng】　梁代著名医药学家和气功养生家陶弘景的称谓。

Mr. Zhen Bai Refers to Tao Hongjing, a great doctor and master of Qigong for nourishing life in Liang Dynasty (502 AD - 557 AD).

针灸大成【zhēn jiǔ dà chéng】　《针灸大成》为针灸学专著,由明代杨继洲所撰,书中除对脏腑、经络、俞穴、针法、灸法等做了全面论述外,还较好地论述了气功对脏腑经络的保健作用及任、督二脉与小周天功法的关系。

Zhenjiu Dacheng (*A Great Compendium of Acupuncture and Moxibustion*)　A monograph of acupuncture and moxibustion entitled *A Great Compendium of Acupuncture and Moxibustion*, written by Yang Jizhou in the Ming Dynasty (1368 AD - 1644 AD). This book not only discussed the five Zang-organs (including the heart, the liver, the spleen, the lung and the kidney), the six Fu-organs (including the gallbladder, the stomach, the small intestine, the large intestine, the bladder and the triple energizer), the meridians and collaterals, the acupoints (acupuncture point), the acupuncture therapy and the moxibustion therapy, but also mentioned the effect of Qigong on the five Zang-organs, the six Fu-organs, the meridians and collaterals as well as the relationship between the conception meridian, the governor meridian and the small celestial circle.

真禅【zhēn chán】　即真静,为意识思维活动的静止状态。

genuine dhyana Refers to genuine tranquility, indicating the tranquil condition of the activities of consciousness and thinking.

真常【zhēn cháng】　指常得清静之境。

genuine constancy Refers to general state of clarity and tranquility.

真道【zhēn dào】　① 指气功景象,即精神和形体保持稳定状态;② 指气功养生法的基本理论。

genuine Dao Refers to the scene of Qigong, indicating stability of the spirit and body as well as the basic theory of Qigong and life cultivation.

真道养神【zhēn dào yǎng shén】① 指排除声色气味的干扰,维持意识思维活动的稳定;② 指避免精神刺激,去智损欲;③ 指闲居静室,以虚为身,以无为意,守神形为一。

nourishing the spirit with genuine Dao Refers to ① either eliminating the disturbance of external voice, color and taste in order to stabilize the activities of consciousness and thinking; ② or avoiding stimulation of the spirit and eliminating wisdom and desires; ③ or idly staying in a quiet room to relax the body, tranquilize the mind and integrate the spirit and body.

真定【zhēn dìng】　指脑神制而无著,放而不逸,处喧无恶,涉事无恼,以无著为真常,以有为应迹,此为真定。

genuine tranquilization Refers to the fact that the brain spirit controls without any command, relieving without any leisure, solving without any evil, involving without any annoyance, regarding non-source as the convention, and conforming possession to the true

Z

state of the mind.

真动真静【zhēn dòng zhēn jìng】 指从无知觉而恍惚有妙觉是为真动，虚静至极则曰真静。

genuine action and genuine tranquility Refers to either practitioners of Qigong without aesthesia but with enlightenment; or being tranquilized to the utmost point.

真法真机【zhēn fǎ zhēn jī】 指神驭气，神行气行，神住气住之法为真法。

genuine principle and genuine opportunity Indicates that the spirit controls Qi and that only when the spirit moves can Qi move and only when the spirit calms down can Qi calm down.

真诰【zhēn gào】《真诰》为道家书，由南朝陶弘景所著，其中论述的气功养生极为繁富。

Zhen Gao A book about Daoism, written by Tao Hongjing in the Nan Dynasty（502 AD‑557 AD），also describing the importance of Qigong and life cultivation.

真功【zhēn gōng】 指意守气海，抱元守一，神形达到相对稳定的功夫。

genuine exercise Refers to concentrating consciousness in the sea of Qi, embracing the origin and defending the integrity, indicating stability of the spirit and body.

真汞【zhēn gǒng】 即青娥，喻真意。

genuine mercury The same as Green Female Immortal in ancient China, comparing to genuine idea.

真候【zhēn hòu】 指呼吸。

genuine state Refers to respiration.

真虎【zhēn hǔ】 指肾气中之水。

genuine tiger Refers to the water in the kidney Qi.

真慧【zhēn huì】 指气功中，虚极静笃而慧生，慧生而能调节意识思维活动。

genuine wisdom Refers to wisdom produced by tranquility in Qigong practice, which regulates the activities of consciousness and thinking.

真火【zhēn huǒ】 ① 指心火；② 指火为精神意识。

genuine fire Refers to ① either heart fire；② or the spirit and consciousness.

真火本无候【zhēn huǒ běn wú hòu】 源自气功专论，主要阐述火候因练功的不同阶段而有不同的火候。

genuine fire originally showing no opportunity Collected from a monograph of Qigong, mainly describing the different situations of fire at different periods in practicing Qigong.

真火候【zhēn huǒ hòu】 指一念不起，一意不散，意念活动虚极静笃。

genuine fire condition Refers to keeping one idea and remaining one consciousness in order to tranquilize the activity of consciousness and thought.

真火起坎宫【zhēn huǒ qǐ kǎn gōng】 指习练气功时，肾阳充足，机体则富有生机。

genuine fire starting from Kan palace Refers to sufficiency of kidney Qi and vital force in practicing Qigong.

真火育【zhēn huǒ yù】 指真火即神，即神运精气以成丹之意。

genuine fire fostering Refers to genuine fire as the spirit, indicating that the spirit moves the essential Qi to develop into Dan（pills of immortality）.

真机【zhēn jī】 指先天、后天二气合一的瞬间。

genuine opportunity Refers to the crucial period during which the innate Qi and postnatal Qi integrate with each other.

真际【zhēn jì】 指脑。

genuine edge Refers to the brain.

真解脱【zhēn jiě tuō】 佛家气功习用语,指断除一切烦恼,而达神形调和的理想境界。

genuine relief A common term of Qigong in Buddhism, referring to eliminating annoyance and reaching the ideal state of coordinated spirit and body.

真金丹【zhēn jīn dān】 指气功炼精气神所结之丹。

genuine golden Dan (pills of immortality) Refers to Dan (pills of immortality) produced by refining the essence, Qi and the spirit in practicing Qigong.

真金鼎【zhēn jīn dǐng】 指身中之一窍,为呼吸交换之所,意念归存之所。

genuine golden cauldron Refers to one orifice in the body, which is the place for the exchange of inhalation and exhalation as well as the entrance of consciousness and thought.

真精【zhēn jīng】 指精中之精,或纯洁明净之精。

genuine essence Refers to essence within essence, or the pure and bright essence.

真景象【zhēn jǐng xiàng】 指气功现象,为形神相合为一的状态。

genuine scene Refers to integration of the spirit and the body, which is the scene of Qigong.

真境界【zhēn jìng jiè】 指神形合一,无思无虑,无喜无恶,意识思维活动处于相对静止状态。

genuine state Refers to integration of the spirit and body without any anxie-ty, happiness and rage, indicating the tranquilized activities of consciousness and thinking.

真君【zhēn jūn】 指脑神为五脏六腑、四肢百骸之君。

genuine immortal Refers to the spirit of the five Zang-organs (including the heart, the liver, the spleen, the lung and the kidney) and the six Fu-organs (the gallbladder, stomach, small intestine, large intestine, bladder and triple energizer) as well as the four limbs and all the skeletons.

真空【zhēn kōng】 指太空,文中意指真空中。

genuine vacuum Refers to the celestial space or vacuum in the literature of Qigong.

真空炼形【zhēn kōng liàn xíng】 指气功习练中神形合一的状态。

refining the body in genuine vacuum Refers to the integration of the spirit and the body in practicing Qigong.

真理六气诀【zhēn lǐ liù qì jué】 源自气功专论,阐述六气分治五脏三焦之疾。

formula for truth and six kinds of Qi Collected from a monograph of Qigong, describing that six kinds of Qi can treat diseases in the five Zang-organs (including the heart, the liver, the spleen, the lung and the kidney) and triple energizer.

真龙【zhēn lóng】 即真龙出自离宫,气功文献认为龙从火里出。

genuine Loong Refers to the fact that the genuine Loong exists in the detached palace. According to the literature of Qigong, Loong appears from fire.

真龙虎【zhēn lóng hǔ】 ① 指真阴、真

Z

阳;② 或指元神、元气。喻身体阴阳两各方面。

genuine Loong and tiger Refers to ① either genuine Yin and genuine Yang;② or the original spirit and the original Qi. Usually it compares to Yin and Yang.

真龙虎九仙经【zhēn lóng hǔ jiǔ xiān jīng】《真龙虎九仙经》为气功学专著，唐罗公远、叶法善注。书及注中具体介绍了观鼻法、仙家睡法、练五脏法、河车运转法、练婴儿法、练地仙法、九等仙侠法等。

Zhenlonghu Jiuxian Jing（*Canon of Genuine Loong and Tiger with Nine Immortals*） A monograph of Qigong entitled *Canon of Genuine Loong and Tiger with Nine Immortals*, explained by Luo Gongyuan and Ye Fashan in the Tang Dynasty（618 AD－907 AD）, the content and explanations of which particularly introduce the exercises for observing the nose, lying of the immortals, refining the five Zang-organs（including the heart, the liver, the spleen, the lung and the kidney）, returning of the river cart, refining baby and refining the earthly immortals.

真念【zhēn niàn】 指气功锻炼中，身心安定，气息调匀，万念俱忘，一灵独存，谓之正念。

genuine thinking Refers to stabilization of the body and heart, harmonization of respiration, loss of all ideas and desires and existence of the single-minded spirit in practicing Qigong.

真七返【zhēn qī fǎn】 指眼不视外色，耳不闻异香，口不食五味，精神内守而不外散，谓之真七返。

seven returning states Refers to the fact that the eyes do not see any external colors, the ears do not listen any abnormal voice, the mouth does not eat five tastes and the spirit concentrates internally without external dispersion.

真气【zhēn qì】 ① 指先天元精之清者;② 指正气;③ 自然之气与谷气之合。

genuine Qi Refers to ① either clarity of innate original essence; ② or healthy Qi; ③ or combination of the natural Qi and grain Qi.

真气还元铭【zhēn qì huán yuán míng】五代梁人所撰，强名子注解，内容为阳气定胎。

Zhenqi Huanyuan Ming（*Inscription of Genuine Qi Returning to the Origin*） A monograph of cultivation Qi and conception entitled *Inscription of Genuine Qi Returning to the Origin*, written by Liang Ren in the Five Dynasties（907 AD－960 AD）and explained by Qiang Mingzi.

真铅【zhēn qiān】 指真阴,亦指真精。

genuine lead Refers to genuine Yin or genuine essence.

真铅入鼎【zhēn qiān rù dǐng】 指元精经河车搬入泥丸的情况。

genuine lead entering cauldron Refers to the situation that the original essence is transmitted to the mud bolus（the brain）by the river cart.

真铅真汞【zhēn qiān zhēn gǒng】① 指太阴之精为真铅，太阳之气为真汞;② 指身体阴阳两个方面。

genuine lead and genuine mercury Refers to ① either essence in Taiyin being genuine lead and Qi in Taiyang being genuine mercury;② or Yin and Yang in the human body.

真铅著意寻【zhēn qiān zhù yì xún】
源自气功专论,主要阐述真铅为炼内丹之本。

genuine lead ensuring consciousness
Collected from a monograph of Qigong, mainly describing that the genuine lead is the root of refining the internal Dan (pills of immortality).

真诠【zhēn quán】《真诠》为气功专著,由清代彭定求校刻,主要阐述修炼之法。

Zhen Quan (*Genuine Reasons*) A monograph of Qigong entitled *Genuine Reasons*, proofread and engraved by Peng Dingqiu in the Qing Dynasty (1636 AD – 1912 AD), mainly describing the exercises for practicing Qigong.

真人【zhēn rén】① 指对道学研究有成就的人;② 指气功锻炼高深的人;③ 指对道家领袖的封号;④ 指金丹;⑤ 指元神。

Genuine man Refers to ① either those who have achieved great successes in studying Daoism; ② or those who have profoundly practiced Qigong; ③ or the title of the Daoism leader; ④ or golden Dan (pills of immortality); ⑤ or the original spirit.

真人常居法【zhēn rén cháng jū fǎ】
为动功。其作法为,不拘时,常常用两手按揉两眉后小穴中,三九过。又以手心及指摩两目,手顺势向上,旋耳三十过。再以手逆从额上三九过,从眉中始上行入发际中。口傍咽液,多少不拘,并用双手顺发轻搓头面部。做毕,以两手按四眦二九过。

exercise of immortal's general living A dynamic exercise, marked by always rubbing the small acupoints behind the eyebrows for three to nine times, rubbing the eyes upwards with the palms and rotating the ears for thirty times, raising the hands from the forehead and along the middle of the eyebrows to the hair line, normally swallowing humor through the mouth, mildly rubbing the head and face with both hands and the four canthus for two or nine times.

真人呼吸处【zhēn rén hū xī chù】
① 指玄关一窍;② 指脐下丹田。

the place for immortal's respiration Refers to ① either an orifice in an important region; ② or the lower Dantian (the region below the navel).

真人秘传火候法【zhēn rén mì zhuàn huǒ hòu fǎ】 一部专著,介绍时中火候、行水方便、真人露火机等。作者不详。

Zhenren Michuan Huohou Fa (*Immortal's Secret Introduction of Fire Opportunity*) A monograph of traditional Chinese culture entitled *Immortal's Secret Introduction of Fire Opportunity*, introducing the secrets of fire condition in the middle period, convenience for moving water and fire advantages shown by immortals. The author was unknown.

真人起居法【zhēn rén qǐ jū fǎ】 为动静相兼功。其作法为,睡前先呵出腹内浊气,或一九止,或五六止。定心闭目,叩齿三十六通,以集心神。然后以大拇指背拭目,大小九过。兼按鼻左右七过。以两手摩令极热,闭口鼻气,然后摩面,不以遍数。

exercise of immortal's getting up and sleeping An exercise combined with dynamic exercise and static exercise, marked by breathing out turbid Qi from the abdomen before sleep for one to nine times or five to six times, stabilizing the heat, closing the eyes, clicking the teeth for thirty-six times in order to concentrate the heart spirit, then pressing the eyes with the thumbs for nine times, then pressing the nose from the left to the right and vice versa for seven times respectively, rubbing the hands hot, closing the mouth, inhaling through the nose and rubbing the face for several times.

真人潜深渊【zhēn rén qián shēn yuān】 指元神守于上丹田。真人指元神,深渊指上丹田。

immortal diving into abyss Refers to concentration of the original spirit in the upper Dantian (the region between the eyes). In this term, immortal refers to the original spirit while abyss refers the upper Dantian (the region between the eyes).

真人潜深渊,浮游守规中【zhēn rén qián shēn yuān fú yóu shǒu guī zhōng】 指存精神于内心,守中抱一。

Immortal dives into abyss and swims according to the principles. Refers to internal concentration of the spirit in the heart with somatic and spiritual balance.

真人食黄气法【zhēn rén shí huáng qì fǎ】 为静功。其作法为,常念脾胃饱,有黄色之气润泽。并意想想有一人像,长三寸,穿黄衣。在人像两手中也各有一人,亦穿黄衣。

exercise of immortal's taking yellow Qi A static exercise, marked by thinking that the spleen and the stomach are full with yellow Qi to moisten, imagining that there is a portrait of man of 3 Cun with yellow clothes that keeps one man in one hand also with yellow clothes.

真人胎息【zhēn rén tāi xī】 指意识稳定,呼吸平和。

immortal's fetal respiration Refers to stability of consciousness and harmonization of respiration.

真人真知法【zhēn rén zhēn zhī fǎ】 指调节饮食起居,调节呼吸,调节精神。

exercise of immortal's real knowledge A dynamic exercise for regulating diet and daily life, regulating respiration and regulating the spirit.

真人之息自游丝【zhēn rén zhī xī zì yóu sī】 指真人呼吸,不分出息入息,绵绵密密,如游丝不断。

Immortal's respiration is natural like gossamer. Indicates that there is no difference between inhalation and exhalation in the respiration of immortals, which is quiet natural and mild, just like gossamer.

真人坐起法【zhēn rén zuò qǐ fǎ】 即真人常居法,为动功。其作法为,不拘时,常常用两手按揉两眉后小穴中,三九过。又以手心及指摩两目,手顺势向上,旋耳三十过。再以手逆从额上三九过,从眉中上行入发际中,口傍咽液,多少不拘,并用双手顺发轻搓头面部。做毕,以两手按四眦二九过。

exercise of immortal's sitting and standing The same as exercise of immortal's general living, is a dynamic exercise, marked by always rubbing the small acupoints behind the eyebrows for three to nine times, rubbing the eyes upwards with the palms and rotating the ears for thirty times, raising the hands from the forehead and along the middle of the eyebrows to the hair line, normally swallowing humor through the mouth, mildly rubbing the head and face with both hands and the four canthus for two or nine times.

真如【zhēn rú】　佛家气功习用语，① 指事物的真实情况；② 指一切现象的本质；③ 指精神境界；④ 指同体异名；⑤ 指调节精神的作用。

genuine fact　A common term of Qigong in Buddhism, referring to ① either the true situation of anything; ② or the essence of anything; ③ or the state of the spirit; ④ or the synonym of anything; ⑤ or the effect of spirit regulation.

真如无为【zhēn rú wú wéi】　佛家气功习用语，指真理，即佛家各派气功所要达到的精神境界。

genuine inaction　A common term of Qigong in Buddhism, referring to truth which is the ideal state of all the schools of Qigong in Buddhism.

真身【zhēn shēn】　指神形相同，合二为一之身。

genuine body　Refers to sameness of the spirit and the body, indicating the integration of the spirit and the body.

真时【zhēn shí】　指药生之时，即习练气功内气发功较明显之时，多为子时。

genuine time　Refers to the time when medicinal is produced, indicating the time when the internal Qi is obviously clear in practicing Qigong, usually referring to Zi (the period of the day from 11 p.m. to 1 a.m.).

真实际【zhēn shí jì】　指性命双修的理论与实践方法。

genuine fact　Refers to the theory and practice for cultivating life.

真水【zhēn shuǐ】　指心生液，以液生于心而不耗散。

genuine water　Refers to humor produced by the heart without any dissipation.

真水真火论【zhēn shuǐ zhēn huǒ lùn】　源自气功专论，主要论述心液为真水，肾气为真火。

idea about genuine water and genuine fire　Collected from a monograph of Qigong, mainly discussing that heart humor is genuine water and kidney Qi is genuine fire.

真思【zhēn sī】　指神思专一，立志学道，认识清静的方法。

genuine thinking　Refers to single-minded spirit and consciousness, earnest study of Dao and understanding the exercise of tranquilization.

真胎【zhēn tāi】　指精气神和合为一，藏于丹田，丹田之精气盈满。

genuine embryo　Refers to integration of the essence, Qi and spirit that are stored in Dantian, exuberating the essence and Qi in Dantian. Dantian is divided into the upper Dantian (the region between the eyes), the middle Dantian (the region below the heart) and the lower Dantian (the region below the navel).

真胎息【zhēn tāi xī】　指调节精神而不注呼吸的功法。

genuine fetal respiration　Refers to the exercise focusing on regulation of the spirit, not on respiration.

真胎息景【zhēn tāi xī jǐng】　指气功中的呼吸景象。

scene of genuine fetal respiration　Refers to the scene of respiration in practicing Qigong.

Z

真土【zhēn tǔ】 ① 指身体内阴阳两个方面；② 指脾之液为真土；③ 指肺之液。

genuine earth Refers to ① either Yin and Yang in the human body；② or humor in the spleen；③ or humor in the lung.

真西山先生卫生歌 【zhēn xī shān xiān shēng wèi shēng gē】《真西山先生卫生歌》为气功专论，主要阐述叩齿、运动水土、养气益津、熨目、擦面、灌溉中岳、修城廓、六字诀(吹、呼、唏、呵、嘘、呬)气功健身却病方法。作者不详。

Zhenxishan Xiansheng Weisheng Ge (*Mr. Zhen Xishan's Health Song*) A monograph of Qigong entitled *Mr. Zhen Xishan's Health Song*, mainly describing the exercises for fortify the body and curing diseases，including clicking the teeth，moving water and earth，nourishing Qi and enriching fluid，ironing the eyes，rubbing the face，irrigating nasal sides，rubbing the ears and reading six Chinese characters，i. e. Chui（blowing），Hu（exhaling），Xi（sighing），Ke（breathing out），Xu（breathing out slowly）and Xi（panting）. The author was unknown.

真息【zhēn xī】 指练功者在入静状态下，出现的均匀、细缓、深长的一种呼吸。

genuine respiration Refers to equal，gentle and deep respiration in practicing Qigong with static exercise.

真息息【zhēn xī xī】 指真息之息，神静息调，绵绵若存，不使其间断。

genuine respiration and respiration Refers to genuine respiration in respiration and regulation of respiration in tranquilizing the spirit，which perpetually exists and never stops.

真仙直指语录【zhēn xiān zhí zhǐ yǔ lù】《真仙直指语录》为气功专著，为元代玄全子集，阐述了内功功法及修心养性。

Zhenxian Zhizhi Yulu (*Pure Quotations of the Genuine Immortals*) A monograph of Qigong entitled *Pure Quotations of the Genuine Immortals*，collected by Xuan Quanzi in the Yuan Dynasty（1271 AD - 1368 AD），describing the exercises to benefit the internal organs and cultivation of the heart and nature.

真先天气【zhēn xiān tiān qì】 指气穴之先天气在动与未动之时称为真先天气。

genuineness of innate Qi Refers to the period of innate Qi that may moves or may not move in the acupoint of Qi.

真心【zhēn xīn】 佛家气功学术语，指真实不妄之心，又指正信无疑之心。意为精神活动协调、稳定。

genuine heart A common term of Qigong Buddhism，referring to the true mind without any delusion or sincerity without any doubt，indicating coordination and stability of the spirit activity.

真心痛【zhēn xīn tòng】 气功适应证，临床上以心悸气短、胸痛彻背为特征，为精神损伤，心脉及心失养所引起。

angina pectoris An indication of Qigong，characterized by palpitation，shortness of breath and radiation of chest pain to the back，caused by injury of the spirit and malnutrition of the heart and heart meridian.

真性【zhēn xìng】 指人体生命的自然本性。

genuine property Refers to the original

nature of human life.

真性命【zhēn xìng mìng**】** 即虚静状态为真性命。性为神,命为气。

genuine nature and life Refers to quietness and tranquility as the real life. In this term, nature refers to the spirit and the life refers to Qi.

真玄【zhēn xuán**】** 指认识阳变阴,阴交阳,阴阳之间的气化作用。

genuine supremeness Means that Yang turns into Yin and Yin turns into Yang, indicating the transformation of Qi between Yin and Yang.

真穴【zhēn xué**】** 指下丹田。下丹田指气海,指脐下。

genuine point Refers to the lower Dantian (the region below the navel). The lower Dantian (the region below the navel) refers to either Qihai (CV 6) located below the navel; or the region below the navel.

真阳初升玉虚内景【zhēn yáng chū shēng yù xū nèi jǐng**】** 为静功。其作法为,于夏历每月初三日卯时(五至七时)在清静的室内坐定,排除一切杂念,叩齿三十六通,意想自己为昆仑山神,慢慢升至山顶,闭息,默念道家"符咒"九遍。

early rise of genuine Yang in the internal scene of jade vacuum A static exercise, marked by sitting in a quiet and clear room in Mao (the period of a day from 5 a.m. to 7 a.m. in the morning) on the third day in every month in summer, eliminating any distracting thought, clicking the teeth for thirty-six times, imagining to become a god in the Kunlun Mountain and slowly reaching the top of Kunlun Mountain, stopping respiration and silently reading

Daoist incantations for nine times.

真阳之精气【zhēn yáng zhī jīng qì**】** 指身内生气之根,藏于丹田,有生视、生听、生言、生动、生思、生虑的作用。

essential Qi in genuine Yang Refers to the root for producing Qi in the body and storing in Dantian, effective for ensuring vision, listening, speech, action, thought and consideration. Dantian is divided into the upper Dantian (the region between the eyes), the middle Dantian (the region below the heart) and the lower Dantian (the region below the navel).

真一【zhēn yī**】** ① 指习练气功,意识活动专一不二;② 指身体阴阳合二为一;③ 指呼吸平和。

one genuineness Refers to ① either concentration of consciousness activity in practicing Qigong; ② or integration of Yin and Yang; ③ or peaceful respiration.

真一处【zhēn yī chù**】** 即祖窍,指位于心与脐之正中。

genuine part The same as ancestral orifice, referring to the central region between the heart and the navel.

真一大略【zhēn yī dà lüè**】** 源自气功专论,阐述气功一分为二、合二为一的变化规律。

genuineness of general idea Collected from a monograph of Qigong, describing the principles of changes in Qigong that one divides into two and two integrates into one.

真一秘要【zhēn yī mì yào**】** 源自气功专论,主要阐述习练气功若达到神气相合、贯通一气、流行上下,则可功成而能长寿。

secretion and importance of genuine

one Collected from a monograph of Qigong, mainly describing the combination of the spirit and Qi as well as the connection with Qi in practicing Qigong, upper and lower flow of which can succeed and prolong life.

真一窍【zhēn yī qiào】 与黄庭相同，① 指中；② 指身体内的中虚空窍；③ 指五脏之中；④ 指脐之后；⑤ 指有名无所；⑥ 指黄八极；⑦ 指黄庭在二肾之中；⑧ 指黄庭在心之下。

genuine orifice The same as Huangting (yellow hall), referring to ① either the center; ② or the middle deficiency and empty orifice in the center of the body; ③ or the center of the five Zang-organs (including the heart, the liver, the spleen, the lung and the kidney); ④ or the region below the navel; ⑤ or a person or something with name but without position; ⑥ or eight yellow extremities; ⑦ or Huangting (yellow hall) located in the region between the kidneys; ⑧ or Huangting (yellow hall) located in the region below the heart.

真一之精【zhēn yī zhī jīng】 指真阴、真阳。

A genuine essence Refers to genuine Yin and genuine Yang.

真一之水【zhēn yī zhī shuǐ】 指肾中之水。

genuine water Refers to water in the kidney.

真一种子【zhēn yì zhǒng zǐ】 同丹，指阴阳两种药物在体内合炼而成丹。

a genuine seed The same as Dan (pills of immortality), refers to the result of Yin and Yang medicinals that have integrated in the body; also It refers to

Qigong, an important appellation of Qigong.

真意【zhēn yì】 指元神。

genuine consciousness Refers to the original spirit.

真阴阳【zhēn yīn yáng】 即真龙虎，① 指真阴、真阳；② 或指元神、元气，喻身体阴阳两各方面。

genuine Yin and Yang The same as genuine Loong and tiger, referring to ① either genuine Yin and genuine Yang; ② or the original spirit and the original Qi. Usually it compares to Yin and Yang.

真阴真阳论【zhēn yīn zhēn yáng lùn】 源自气功专论，主要以人生胞胎发生为喻而述真阴、真阳及其相互关系。

idea about genuine Yin and genuine Yang Collected from a monograph of Qigong, mainly describing the relation between genuine Yin and genuine Yang according to embryo conceived in the human body.

真元【zhēn yuán】 指元气。

genuine origin Refers to the original Qi.

真源反此【zhēn yuán fǎn cǐ】 即还精补脑。

returning of the genuine origin Refers to returning the essence in order to tonify the brain.

真宰【zhēn zǎi】 指天为万物的主宰，喻人之脑为身之主宰。

genuine dominator Refers to the sky as the dominator of all the things in the universe. In Qigong, it refers to the brain as the dominator of the body.

真则守真渊【zhēn zé shǒu zhēn yuān】 精神内守，不染杂念则泰和含真，神形相随，神识明澈湛然。

Z

**Only the genuine element keeps the genu-
ine source.** This is a celebrated dic-
tum，referring to internally concentrating the spirit，eliminating distracting
thought for harmonizing the body and
realizing truth，coordinating the spirit
and body and purifying the mind.

真宅【zhēn zhái】 指脑。

genuine chamber Refers to the brain.

真中【zhēn zhōng】 指无极。

genuine center Refers to non-polar.

真种【zhēn zhǒng】 指父之精，母之
血，交媾合成。喻气功中，神气凝合
一处。

genuine essence Refers to paternal semen and maternal blood，intercourse of
which has achieved conception. In
Qigong，it refers to integration of the
spirit and Qi.

真种子【zhēn zhǒng zi】 指气功锻炼
中精气神合一所结之丹头为真种子。

genuine seed Indicates that，in Qigong
practice，integration of the essence，Qi
and spirit forms Dantou（the synthetic
medicinal）which is the so-called genuine seed.

真宗【zhēn zōng】 指元神、元气，是身
体之本。

genuine ancestor Refers to the original
spirit and original Qi which are the origins of the human body.

枕骨【zhěn gǔ】 指骨名，也指足少阳
胆经上的一个穴位，位于乳突后上方。
这一穴位为气功运行的一个常见部位。

occipital bone Refers to either a special kind of bone；or an acupoint in the
gallbladder of foot Shaoyang，located
in the upper of mastoid process back.
This acupoint is a region usually used
for keeping the essential Qi in practice

of Qigong.

枕上坐卧诀法【zhěn shàng zuò wò
jué fǎ】 为静功。① 指静坐；② 指闭口；
③ 指导引。

exercise of sitting and lying on bed A
static exercise，referring to ① either
sitting quietly；② or closing the mouth；
③ or Daoyin in practicing Qigong.

枕中记【zhěn zhōng jì】 《枕中记》为
气功养生专著，阐述气功的习练方法和
效果，作者不详。

**Zhenzhong Ji（Record of Practice with
Pillow）** A monograph of Qigong entitled Record of Practice with Pillow，de-
scribing the methods and effects of
Qigong practice. The author was unknown.

朋【zhèn】 指脊背上的肌肉。

muscle Refers to the fleshes in the
spine and back of the human body.

振腹【zhèn fù】 即用口吸气，使充满
腹部而鼓起，然后用鼻慢慢呼出，同时腹
部恢复原状。

vibrating the abdomen Refers to inhaling through the mouth in order to enrich Qi in the abdomen，then exhaling
slowly through the nose and normalizing the abdomen.

震【zhèn】 ① 指卦名，其象为雷；② 指
引起情志损伤；③ 指取象比类；④ 指方
向；⑤ 指长男。

quake Refers to ① either Zhen Tri-
gram，the image of which is thunder；
② or damage of emotion；③ or analo-
gy；④ or direction；⑤ or the eldest
man. Zhen Trigram is in the Eight Trigrams from Yijing（Canon of Simplifi-
cation，Change and No Change）.

震旦三圣【zhèn dàn sān shèng】 指
中国古代三圣，即老子、孔子、颜回。

three great sages Refers to Lao Zi, Confucius and Yuan Hui in ancient China.

震宫青气【zhèn gōng qīng qì**】** 震宫为八卦之位，即东方；青气即自然之气。

green Qi in Zhen Trigram In this term Zhen Trigram refers to the east, which is one of the locations in the Eight Trigrams; green Qi refers to natural Qi. Zhen Trigram is in the Eight Trigrams from Yijing (*Canon of Simplification, Change and No Change*).

震眩【zhèn xuàn**】** 指精神不稳定协调所产生的身震颤眩晕。

severe dizziness Refers to tremble and vertigo in regulation due to unstable spirit.

镇静心田【zhèn jìng xīn tián**】** 指震慑邪念，导引入静，和平意识活动。

tranquilizing the heart Refers to eliminating evil thought, tranquilizing the body and harmonizing the mind.

正月中导引法【zhēng yuè zhōng dǎo yǐn fǎ**】** 为动功。其作法为，正月中，每日子丑时，手按臀部转身，左右各十五次，以疏通三焦气机，身体轻便。

exercise of Daoyin in the middle of January A dynamic exercise, marked by pressing the buttocks and turning the body with both hands from the left to the right for fifteen times in Zi (the period of the day from 11 p.m. to 1 a.m.) and Chou (from 1 a.m to 3 a.m. in the early morning) every day in the middle of January in order to unobstruct the activity of Qi in the triple energizer and to relax the body.

正定【zhèng dìng**】** 佛家气功习用语，指意识活动专注于一境。

genuine concentration A common term of Qigong in Buddhism, refers to concentration of consciousness on just one state.

正观【zhèng guān**】** 指练功时眼神集中在"玄牝"。

genuine vision Refers to concentration of the ocular spirit in the chamber of morality.

正果【zhèng guǒ**】** 佛家气功习用语，指练气功取得成绩。

genuine result A common term of Qigong in Buddhism, referring to the achievement in practicing Qigong.

正己【zhèng jǐ**】** 指精神意识思维活动的稳定，正己情性、道德、行为。

self-restriction Refers to stabilizing the activities of the spirit, consciousness and thinking in order to rectify self-temperament, self-morality and self-action.

正觉【zhèng jié**】** 指正之觉，不经思考，原本具有悟性。

genuine consciousness Refers to genuine awareness without any thinking.

正精进【zhèng jīng jìn**】** 佛家气功习用语，指勤修佛家气功，使之通向精神思维活动的理想境界。

genuine progression A common term of Qigong in Buddhism, referring to diligently practicing Qigong in Buddhism in order to reach the ideal state of the spirit and consciousness activities.

正静定【zhèng jìng dìng**】** 指圣人调节精神思维活动的方法。

genuine tranquilization Refers to the method of sages for regulating the spirit and consciousness activities.

正念【zhèng niàn**】** 指练功时杂念易经排除，头脑保持清净的状态。

genuine thought Refers to elimination

of distracting thought and stabilization of the brain in practicing Qigong.

正平【zhèng píng**】** 指神形和合,保持稳定状态。

stability Refers to harmonizing the spirit and the body in order to stabilize the body.

正气【zhèng qì**】** ① 指精神活动;② 指身体的元气;③ 指真气。

genuine Qi Refers to ① either spiritual activity; ② or the original Qi in the body; ③ or the genuine Qi.

正日【zhèng rì**】** 指农历正月初一,又名正旦。

genuine day Refers to New Year's Day of the Chinese lunar calendar.

正身【zhèng shēn**】** 指端正神形。

genuine body Refers to rectifying the spirit and the body.

正室【zhèng shì**】** 指脑内九宫。

genuine chamber Refers to the nine chambers in the brain.

正位【zhèng wèi**】** 指端身正坐,不倾不斜,正坐其中。

right way Refers to sitting in the right way without any deflection.

正位居中【zhèng wèi jū zhōng**】** 指身体居端正之位,喻身体端方正直,意识活动内存于心。

right state Refer to maintaining the body in the right way and concentrating the consciousness activity on the heart.

正卧行气法【zhèng wò xíng qì fǎ**】** 为静功。其作法为,正卧时,以鼻微微纳气,徐徐引之,勿令太极满。

method for regulating Qi in lying on the back A static exercise, referring to mild inhalation through the nose and slowly exhalation without extreme respiration.

正邪【zhèng xié**】** 指干扰刺激身心正常活动的各种因素。

Interfering factor Refers to various factors that disturb and irritate the normal activities of the body and the heart.

正心【zhèng xīn**】** 指意识思维活动端正在中,不偏不倚。

genuine heart Refers to correct activity of consciousness and thought.

正心复性【zhèng xīn fù xìng**】** 指守中抱一,复其本性,自然神形协调平衡,保持稳定。

genuine balance Refers to somatic and spiritual balance, recovering natural property, regulating, balancing and stabilizing the spirit and body.

正信【zhèng xìn**】** 佛家气功习用语,指意识活动不受杂念干扰。

genuine faith A common term of Qigong in Buddhism, referring to the fact that the activity of consciousness cannot be disturbed by distracting thought in practicing Qigong.

正性【zhèng xìng**】** 指人体的精神意识思维活动。

genuine property Refers to the activities of the spirit, consciousness and thinking.

正阳朝拜灵辉内景【zhèng yáng cháo bài líng huī nèi jǐng**】** 为静功。于夏历每月十五日在清净的室内静坐,默诵。

internal scene of celestial visiting imagination A static exercise, marked by sitting quietly in a clear room on 15th in every month in summer, and silently reading.

正阳灵光通明内景【zhèng yáng líng guāng tōng míng nèi jǐng**】** 为静功。

Z

其作法为,于夏历每月十七日午时,净室静坐,排除杂念,调匀呼吸,叩齿三十六通,咽下津液。

scene of celestial imagination A quiet room in the noon in the seventeenth day in every month in summer, eliminating distracting thought, regulating respiration, clicking teeth for thirty-six times and swallowing fluid and humor.

正药【zhèng yào**】** 指元气、元精、元神。

genuine medicinal Refers to the original Qi, the original essence and the original spirit.

正业【zhèng yè**】** 佛家气功学习用语。① 指习练气功,身心清净,排除一切杂念;② 佛为觉悟之意,指口中念"佛",以排除杂念。

regular occupation A common term of Qigong in Buddhism, referring to ① either tranquilizing the body and the heart in practicing Qigong in order to eliminate distracting thought; ② or reading Buddhism when practicing Qigong in order to eliminate distracting thought.

正一【zhèng yī**】** ① 指意念纯正,集中统一;② 指行功中意念活动协调,神形维持相对稳定状态。

right one Refers to ① either concentrated unity; ② or regulation of mental activities in movement in order to stabilize the condition of consciousness.

正一法文修真旨要【zhèng yī fǎ wén xiū zhēn zhǐ yào**】** 《正一法文修真旨要》为气功专著,成书于南北朝时期,作者不详。

Zhengyi Fawen Xiuzhen Zhiyao(*Essentials of Righteous Law for Cultivating Genuineness*) A monograph of Qigong entitled *Essentials of Righteous Law for Cultivating Genuineness*, compiled in the Northern and Southern Dynasties (420 AD – 589 AD). The author was unknown.

正一服日月精华法【zhèng yī fú rì yuè jīng huá fǎ**】** 为静功。晨起或夜半生气时,仰卧,觉腹空即服,不限时节,四肢自然,行住坐卧皆可。

exercise for inhaling natural essence A static exercise, marked by lying on the back, inhaling essence in the early morning or at night when Qi is increasing and naturally keeping the four limbs at any side. In such a static exercise, walking, staying, sitting and lying are all necessary for practicing Qigong.

正一服元和正气法【zhèng yī fú yuán hé zhèng qì fǎ**】** 为静功。全自动为,不拘时,闲即可作。每一二时服三五十咽,令腹中常有元气在气海中。

exercise for inhaling primordial and normal Qi A static exercise, marked by practicing Qigong at any free time without any restraint, and swallowing in one or two periods for thirty or fifty times in order to promote the original Qi in the abdomen and to enter it into the sea of Qi.

正一服元气法【zhèng yī fú yuán qì fǎ**】** 为静功。指不论早晚,得服则服,强身健体,预防疾病。

method for genuine inhalation of original Qi A static exercise, referring to the fact that respiration must be regulated in daytime and nighttime in order to strengthen the body, to cultivate health and to prevent diseases.

正意【zhèng yì**】** 佛家气功习用语,指意识活动端正而无邪念。

Z

genuine mind A common term of Qigong in Buddhism, refers to righteous mental activity without any distracting thought.

正直舍方便法【zhèng zhí shě fāng biàn fǎ**】** 佛家气功功法。意守"正直",排除偏旁,曲折念头。

method for maintaining genuine consciousness A method for practicing Qigong in Buddhism, referring to concentration of the mind and elimination of distracting thought.

正祖宗【zhèng zǔ zōng**】** 指元精,以其为炼丹的基础物质。

genuine ancestor Refers to original essence which is the basic substance for alchemy.

证道秘言【zhèng dào mì yán**】** 《证道秘言》为气功丛书,为清代付金铨所辑,该书收载了自撰的五种气功专著。

Zhengdao Miyan（*Secret Discussions about Proving Truth***）** A series of Qigong entitled *Secret Discussions about Proving Truth*, compiled by Fu Jinquan in the Qing Dynasty（1636 AD－1912 AD）, including five monographs written by Fu Jinquan.

证真【zhèng zhēn**】** 指气功中神形相互作用,相顾、相并、相入、相抱,逐步进入俱妙、双舍的境界。

proving truth Refers to mutual effect of the spirit and the body, including mutual support, mutual combination, mutual entrance and mutual integration, eventually developing into the wonderful and double alms state.

郑卫【zhèng wèi**】** 指春秋战国时期的郑国和卫国的民间音乐,后为淫靡之乐的代称。气功学中认为证卫之音能引起精神紊乱。

Zheng Wei Refers to the popular music in the Zheng State and Wei State in the Spring and Autumn Period（770 BC－476 BC）and Warring States Period（475 BC－221 BC）, which was called decadent and extravagant music. In Qigong, it is deemed to be the cause of the spirit disorders.

癥瘕候导引法【zhèng jiǎ hòu dǎo yǐn fǎ**】** 动静相兼功。其作法为,凌晨,去枕,正仰卧,伸展四肢,合目闭口,闭气不息,尽力鼓腹,两脚用力。然后再呼吸,过一会收腹,仰两足,反向蹉屈,待呼吸平静后再作。

exercise of Daoyin fair abdominal mass An exercise combined with dynamic exercise and static exercise, marked by lying on the back in the early morning without a pillow, stretching the four limbs, closing the eyes and mouth, stopping respiration, instigating the abdomen, stretching the feet forcefully, then breathing again, keeping the abdomen, raising the feet, bending to the opposite side and continuing to practice after quieted respiration.

支饮【zhī yǐn**】** 气功适应证,指饮停留胸膈。症见胸闷短气,咳逆喘满不得卧,甚则面浮跗肿,或头晕目眩,痰多、食少。

thoracic retention of fluid An indication of Qigong, refers to retention of water in the chest and diaphragm characterized by chest tightness, shortness of breath, inability to sleep due to cough and asthma or even facial edema, tarsal swelling, dizziness and dazzling, causing excessive sputum and reduced appetite.

只闲而少欲【zhī xián ér shǎo yù**】** 指心志安闲,少有欲望,保持人体情绪安

Z

定,气血流畅,内环境协调平衡。

leisure with less desire A celebrated dictum, referring to the leisurely mind and the heart that stabilize the emotion, circulate Qi and blood as well as coordinate and balance the internal environment.

只要凝神入气穴 【zhī yào níng shén rù qì xué】 《只要凝神入气穴》为气功专论,作者不详。

Zhiyao Ningshen Ru Qixue (*Concentration Ensuring the Spirit to Enter Qi Point*) A monograph of Qigong entitled *Concentration Ensuring the Spirit to Enter Qi Point*. The author was unknown.

只知修性不修命,此是修行第一病 【zhǐ zhī xiū xìng bù xiū mìng cǐ shì xiū xíng dì yī bìng】 性指的是阴,命指的是阳。只修阴气,不修阳气,自然致病。

Only clear about cultivating property but not clear about cultivating life, this is the first disease caused in practicing Qigong. Property refers to Yin while life refers to Yang. Only when Yin Qi is cultivated but Yang Qi is not cultivated can disease certainly be occurred.

知 【zhī】 ① 指认识事物的变化,以协调情志活动;② 为佛家气功习用语,指了了自觉。

cognition Refers to ① either the changes of understanding anything in order to regulate consciousness activity; ② or the common term of Qigong in Buddhism, referring to awareness.

知白守黑 【zhī bái shǒu hēi】 即内守精神而不外散。

cognizing white and keeping black Refers to internal concentrating the essence and spirit and avoiding any dispersion.

知法 【zhī fǎ】 即知十二部经能诠之法。

cognizing laws Means to understand the principles of twelve meridians.

知防 【zhī fáng】 指知道自然环境和四时气化变化,防治六淫贼邪侵袭而致病。

cognizing prevention Means to understand natural environment and changes of weather in the four seasons in order to prevent disease caused by invasion of pathogenic factors.

知节 【zhī jié】 指节嗜欲、节烦恼、节忿怒、节辛勤、节思虑、节悲哀,以防情志变化、思虑过度而致病。

mental control Refers to control craving, annoyance, anger, hardness, contemplation, and sorrow in order to prevent disease caused by emotional changes and excessive contemplation.

知觉 【zhī jué】 指人体形成之后才有精神意识,有精神意识作用才具感觉和知觉。

cognizing consciousness Refers to the fact that only when only there is the manifestation of the essence, the spirit and the mentality after the formation of the body can a person contain sensation and consciousness.

知乃止 【zhī nǎi zhǐ】 指精气运行与意识活动之间的关系。知为神,止为行止,即神行则气行,神住则气止。

cognition with stop Refers to the relationship between the essential Qi activity and consciousness activity. In this term, cognition refers to the spirit and stop refers to end of activity, indicating that the spirit movement ensures Qi movement and the end of the spirit movement stops the Qi movement.

知时【zhī shí】　指可修寂静、精进、舍定、般若等。

cognizing time　Means to cultivate mind and spirit and to understand officials and wisdom.

知位【zhī wèi】　指阴阳变化规律。

cognizing position　Refers to principles of Yin and Yang changes.

知信【zhī xìn】　指区别于不信。

Cognizing belief　Means to be different from unbelief.

知一【zhī yī】　指认识事物发展变化的规律。

principle of cognition　Refers to the principle for understanding the development and change of anything.

知止而后有定【zhī zhǐ ér hòu yǒu dìng】　指知道满足及适可而止,不贪名货钱财,即可避免干扰,稳定精神,健康延年。

Only when the acme of perfection is attained can a man decide his ambitions.　Indicates that only when a man is satisfied without any avarice can he avoid any disturbance, stabilizing this spirit, cultivating heath and prolonging life.

知众【zhī zhòng】　指了解其他人物和事物。

cognizing others　Means to understand other people and things.

知自【zhī zì】　指知悉自己之戒,多闻、慧正念、善行等。

Self-cognition　Means to understand self-exhortation, to listen more, to purify the idea and activity.

知足【zhī zú】　即对饮食、衣、药、行、住、坐、卧等知止知足。

cognizing satisfaction　Means to really understand how to take food, to dress clothes, to take medicine and to start the activities of walking, staying, sitting and lying.

脂瘤【zhī liú】　气功学适应证,多因湿痰凝滞于皮肤间所致。

lipoma　An indication of Qigong, usually caused by stagnation of dampness and phlegm in the skin.

执中【zhí zhōng】　指习练儒家气功,控制意识思维活动,使其不疾不徐,不浮不躁,稳定在形体之中。

mental control　Refers to controlling consciousness activity in practicing Qigong in Confucianism in order to balance, to tranquilize and to stabilize the body.

止【zhǐ】　佛家气功习用语。① 指精神集中于事或物,或景象,或念头,不分散注意力;② 指禅定之意。

concentration　A common term of Qigong in Buddhism, referring to ① either concentration of the spirit and the essence on anything in order to avoid dispersing anything; ② or Jhana.

止观【zhǐ guān】　指精神思维活动集中于所意守的事物。

concentrated observation　Refers to concentrating the activities of the spirit and thinking to a certain thing or a certain activity in order to tranquilize the mind.

止观法【zhǐ guān fǎ】　为静功。主要是"念念归一为止,了了分明为观",调身、调神、调气。

concentrated observation exercise　A static exercise, referring to concentration and clarification mainly with regulation of the body, Qi, spirit, mind, and health cultivation.

止火【zhǐ huǒ】　指炼精化气阶段的了手功夫,必须止火转入炼气化神阶段。

Z

stopping fire Refers to stopping fire for refining Qi and transforming the spirit with the skills at this stage.

止能止众止 【zhǐ néng zhǐ zhòng zhǐ】指静止的水，照见静止的人影。唯有相对静止的意识，才能止住各种妄念。

total calmness depending on entire tranquilization Refers to the fact that only when water is tranquilized can the body be quiet. That means only when the mind is tranquilized can various distracting thoughts be eliminated.

止念 【zhǐ niàn】 指习练气功，首先要精神内守，排除妄念。

elimination of avarice Refers to internal concentration of the spirit and elimination of wild fancy in practicing Qigong.

止念法 【zhǐ niàn fǎ】 指意识思维活动集中在所观、理的景物，或身体的某一部分。

focused contemplation exercise Refers to concentrating the activities of consciousness and thinking to an imagined scene and a certain part of the body.

止水空壶 【zhǐ shuǐ kōng hú】 指习练气功时，意识思维活动宁静，脑神无一毫杂念。

tranquilized vacuum Refers to tranquilizing the activities of consciousness and thinking and eliminating any distracting thought in the brain in practicing Qigong.

止泻法 【zhǐ xiè fǎ】 为动功。意念守脐，两手心复按脐部，两眼内视脐中。

stopping diarrhea exercise A dynamic exercise, referring to concentration of thought on the navel, pressing the navel with palms and internal observation of the navel with the eyes.

纸舟先生全真直指 【zhǐ zhōu xiān shēng quán zhēn zhí zhǐ】《纸舟先生全真直指》为气功专著，由元代金月岩编，记述了入室静坐功夫，以及多种气功效应及气功修炼的七个阶段。

Zhizhou XIansheng Quanzhen Zhizhi (*Direct Guidance of Mr. Zhi Zhou with Perfect Truth*) A monograph of Qigong entitled *Direct Guidance of Mr. Zhi Zhou with Perfect Truth*, compiled by Jin Yueyan in the Yuan Dynasty (1271 AD–1368 AD), mainly recording the function of sitting quietly in a clean room, various effects of Qigong and seven stages of Qigong practice.

趾 【zhǐ】 足厥阴肝经循行线经大趾，气功排肝经毒气常从此出。

large toe The area through which the liver meridian of foot Jueyin moves around and pathogenic factors in the liver meridian are expelled.

至道 【zhì dào】 气功养生法的理论知识和操作方法。

supreme theory Refers to the theoretical knowledge and practical methods in practicing Qigong for nourishing life.

至道之精 【zhì dào zhī jīng】 指气功的上乘境界，即神形合一的状态，亦指合二而一。

best essential state Refers to the best state of Qigong, indicating the integration of the spirit and body.

至忌死气 【zhì jì sǐ qì】 指习练气功，忌在污秽之处。

avoidance of dead Qi Refers to avoiding foul place when practicing Qigong.

至静 【zhì jìng】 佛家气功习用语，指极静。

complete tranquilization A common

term of Qigong in Buddhism, referring to extreme tranquility.

至静真机【zhì jìng zhēn jī】 指神形静极之时,即亥末子初之时为真时;阴静极必有阳动,阳功之时即为真机。

best tranquilized genuine mechanism Refers to extreme tranquilization of the spirit and body. That means the time at the end of Hai（the period of the day from 21 p.m. to 23 p.m. at night）and at the beginning of Zi（the period of the day from 11 p.m. to 1 a.m. in the afternoon）is the genuine time. When Yin is best tranquilized, Yang must move; when Yang is moving, there must be genuine mechanism.

至人【zhì rén】 ① 指神意聪敏,情绪稳定的人;② 指气功造诣精深的人。

lofty man Refers to ① either a wise and stable person; ② or a man with great accomplishments in practicing Qigong.

至人呼吸【zhì rén hū xī】 与踵息相同,① 指息归命门;② 指息直达足跟。

immortal respiration Same as the deep respiration, referring to either respiration returning to life gate; or respiration directly reaching the heel.

至善之地【zhì shàn zhī dì】 为"祖窍"之异名,位于心与脐之正中。

best place A synonym of Zuqiao which is an acupoint located in the region between the heart and the navel.

至神【zhì shén】 指精神守于内,神形和调,情绪稳定,安于自然,和于社会。

sincere spirit Refers to internal concentration of the spirit, regulation of the spirit and the body, stabilization of the mind, pacifying in the natural world and harmonizing in the society.

至心【zhì xīn】 指至诚的意识思维活动。

sincere heart Refers to sincere activities of consciousness and thought.

至阳【zhì yáng】 督脉中的一个穴位,位于后正中线。这一穴位为气功运行的一个常见部位。

Zhiyang（GV 9） An acupoint in the governor meridian, located in the midline on the back. This acupoint is a region usually used for keeping the essential Qi in practice of Qigong.

至一【zhì yī】 指人与自然、社会高度的协调统一。

wholeness Refers to perfect regulation and unity of man with the natural and social environments.

至一真人【zhì yī zhēn rén】 唐代气功家崔希范的另外一个称谓。

Zhiyi Zhenren Another name of Cui Xifan, a great master of Qigong in the Tang Dynasty（618 AD - 907 AD）.

至阴肃肃,至阳赫赫【zhì yīn sù sù zhì yáng hè hè】 至阴即阴中之阴,至阳即阳中之阳。指习练气功,应认识至阴至阳的性质及其相互关系。

Supreme Yin is respectful and supreme Yang is conspicuous. This is a celebrated dictum, in which supreme Yin is Yin within Yin while supreme Yang is Yang within Yang. It refers to understanding the nature and interrelation of supreme Yin and supreme Yang in practicing Qigong.

至游子【zhì yóu zǐ】 南宋诗人兼气功家曾慥的另外一个称谓。

Zhi Youzi Another name of Zeng Zao, a great poet and master of Qigong in the South Song Dynasty（1127 AD - 1279 AD）.

Z

至游子坐忘法【zhì yóu zǐ zuò wàng fǎ**】** 为静功,指调身、调气、调神,用于养生,强健体魄,开发智力。

ideal travelling exercise for sitting and overlooking A static exercise, referring to regulation of the body, Qi and the spirit in order to nourish life, to cultivate health and to develop wisdom.

至真诀【zhì zhēn jué**】**《至真诀》为气功专论,刘海蟾著,主要阐述内丹修炼以养元神、息真息为关键。

Zhizhen Jue（*Perfect and Genuine Formula***）** A monograph of Qigong entitled *Perfect and Genuine Formula*, written by Liu Haichan, mainly describing the way for nourishing the original spirit and regulating respiration in practicing Qigong with internal Dan (pills of immortality).

志念除妄【zhì niàn chú wàng**】** 指加强道德修养,避免有害精神刺激,除去妄想,保持身心安静。

cultivating mind to expel avarice Refers to strengthening moral cultivation, avoiding stimulation that injures the essence and spirit, eliminating distracting thought and tranquilizing the heart and mind.

志气【zhì qì**】** 气功中,志为精神意识活动,气为呼吸之气。

will Qi In Qigong, the so-called will refers to the activities of the spirit and consciousness and the so-called Qi refers to air in respiration.

制伏睡魔法【zhì fú shuì mó fǎ**】** 为静功。其作法为,静坐,凝我微细之神于气穴,心目所在,坦坦然然,惟当此理欲相争,不能无妄念发生,但念一生,即以朗朗性光照之,亦自随生随灭,每一生一

照,一照一灭,使生无所生,照无所照,则睡魔无所用力,始获入大静。

exercise for controlling demon in sleep A static exercise, marked by sitting quietly, concentrating the spirit on the acupoint, purifying the heart and the mind with efforts but without distracting thought, shining the whole body with purity and sincerity all the time without vulgar light and efforts. Such a way of practice can eliminate demon in sleep and enable the practitioners to enter the tranquil state.

制魂魄【zhì hún pò**】** 指调节阴神与阳神,并制伏之。

controlling the ethereal soul and corporeal soul Refers to regulating and controlling Yin spirit and Yang spirit.

制七魄法【zhì qī pò fǎ**】** 为静功。其作法为,于月朔、月望、月晦傍晚,正卧去枕,伸展下肢,两手掌心掩耳,两手指端向后相接交于后项中。闭气不息,至极限时慢慢呼出,作七遍,叩齿七遍。静心存想鼻尖有白气如小豆大,不一会,渐渐变大,下至两足,上至头上覆盖周身九层。

exercise for controlling seven corporeal souls A static exercise, marked by practice in the evening on the first day, the fifteenth day and the last day in every month, lying on the back without pillow, stretching the lower limbs, covering the ears with palms, connecting with the back of the neck with two fingers, closing respiration to a certain stage and then slowly exhaling for seven times, clicking teeth for seven times, tranquilizing the heart and imagining white Qi like a small bean in the nose tip which eventually becomes large, flowing downwards to the feet and upwards to the head for nine times to cover the whole body.

制外养中【zhì wài yǎng zhōng**】** 指习练气功,调节精神并意守之,保养形体。

controlling the external and nourishing the internal Refers to regulating the essence and the spirit with consciousness in order to nourish the body.

治齿疾法【zhì chǐ jí fǎ**】** 为静功。其作法为,晨起,叩齿四十九下,纳气三口,出气念呼音。食后漱口刷牙,小便时闭口,齿紧咬。

exercise for treating dental disease A static exercise, marked by clicking the teeth for forty-nine times in the early morning, inhaling for three times, exhaling with sound, rinsing the mouth and brushing the teeth after taking food, closing the mouth and gritting the teeth during defecation.

治胆吐纳法【zhì dǎn tǔ nà fǎ**】** 为静功。其作法为,以鼻微引气,以口嘻之。能急去胆病并肾脏一切冷,阴汗盗汗,面无颜色,小腹胀满,脐下冷痛。

exercise for curing gallbladder and respiration A static exercise, marked by mildly inhaling through the nose, exhaling through the mouth, quickly curing gallbladder disease, expelling coldness in the kidney, stopping night sweating, improving colorless complexion, and relieving lower abdominal distension and fullness as well as coldness and pain in the region below the navel.

治肺六气法【zhì fèi liù qì fǎ**】** 为静功。其作法为,吐纳用咽法,以鼻微长引气,以口咽之,勿令耳闻。皆先须调气令和,然后咽之。

exercise for curing the lung with six kinds of Qi A static exercise, marked by respiration with panting exercise, mildly inhaling through the nose and panting through the mouth without any listening. Such a way of practice should regulate Qi and harmonize the body first and then swallow Qi.

治肺脏吐纳法【zhì fèi zàng tǔ nà fǎ**】** 为静功。其作法为,以鼻微长引气,以口呬之,肺病用大呬三十遍,细呬十遍。去肺家房热,上气咳嗽,皮肤疮痛,四肢烦疼,鼻塞、胸背痛。数数呬之,疾愈止,过度则损。

exercise of respiration for curing the lung A static exercise, marked by inhaling mildly and continuously through the nose, breathing out through the mouth heavily for thirty times and mildly for ten times for curing lung disease. This way of Qigong practice can relieve heat in the lung, cough, sore and pain in the skin, pain in the four limbs, nasal congestion and pain in the chest and back. To exhale continuously for several times can cure disease. When the disease is cured, the practice should be stopped, otherwise damage will be caused.

治肝脏吐纳法【zhì gān zàng tǔ nà fǎ**】** 为静功。其作法为,以鼻微引气,以口嘘之,肝病用大嘘三十遍,细嘘十遍。能去肝家虚热、眼暗,一切热,数数嘘之,绵绵不绝。

exercise of respiration for curing the liver A static exercise, marked by mildly inhaling through the nose, exhaling through the mouth for heavily for thirty times and mildly for ten times for curing liver disease. This way of Qigong

Z

practice can eliminate deficiency heat in the liver and obscurity in the eyes. If there is serious heat, exhalation should be continued for several times to expel it.

治脾脏吐纳法【zhì pí zàng tǔ nà fǎ】为静功。其作法为,以鼻微长引气,以口呼之。脾病用大呼三十遍,细呼十遍。能去脾家一切冷气,发热,霍乱,宿食不消,偏风顽痹,腹内结块。数数呼之,相次勿绝,疾退则止,勿过度。

exercise of respiration for curing the spleen A static exercise, marked by mildly and continuously inhaling through the nose, exhaling through the mouth heavily for thirty times and mildly for ten times for curing spleen disease. This way of Qigong practice can relieve coldness in the spleen, fever, cholera, indigestion, severe impediment with slanting wind and abdominal mass. To exhale continuously for several times can cure disease. When the disease is cured, the practice should be stopped, otherwise damage will be caused.

治其内,不识其外【zhì qí nèi bù shí qí wài】 指控制精神于内而不散于外。

Keep it inside and avoid dispersion. Indicates that the essence and the spirit are controlled in the body and cannot be dispersed.

治气养心法要【zhì qì yǎng xīn fǎ yào】 气功治法,按照气质、性情、意识、行为的不同,确定不同的治则,应用不同的功法,如和法、一法、顺法、节法、动法、广法、友法、乐法等。

essential exercise for controlling Qi and cultivating the heart A treatment exercise in Qigong, indicating different exercises for different nature, temperament, consciousness and action, such harmonious exercise, single exercise, smooth exercise, controlling exercise, active exercise, general exercise, moral exercise and joyful exercise.

治肾脏吐纳法【zhì shèn zàng tǔ nà fǎ】 为静功。其作法为,以鼻微长引气,以口吹之,肾病用大吹三十遍,细吹十遍。去肾家一切冷,腰疼,膝沉重,久立不得,阳道衰弱,耳中蝉鸣及口中有疮。数数吹之,相次勿绝,病愈止,过度则损。

exercise of respiration for curing the kidney A static exercise, marked by inhaling mildly and continuously through the nose, blowing through the mouth heavily for thirty times and mildly for ten times for curing kidney disease. This way of Qigong practice can relieve coldness in the whole body, pain in the waist, heaviness of the knees, inability to stand for a long time, weakness of semen, tinnitus like the chirping of a cicada and sore in the mouth. To exhale continuously for several times can cure disease. When the disease is cured, the practice should be stopped, otherwise damage will be caused.

治睡觉口干舌涩法【zhì shuì jiào kǒu gān shé sè fǎ】 为静功。其作法为,睡觉起后,盘膝正坐,大开口,微呵数十遍,候喉中津液出。

exercise for curing dry and inflexible tongue in sleeping A static exercise, marked by sitting upright with crossed legs after getting up, opening the mouth, mildly exhaling for dozens of times and blowing fluid and humor from the mouth.

治万病坐功法【zhì wàn bìng zuò gōng fǎ】 为动功,方法多样,如口出气鼻吸气为泻,闭口温气咽之为补。台头疾则仰头,治腰脚病仰足十趾,治胸中病牵引足十趾,治腹中寒热诸疾则闭气鼓腹。

exercise of sitting for curing all diseases A dynamic exercise with various methods, such as treating diarrhea by exhaling through the mouth and inhaling through the nose; tonifying the body by closing the mouth warming Qi and swallowing saliva; curing the brain disorder by raising the head; relieving pain of the waist and feet by raising the ten toes; curing disease in the chest by stretching the ten toes; curing various diseases with coldness and heat in the abdomen by closing respiration and bulging the abdomen.

治心在中【zhì xīn zài zhōng】 指控制意识思维活动,稳定在形体之中。

controlling heart in the center Refers to controlling the activities of consciousness and thinking in order to stabilize it in the body.

治心脏吐纳法【zhì xīn zàng tǔ nà fǎ】 为静功。其作法为,以鼻微引气,以口嘘之。心病用大呵三十遍,细呵十遍。本法去心劳热,一切烦闷、心疾。病愈即止,过度则损。

exercise of respiration for curing the heart A static exercise, marked by mildly inhaling through the nose and exhaling through the mouth heavily for thirty times and mildly for ten times for curing heart disease. This way of Qigong practice can eliminate dysphoria, irritancy and heart disease. When the disease is cured, the practice should be stopped, otherwise damage will be caused.

治腰痛法【zhì yāo tòng fǎ】 动静相兼功。其作法为,卧时坐于床,垂足解衣,闭息,舌舐上腭,目视顶门,提缩谷道,两手摩两肾脯,各一百二十次,多多益善。极能生精固阳,防治腰痛。

exercise for curing lumbago An exercise combined with dynamic exercise and static exercise, marked by sitting on the bed when lying, drooping the feet and taking off clothes, stopping respiration, licking the upper palate with the tongue, raising the head to see the top, lifting and shrinking the grain trail (anus), rubbing the kidney regions with both hands for one hundred and twenty times. Such a way of practice can produce essence, stabilize Yang, prevent and cure lumbago.

治阴虚无上妙方【zhì yīn xū wú shàng miào fāng】 为静功,是一种用气功治疗真阴亏损,不能制火,心火上炎而克肺金所引起的发热、咳嗽、吐痰的方法。

fine exercise for curing severe Yin deficiency A static exercise, referring to treating insufficiency of genuine Yin which cannot control fire, making heart fire rise up to restrict lung-metal, causing fever, cough and expectoration.

栉髪去风【zhì fà qù fēng】 为动功。其作法为,多梳髪,可使头部气血流通,头发坚固不易脱落,祛头风。

eliminating wind by combing hair A dynamic exercise, marked by repeatedly combing hair in order to promote circulation of Qi and the blood in the head. Only when the hair is firm can head wind (headache) be expelled.

Z

致虚极【zhì xū jí】 指行功中精神意识活动处于静谧安宁的状态。

extreme tranquilization Refers to tranquilized and pacified activities of the spirit and consciousness in practicing Qigong.

痔【zhì】 气功适应证,多因湿热内蕴、过食辛辣厚味、久坐久立、便秘,或久泻久病等因素而湿热、瘀血、浊气下注肛门而发病。

hemorrhoids An indication of Qigong, caused by internal accumulation of dampness heat, eating deliciously pungent food, siting and standing for a long time, constipation, or chronic diarrhea and chronic disease that have caused dampness heat, blood stasis and turbid Qi flowing downwards to the anus.

痔疮导引法【zhì chuāng dǎo yǐn fǎ】 为动功。其作法为,尾闾部捏擦数十次,心静调息,用吸提清气,呵除浊气。治痔疮。

exercise of Daoyin for hemorrhoids A dynamic exercise, marked by rubbing the coccyx for ten times, tranquilizing the heart, regulating respiration, inhaling clear Qi and exhaling turbid Qi. This dynamic exercise can cure hemorrhoids.

智【zhì】 佛家气功习用语,指决断事理的能力。

wisdom A term of Qigong, referring the ability to decide anything and any reason.

智慧【zhì huì】 佛家气功习用语,① 指破除迷惑、证实真理、平和形神的能力;② 指才智,认识事物的能力。

wisdom and intelligence A common term of Qigong in Buddhism, referring to ① either eliminating confusion, proving truth and pacifying the body and the spirit; ② or intelligence for understanding anything.

智慧观【zhì huì guān】 为静功。其作法为,以清静之智慧,观察物性而使之稳定情性。

wisdom view A static exercise, marked by observing properties of anything to stabilize emotion based on quietness and wisdom.

智境冥一【zhì jìng míng yī】 佛家气功习用语,指意想与意想对象(境)高度结合。

wisdom state and obscure one A common term of Qigong Buddhism, referring to high combination of imagination and imagination state.

智识【zhì shí】 即识别能力,为意识之一,指意识稳定,情绪才能和平。

wisdom and knowledge Refers to ability to recognize, as a sort of consciousness. Only when consciousness is stabilized can emotion be harmonized.

智养恬【zhì yǎng tián】 指恬静涵养智慧,智慧又育养恬静。

wisdom preserving quietness Refers to quietness increasing wisdom and wisdom keeping quietness.

智圆【zhì yuán】 指一切智慧在中道。

wisdom cycle Refer to all wisdom existing in the central Dao (madhyamāmārga).

智圆行方【zhì yuán xíng fāng】 指习练气功中,智识圆和,平静,行为才能方正自如。

pacifying wisdom and rectifying activity Indicates that only when wisdom is pacified and the mind is tranquilized can the activity be normal and natural in practicing Qigong.

滞碍【zhì ài】 指意生杂念,形体紧张。

distracted tension Refers to distracting thought that makes the mind nervous.

中【zhōng】 ① 指不上不下,不左不右,恰在其中;② 指精神稳定;③ 指静以制动;④ 指生化之根;⑤ 指里面或内里。

middle Refers to ① either staying in the center; or mental activity inside the body; ② or stability of spirit; ③ or tranquility to control activity; ④ or the root of life; ⑤ or the internal side; or the viscera.

中不静,心不治【zhōng bù jìng xīn bù zhì】 指意识紊乱,杂念横生。

No tranquility of the center and no pacification of the heart Refers to disorder of distracting thought and excessive avarice.

中部八景【zhōng bù bā jǐng】 指肺神、心神、肝神、脾神、左肾神、右肾神、胆神、喉神。

eight central sceneries Refer to the lung spirit, the liver spirit, the spleen spirit, the left kidney spirit, the right kidney spirit, the gallbladder spirit and the throat spirit.

中池【zhōng chí】 指胆或元海。

central pool Refers to either gallbladder; or the palace of immortals.

中池立【zhōng chí lì】 指心神统四脏之气而立于心之上。言四脏之中,以心为主。

cardiac spirit Refers to the fact that the heart spirit controls Qi in the other four viscera (including the liver, the spleen, the lung and the kidney).

中冲【zhōng chōng】 手厥阴心包经的一个穴位,位于中指桡侧,为气功常用意守部位。

Zhongchong(PC 9) An acupoint in the pericardium meridian of hand Jueyin, located in the radialis side of the middle finger, a region usually used for keeping essential Qi in practicing Qigong.

中春【zhōng chūn】 ① 指农历二月十五日;② 指春季三月的第二个月。

middle spring Refers to ① either February fifteen in traditional Chinese calendar; ② or the second month in the spring.

中丹田【zhōng dān tián】 ① 指心;② 指心脐之间。

central Dantian Refers to ① either the heart; ② or the area between the heart and navel. Dantian is divided into the upper Dantian (the region between the eyes), the middle Dantian (the region below the heart) and the lower Dantian (the region below the navel).

中道【zhōng dào】 佛教气功用语,指弃两边而取中。

central cognition A common term of Qigong in Buddhism, referring to abandoning both sides and keeping the middle.

中得【zhōng dé】 指不受自然及社会各方面的影响而能"内外两忘"。

intrinsic achievement Refers to psychological stability without being affected by factors from the natural environment and social situation.

中渎之腑【zhōng dú zhī fǔ】 指三焦。

organ in the middle Refers to triple energizer.

中孚【zhōng fú】 研究思想活动的卦象。

Zhongfu Trigram Refers to the Trigram for analyzing thought.

中府【zhōng fǔ】 手太阴肺经的一个穴位,位胸壁之外上部,为气功常用意守部位。

Zhongfu（LU 1） An acupoint in the lung meridian of hand Taiyin, located in the upper part of the walls of the chest, a region usually used for keeping the essential Qi in practice of Qigong.

中宫【zhōng gōng】 指北极星所处的天域。

central paradise Refers to the place where Polaris is located.

中宫之窍【zhōng gōng zhī qiào】 指肺,为"四象五行全聚土"。

orifice in the central palace Refers to the spleen which is the concentration of the weather in the four seasons and the movement of the five elements（including wood, fire, earth, metal and water）.

中合于人事【zhōng hé yú rén shì】 指人与社会相合,要稳定神形,即应调节人际关系。

combination of men and community Refers to regulating the relationship between different people in order to stabilize the spirit and the body.

中和【zhōng hé】 ①指正中;②指修养神形;③指思维意识活动处于不偏不倚。

central balance Refers to ① either normal center; ② or cultivation of the spirit and body; ③ or balanced mental activity.

中和集【zhōng hé jí】 《中和集》为气功学专著,由元代李道纯所撰,全书以守中为要诀。

Zhonghe Ji（*Collection of Central Harmony*） A monograph of Qigong enti-

tled *Collection of Central Harmony*, written by Li Daochun in the Yuan Dynasty（1271 AD – 1368 AD）, mainly describing the importance of concentrating the center.

中和集·论内丹【zhōng hé jí lùn nèi dān】 《中和集·论内丹》为气功专论,简明论述了内丹修炼。作者不详。

Zhonghe Ji and Lun Neidan（*Collection of Central Harmony and Discussion of Internal Dan*） A monograph of Qigong entitled *Collection of Central Harmony and Discussion of Internal Dan*（*Pills of Immortality*）, mainly describing about how to practice internal Dan（pills of immortality）. The author was unknown.

中黄【zhōng huáng】 指天神,喻脑神。

celestial spirit Refers to the celestial spirit, comparing to the celebral spirit.

中黄八极【zhōng huáng bā jí】 指行功中阴阳交会而平秘的枢纽作用,为脑神及其功能作用。

eight poles in the central palace Refers to the coordinative effect of Yin and Yang, and the function of the celebral spirit.

中黄宫【zhōng huáng gōng】 指心与脐中之位。

middle yellow palace Refers to the region between the heart and the navel.

中黄之气【zhōng huáng zhī qì】 指胆气。

Qi of the central palace Refers to gallbladder Qi.

中极【zhōng jí】 任脉的一个穴位,位于脐下四寸,为气功常用意守部位。

Zhongji（CV 3） An acupoint in the conception meridian, located 4 Cun below the navel, a region usually used for keeping the essential Qi in practice of Qigong.

中焦【zhōng jiāo】　指人体的三焦之一,助脾胃腐熟水谷。

middle energizer　One of the triple energizer, supporting the spleen and the stomach to digest food.

中焦如沤【zhōng jiāo rú ōu】　形容中焦脾胃腐熟水谷。

middle energizer like bubble　Refers to the function of the middle energizer to digest food and water in the stomach and the spleen.

中节【zhōng jié】　指精神意识活动合乎规律。

Reasonability　Refers to the principle for the activities of the spirit and consciousness.

中精之腑【zhōng jīng zhī fǔ】　指胆。

organ of the central essence　Refers to gallbladder.

中论【zhōng lùn】　《中论》指书名,汉代徐幹所著,提倡调节精神,稳定情绪。

Zhonglun（*Concentrated Discussion*）　A monograph entitled *Concentrated Discussion*, written by Xu Gan in the Han Dynasty（202 BC - 263 AD）, suggesting regulation of the spirit and stabilizing the emotion.

中门【zhōng mén】　指身有七门,即泥丸为天门,尾闾为地门,夹脊为中门,明堂为前门,玉枕为后门,重楼为楼门,绛宫为房门。

middle gate　Refers to the mud bolus（the brain）known as the celestial gate, the coccyx known as the earthly gate, the back and the waist known as the middle gate, the nose known as the front gate, the posterior hairline known as the back gate, the trachea as the building gate and the precordium known as the house gate.

中男【zhōng nán】　指坎卦。

central male　Refers to Kan Trigram in Bagua（Eight Trigrams）.

中南山【zhōng nán shān】　终南山之别称,为秦岭主峰之一,相传为全真派北五祖中的吕洞宾、刘海蟾修炼之处。

Zhongnan Mountain　A synonym of Zhongnan Mountain in Shaanxi Province where Lǚ Dongbin and Zhang Haichan, two important immortals in ancient China and founder of entire genuine school, practiced Qigong.

中秋【zhōng qiū】　① 指农历八月十五日;② 指秋季三月的第二个月。

middle autumn　Refers to ① either August fifteen in traditional Chinese calendar; ② or the second month in the autumn.

中寿【zhōng shòu】　中寿说法不一。一说中寿为百岁,一说中寿为八十岁,一说中寿为七十岁,一说中寿为六十岁。

intermediate longevity　Refers to either one hundred years of life; or eighty years of life; or seventy years of life; or sixty years of life.

中体【zhōng tǐ】　指中焦。

central aspect　Refers to the middle energizer.

中外相距重闭之【zhōng wài xiāng jù zhòng bì zhī】　指内以外为寇,外以内为仇,重重闭户,不使其相通,以维持内外之间的稳定状态。

distance between the middle and external causing serious obstruction　Refers to the maintenance of internal and external stability by preventing thorough communication with each other because the internal should avoid the external

Z

and the external should deviate from the internal.

中脘【zhōng wǎn】　任脉中的一个穴位,位于前正中线,脐下 4 寸,为气功常用意守部位。

Zhongwan（**CV 12**）　An acupoint in the conception meridian, located in the anterior midline and 4 Cun below the navel, a region usually used for keeping the essential Qi in practice of Qigong.

中夏【zhōng xià】　① 指夏季之中,农历五月;② 指夏季的第二个月,同仲夏。

middle summer　Refers to ① either March in traditional Chinese calendar; ② or the second month in the summer.

中霄【zhōng xiāo】　指中夜之半,即子时。

midnight　Refers to half of midnight, i. e. the period of the day from 11 p. m. to 1 a. m.

中心【zhōng xīn】　指精神意识活动。

concentration　Refers to activities of the spirit and consciousness.

中央【zhōng yāng】　① 指四方之中;② 指中心位置。

center　Refers to ① either the center among the four directions, ② or the central position.

中央黄老君胎息法 【 zhōng yāng huáng lǎo jūn tāi xī fǎ】　为静功。其作法为,习练气功在于能否排除杂念,内守精神。若不能入静时,应静坐,情绪稳定,神栖泥丸。

immortal's exercise for fetal respiration A static exercise. In practicing Qigong, distracting thought must be eliminated and the spirit must be stabilized. If the mind is not tranquilized, sitting must be quiet in order to stabilize the mind and concentrate the spirit on the mud bolus

(the brain).

中庸【zhōng yōng】　① 指不偏,正中;② 指平平常常;③ 指精神的最高境界。

impartial doctrine　Refers to ① psychological stability, ② normality and ③ the high state of the spirit.

中有阴阳夫妻仙【zhōng yǒu yīn yáng fū qī xiān】　指人体左右乳。左乳为阳,右乳为阴。

existence of Yin-Yang and parents in the center　Refers to the right breast and the left breast in the human body, in which the left one is Yang and the right one is Yin.

中元【zhōng yuán】　指农历七月十五日。

central prime　Refers to July 15th in traditional Chinese calendar.

中岳【zhōng yuè】　指鼻。

central mountain　Refers to the nose.

中岳郄检食气法【zhōng yuè xì jiǎn shí qì fǎ】　为静功。平旦四十九咽,日出二十六咽,食时二十五咽,禺中一十六咽,日中八十一咽,哺时四十九咽,日入三十六咽,黄昏二十五咽,人定一十六咽。

exercise for absorption Qi　A static exercise, marked by absorbing Qi for forty-nine times in the early morning, twenty-six times during sunrise, twenty-five times when taking food, sixteen times when looking up, eighty-one times in the noon, forty-nine times when chewing, thirty-six times during sunset, twenty-five times in the dusk and sixteen times in the midnight.

中运【zhōng yùn】　为十干所统运的通称。因天气在上,地气在下,运居于天地之中,气交之分,统司一岁之气。

central motion　A term of Qi motion

and the general description about the movement of ten Heavenly Stems，mainly referring to movement in the middle of the sky and the earth because the celestial Qi is in the upper and the earthly Qi is in the lower.

中正之官【zhōng zhèng zhī guān**】**指胆，位于体中而主决断。

fair organ　Refers to the gallbladder，located in the center of the body and responsible for making decision.

中之守【zhōng zhī shǒu**】**　指五脏藏精气，藏而不泻，宜守之不失之意。

central protection　Refers to the essential Qi in the five Zang-organs (including the heart, the liver, the spleen, the lung and the kidney) that is stored and not leaked.

中注【zhōng zhù**】**　足少阴肾经的一个穴位，位脐下 1 寸，为气功常用意守部位。

Zhongzhu（KI 15）　An acupoint in the kidney meridian of foot Shaoyin，located 1 Cun below the navel，a region usually used for keeping the essential Qi in practice of Qigong.

终南山【zhōng nán shān**】**　秦岭主峰之一，相传为全真派北五祖中的吕洞宾、刘海蟾修炼之处。

Zhongnan Mountain　In Shaanxi Province where Lǚ Dongbin and Zhang Haichan，two important immortals in ancient China and founder of entire genuine school，practiced Qigong.

终脱胎，看四正【zhōng tuō tāi kàn sì zhèng**】**　指习练气功，到炼神还虚时，阳神出现，通达无碍，东西南北，无所不往。

emergence for seeing four directions　Indicates that Yang spirit appears when

refined spirit is weak in practicing Qigong，making it quite normal for the essence，Qi and spirit to move in any parts of the body.

钟离权【zhōng lí quán**】**　唐代气功学家，传说为八仙之一，著有多部气功专著。

Zhong Liquan　A master of Qigong in the Tang Dynasty (618 AD - 907 AD)，who was one of the eight immortals and wrote several monographs of Qigong.

钟离仙聪耳法【zhōng lí xiān cōng ěr fǎ**】**　为动静相兼功。其作法为，端坐咬牙闭息，两手掩两耳，击天鼓三十六通。存想精气神入泥丸。

Zhong Lixian's exercise for improving ears　An exercise combined with dynamic exercise and static exercise，marked by sitting upright，clicking the teeth，stopping respiration，covering the ears with both hands，touching the occipital for thirty-six times and imagining to keep the essence，Qi and spirit in the mud bolus (the brain).

钟离云房摩肾【zhōng lí yún fáng mó shèn**】**　为动功。其作法为，端坐，两手擦热，以双拳置于两肾俞穴运气二十四口。主治虚冷、腰腿疼。

Zhongli's exercise for rubbing the kidney in cloud room　A dynamic exercise，marked by sitting upright，rubbing the hands warm，and putting the fists on the acupoints located in the nephric regions for twenty-four times. Such a dynamic exercise can cure deficiency-cold，lumbago and leg pain.

钟吕传道记【zhōng lǚ chuán dào jì**】**　《钟吕传道记》为气功专著，由唐代施肩吾所著，阐述了气功养生的基本理论和方法。

Z

Zhonglǔ Chuandao Ji（*Zhonglǔ's Record about Inheritance of Daoism*） A monograph of Qigong entitled *Zhonglǔ's Record about Inheritance of Daoism*, written by Shi Jianwu in the Tang Dynasty（618 AD－907 AD）, describing the basic theory and practice of Qigong and life cultivation.

钟律【zhōng lǜ】 古代音律名词,气功文献中借以协调阴阳,阐述阴阳的变化。

bell temperament A term of phonetic principle in ancient China. In the literature of Qigong, it is used to regulate Yin and Yang and to describe the changes of Yin and Yang.

钟云房【zhōng yún fáng】 唐代气功学家钟离权的另外一个称谓,传说为八仙之一,著有多部气功专著。

Zhong Yunfang Another name of Zhong Liquan, a master of Qigong in the Tang Dynasty（618 AD－907 AD）, who was one of the eight immortals and wrote several monographs of Qigong.

种性外道【zhǒng xìng wài dào】 即左道旁门,没有理论指导,亦无实践基础的邪本。

abnormal external way Refers to left postern without any theory and practical foundation.

种子【zhǒng zi】 佛家气功习用语,指产生世界各种现象的精神因素。

seed A common term of Qigong in Buddhism, referring to spiritual factors related to various phenomena in the world.

踵息【zhǒng xī】 ① 为命门,为息归命门之意;② 指气息直达足跟。

deep respiration Refers to ① either respiration entering the life gate; ② or respiration entering the heels.

踵息论【zhǒng xī lùn】 源自气功专论,说明踵息即胎息,人能睡息,才可减少身体能源的消耗,轻身延年。

discussion about deep respiration Collected from a monograph, referring to fetal respiration. Only respiration in sleep can reduce consumption of energy, relax the body and prolong life.

中风【zhòng fēng】 气功适应证,① 指卒然昏仆,不省人事;② 指外感风邪的病证。

apoplexy An indication of Qigong, refers to ① either sudden faint and unconsciousness; ② or external contraction of pathogenic wind.

中风治法【zhòng fēng zhì fǎ】 为动静相兼功,方法多种。① 如可正立靠墙,不息行气;② 可仰起两脚趾,引气至要背,五息而止;③ 可用背正靠,展开两脚及趾,安定精神;④ 可端正靠坐,不息行气,意念导引内气。

exercise for apoplexy An exercise of Qigong combined with dynamic exercise and static exercise, referring to various methods in practicing Qigong for expelling apoplexy, such as ① standing against the wall to promote circulation of Qi without breath; ② raising the feet and toes to move Qi to the back; ③ standing against the wall with the back to stretch the feet and toes in order to stabilize the spirit; ④ sitting upright to mentally move Qi without breath.

中暑导引法【zhòng shǔ dǎo yǐn fǎ】 为动功。其作法为,先饮热茶或热汤,颈项伸直,舌卷托上腭,两手握拳,两足趾紧缩屈曲,自然发汗,暑从汗解。

exercise of Daoyin for summer stroke A dynamic exercise, marked by drinking

Z

hot tea or hot soup first, stretching the neck and the nape, raising the tongue to the palate, holding the hands with each other, retrenching and buckling the feet and toes, naturally sweating and relieving sunstroke after sweating.

众妙归根【zhòng miào guī gēn】 即胎息之真功夫,气归藏气穴。

mysterious ways returning to the origin Refers to genuine function of the fetal respiration and Qi returning to Qi point.

众生【zhòng shēng】 佛家气功习用语,① 指世间众生共生;② 指各种法(含气功法)通过比较而存在;③ 指生命。

all living creatures A common term of Qigong in Buddhism, referring to ① either all creatures in this world living together; ② or existence of all methods related to Qigong; ③ or the life.

重积德【zhòng jī dé】 指七窍内观,意识思维活动安静,精神内守,和气在身。

great concentration of virtue Refers to internal observation of the seven orifices, tranquilization of the activities of consciousness and thinking, internal concentration of the spirit and harmonization of Qi in the body.

重舌【zhòng shé】 气功适应证,指舌下血络肿起,形如又生一小舌。多因心脾积热,复感外邪,循经上冲所致。

swollen tongue An indication of Qigong, referring to swelling of the blood collateral below the tongue like production of a small tongue. It is usually caused by accumulation of heat in the heart and spleen like external pathogenic factors that rise up along the meridians.

重舌导引法【zhòng shé dǎo yǐn fǎ】 为动功。其作法为,用手指从舌下筋脉上(舌下静脉)到舌尖揉擦至舌根。

exercise of Daoyin for sublingual swelling A dynamic exercise, marked by rubbing the tongue root from the vein below the tongue to the tip of the tongue.

重堂【zhòng táng】 ① 指喉咙;② 指内外明堂。

great chamber Refers to ① either the throat; ② or the external and internal sides of the nose.

周荆盛【zhōu jīng shèng】 清代中医学家周学霆的另外一个称谓。周学霆也精于气功实践。

Zhou Jingsheng Another name of Zhou Xueting, a doctor of traditional Chinese medicine in the Qing Dynasty (1636 AD – 1912 AD) who was also quite familiar with the practice of Qigong.

周履靖【zhōu lǚ jìng】 明代气功学家,其精研气功导引,对气功的发展有一定的贡献。

Zhou Lǚjing A master of Qigong in the Ming Dynasty (1368 AD – 1644 AD) who was very proficient in Qigong and Daoyin, making certain contribution to the development of Qigong.

周南山【zhōu nán shān】 终南山之别称,为秦岭主峰之一,相传为全真派北五祖中的吕洞宾、刘海蟾修炼之处。

Zhounan Mountain A synonym of Zhongnan Mountain in Shaanxi Province where Lü Dongbin and Zhang Haichan, two important immortals in ancient China and founder of entire genuine school, practiced Qigong.

周天【zhōu tiān】 指太阳每日转一周。

Z

气功学文献中,有小周天和大周天之别。人体精气的运行从任脉到督脉,而又回归于任脉,此为一周,称为小周天。精气从手太阴肺经开始,到足厥阴肝经终止,循环往复,昼夜不舍,称为大周天。

circulatory cycle Refers to turnover of the sun in one day. In the literature of Qigong, there are small circulatory cycle and large circulatory cycle. According to Qigong theory, small circulatory cycle refers to the movement of the essential Qi from the conception meridian to the governor meridian and finally returning to the conception meridian; while large circulatory cycle refers to the movement of the essential Qi from the lung meridian of hand Taiyin to the liver meridian of foot Jueyin with movement in circles and continuity in daytime and at nighttime.

周天火候说【zhōu tiān huǒ hòu shuō】源自气功专论,主要阐述小周天功的精气运行及其注意事项。

discussion about duration of heating Collected from a monograph of Qigong, mainly describing the movement of and attention to the essential Qi in small circulatory cycle.

周小颠【zhōu xiǎo diān】 清代中医学家周学霆的另外一个称谓。周学霆也精于气功实践。

Zhou Xiaodian Another name of Zhou Xueting, a doctor of traditional Chinese medicine in the Qing Dynasty (1636 AD - 1912 AD) who was also quite familiar with the practice of Qigong.

周学霆【zhōu xué tíng】 清代中医学家,也精于气功实践。

Zhou Xueting A doctor of traditional Chinese medicine in the Qing Dynasty (1636 AD - 1912 AD) who was also quite familiar with the practice of Qigong.

周易参同契【zhōu yì cān tóng qì】《周易参同契》为气功学经典著作,由东汉魏伯阳所撰,自唐代推为内丹要籍。

Zhouyi Cantongqi(*Essential Analysis and Discussion of Zhouyi*) A classic canon of Qigong entitled *Essential Analysis and Discussion of Zhouyi*(*Simplification, Change and No Change*), written by Wei Boyang in the East Han Dynasty(25 AD - 220 AD), which was taken as the key book of internal Dan(pills of immortality).

周易参同契解【zhōu yì cān tóng qì jiě】 为《易经》研究专著,由宋代陈显微解。书中解释说,乾坤为神室,日月为运用,六十四卦为行火,以升降往来为枢毂。

Zhouyi Cantong Qijie(*Essential Explanation, Analysis and Discussion of Zhouyi*) A monograph about explanation of Yijing(*Simplification, Change and No Change*), entitled *Essential Explanation, Analysis and Discussion of Zhouyi*(*Simplification, Change and No Change*), compiled by Chen Xianwei in the Song Dynasty(960 AD - 1279 AD). According to the explanation, analysis and discussion in this book, Qian Trigram and Kun Trigram are the chambers of the spirit, based on which the sun and the moon move; and the all sixty-four Trigrams in Yijing(*Simplification, Change and No Change*)all move fire upwards and downwards.

周易大传【zhōu yì dà zhuàn】《周易

大传》为哲学专著,成书于春秋战国时期,是对《易经》最古的注释,其中也涉及气功养生法的论述。作者不详。

Zhouyi Dachuan(*Great Inheritance of Zhouyi*) A monograph of philosophy entitled *Great Inheritance of Zhouyi*(*Simplification*, *Change and No Change*), compiled in the Spring and Autumn Period(770 BC－476 BC)and Warring States Period(475 BC－221 BC). This is first explanation of Yijing(*Simplification*, *Change and No Change*), also containing the theory and practice of Qigong and life cultivation. The author was unknown.

周逸之【zhōu yì zhī】 明代气功学家周履靖的另外一个称谓,其精研气功导引,对气功的发展有一定的贡献。

Zhou Yizhi Another name of Zhou Lǚjing, a master of Qigong in the Ming Dynasty(1368 AD－1644 AD)who was very proficient in Qigong and Daoyin, making certain contribution to the development of Qigong.

周庄蝴蝶梦【zhōu zhuāng hú dié mèng】 为静功。其作法为,右侧卧,右手枕子头部,左腿伸直,右腿屈膝,左手自然置于左腿上。存想运气二十四口。

Zhou Zhuang's dream of butterfly A static exercise, marked by lying on the right side, putting the right hand underneath the head, stretching directly the left leg, bending the right knee, putting the left hand on the left leg, and imagining to circulate Qi for twenty-four times.

肘后飞金晶【zhǒu hòu fēi jīn jīng】 源自气功专论,主要阐述精气自尾间,经夹脊、玉枕而上至泥丸的运动过程。

golden brilliance flying behind the el-bow Collected from a monograph of Qigong, mainly describing the movement of the essence and Qi that flow from the coccyx, bilateral sides of vertebrae and occipital bone to the mud bolus(the brain).

朱本中【zhū běn zhōng】 气功养生家,生活于清代康熙年间,在书中介绍了较多的气功功法。

Zhu Benzhong A master of Qigong for nourishing life in the Qing Dynasty(1636 AD－1912 AD), introducing most of the methods for practicing Qigong and nourishing life.

朱里汞【zhū lǐ gǒng】 ① 喻心,属火,为正阳之精;② 指神气。

scarlet mercury Refers to ① the heart that belongs to fire;② or spiritual Qi.

朱鸟【zhū niǎo】 指舌象。

scarlet bird Refers to manifestations of the tongue.

朱鸟吐缩白石源【zhū niǎo tǔ suō bái shí yuán】 指舌沿齿龈跟上下来回运动,有导引津液,使阴阳气津流通不绝的作用。

Scarlet bird exhales and shrinks the white stone origin. This is a celebrated dictum, referring to the tongue moving upwards and downwards along the gingiva for leading fluid and humor, enabling Yin, Yang, Qi and fluid to circulate continuously.

朱权【zhū quán】 明代戏剧家,对气功养生很有研究,并著有气功养生专著。

Zhu Quan A dramatist in the Ming Dynasty(1368 AD－1644 AD)who studied Qigong for nourishing life and wrote several monographs about Qigong and life cultivation.

朱砂鼎内水银平【zhū shā dǐng nèi

shuǐ yín píng】 指头中朱砂鼎为阳鼎，阳中有一阴生，而曰水银平。

Peaceful mercury in cinnabar cauldron
Refers to cinnabar cauldron as Yang cauldron. Usually there is Yin within Yang. That is why it is called peaceful mercury.

朱子调息签【zhū zǐ tiáo xī qiān】 源自气功专论，主要阐述习练气功调息入静的方法以及习练过程中出现的气功景象。

Zhuzi's autograph for regulating respiration Collected from a monograph of Qigong, mainly describing the method for regulating respiration in order to tranquilize the mind in practicing Qigong and the manifestations of Qigong during the procedure of practice.

诸病源候论【zhū bìng yuán hòu lùn】《诸病源候论》由隋代巢元方所著，为中医现存的第一部病因学专著。

Zhubing Yuanhou Lun（*Discussion about the Causes of Various Diseases*） The first monograph about aetiology of traditional Chinese medicine entitled *Discussion about the Causes of Various Diseases*, written by Chao Yuanfang in the Sui Dynasty（581 AD - 618 AD）.

诸恶疮候导引法【zhū è chuāng hòu dǎo yǐn fǎ】 为静功。其作法为，低头向下看，闭气不息，至极限时慢慢呼出，作十二次。清热解毒，凉血消肿，治疮肿。

exercise of Daoyin for various ulcerations
A static exercise, marked by lowering the head to see the underground, stopping respiration and slowly exhaling for twelve times when respiration is stopped to the maximum. Such a static exercise for practicing Qiong can clear heat to remove toxin, cool the blood to subdue swelling and cure swollen sores.

诸否候导引法【zhū fǒu hòu dǎo yǐn fǎ】 为动功。其作法为，正坐挺腰，昂胸抬头，两手指相对，向前按地，身体及头、胸向下，接近地面时即回身向上，作十四次。宽胸消痞积，温脏通络。治臂痛不舒，腰脊不适，去胸胁痞块。

exercise of Daoyin for distension A dynamic exercise, marked by sitting with stretched waist, chest and head, keeping the hands near each other to press the ground in the front, lowering the head and chest and turning upwards when nearing the ground for fourteen times, relaxing the chest to expel accumulation of lump, warming the viscera to open the collaterals. Such a static exercise can relieve pain of the shoulders, waist and spine as well as mass in the chest and rib-sides.

诸根【zhū gēn】 佛家气功习用语，指信、勤、念、定、慧之五根。

various roots A common term of Qigong in Buddhism, referring to the five roots, i. e. the root of belief, the root of diligence, the root of emotion, the root of tranquility and the root of wisdom.

诸淋【zhū lín】 气功适应证，指小便频数短涩，欲出不尽，滴沥刺痛，痛引腰腹一类的疾病。

stranguria An indication of Qigong, referring to frequent scanty urination with stabbing pain that causes waist pain and abdominal pain.

诸淋候导引法【zhū lín hòu dǎo yǐn fǎ】 为动功。其作法为，仰卧，两手放膝头，两足跟放臀下，用口服气，鼓腹，待气充满腹部时，用鼻慢慢呼出，利水通淋。治淋病，小便频数。

exercise of Daoyin for various gonorrhea
A dynamic exercise，marked by lying on the back，putting both hands on the knees，keeping the heels below the buttock，inhaling Qi through the mouth，increasing the abdomen，slowly exhaling when Qi is enriched in the abdomen，promoting urination to relieve stranguria. Such a dynamic exercise can cure stranguria and frequent urination.

诸阳会【zhū yáng huì】 指阳维脉所交会的头肩部各穴。此穴位为气功习练之处。

various Yang intersections Refers to the acupoints in the head and shoulders associated with the Yang link vessel. These acupoints are the regions usually used in practice of Qigong.

诸阴交【zhū yīn jiāo】 指阴维脉所交会的胸腹部各穴。此穴位为气功习练之处。

various intersections of Yin Refers to the acupoints in the chest and abdomen associated with the Yin link vessel. These acupoints are the regions usually used in practice of Qigong.

诸饮候导引法【zhū yǐn hòu dǎo yǐn fǎ】 为静功。其作法为，左侧或右侧而卧，闭目、闭气不息十二遍，肖痰饮。右有饮病，左侧卧、闭气不息，并以意引气而排除。

exercise of Daoyin for fluid distension A static exercise，marked by lying on the right side or left side，closing the eyes and stopping respiration for twelve times for relieving phlegm and fluid；or lying on the left side and stopping respiration for eliminating fluid disorder in the right.

诸真内丹集要【zhū zhēn nèi dān jí yào】《诸真内丹集要》为气功专著，成书于元代，主要论述气功内练之法，作者不详。

Zhuzhen Neidan Jiyao（*Collection of Various Genuine Internal Dan*） A monograph of Qigong in the Yuan Dynasty（1271 AD‑1368 AD）entitled *Collection of Various Genuine Internal Dan*（*Pills of Immortality*），mainly describing the exercises for practicing Qigong. The author was unknown.

诸真圣胎神用诀【zhū zhēn shèng tāi shén yòng jué】《诸真圣胎神用诀》为气功学专著，内容包括御气之法及二十九家胎息。作者不详。

Zhu Zhensheng Taixi Yongjue（*Formula of Various Genuine Sages' Fetal Spirit*） A monograph of Qigong entitled *Formula of Various Genuine Sages' Fetal Spirit*，describing the exercises for promoting Qi and twenty-nine kinds of fetal respiration. The author was unknown.

诸真玄奥集成【zhū zhēn xuán ào jí chéng】《诸真玄奥集成》为气功学专著，由明代朱载玮所编，其中收录了多部气功著作。

Zhuzhen Xuan'ao Jicheng（*Collection of Various Genuine and Supreme Abstruseness*） A monograph of Qigong entitled *Collection of Various Genuine and Supreme Abstruseness*，compiled by Zhu Zaiwei in the Ming Dynasty（1368 AD‑1644 AD），including several monographs of Qigong written by other masters.

诸痔候导引法【zhū zhì hòu dǎo yǐn fǎ】 为动功，方法多样。如一足踏地，一足膝关节弯曲,两手抱膝关节处,使之尽量向上身牵引,左右交替各二十八次。舒筋通络,治痔疮,虚劳病,下肢经络不利。

exercise of Daoyin for various Hemorrhoids A dynamic exercise with various methods, such as treading on the ground with one foot, bending one knee, holding upwards the knee joints with both hands from the left to the right and vice versa for twenty-eight times respectively. Such a dynamic exercise can soothe sinews, to activate collaterals, and to cure hemorrhoids, consumptive disease and obstructed meridians and collaterals in the legs.

诸痔治法【zhū zhì zhì fǎ】 动静相兼功,方法多样。如高枕仰卧,心平气定的调息。或一脚踏地,一脚屈膝,两手抱犊鼻穴向下,快速尽力向上牵引,左右交换各作二十八次。

treatment of various hemorrhoids An exercise combined with dynamic exercise and static exercise with various methods, such as lying on the back with a high pillow, tranquilizing the heart and stabilizing Qi, or one foot treading on the ground, the other foot bending the knee, holding Dubi (ST 35) acupoint downwards with both hands, and then quickly raising up to exchange from the left to the right and vice versa for twenty-eight times respectively.

主不明则十二官危【zhǔ bù míng zé shí èr guān wēi】 出自《黄帝内经》。主指心,心在人身中处于统帅地位。心神安宁,则一身得安。心神不宁,则一身失调,各不相安。

If the monarch (the heart) **is not wise** (abnormal in function), **all the twelve organs will be in danger and cannot function well.** This is a celebrated dictum from Huangdi Neijing (entitled *Yellow Emperor's Internal Canon of Medicine*). In this sentence, the monarch refers to the heart that controls the whole body. Only when the heart spirit is stabilized can the body be balanced. If the heart spirit is not stabilized, the body is in disorder.

主客【zhǔ kè】 在下为客,在上为主;主指命,客指性。

host and guest Traditionally the so-called guest refers to either the lower position or the property and the so-called host refers to either the upper position or the life.

主明则下安【zhǔ míng zé xià ān】 主即心。心神清净则一身安和,心虚净则明,心为七情六欲所干扰则不明。

If the monarch (the heart) **is wise** (normal in functions), **the subordinates** (the other organs) **will be peaceful** (normal in function). This is a celebrated dictum in *Yellow Emperor's Internal Canon of Medicine*. In this sentence, the so-called monarch refers to the heart. Only when the heart spirit is normal and stable can the body be stabilized and harmonized. Usually the so-called seven emotions and six desires disturb the heart.

主人【zhǔ rén】 上关的一个别称,为足少阳胆经中的一个穴位,位于颧弓上缘,距耳郭前缘约1寸处,为气功常用意守部位。

Zhuren A synonym of Shangguan (GB 3), which is an acupoint in the gallbladder of foot Shaoyang, located on the upper of the zygoma and about 1 Cun to the upper of the auricle. This acupoint is a region usually used in practice of Qigong.

主适寒热荣卫和【zhǔ shì hán rè róng wèi hé】 出自《黄帝内经》,指心的功能作用是调适寒热,和顺荣卫之气。

It is the monarch that regulates cold and heat as well as the nutrient aspect and defense aspect. This is a celebrated dictum in Huangdi Neijing (entitled *Yellow Emperor's Internal Canon of Medicine*), referring to the function of the heart that regulates cold and heat as well as Qi in the nutrient aspect and defense aspect.

主翁【zhǔ wēng】 指心,人体中最为重要的脏腑。

host Refers to the heart, the most important viscus in the body.

住【zhù】 住在气功文献中的含义有二,① 指到或止之意;② 指相对稳定。

Stop In the literature of Qigong, stop refers to ① either reach or termination;② or comparative stability.

住势【zhù shì】 指将导引姿势保留一会儿。

suspended posture Means to keep the posture of Daoyin for a whole.

住心一神【zhù xīn yī shén】 指以意念稳定精神意识思维活动之意。

stabilizing the heart tranquilizing the spirit Refers to stabilization of the activities of the essence, the spirit, the thought and the consciousness.

住缘一境【zhù yuán yī jìng】 指意识思维活动集中于一处,或一景物。

stabilization of an edge in a state Refers to concentrating the activities of consciousness and thought in a position

or in a scenery.

注心一神【zhù xīn yī shén】 指精神思维意识活动高度集中统一。

Supreme concentration with one spirit Refers to concentration and unification of the activities of the spirit, thinking and consciousness.

柱骨【zhù gǔ】 ① 指锁骨;② 指颈椎;③ 指第七颈椎棘突。

styloideum Refers to ① either clavicle;② or cervical vertebra;③ or furcella of cervical vertebra.

祝融峰【zhù róng fēng】 指脑。

Fire god peak Refers to the brain.

祝由【zhù yóu】 即祝说病由,转移病人精神的方法,以改变病人脏气紊乱状况,使之精神内守而病自愈的精神疗法。

wishing causes Refers to hoping to understanding the causes of diseases, indicating to turn the spirit of patients in order to change the disorders of the visceral Qi in the patients, to concentrate the spirit inside and to cure the disease naturally.

贮香导引法【zhù xiāng dǎo yǐn fǎ】 为动功,共有六法,即心病导引,正坐,两手握拳,用力左右相等,各六度;肝病导引,正坐,两手相重按胜下,徐缓身,左右各三五度;肾病导引,正坐,两手从耳左右引肋三五度;肺病导引,正坐,两手据地,缩身曲脊,向上五拳;脾病导引,大坐伸一足,屈足,二手放后反擎,各三五度;胆病导引,平坐,合两脚掌,仰头,两手挽脚腕起,摇动为之三五度。本法治疗五脏各种疾病。

exercise of Daoyin for storing fragrance A dynamic exercise with six ways of Daoyin. Daoyin for heart disease is marked by sitting upright, holding the fists with both hands and enforcing the same in the left and right for six degrees respectively; Daoyin for liver disease is marked by sitting upright, pressing the fleshes with both hands and relaxing the body from the left to the right and vice versa for three and five degrees respectively; Daoyin for kidney disease is marked by sitting upright and pressing the ribs from the left and right ears with both hands for three and five degrees respectively; Daoyin for lung disease is marked by sitting upright, pressing the ground with both hands, shrinking the body and bending the spine upward with five fists; Daoyin for spleen disease is marked by sitting fully, stretching one foot, bending the other foot, putting the hands backwards and returning for three and five degrees respectively; Daoyin for gallbladder disease is marked by sitting down, concentrating the feet, raising the head, pulling the ankles with both hands and shaking for three and five degrees. This exercise can be used to treat diseases in the five Zang-organs (including the heart, the liver, the spleen, the lung and the kidney).

贮香小品【zhù xiāng xiǎo pǐn】《贮香小品》为导引专著,由明代万后贤所著,书中介绍了五脏病导引法,对辨证施功有一定的使用价值。

Zhuxiang Xiaopin (*Essay for Storing Fragrance*) A monograph of Qigong entitled *Essay for Storing Fragrance*, written by Wan Houxian in the Ming Dynasty (1368 AD – 1644 AD) describing the exercise of Qigong for treating diseases in the five Zang-organs (inclu-

ding heart, liver, spleen, lung and kidney), quiet effective for differentiation of syndromes and practicing Qigong.

筑宾【zhù bīn】 足少阴肾经中的一个穴位,位于内踝尖与跟腱水平连线中点直上 5 寸,为气功中常用的意守部位。

Zhubin (KI 9) An acupoint in the kidney meridian of foot Shaoyin, located 5 Cun above the middle line between the tip of the medial malleolus and the heel tendon, which is the region for concentrating consciousness in practicing Qigong.

筑基【zhù jī】 习练气功的基础。

construction base Refers to the foundation for practicing Qigong.

筑空【zhù kōng】 指手向前击。

construction space Indicates that the hands are stretching forward.

专闭御景法【zhuān bì yù jǐng fǎ】 动静相兼功。其作法是常以日初出,面向东方,叩齿就此。叩毕即默意念,咽液九次,补身中之阳,调节全身阴阳。

combination of activity and tranquility An exercise combined with dynamic exercise and static exercise, marked by standing to the east in sunrise, clicking the teeth, silencing consciousness after clicking teeth, swallowing humor for nine times. Such an exercise combined with dynamic exercise and static exercise can tonify Yang and regulate Yin and Yang in the whole body.

专气至柔神久留【zhuān qì zhì róu shén jiǔ liú】 源自气功专论。全诗精辟阐述明神,息悠然就是炼内丹。

mansuetude of special Qi and long-term remain of spirit Collected from a monograph of Qigong, the poems in which have discussed and analyzed the spirit for refining the internal Dan（pills of immortality）.

专气致柔【zhuān qì zhì róu】 指行功中,呼吸出入之气在意识的作用下柔和自然。

softened inhalation Refers to Qi in the respiration gentle and natural in practice of Qigong under the guidance of consciousness.

专想【zhuān xiǎng】 佛家气功习用语,指行功中,意念活动观一境而不分散。

special thought A commonly used term of Qigong in Buddhism, referring to concentrated mind without any disorder.

专行【zhuān xíng】 指意识活动专一。

special movement Refers to concentrated activity of consciousness.

专修静定身如玉【zhuān xiū jìng dìng shēn rú yù】 指习练气功,内绝所思,外绝所欲,可使元气自足,身体健康。

Special tranquilization will cultivate the body like a jade. Refers to relieving thought and eliminating avarice in order to enrich original Qi and to cultivate health in practicing Qigong.

专于意【zhuān yú yì】 指的是精神守一而不散,则意识在中,行为端正。

special consciousness Refers to concentration of the essence and the spirit with the consciousness in the middle and the activities correct.

转法论【zhuǎn fǎ lùn】 即周天功。道家周天功即佛家转法论,理论相同,功法各异。

exercise for circulatory cycle Refers to celestial circuit of Qigong which is the concept in Daoism. In Buddhism, it is called turn of the wheel of the law

（Sanskrit Dharmacakra）. The theory in Daoism and Buddhism is the same, but the exercise for practicing Qigong is different.

转胁舒足【zhuǎn xié shū zú】 为动功,即人睡时气停留于全身关节处,所以养生的人睡时当蜷缩身体,睡醒时当伸舒肢体。到阳气生发的子时身体当侧身舒足而卧,这样可以使荣卫气血周流不息。

turning the flank and stretching the foot A dynamic exercise, marked by remaining Qi in the joints of the whole body in sleeping, huddling up the body in sleeping in order to cultivate life and stretching the body when waking up, lying on the right side to stretch the feet in Zi period（the period of the day from 11 p. m. to 1 a. m.）when Yang Qi begins to grow in order to circulate nutrient Qi, defense Qi, Qi and the blood normally.

转筋【zhuàn jīn】 气功适应证,指抽筋。

change of sinew An indication of Qigong, referring to spasm of the lower limbs.

转筋候导引法【zhuàn jīn hòu dǎo yǐn fǎ】 为动功,方法多样。如仰卧,舒展手脚,足跟向外,趾相对,用鼻吸气至极限时慢慢呼出,作七息。温经散寒,活血通络,治膝寒,小腿疼,转筋。

exercise of Daoyin for turning sinews A dynamic exercise with several methods, such as lying on the back, stretching the hands and feet, turning the heels laterally, corresponding the toes from two feet, inhaling through the nose and then slowly exhaling for seven times. Such a way of Qigong practice can

Z

warm the meridians and expel cold, activate the blood, promote the collaterals, treat coldness of the knees and pain of the shanks, and turn the sinews.

馔食【zhuàn shí】　本意指饮食,气功指吞咽津液。

Diet　Refers to swallowing fluid and humor in Qigong practice.

庄周气诀解【zhuāng zhōu qì jué jiě】《庄周气诀解》为气功专论,作者及成书年代不详,说明要增进健康,延年益寿,就应平素珍惜时间,节欲去嗔,调节饮食,心意坦然,安定形神。

Zhuangzhou Qijue Jie(*Inscription of Qi Circulation with Jade Pendant*)　A monograph of Qigong entitled *Explanation of Zhuang Zhou's Qi Formula*, explaining that only the time is cherished, desire is restricted, diet is regulated, mind is purified, the body and spirit are stabilized can health be cultivated and life be prolonged. The author and the time to compile this book were unknown.

庄子【zhuāng zǐ】　战国时期的哲学家和气功学家。

Zhuang Zi　A great philosopher and a great master of Qigong in the Warring States Period.

庄子达生法【zhuāng zǐ dá shēng fǎ】为静功,指守纯和之气以养其气;指守精神之和以一其性。

Zhuang Zi' exercise for cultivating life　A static exercise, referring to either purifying Qi in order to nourish Qi; or stabilizing the normal function of the spirit in order to perfect the property.

庄子体道法【zhuāng zǐ tǐ dào fǎ】　为

静功,指虚静纯一;指合于自然;指调节阴阳;指安时处和;指内守精神。

Zhuang Zi's exercise for experiencing Daoism　A static exercise, referring to either purification of quietness; or combination with the natural world; or regulating Yin and Yang; or pacifying anything and balancing any activities; or internal concentration of the spirit.

撞三关【zhuàng sān guān】　指交通任督二脉的一种运气方法。

bumping three passes　Refers to a method for moving Qi in the conception meridian and the governor meridian.

准提求愿观想法【zhǔn tí qiú yuàn guān xiǎng fǎ】　佛家气功功法,方法多样。如若求无分别,当精神集中;若秋无相无色,当意想文字;若求不二法门,当意想观两臂等。

exercise for desire and contemplation　An exercise of Qigong in Buddhism with various methods, such as concentrating the spirit for indifference, imagining Chinese characters for no desires and no hopes and observing the shoulders for keeping one way.

准提陀罗尼布字法【zhǔn tí tuó luó ní bù zì fǎ】　佛家气功功法,方法多样。如唵,意想安在自身头顶上,其色白如月,放出无量光,功在灭除一切障消除烦恼,稳定情绪。

exercise for distributing dharani words　An exercise of Qigong in Buddhism with various methods, such as silent reading the Chinese character An (Sanskrit) and imagining to keep it on the top of the head which appears as white as the moon with immeasurable light in order to eliminate annoyance and to stabilize emotion.

准胝法【zhǔn zhī fǎ】　佛家气功功法。其作法为,结跏趺坐,意想观身体前面金刚墙内有大海,大海中有大宝山,山上有楼阁,阁中有八叶莲花台,莲花上有月轮。主要是默念。

exercise for solving callus An exercise of Qigong in Buddhism, marked by sitting in lotus position and imagining that there is a large sea in the diamond wall at the front, a large mountain in the sea, a pavilion in the mountain, a lotus platform in the pavilion and a moon over the lotus, indicating that imagination is the way to practice Qigong.

顿【zhuō】　① 指人体部位名,即眼眶下面的骨,包括上颌骨与颧骨参与构成眼眶下面的部分;② 指经穴别名,即禾髎。

malar bone Refers to ① either the bone below the orbital cavity, including maxilla and cheekbone; ② or synonym of the acupoint Huoliao (LI 19), which is an acupoint in the large intestine meridian of hand Taiyang.

浊恶【zhuó è】　佛家气功习用语,指影响神形失调的言语和行为。

wrong behavior A common term of Qigong in Buddhism, referring to imbalance of the spirit and the body due to abnormal speech and action.

浊阳【zhuó yáng】　指天气晦暗不明,浑浊不清。

turbid Yang Refers to tarnish and turbidity of air.

琢齿【zhuó chǐ】　即叩齿,为动功,指上下牙互相叩击。

pondering teeth The same as clicking teeth, is a dynamic exercise, referring to the upper teeth and the lower teeth

clicking each other.

子丹【zǐ dān】　指心神。

zidan Refers to the heart spirit.

子断【zǐ duàn】　佛家气功习用语,指弃除烦恼,稳定情绪。

tranquilization A term of Qigong in Buddhism, referring to elimination of annoyance and stabilization of emotion in practicing Qigong.

子房祠【zǐ fáng cí】　在白云山上,相传张良(张子房,名良)辟谷来隐于此。

Zifang's temple Refers to the temple in Baiyun Mountain where Zhang Liang, a great minister in the Han Dynasty (202 BC - 263 AD), lived in seclusion for inedia.

子缚【zǐ fù】　佛家气功习用语,指烦恼缚身,神形不调。

troubled mind A term of Qigong in Buddhism, referring to disturbance of the body and disharmony of the body and spirit.

子户【zǐ hù】　① 指女外生殖器;② 指气穴,即足少阴肾经中的一个穴位。

Zihu Refers to ① either female external genital; ② or Qixue (KI 13), an acupoint in the kidney meridian of foot Shaoyin.

子母【zǐ mǔ】　指阳气和阴气。

son and mother Refers to Yang Qi and Yin Qi.

子母分胎路【zǐ mǔ fēn tāi lù】　指任买和督脉的交接之处。

converging point of son and mother Refers to converging point of the conception meridian and governor meridian.

子母会合【zǐ mǔ huì hé】　① 指先天祖气谓之母,后天呼吸谓之子;② 指神与气合,即神气合一。

son and mother joining together Refers

to ① either the innate ancestral Qi as mother and the postnatal respiration as son; ② or combination of the spirit and Qi, indicating integration of the spirit and Qi.

子时【zǐ shí】 指一日十二时辰中,以子时为六阳时之开始时辰。

midnight Refers to the period of the day from 11 p.m. to 1 a.m.

子午【zǐ wǔ】 ① 指子时、午时;② 指日月、心肾、坎离;③ 指子为阳之首,午为阴之首。

midnoon and midnight Refers to ① either Zi (the period of the day from 11 p.m. to 1 a.m.) and Wu (the period of the day from 11 a.m. to 1 p.m.); ② or the sun and the moon, the heart and the kidney; ③ or Kan Trigram and Li Trigram; or Zi (the period of the day from 11 p.m. to 1 a.m.) is the head of Yang and Wu (the period of the day from 11 a.m. to 1 p.m.) is the head of Yin.

子午固关元【zǐ wǔ gù guān yuán】 为静功,子时一阳生,属肾。午时一阴生,属心。其作法为,子午二时洗心静坐,鼻吸调匀,反观内顾于关元之处。能补益元气,延年益寿。

dhyana in midnoon and midnight A static exercise, referring to Yang growth in Zi (the period of the day from 11 p.m. to 1 a.m.) which pertains to the kidney and Yin growth in Wu (the period of the day from 11 a.m. to 1 p.m.) which pertains to the heart; usually marked by purifying the heart and sitting quietly in Zi (the period of the day from 11 p.m. to 1 p.m.) and Wu (the period of day from 11 a.m. to 1 a.m.), breathing in normally through the nose and internally observing Guanyuan (CV 4). Such a static exercise can tonify and replenish the original Qi, prolonging life and nourishing health.

子午教合三戊己号称五【zǐ wǔ jiào hé sān wù jǐ hào chēng wǔ】 根据五行学说,指子居北,坎水之正位;午属南,离火之正位。

coordination of water and fire with five elements in midnoon and midnight Refers to the fact that Zi means the normotopia of water in the north and Wu means the normotopia of fire in the south which are formed according to the five elements.

子午流注【zǐ wǔ liú zhù】 子午代表时间,流注指气血流注。

midnight-noon ebb-flow Refers to flow of Qi and the blood in Zi (the period of the day from 11 p.m. to 1 a.m.) and Wu (the period of the day from 11 a.m. to 1 p.m.).

子午卯酉【zǐ wǔ mǎo yǒu】 子为六阳之首,以应冬至;午为六阴之首,为阳极阴生之际;卯酉为心肾二气交分之际,应春秋二分。

Zi Wu Mao You Zi refers to the head of the six kinds of Yang, related to winter; Wu is the head of the six kinds of Yin, indicating the growth of Yin when Yang has developed to the extreme; Mao and You are connected with Qi in the heart and the kidney, related to spring and autumn.

子英捕鱼【zǐ yīng bǔ yú】 为动功。其作法为,自然站立,弯腰,以左手握右脚,右手握左脚。

Ziying' fishing exercise A dynamic exercise, marked by naturally standing up，bending the waist，holding the right foot with the left hand and holding the left foot with the right hand.

子主披发鼓琴【zǐ zhǔ pī fā gǔ qín**】**为动功。其作法为，身体盘端坐，先用两手擦抹脚心令热，然后趁热，两手按于两膝上。可以调理血脉，治三焦不和，眼目昏花，身体虚弱。

cross-legged dhyana A dynamic exercise，marked by sitting with crossed knees，rubbing the soles hot with the hands，pressing the knees with the hands. Such a dynamic exercise can regulate the blood and treat disorder of the triple energizer，dim-sightedness and weakness of the body.

紫房【zǐ fáng**】** 即心的别称。

Purple room A synonym of the heart.

紫房帏幕【zǐ fáng wéi mù**】** 指心和心包。

purple room with curtain Refers to the heart and pericardium.

紫府【zǐ fǔ**】** 指真气归藏之所，即丹田。

purple mansion Refers to the place storing genuine Qi，which is Danian. Dantian is divided into the upper Dantian（the region between the eyes），the middle Dantian（the region below the heart）and the lower Dantian（the region below the navel）.

紫河车【zǐ hé chē**】** 指真气生，阳神就，化圣离俗。

purple river cart Refers to generating genuine Qi，perfecting Yang spirit and leaving the external world.

紫极宫【zǐ jí gōng**】** 即胆。

purple and utmost palace Refers to the gallbladder.

紫金城【zǐ jīn chéng**】** 指脑，亦指脑

内泥丸宫。

purple golden city Refers to the brain，also referring to the mud bolus（the brain）chamber in the brain.

紫金丹【zǐ jīn dān**】** ① 指金丹成就；② 指身体阴阳和合，即稳定状态。

Purple golden Dan（pills of immortality） Refers to ① either achievement of golden Dan（pills of immortality）；② or balance of Yin and Yang，indicating stable state.

紫金霜【zǐ jīn shuāng**】** 即白虎、青龙相互作用后形成的金丹大药。

purple golden frost Refers to golden Dan（pills of immortality）medicinal formed by mutual role of the white tiger and green Loong.

紫清宫【zǐ qīng gōng**】** 指泥丸宫。

purple clear chamber Refers to the mud bolus（the brain）chamber.

紫团丹经【zǐ tuán dān jīng**】** 《紫团丹经》为气功专著，由宋代紫团真人撰，倡导内修，运炼精、气、神而成丹药。

Zituan Danjing（*Canon of Purple Group Dan***）** A monograph of Qigong entitled *Canon of Purple Group Dan*，written by the immortal in the purple group，suggesting to cultivate the internal parts of the body and to move and to refine the essence，Qi and the spirit for producing Dan（pills of immortality）medicinal.

紫微【zǐ wēi**】** 指脑内部分结构，亦指脑。

purple subtlety Refers to either one part in the brain；or the brain.

紫微宫【zǐ wēi gōng**】** 位于河南怀庆王屋山下，为唐代气功家司马承祯的居住地。

Purple Subtle Palace Located below

Z

the Palace of Huaiqing King in the Henan Province, where Ma Chengzhen, the master of Qigong in the Tang Dynasty (618 AD – 907 AD), lived.

紫贤真人【zǐ xián zhēn rén】 是对宋代气功家薛道光的赞美,其著有两部气功专著。

Purple Virtuous Immortal The celebration of Xue Daoguang, a great master of Qigong in the Song Dynasty (960 AD – 1127 AD) who wrote two monographs about Qigong.

紫烟【zǐ yān】 指目神精妙之气。

purple smoke Refers to ingenious Qi in the ocular spirit.

紫阳宫【zǐ yáng gōng】 位于山西翼城,相传为宋代紫阳真人张伯端修养处。

Ziyang Palace Located in Yicheng County in Shanxi Province. It was said that the immortal Zhang Borui in the Song Dynasty (960 AD – 1279 AD) practiced Qigong and cultivated life there.

紫阳真人【zǐ yáng zhēn rén】 是对北宋气功学家张伯端的赞美,其著有气功专著,分析研究了气功的基本理论和方法。

purple Yang Immortal The celebration of Zhang Boduan, a great master of Qigong in the North Song Dynasty (960 AD – 1127 AD), who wrote a monograph of Qigong, analyzing and studying the basic theory and practice of Qigong.

自汗盗汗导引法【zì hàn dào hàn dǎo yǐn fǎ】 为静功。其作法为,先意念守脐,想火于脐内旋转,以手复脐,想脐下一条水入膀胱,上尾闾,至背穿出心头而洗之。治自汗、盗汗、兼遗精。

exercise of Daoyin for spontaneous swea- ting and night sweating A static exercise, marked by concentrating the navel with consciousness, imaging that fire is rotating in the navel, pressing the navel with the hands, imagining that water below the navel enters the bladder, flows to the coccygeal end, runs up to the back and head in order to wash the body. Such a way of practice can relieve spontaneous sweating, night sweating and spermatorrhea.

自己元神【zì jǐ yuán shén】 ① 指自体的本神;② 指神气的聚合。

self-original spirit Refers to ① either the original spirit in the human body; ② or combination of the spiritual Qi.

自家精血自交媾【zì jiā jīng xuè zì jiāo gòu】 指习练气功,能融合精神气血。

Personal coitus with personal essence and blood Refers to integration of the essence, the spirit, Qi and the blood in practicing Qigong.

自然【zì rán】 ① 指华池;② 指太和自然之气。

natural side Refers to ① either the mouth; ② or natural Qi.

自然之道静【zì rán zhī dào jìng】 指自然界的变化有序而规律。

natural tranquility Refers to the procedure and principle of changes in the natural world.

自然之术【zì rán zhī shù】 指事物本身的内在变化规律。

natural technique Refers to the internal change regulations of anything.

自柔【zì róu】 指呼吸之气均匀缓和。

natural softening Refers to natural and relaxed respiration.

自心感现【zì xīn gǎn xiàn】 指一切

智慧、感应、知识、灵明、觉悟，都是脑神精神意识思维活动的外在表现。

Manifestation of the heart A term of Qigong, refers to wisdom, telepathic response, knowledge, brilliance and consciousness which are all the manifestations of the activities of the spirit, consciousness and emotion in the brain.

自性禅【zì xìng chán】 佛家气功功法，指思维意识集中于一，意识内守不散，逐步相对静止。

personal meditation An exercise of Qigong in Buddhism, referring to concentration of consciousness and emotion without any dispersion in order to tranquilize the mind and body.

自知不自见【zì zhī bù zì jiàn】 指气功中一种稳定精神的方法。

personal knowledge without personal opinion Refers to the method that stabilizes the spirit in practicing Qigong.

眦㿏【zì wēi】 指按摩。

nice canthus Refers to Tuina, an important way to press and to rub any part of the body, much better than the so-called massage.

宗筋【zōng jīn】 指阴茎和睾丸。

ancestral sinew Refers to penis and testicle

宗气【zōng qì】 指积于胸中之气，由肺吸入的清气和脾胃化生的水谷精气结合而成。

ancestral Qi Refers to Qi in the chest, which is produced by combination of clear Qi inhaled by the lung and essential Qi from water and grain made by the spleen and stomach.

宗气泄【zōng qì xiè】 气功适应证，指宗气失藏而外泄的病证，表现为气喘，虚

里部位（左乳下心尖搏动处）跳动甚剧而振衣，伴有胸闷、心悸、气短、自汗出、形寒肢冷、舌淡、脉迟无力等心功能不全的症状。

diarrhea of ancestral Qi An indication of Qigong, caused by dispersion of ancestral Qi that fails to keep inside. The symptoms of this disease include panting and beating of the deficient region (the throbbing region below the left breast and above the heart) that shakes the clothes, accompanied by chest oppression, palpitation, shortness of breath, sweating, coldness of the body and limbs, pale tongue and weakness of the vessels and meridians.

总持门【zǒng chí mén】 指脑。

general controlling gate Refers to the brain.

总有一毫之不定，命非己有【zǒng yǒu yī háo zhī bú dìng mìng fēi jǐ yǒu】指习练气功调节呼吸时，如不能达到"伏其气于脐下，守其神于身内"的稳定状态，要想获得成功是不可能的。

If a small bit is unsteady, how can life be protected? Indicates that it is impossible to succeed if one fails to "move Qi to the region below the navel and keep the spirit inside the body" in practicing Qigong.

纵息【zòng xī】 指深呼吸。

longitudinal breath Refers to deep respiration.

邹铉【zōu hóng】 元代医学家和气功学家邹铉的另外一个称谓。

Zou Hong Another name of Zou Xuan, a great doctor and master of Qigong in the Yuan Dynasty (1271 AD – 1368 AD).

邹铉【zōu xuàn】 元代医学家和气功

Z

学家。

Zou Xuan A great doctor and master of Qigong in the Yuan Dynasty（1271 AD－1368 AD）.

足大趾【zú dà zhǐ】 即踇趾。足厥阴肝经循行线经大趾，气功排肝经毒气常从此出。

large toe The area through which the liver meridian of foot Jueyin moves around and pathogenic factors in the liver meridian are expelled.

足跗【zú fū】 即足背，为习练气功时所必须运用的一个部位。

acrotarsium Refers to the dorsal region of the foot that is often used in practicing Qigong.

足功【zú gōng】 为动功。其作法为，正坐，伸足低头，以两手用力攀足心十二次。高坐垂足，将两足跟相对扭向外，复将两足尖相对扭向内，各二十四遍。可除两脚风气，可除湿热，可除两肩邪，可治股膝肿痛。

foot exercise A dynamic exercise, marked by sitting upright, stretching the feet, lowering the head and climbing the soles with both hands for twelve times; then sitting high, drooping the feet, turning the heels laterally and internally for twenty-four times respectively. Such a way of practice Qigong can expel wind Qi in the feet, relieve damp heat, eliminate pathogenic factors in the shoulders and cure swelling and pain of the thighs and knees.

足厥阴【zú jué yīn】 足厥阴肝经，其循行从大趾背毫毛部开始，向上沿着足背内侧，离内踝一寸，上行小腿内侧，离内踝八寸处交出足太阴脾经之后，上膝胭内侧，沿着大腿内侧，进入阴毛中，与督脉交会于头顶。此经脉为气功习练之处。

foot Jueyin Refers to the liver meridian of foot Jueyin. It starts from the dorsal hair of the great toe, runs upward along the dorsum of the foot, and passes through a point, 1 Cun in front of the medial malleolu. It ascends to the area 8 Cun above the medial malleolus, where it runs across and behind the spleen meridian of foot-Taiyang. Then it runs upward to the medial aspect of the knee, and along the medial aspect of thigh into the pubic hair region, finally meets with the governor meridian at the vertex. This meridian is a region usually used in practice of Qigong.

足厥阴肝经【zú jué yīn gān jīng】 从大趾和背毫毛部开始循行，向上沿着足背内侧，离内踝一寸，上行小腿内侧，离内踝八寸处交出足太阴脾经之后，上膝胭内侧，沿着大腿内侧，进入阴毛中，与督脉交会于头顶。此经为气功习练之处。

liver meridian of foot Jueyin Starts from the dorsal hair of the great toe, runs upward along the dorsum of the foot, and passes through a point, 1 Cun in front of the medial malleolu, it ascends to the area 8 Cun above the medial malleolus, where it runs across and behind the spleen meridian of foot-Taiyang. Then it runs upward to the medial aspect of the knee, and along the medial aspect of thigh into the pubic hair region, finally meets with the governor meridian at the vertex. This meridian is a region usually used in practice of Qigong.

足厥阴络脉【zú jué yīn luò mài】 脉

循行在离内踝上五寸处蠡沟穴分出，走向足少阳经脉。此络为气功习练之处。

collateral of foot Jueyin Derives from Ligou (LR 5), 5 Cun above the medial malleolus, and runs to the gallbladder meridian of foot Shaoyang. This collateral is a region usually used in practice of Qigong.

足厥阴之别【zú jué yīn zhī bié】 即足厥阴络脉，脉循行在离内踝上五寸处蠡沟穴分出，走向足少阳经脉。此经别为气功习练之处。

branch of foot Jueyin Derives from Ligou (LR 5), 5 Cun above the medial malleolus, and runs to the gallbladder meridian of foot Shaoyang. This branch is a region usually used in practice of Qigong.

足窍阴【zú qiào yīn】 足少阳胆经中的一个穴位，位于第四趾的外侧。这一穴位为气功运行的一个常见部位。

Zuqiaoyin（GB 44） An acupoint in the gallbladder meridian of foot Shaoyin, located on the lateral side of the fourth toe. This acupoint is a region usually used for keeping the essential Qi in practice of Qigong.

足三里【zú sān lǐ】 足阳明胃经中的一个穴位，位于犊鼻穴下三寸。本穴常为气功的意守部位。

Zusanli（ST 36） An acupoint in the stomach meridian of foot Yangming, located 3 Cun below Dubi（ST 35）, which is a region to concentrate consciousness in practicing Qigong.

足三阳经【zú sān yáng jīng】 指足阳明胃经，足太阳膀胱经和足少阳胆经，为十二经脉中循行于下肢前、外和后侧的三条阳经。此经脉为气功习练之处。

three Yang meridians of foot Refer to the stomach meridian of foot Yangming, bladder meridian of foot Taiyang and gallbladder meridian of foot Taiyang, which are the three ones among the twelve meridians that circulate along the front, lateral sides and back of the legs. These meridians are the region usually used in practice of Qigong.

足三阴经【zú sān yīn jīng】 指足太阴脾经、足少阴肾经和足厥阴肝经，为十二经脉中循行于下肢内侧的三条阴经。此经脉为气功习练之处。

three Yin meridians of foot Refer to the spleen meridian of foot Taiyin, kidney meridian of foot Shaoyin and liver meridian of foot Jueyin, which are the three ones among the twelve meridians that circulate along the internal side of the legs. These meridians are the region usually used in practice of Qigong.

足少阳【zú shào yáng】 指足少阳胆经，为十二经脉之一，起于目外眦，上行到额角，转后下行至耳后。此经脉为气功习练之处。

foot Shaoyang Refers to gallbladder meridian of foot Shaoyang, one of the twelve meridians, starting from the outer canthus, running to the forehead and turning downwards to the ear. This meridian is a region usually used in practice of Qigong.

足少阳胆经【zú shào yáng dǎn jīng】 十二经脉之一，起于目外眦，上行到额角，转后下行至耳后。沿颈后行手少阳三焦经的前面，至肩上交出手少阳经的后面，在大椎穴处与督脉相会，向前入缺盆。此经为气功习练之处。

bladder meridian of foot Shaoyang One

Z

of the twelve meridians，starts from the outer canthus and runs to the forehead and turning downwards to the ear. From the back of the neck，it moves in front of the triple energizer meridian of hand Shaoyang，reaching the shoulder behind the triple energizer meridian of hand Shaoyang，meeting the governor meridian at the acupoint of Dazhui（GV 14），and finally moving forward into Quepen（ST 12）. This meridian is a region usually used in practice of Qigong.

足少阳经别【zú shào yáng jīng bié】从足少阳胆经分出，绕过大腿前侧进入外阴部，同足厥阴经别会合。此经别为气功习练之处。

branch of foot Shaoyang Derives from the gallbladder meridian of foot Shaoyang，and curves around the anterior aspect of the thigh. Then it enters the external genitalia region to meet the liver meridian of foot Jueyin. This branch is a region usually used in practice of Qigong.

足少阳络脉【zú shào yáng luò mài】在距离外踝上五寸光明穴处分出，走向足厥阴经脉，向下联络足背。此络为气功习练之处。

collateral of foot Shaoyang Derives from Guangming（GB 3），5 Cun above the external malleolus，and goes to the liver meridian of foot-Jueyin to run downwards and connect with the dorsum of the foot. This collateral is a region usually used in practice of Qigong.

足少阳之别【zú shào yáng zhī bié】指足少阳络脉，在距离外踝上五寸光明穴处分出，走向足厥阴经脉，向下联络足背。此经别为气功习练之处。

branch of foot Shaoyang Refers to the collateral of bladder meridian of foot Shaoyang. It derives from Guangming（GB 3），5 Cun above the external malleolus，and goes to the liver meridian of foot-Jueyin to run downwards and connect with the dorsum of the foot. This branch is a region usually used in practice of Qigong.

足少阴【zú shào yīn】足少阴肾经，其循行从足少趾下边开始，斜向足底心，出于舟骨粗隆下。此经脉为气功习练之处。

foot Shaoyin Refers to the kidney meridian of foot-Shaoyin. It starts from the inferior aspect of the small toe，runs obliquely towards the sole and emerges from the lower aspect of the tuberosity of the navicular bone. This meridian is a region usually used in practice of Qigong.

足少阴经别【zú shào yīn jīng bié】从本经脉在腋窝部分出后，与足太阳经别相合并行，上至肾脏，在十四椎处分出来，归属于带脉。此经别为气功习练之处。

branch of foot Shaoyin Derives from its own regular meridian at the popliteal fossa，then running together with the branch of the bladder meridian of foot Taiyang，ascending to the kidney and emerging from the 14th vertebra to the belt meridian it pertains to. his branch is a region usually used in practice of Qigong.

足少阴络脉【zú shào yīn luò mài】在内踝后足跟部大钟穴分出，走向足太阳经。其支脉与本经相并上行，走到心包下，外行通过腰脊部。此络为气功习练之处。

collateral of foot Shaoyin Derives from Dazhong (KI 4) at the heel posterior to the medial malleolus, and running to join the bladder meridian of foot Taiyang. The branch goes upwards parallel to its own meridian to the region below the pericardium, and runs outwards through the part of the loin and spine. This collateral is a region usually used in practice of Qigong.

足少阴肾经【zú shào yīn shèn jīng】 其循行从足少趾下边开始，斜向足底心，出于舟骨粗隆下，沿内踝之后，分支进入足跟中。此经为气功习练之处。

kidney meridian of foot Shaoyin Starts from the inferior aspect of the small toe, running obliquely towards the sole and emerging from the lower aspect of the tuberosity of the navicular bone, along the region posterior to the medial malleolus, one branch entering the heel. This meridian is a region usually used in practice of Qigong.

足少阴之别【zú shào yīn zhī bié】 指足少阴络脉，在内踝后足跟部大钟穴分出，走向足太阳经。其支脉与本经相并上行，走向心包下，外行通过腰脊部。此经别为气功习练之处。

branch of foot Shaoyin Refers to the kidney meridian of foot Shaoyin. It derives from Dazhong (KI 4) at the heel posterior to the medial malleolus, and running to join the bladder meridian of foot Taiyang. The branch goes upwards parallel to its own meridian to the region below the pericardium, and runs outwards through the part of the loin and spine. This branch is a region usually used in practice of Qigong.

足太阳【zú tài yáng】 指足太阳膀胱经，为十二经脉之一。其循行从内眼角开始，上行额部，与督脉交会于头顶。此经脉为气功习练之处。

foot Taiyang Refers to the bladder meridian of foot Taiyang, one of the twelve meridians, starting from the inner canthus and ascending to the forehead and joining the governor meridian at the vertex. This meridian is a region usually used in practice of Qigong.

足太阳经别【zú tài yáng jīng bié】 在腘窝部从足太阳经分出，其中一条在骶骨下五寸处别行进入肛门，向里属于膀胱，散布联络肾脏，沿着脊柱两旁的肌肉，到心脏部进入散布在心内。此经别为气功习练之处。

branch of foot Taiyang Derives from the bladder meridian of foot Taiyang in the popliteal fossa, one branch entering the anus from the region 5 Cun below the sacral bone, running into the pertaining organ, the bladder, distributing in and connecting with the kidney, running upwards in the muscles alongside the spine to the heart. This branch is a region usually used in practice of Qigong.

足太阳络脉【zú tài yáng luò mài】 在外踝上七寸处飞扬穴分出，走向足少阴经。此络为气功习练之处。

collateral of foot Taiyang Derives from Feiyang (BL 58), 7 Cun above the externl malleolus and running towards the kidney meridian of foot Shaoyin. This collateral is a region usually used in practice of Qigong.

足太阳膀胱经【zú tài yáng páng guāng jīng】 为十二经脉之一。其循行从内眼角开始，上行额部，与督脉交会于头顶。此经为气功习练之处。

Z

bladder meridian of foot Taiyang One of the twelve meridians, starts from the inner canthus, ascending to the forehead and joining the governor meridian at the vertex. This meridian is a region usually used in practice of Qigong.

足太阳之别【zú tài yáng zhī bié】 指足太阳络脉,其脉在外踝上七寸处飞扬穴分出,走向足少阴经。

branch of foot Taiyang Refers to the collateral of the bladder meridian of foot Taiyang. It derives from Feiyang (BL 58),7 Cun above the external malleolus, and runs towards the kidney meridian of foot-Shaoyin.

足太阴【zú tài yīn】 ① 指足太阴脾经,为十二经脉之一;② 指穴位别名,如地机穴、三阴交穴、公孙穴。这些穴位为气功精气运行之重要部位。此经脉为气功习练之处。

foot Taiyin Refers to ① either the spleen meridian of foot Taiyin which is one of the twelve meridians; ② or another name of Diji (SP 8), Sanyinjiao (SP 6) and Songsun (SP 4). These acupoints are the regions usually used in practice of Qigong. This meridian is a region usually used in practice of Qigong.

足太阴经别【zú tài yīn jīng bié】 从足太阴经脉分出后到达大腿前面,和足阳明经的经别相合行,向上结于咽喉,贯通到舌本。此经别为气功习练之处。

branch of foot Taiyin Derives from the spleen meridian of foot Taiyin and reaches the anterior side of the thigh, joining the stomach meridian of foot Yangming, running side by side with it upward to amass at the throat and passing through the root of the tongue. This branch is a region usually used in practice of Qigong.

足太阴络脉【zú tài yīn luò mài】 在距离足大趾本节后方一寸处公孙穴分出,走向足阳明胃经,其支脉进入腹腔,与肠胃联络。此络为气功习练之处。

collateral of foot Taiyin Derives from Gongsun (SP 4) 1 cun posterior to the 1st metatarsodigital joint, and runs towards the Stomach Meridian of Foot-Yangming. Its branch enters the abdominal cavity to connect with the intestines and stomach. This collateral is a region usually used in practice of Qigong.

足太阴脾经【zú tài yīn pí jīng】 从大趾末端开始循行,大趾足内侧赤白肉际,经核骨,上向内踝前边,上小腿内侧,沿胫骨后,交出足厥阴肝经之前,上膝股内侧前边,进入腹部,属于脾,络于胃。此络为气功习练之处。

spleen meridian of foot Taiyin Starts from the tip of the big toe, runs along the medial aspect of the big toe at the junction of red and white skin, passing through the nodular process on the medial aspect of the 1st metatarsophalangeal joint, ascending to the front of the medial malleolus and further up to the medial aspect of the leg, following the posterior aspect of the tibia and passing through the front of the liver meridian of foot Jueyin. Going on along the anterior medial aspect of the knee and then the thigh, it enters the abdomen, reaches the spleen it pertains to and connects with the stomach. This collateral is a region usually used in practice of Qigong.

Z

足太阴之别【zú tài yīn zhī bié】 指足太阴络脉,在距离足大趾本节后方一寸处公孙穴分出,走向足阳明胃经,其支脉进入腹腔,与肠胃联络。此经别为气功习练之处。

the branch of foot Taiyin Refers to the collateral of the spleen meridian of foot Taiyin. It derives from Gongsun (SP 4) 1 cun posterior to the 1st metatarsodigital joint, and runs towards the Stomach Meridian of Foot-Yangming. Its branch enters the abdominal cavity to connect with the intestines and stomach. This branch is a region usually used in practice of Qigong.

足阳明【zú yáng míng】 足阳精及足阳明胃经,其循行从鼻旁开始,交会鼻根中,旁边会足太阳经,向下沿鼻外侧,进入上齿槽中。此经脉为气功习练之处。

foot Yangming Refers to the stomach meridian of foot Yangming. It starts from the lateral side of ala nasi and ascends to the bridge of the nose, where it meets the bladder meridian of foot Taiyang. Turning downwords along the lateral side of the nose, it enters the upper gum. This meridian is a region usually used in practice of Qigong.

足阳明经别【zú yáng míng jīng bié】 在大腿前面从足阳明分出,进入腹腔之内,属于胃腑,散布到脾脏,向上通连心脏,沿着食道浅出于口腔,上达于鼻根和眼眶下部,会合于足阳明经。此经别为气功习练之处。

branch of foot Yangming Derives from the Meridian of Foot-Yangming anterior to the thigh, enters the abdominal cavity. It pertains to the stomach and distributes in the spleen. Then it runs upward to connect with the heart, emerging from the mouth cavity along the esophagus, reaching the root of the nose and the infra-orbital region and combining with the stomach meridian of foot Yangming. This branch is a region usually used in practice of Qigong.

足阳明络脉【zú yáng míng luò mài】 在距离外踝上八寸丰隆穴处分出,走向足太阴经。此络为气功习练之处。

collateral of foot Yangming Refers to the collateral of foot Yangming, deriving 8 Cun above the lateral malleolus and running towards the spleen meridian of foot Taiyin. This collateral is a region usually used in practice of Qigong.

足阳明胃经【zú yáng míng wèi jīng】 从鼻旁开始循行,交会鼻根中,旁边会足太阳经,向下沿鼻外侧,进入上齿槽中,回出来夹口旁环绕口唇,至额颅中部。此经为气功习练之处。

stomach meridian of foot Yangming Refers to the stomach meridian of foot Yangming. It starts from the lateral side of ala nasi and ascends to the bridge of the nose, where it meets the bladder meridian of foot Taiyang. Turning downwords along the lateral side of the nose, it enters the upper gum, curving round the lips and finally reaching the forehead. This meridian is a region usually used in practice of Qigong.

足阳明之别【zú yáng míng zhī bié】 指足阳明络脉,在距离外踝上八寸丰隆穴处分出,走向足太阴经。此经别为气功习练之处。

branch of foot Yangming Refers to the collateral of foot Yangming, deriving 8

Z

Cun above the lateral malleolus and running towards the spleen meridian of foot Taiyin. This branch is a region usually used in practice of Qigong.

祖气【zǔ qì】 指禀先天父母之气。

ancestral Qi Refers to Qi from parents.

祖窍【zǔ qiào】 指位于心与脐之正中。

ancestral orifice Refers to the central region between the heart and the navel.

最高峰【zuì gāo fēng】 指百会穴,亦指头。

highest peak Refers to either Baihui (CV 20), which is an acupoint in the conception meridian; or the head.

尊生导养编【zūn shēng dǎo yǎng biān】《尊生导养编》为气功养生学专书,由清代张映汉所著,介绍了导引气功按摩术,并介绍了具体方法及注意事项。

Zunsheng Daoyang Bian(*Compilation of Life Respect and Cultivation Improvement*) A monograph of Qigong entitled *Compilation of Life Respect and Cultivation Improvement*, written by Zhang Yinghan in the Qing Dynasty (1636 AD - 1912 AD), introducing Daoyin, Qigong and Tuina techniques as well as the exercises, methods and points for attention.

尊生老人【zūn shēng lǎo rén】 即沈金鳌,为清代中医学家,精通气功养生,对后世医学气功的推广产生了一定的影响。

old man respecting life Celebration of Shen Jin'ao, a scientist of traditional Chinese medicine in the Qing Dynasty (1636 AD - 1912 AD). He was also proficient in studying Qigong and life

cultivation, influencing the later generations in a certain extent.

遵生八笺【zūn shēng bā jiān】《遵生八笺》为养生学专著,兼论气功,由明代高濂所著,重点阐述精、气、神、形之间的关系及对人体的重要性。

Sunsheng Bajian(*Eight Explanations of Complying Life*) A monograph of cultivation life with Qigong entitled *Eight Explanations of Complying Life*, written by Gao Lian in the Ming Dynasty, mainly describing the relations and importance of the essence, Qi, spirit and body.

左慈【zuǒ cí】 东汉的一位气功学家,生卒岁月不详。为葛玄之师,善道术。

Zuo Ci A master of Qigong in the East Han Dynasty (25 AD - 220 AD), the years of birth and death were unknown. He was the teacher of Ge Xuan, a great Daoist in the East Han Dynasty (25 AD - 220 AD).

左神公子【zuǒ shén gōng zǐ】 指肝神无英。

left spiritual lord Refers to intelligence of the spirit of the liver.

左右开弓【zuǒ yòu kāi gōng】 为动功,其作法为,一手侧平举,一手在胸前屈曲,去臂腋疾病。

drawing the bow both on the left and right A dynamic exercise, marked by one hand lifting up and the other hand turning to the front of the chest to expel diseases in the shoulders and the armpits.

左右视不并见【zuǒ yòu shì bù bìng jiàn】 指一时只能有一个注意中心,只有精神意识活动的高度集中,才能有所成功。

mutual observation of the left and right

Z

visions Refers to the fact that only when there is one central attention and one concentration of the spirit and consciousness activities in a period of time can any practice of Qigong be successful.

左元放【zuǒ yuán fàng】 东汉气功学家左慈的另外一个称谓,为葛玄之师,善道术。

Zuo Yuanfang Another name of Zuo Ci, a great master of Qigong in the East Hand Dynasty (25 AD – 220 AD), the years of birth and death were unknown. He was the teacher of Ge Xuan, a great Daoist in the East Han Dynasty (25 AD – 220 AD).

作念【zuò niàn】 指气功医师集中意念,运气攻逐病者患处。

maintaining contemplation Refers to the fact that doctors of Qigong concentrate ideas and circulate Qi to attack the location of diseases.

坐禅【zuò chán】 佛家气功学习用语,指习练佛家气功功法。

sitting dhyana A common term of Qigong in Buddhism, referring to the methods of practicing Qigong in Buddhism.

坐禅法【zuò chán fǎ】 为静功。其作法为,正坐,顶脊端直,胁不拄床,不委不倚,不动不摇,调节呼吸,使之平静安适。

exercise of dhyana sitting A static exercise, marked by sitting upright, quietly straightening the spine without any rotation and regulating respiration in order to tranquilize and to stabilize the body.

坐驰【zuò chí】 指精神意识活动外散,杂念不绝。

sitting distraction Refers to disorder of the activities of the spirit and consciousness with various distracting thought.

坐功诀【zuò gōng jué】 为静功。其作法为,两足曲盘,气由尾闾上达泥丸,下注丹田者九次;气由左右两臂,达于手指者七次;由左右两股,达于足趾者七次。

sitting exercise formula A static exercise, marked by crossing the feet in sitting, promoting Qi to flow from the coccyx to the mud bolus (the brain) and descending to Dantian for nine times, from the shoulders to the fingers for seven times, from the thighs to the toes for seven times. Dantian is divided into the upper Dantian (the region between the eyes), the middle Dantian (the region below the heart) and the lower Dantian (the region below the navel).

坐功十段【zuò gōng shí duàn】 为动功,方法多样,如跌坐、擦热两掌,作洗面状,眼眶、鼻梁、耳根各处周到,面觉微热为度。

ten courses of sitting exercise A dynamic exercise with various methods, such as sitting quietly, rubbing the hands warm, wiping the face like washing, and kneading the orbital cavity, bridge of the nose and roots of ears (sulcus auriculae posterior) till the face feels warm.

坐忘【zuò wàng】 为静功。其作法为,坐势为遗忘自己的肢体,除去自己的聪明,离弃自己的形体,稳定自己的意识,与自然社会融为一体。

quiet sitting A static exercise, marked by forgetting self-limbs, eliminating self-wisdom, abandoning self-body, stabilizing self-consciousness and coor-

Z

dinating with the natural society.

坐忘论【zuò wàng lùn】《坐忘论》为气功专著,由唐代司马承祯著,主要论述坐忘安心、修炼形气、养和心灵。认为身体健康长寿在于静定功夫。

Zuowang Lun (*Discussion about Quiet Sitting*) A monograph of Qigong entitled *Discussion about Quiet Sitting*, written by Sima Chengzhen in the Tang Dynasty (618 AD－907 AD), mainly describing stabilization of the heart in quiet sitting, cultivation of physical Qi and fortification of the heart spirit. It believes that health and longevity depend on tranquilization in practicing Qigong.

坐在金台【zuò zài jīn tái】 为静功。其作法为,坐势,意念存精神活动于脾中,不使其外越。金台指脾。

sitting on golden platform A static exercise, marked by sitting upright, keeping the activity of consciousness with the spirit in the spleen and avoiding any external dispersion. In this term, the so-called golden platform refers to the spleen.

Z